U S M G NATO ASI

LES HOUCHES
Session XXXIII
1979

MEMBRANES
ET COMMUNICATION INTERCELLULAIRE

MEMBRANES
AND INTERCELLULAR COMMUNICATION

USMG NATO ASI

LES HOUCHES

SESSION XXXIII

30 Juillet–30 Août 1979

MEMBRANES ET COMMUNICATION INTERCELLULAIRE

MEMBRANES AND INTERCELLULAR COMMUNICATION

édité par

ROGER BALIAN, MARC CHABRE, PHILIPPE F. DEVAUX

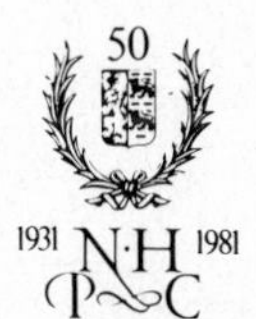

NORTH-HOLLAND PUBLISHING COMPANY
AMSTERDAM · NEW YORK · OXFORD

ISBN 0 444 85469 X

Published by:
NORTH-HOLLAND PUBLISHING COMPANY
AMSTERDAM · NEW YORK · OXFORD

Sole distributors for the USA and Canada:
ELSEVIER NORTH-HOLLAND, INC.
52 VANDERBILT AVENUE
NEW YORK, N.Y. 10017

Library of Congress Cataloging in Publication Data
Main entry under title:

Membranes et communication intercellulaire = Membranes and intercellular communication.

At head of title: USMG. NATO ASI.
Lecture notes delivered at the 33rd session of Les Houches Summer School.
Texts in English with preface in French and English.
Includes bibliographical references.
1. Cell membranes--Congresses. 2. Cell interaction --Congresses. I. Balian, Roger. II. Chabre, Marc. III. Devaux, Philippe. IV. Université scientifique et médicale de Grenoble. École d'été de physique théorique. V. Title: Membranes and intercellular communication.

QH601.M482 574.87'5 80-20464
ISBN 0-444-85469-X

Printed in The Netherlands

CONFÉRENCIERS

Philippe ASCHER
Claude BERGMAN
Jean-Pierre CHANGEUX
Michel FOUGEREAU
Richard HENDERSON
Serge JARD
Martin KARPLUS
Peter LÄUGER
Harden M. McCONNELL
Hans MEVES
Martin RODBELL
Joachim SEELIG
Nathan SHARON
S. Jonathan SINGER

E. L. Benedetti, J. Bockaert, M. Chabre, Ph. F. Devaux, L. Dorland, Y. Dupont, S. Fermandjian, B. de Kruijff, J. Miller, B. Neumcke, J. Parello, J.-L. Popot

SESSIONS PRÉCÉDENTES

I	1951	Mécanique quantique. Théorie quantique des champs
II	1952	Quantum mechanics. Mécanique statistique. Physique nucléaire
III	1953	Quantum mechanics. Etat solide. Mécanique statistique. Elementary particles
IV	1954	Mécanique quantique. Théorie des collisions; two-nucleon interaction. Electrodynamique quantique
V	1955	Quantum mechanics. Non-equilibrium phenomena. Réactions nucléaires. Interaction of a nucleus with atomic and molecular fields
VI	1956	Quantum perturbation theory. Low temperature physics. Quantum theory of solids; dislocations and plastic properties. Magnetism; ferromagnetism
VII	1957	Théorie de la diffusion; recent developments in field theory. Interaction nucléaire; interactions fortes. Electrons de haute énergie. Experiments in high energy nuclear physics
VIII	1958	Le problème à *N* corps (Dunod, Wiley, Methuen)
IX	1959	La théorie des gaz neutres et ionisés (Hermann, Wiley)*
X	1960	Relations de dispersion et particules élémentaires (Hermann, Wiley)*
XI	1961	La physique des basses températures. Low-temperature physics (Gordon and Breach, Presses Universitaires)*
XII	1962	Géophysique extérieure. Geophysics: the earth's environment (Gordon and Breach)*
XIII	1963	Relativité, groupes et topologie. Relativity, groups and topology (Gordon and Breach)*
XIV	1964	Optique et électronique quantiques. Quantum optics and electronics (Gordon and Breach)*
XV	1965	Physique des hautes énergies. High energy physics (Gordon and Breach)*
XVI	1966	Hautes énergies en astrophysique. High energy astrophysics (Gordon and Breach)*
XVII	1967	Problème à *N* corps. Many-body physics (Gordon and Breach)*
XVIII	1968	Physique nucléaire. Nuclear physics (Gordon and Breach)*
XIX	1969	Aspects physiques de quelques problèmes biologiques. Physical problems in biology (Gordon and Breach)*
XX	1970	Mécanique statistique et théorie quantique des champs. Statistical mechanics and quantum field theory (Gordon and Breach)*
XXI	1971	Physique des particules. Particle physics (Gordon and Breach)*
XXII	1972	Physique des plasmas. Plasma physics (Gordon and Breach)*
XXIII	1972	Les astres occlus. Black holes (Gordon and Breach)*
XXIV	1973	Dynamique des fluides. Fluid dynamics (Gordon and Breach)
XXV	1973	Fluides moléculaires. Molecular fluids (Gordon and Breach)*
XXVI	1974	Physique atomique et moléculaire et matière interstellaire. Atomic and molecular physics and the interstellar matter (North-Holland)*
June Inst.	1975	Structural analysis of collision amplitudes (North-Holland)
XXVII	1975	Aux frontières de la spectroscopie laser. Frontiers in laser spectroscopy (North-Holland)*
XXVIII	1975	Méthodes en théorie des champs. Methods in field theory (North-Holland)*
XXIX	1976	Interactions électromagnétiques et faibles à haute énergie. Weak and electromagnetic interactions at high energy (North-Holland)*
XXX	1977	Ions lourds et mésons en physique nucléaire. Nuclear physics with mesons and heavy ions (North-Holland)*
XXXI	1978	La matière mal condensée. Ill-condensed matter (North-Holland)*
XXXII	1979	Cosmologie physique. Physical cosmology (North-Holland)*
XXXIII	1979	Membranes et communication intercellulaire. Membranes and intercellular communication (North-Holland)*

En préparation

XXXIV	1980	Interaction laser-plasma
XXXV	1980	Physique des défauts*

*Sessions ayant reçu l'appui du Comité Scientifique de l'OTAN.

LES HOUCHES,
ÉCOLE D'ÉTÉ DE PHYSIQUE THÉORIQUE

ORGANISME D'INTÉRÊT COMMUN DE L'UNIVERSITÉ SCIENTIFIQUE ET MÉDICALE DE GRENOBLE ET DE L'INSTITUT NATIONAL POLYTECHNIQUE DE GRENOBLE

AIDÉ PAR LE COMMISSARIAT À L'ÉNERGIE ATOMIQUE

SESSION XXXIII

INSTITUT D'ÉTUDES AVANCÉES DE L'OTAN
NATO ADVANCED STUDY INSTITUTE
30 Juillet–30 Août 1979

Directeurs scientifiques de la session: Marc Chabre, Laboratoire de biophysique moléculaire et cellulaire, CEA, CENG, 85X, 38041 Grenoble, et Philippe F. Devaux, Institut de biologie physico-chimique, 13 rue Pierre et Marie Curie, 75005 Paris

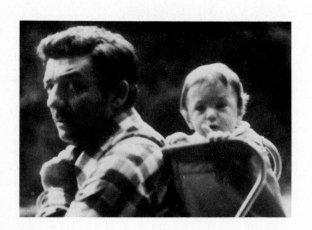

PARTICIPANTS

Allegrini, Peter, Institut fuer Biochemie, Freiestr. 3, CH-3012 Berne, Switzerland.

Barberis, Claude, Laboratoire de Physiologie Générale, Université Nancy 1, C.O. 140, 54037 Nancy Cedex, France.

Besançon, Françoise, Institut de Biologie Physico-Chimique, 13 rue Pierre et Marie Curie, 75005 Paris, France.

Bloom, Myer, Dept. of Physics, University of British Columbia, Vancouver, B.C., VGT IW5, Canada.

Boulanger, Yvan, Conseil National de Recherche, 100 Sussex Dr., 2109 Ottawa, Ont., Canada.

Bratko, Filipic, Fabijanijeva 23, 61000 Ljubljana, Yugoslavia.

Canciglia, Paolo, Inst. of General Physiology, Faculty of Science, University of Messina, via del Vespro, 5, 98100 Messina, Italy.

Charcosset, Jean-Yves, Unité de Biochimie-Enzymologie, Institut Gustave Roussy, 16 bis av. Paul-Vaillant Couturier, 94 Villejuif, France.

Christen, Richard, Station Zoologique, 06230 Villefranche/Mer, France.

Dalton, Lauraine A., Department of Chemistry, State University of New York, Stoney Brook, New York 11794, USA.

Dautry, François, D. Ph. T. C. E. N Saclay, 91191, Gif-sur-Yvette, France.

Davoust, Jean, I. B. P. C., 13 rue Pierre et Marie Curie, 75005 Paris, France.

Delaye, Mireille, Laboratoire de Physique des Solides, Bat. 510, Université de Paris-sud, 91405 Orsay, France.

Delia, Domenico, Imperial Cancer Research Fund, Membrane Immunology Lab., Lincoln's Inn Fields, London WC2, England.

Deugnier, Marie-Ange, Laboratoire de Microscopie Quantitative, UER Biomédicale, 74 rue Marcel Cachin, 93000 Bobigny, France.

Di Virgilio, Francesco, Institute of General Pathology, Via Loredan 6, 35 100 Padova, Italy.

Duperray, Alain, Biochimie Endocrinienne, CERMO-USMG, BP. 53 X, Saint-Martin d'Hères, France.

Edelman, Alexandre, INSERM U. 30, Hôpital Necker, Tour Technique, 6ème étage, 149 rue de Sèvres, 75730 Paris Cedex 15, France.

Fischmeister, Rodolphe, Laboratoire Physiologie Comparée (bat. 443), Université Paris XI, 91405 Orsay, France.

Gresh, Nohad, Institut de Biologie Physico-Chimique, 13 rue Pierre et Marie Curie, 75005 Paris, France.

Haranczyk, Hubert, Institute of Physics, Jagellonian University, Cracow, Reymonta 4, Poland.

Ince, Can, Department of Physiology, University of Leiden, Leiden, The Netherlands.

Kay, Alan Robert, Physiological Laboratory, University of Cambridge, Cambridge, CB2 3EG, England.

Krishnan, K. S., Molecular Biology Unit. Tata Inst. Fundamental Res. Colaba, Homi Bhabha Road, Bombay 400 005, India.

Lahav, Judith, Center for Cancer Research, Blvd. E17-227 M.I.T., Cambridge, MA, USA.

Lang, Robert, National Institute for Medical Research, the Ridgeway, Mill Hill, London NW7 1AA, England.

Maraviglia, Bruno, Istituto di Fisica, Università di Roma, 00185 Rome, Italy.

Methfessel, Christoph, Institut für Experimentalphysik VI, Ruhr-Universität Bochum, D-463 Bochum, Querenburg, Germany.

Minetti, Maurizio, Lab. Cell Biology and Immunology, Istituto Superiore di Sanita, V. Regina Elena, 299 Rome, Italy.

Perret, Joël, IRBM, SCE Génétique et Membranes, 2 place Jussieu, Tour 43–44, 5ème étage, 75021 Paris Cedex 05, France.

Pfister, Claude, CENG–DRF/BMC, BP. 85 X, 38041 Grenoble Cedex, France.

Prujansky-Jakobovits, Aya, Biophysics Dept. The Weismann Institute of Science, Rehovot, Israel.

Pop, Victor, I., Medical and Pharmaceutical Institute, Faculty of Medicine, Dept. of Cell Biology, 6st. Pasteur, 3400 Cluj-Napoca, Romania.

Reidl, Helwig, Institut Für Biophysik und Strahlenbiologie, Albertstr. 23, D 7800 Freiburg, Germany.

Saint-Yves, André, E.R. 140, Bat. Chimie Ext., U.S.T.L., Place Eugène Bataillon, 34060 Montpellier, France.

Sakmar, Tom, c/o Heinrikson, University of Chicago, Dept. of Biochem., 920 E. 58th St., Chicago, IL 60637, USA.

Sansonetty Goncalves, Alberto Filipe, Centre de Cytologie Expérimentale, 1021 Rua do Campo Alegre, 4200 Porto, Portugal.

Scherman, Daniel, Institut de Biologie Physico-Chimique, 13 rue Pierre et Marie Curie, 75005 Paris, France.

Simopoulos, Athanassios, Nuclear Research Center Democritos, Aghia Paraskevi, Attiki, Greece.

Tan, Yusuf Plamenko, Middle East Technical University, Dept. of Life Sciences, Ankara, Turkey.

Tatischeff, Irène, Institut Curie, Laboratoire Curie, 11 rue Pierre et Marie Curie, 75231 Paris, Cedex 05, France.

Tetteroo, Pedro, Laboratory of Zoology, Dept. of Cell Biology, Kaiserstraat 63, Leiden, The Netherlands.

Tiedge, Joachim, Institut für Theoretische Physik D, RWTH Aachen, Melaten Nord 26, D-51 Aachen, Germany.

Trevisani, Agostino, Institute of General Physiology, University of Ferrara, via Borsari 46, 44100 Ferrara, Italy.

Uribe, Salvador, Universidad Nacional A. de Mexico, Centro de Investigaciones en Fisiologia-Celular, Apdo postal 70600, Mexico 21, D.F. Mexico.

Valiron, Odile, Laboratoire de Physiopathologie des Facteurs d'Ambiance, Université Bordeaux II, 146 rue Léo-Seignat, 33076 Bordeaux Cedex, France.

Verlinden, Josse, Centrum Voor Menselijke Erfelijkheid, Minderbroederstraat 12, 3000 Leuven, Belgium.

Weinstein, Harel, Dept. of Pharmacology, Mount Sinai School of Medecine of the City University of New York, 1 Gustave L. Levy Place, New York, N.Y. 10029, USA.

PRÉFACE

Ce volume tient une place un peu particulière dans la série des cours des Houches . . . bien loin de la physique théorique: il traite en effet de biologie, et ne se rattache à la physique, domaine traditionnel de l'Ecole, que par l'intermédiaire de la biophysique. Celle-ci est d'ailleurs une discipline aux contours difficiles à cerner. Il existe une biophysique médicale, centrée sur les applications de la physique à la médecine; sa raison d'être est essentiellement technique. Quant à la biophysique dite moléculaire, son champ d'application est celui de la biologie moléculaire, et ses frontières avec la biochimie sont assez floues. Le but de cette session était de comprendre certains des mécanismes moléculaires à la base du fonctionnement des organismes vivants. C'est par une référence constante au langage de la physico-chimie ainsi que par l'emploi dominant des techniques physiques que s'en révèle la coloration biophysique.

La membrane cellulaire, cette barrière moléculaire essentielle à la définition même de la cellule biologique qu'elle délimite, a focalisé depuis une douzaine d'années l'attention et les efforts de nombreux biologistes et physico-chimistes. Les membranes artificielles, qu'elles soient constituées de lipides purs ou qu'elles contiennent de plus des protéines, ont joué un rôle essentiel dans l'établissement des caractéristiques fondamentales des membranes biologiques. Etudiées par des techniques physiques très élaborées, diffraction, spectroscopie, mesures électriques, microscopie, ces membranes modèles ont permis une description de l'aspect statique et dynamique des interactions entre leurs constituants. Mais le vrai problème reste l'intégration de ces connaissances moléculaires dans la compréhension des diverses fonctions membranaires. Ces fonctions sont multiples et ne peuvent être groupées en un thème unique: c'est en effet la membrane qui contrôle tous les échanges entre cellule et milieu extérieur, qui définit les flux, établit des gradients électriques et ioniques. Elle constitue le support d'ancrage des édifices multimoléculaires qui interviennent dans les mouvements cellulaires, dans la synthèse protéique, dans les processus bioénergétiques . . . On peut à partir de la membrane faire l'inventaire de pratiquement toutes les grandes fonctions cellulaires.

Dans les systèmes pluricellulaires, vers lesquels se développe de plus en plus la biologie moléculaire, la coordination entre les cellules et donc la communication d'information entre elles devient un problème fondamental. Elle peut dans certains cas s'exprimer en termes d'interaction au niveau de la membrane cellulaire d'un nombre limité de molécules, qui fonctionnent comme émetteurs, transmetteurs et récepteurs. Les molécules messagères sont généralement petites, et leur structure souvent connue avec une grande précision. Malheureusement la méconnaissance de la structure des récepteurs limite sévèrement les études physico-chimiques.

C'est sur ce thème de la communication intercellulaire que nous avons néanmoins voulu focaliser la session. Le but visé était d'approcher à l'échelle moléculaire les principaux systèmes de communication et de transfert d'information intercellulaire en partant de nos connaissances actuelles sur la structure et la dynamique des membranes. Pour limiter le sujet, ont été exclus l'émission et la traduction des messages au niveau intracellulaire; tout le couplage avec l'information génétique est donc laissé de côté. Malgré cela, le domaine reste large, et n'a pu être couvert que partiellement.

Le cours a commencé par une introduction générale sur les membranes donnée par S. J. Singer, qui en 1972 lia son nom et celui de G. Nicolson au concept de la mosaïdque fluide. Cette présentation avait pour but de fixer pour les participants le cadre des cours ultérieurs, et seul un plan détaillé en figure ici.

L'ensemble du volume s'articule ensuite en deux parties. La première met l'accent sur la description physico-chimique des composants membranaires (lipides, protéines et glyco-conjugués), tandis que la seconde est orientée vers le fonctionnement biologique.

La structure des bicouches phospholipidiques a été décrite par J. Seelig, qui s'est appuyé sur les méthodes classiques en physique de la matière con-densée (diffraction, RMN, RPE) d'un apport considérable dans ce domaine. Le cours suivant étudie les glyco-conjugués, constituants complexes au rôle encore mal compris: à travers le dédale des schémas à multiples branchements, N. Sharon a su dégager la systématique et la logique de leur organisation structurale riche en information.

On passe enfin aux protéines, macromolécules "actives" de la membrane. Les conformations des protéines solubles ont été présentées par M. Karplus, qui a joué au cours des dernières années un rôle essentiel dans l'étude quantitative de leur dynamique (son cours est représenté dans ce livre par un bref résumé accompagné d'une bibliographie). Mais les protéines membranaires intrinsèques ont des structures particulières liées à leur insolubilité dans la phase aqueuse. Il revenait à R. Henderson d'exposer les idées actuelles (encore fragmentaires) sur ce problème: lui-même et N. Unwin sont en effet les seuls à avoir réussi à résoudre la structure d'une protéine membranaire (la bactériorhodopsine).

La contribution à l'Ecole de H. M. McConnell, qui fut à l'origine de la notion de fluidité membranaire, sert de transition vers l'étude fonctionnelle des membranes. Il présente en effet dans la première partie de son cours des données récentes sur la mobilité latérale des composants lipidiques et protéiques, basées sur des expériences d'optique particulièrement élégantes, tandis qu'il aborde ensuite le problème de la reconnaissance immunologique.

La deuxième partie du livre est consacrée à l'étude de trois systèmes de communication intercellulaire, qui relèvent de trois branches importantes de la biologie: la reconnaissance immunologique au niveau membranaire (un aspect de ce vaste domaine qu'est l'immunologie), la transmission hormonale (branche de l'endocrinologie), la transmission nerveuse et synaptique (branche de la neurobiologie). Ces trois sujets d'études sont habituellement enseignés en tant que spécialités indépendantes, et l'ambition des organisateurs en les rassemblant dans une même session pédagogique était d'essayer de retrouver leurs aspects moléculaires communs au niveau de la membrane.

Des visions différentes, mais complémentaires, de la reconnaissance immunologique sont proposées par H. M. McConnell, J. Miller et M. Fougereau. Ce dernier réussit à présenter de manière brève et pédagogique l'immense domaine encore mal débrouillé de l'immunologie.

En ce qui concerne la transduction hormonale, l'explication moléculaire des mécanismes de communication se heurte à un problème qui vient paradoxalement de l'extraordinaire efficacité du système. Les édifices moléculaires en jeu, encore non identifiés, n'existent qu'en très faibles quantités. L'économie des récepteurs hormonaux dans les membranes plasmiques rend ainsi problématique l'isolement et la caractérisation des molécules impliquées. Ces difficultés sont au centre des cours de S. Jard et M. Rodbell, qui ont su montrer qu'il était néanmoins possible de dégager des modèles fonctionnels multimoléculaires.

Avec le cours de P. Läuger a été abordé le fonctionnement des membranes en tant que barrière sélective aux ions; il faut encore se contenter pour cela de systèmes modèles, les films lipidiques (dits "films noirs") dans lesquels sont introduits des ionophores. La transmission axonale proprement dite a été décrite phénoménologiquement de façon remarquable il y a près de trente ans. C. Bergman et H. Meves présentent les résultats actuels concernant les canaux ioniques des nerfs, dont l'ouverture est fonction du voltage: les connaissances, obtenues essentiellement par des techniques électrophysiologiques, restent malheureusement encore loin de l'explication moléculaire. En effet, les même problèmes qu'en endrocrinologie se posent ici: les canaux n'existant qu'en très faible quantité, leur isolement et leur caractérisation biochimique n'ont toujours pas été possible. La nature fut plus généreuse dans le cas des synapses, tout au moins pour les synapses cholinergiques présentes en très forte densité dans l'organe électrique de certains poissons: la structure de ces synapses, aussi bien que leurs mécanismes fonctionnels, sont actuellement abordés par des méthodes couvrant la biophysique, la biochimie structurale, l'électrophysiologie et la pharmacologie. Ph. Ascher expose les difficultés et les brillants succès de ces approches. Dans deux conférences de clôture, J.-P. Changeux a abordé le thème du développement du système nerveux, qui dépend de manière essentielle de la reconnaissance sélective entre cellules, ellemême liée aux contacts membranaires.

Ces cours ont été illustrés par des séminaires mettant un accent sur les techniques d'étude, et présentant souvent des points de vue contradictoires menant à des discussions intéressantes. Mentionnons plus particulièrement la contribution de L. Benedetti, qui a décrit avec maestria un système de communication intercellulaire de type particulier, les "gap-junctions". On trouvera dans ce volume le texte des séminaires, dont nous tenons à remercier ici les auteurs pour avoir contribué, à côté des conférenciers principaux, à maintenir une atmosphère stimulante tout au long de la session.

Remerciements

L'organisation et la tenue de cette session XXXIII de l'Ecole d'Eté de Physique Théorique des Houches et la production de ce livre n'ont été rendus possibles que grâce à de nombreuses contributions:

-le soutien financier apporté par l'Université Scientifique et Médicale de Grenoble, et par la Division des Affaires Scientifiques de l'OTAN, qui a inclus cette session dans son programme d'Instituts d'Etudes Avancées, ainsi que la subvention du Commissariat à l'Energie Atomique;

-l'orientation donnée par le Conseil de l'Ecole;

-la frappe de plusieurs manuscrits par Lauris Balian;

-le rôle joué par Nicole Coiffier et Annie Battendier dans la préparation et l'administration de cette session;

-la part qu'Henri Coiffier et l'ensemble de son équipe ont prise dans la résolution de nos problèmes matériels;

-la coopération de tous les participants, qui ont enrichi les cours donnés pendant la session grâce à leurs questions vivantes et leurs commentaires.

Nous tenons enfin à remercier encore les conférenciers pour les nombreuses heures passées à préparer leurs cours et pour la qualité de leurs manuscrits, qui nous l'espérons feront de ce livre un outil utile à la communauté scientifique.

Roger Balian
Marc Chabre
Philippe F. Devaux

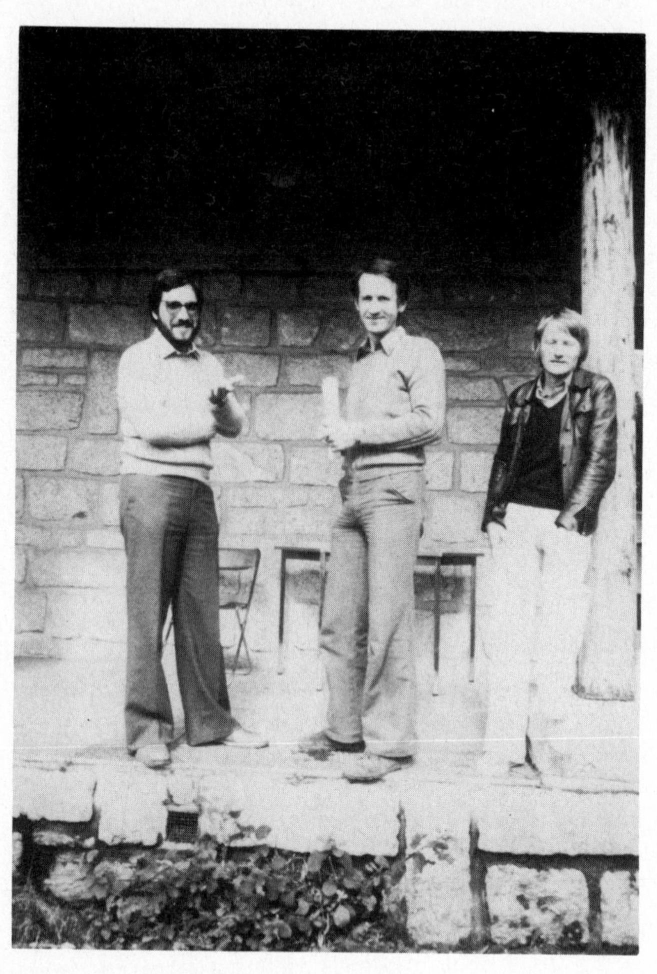

PREFACE

This volume occupies a rather special place in the series of Les Houches courses . . . quite far from theoretical physics: it deals with biology, and is connected to physics, the traditional field of the School, only through biophysics. This is a vast discipline, without well-defined boundaries. There exists a medical biophysics, focusing on applications of physics to medicine, with an essentially practical justification. The field of molecular biophysics is that of molecular biology, with an inevitable overlap with biochemistry. The aim of the present session was to grasp some of the molecular mechanisms which underlie the functioning of living organisms. Its biophysical flavour is evidenced both by a constant use of the language of physical chemistry and by the predominance of physical techniques.

The plasma membrane, a molecular barrier essential to the very definition of a biological cell, has been the focus of research efforts of many biologists and physical chemists during the past decade. Artificial membranes, whether prepared from pure lipids or containing additional proteins, have played an essential role in establishing the fundamental properties of biological membranes. The static and dynamic aspects of the interactions between the components of these model membranes have been elucidated through the use of elaborate physical techniques, diffraction, spectroscopy, electrical measurements, and microscopy. The major goal however consists of setting up this knowledge at a molecular level to understand the functions of biological membranes. Such functions are of course multiple, and are not expected to be grouped into a unique theme. Indeed, the plasma membrane controls all exchanges between the cell and its environments, it defines fluxes, establishes electrical and chemical gradients. It also provides the scaffolding on which the macromolecular assemblies responsible for cell movements, protein synthesis or bioenergetical processes fasten themselves. Actually, most of the major cellular functions can be studied at the membrane level.

For multicellular systems, towards which molecular biology is developing, the coordination between cells, and therefore their exchanges of information are crucial. In some cases, they are performed through the interaction at the level of the plasma membrane of a limited number of molecules, acting as emitters, messengers, and receptors. Messenger molecules are often small, and their structure may then be known precisely; unfortunately, our lack of knowledge on the structure of receptors severely hinders the physical-chemical analysis of their function.

We have nevertheless chosen intercellular communication as a theme for the session. Our purpose was to approach on the molecular scale the main systems involved in the transfer of information between cells, starting from our current understanding of the structures and dynamics of membranes. To limit the subject matter, we have excluded the emission and transduction of intracellular signals, and thus regulation at the level of the genetic information is not considered. Even so, the field is wide and could be covered only in part.

The session begins with a general introduction to biological membranes, presented by S. J. Singer, who along with G. Nicolson has articulated, in 1972, the notion of fluid-mosaic membrane. The aim of this introduction was to provide a framework for the subsequent courses; it has been found suitable to include its detailed outline in the present book.

The contents of the volume may be divided into a first part emphasizing the physical-chemical description of the membrane components, and a second part devoted to biological functions.

The structure of phospholipidic bilayers is described by J. Seelig, who reviews the considerable information provided by the standard techniques used in the physics of condensed phases (diffraction, NMR, EPR). The following course studies the glycoproteins, complex components with a role not yet well understood: N. Sharon has succeeded in extracting the systematics and the logic of their rich structural organization amidst the maze of twisting paths and multiple branch points. Finally, proteins, the "active" macromolecules of the membrane, are studied. The conformation of soluble proteins have been presented at the School by M. Karplus, who has played an essential role in the quantitative study of their dynamics (his course is represented in this book by a short review summary with references). Intrinsic membrane proteins, however, have special structures related to their insolubility in water. R. Henderson was most qualified to present the current ideas (still fragmentary) on this problem, since to date only he and N. Unwin have solved the structure of a membrane protein (bacteriorhodopsin).

The contribution to the School of H. M. McConnell, who originally introduced the concept of membrane fluidity, appears as a transition toward the functional study of membranes: he first presents recent results concerning the lateral mobility of membrane proteins and lipids, based on the use of elegant optical techniques, then tackles the problem of immunologic recognition.

The second part of the book is devoted to the study of three systems involved in intercellular communication, which are part of three important areas of biology: antigen-antibody recognition at the level of the membrane (an aspect of the wide field of immunology), hormonal transmission (a branch of endocrinology), axonal conduction, and synaptic transmission (a branch of neurobiology). These three topics are usually taught as independent specialties and the organizers' aim in combining them into a single pedagogical session was to exhibit their common molecular aspects at the level of the membrane.

Different but complementary views on immunological recognition are proposed by H. M. McConnell, J. Miller and M. Fougereau. The latter succeeds in presenting in a concise and pedagogical way the vast and as yet tangled domain of immunology.

Concerning hormonal transduction, the molecular explanation of communication mechanisms encounters a problem which paradoxically arises from the extraordinary efficiency of the system. The molecular assemblies involved in hormonal receptors, yet unidentified, need only be present in very small quantities. This limited concentration has so far hindered their isolation and characterization. Such difficulties lie at the heart of the courses of S. Jard and M. Rodbell, who show how it is nevertheless possible to build multimolecular, functional models consistent with the known drug-receptor interactions.

With the course of P. Läuger, membrane function is addressed in terms of selective permeability to ions; it is still necessary to rely on model systems, the lipidic bilayers (called "black films") into which peptid ionophores are added. Axonal transmission proper has been described phenomenologically with precision nearly thirty years ago. C. Bergman and H. Meves state our present information about the ion channels of nerve, which are voltage sensitive: the understanding gained mainly through the use of electrophysiological techniques unfortunately remains far from a molecular explanation. Indeed, the same problems as in endocrinology arise: since channels exist only in very small quantities, their isolation and biochemical characterization have not yet been carried out. Nature was more generous in the case of synapses, or at least the cholinergic synapses present at very high densities in the electric organs of some fishes: the structure of these synapses as well as their mechanism of function are being tackled by approaches including biophysics, structural biochemistry, electrophysiology and pharmacology; both the great successes and the limitations inherent in these various approaches are presented by Ph. Ascher. Finally, in two concluding lectures, J.-P. Changeux approaches the theme of the development of the nervous system, which depends critically on the selective recognition between cells, resulting from membrane contacts.

These courses have been accompanied by seminars, stressing the study techniques, and often offering contradictory viewpoints leading to interesting discussions. A special mention should be made of the contribution of L. Benedetti, who described with brio a special system of intercellular communication, the gap-junction. This volume includes the texts of these seminars. We wish to thank here both the seminar speakers and the main lecturers for having contributed so much to create a stimulating atmosphere throughout the session.

Acknowledgements

The XXXIII session of Les Houches Summer School and this volume of lecture notes would not have been possible without:

-the financial support from the Université Scientifique et Médicale de Grenoble, from the NATO Scientific Affairs Division (who included this session in its Advanced Study Institutes Programme) and from the Commissariat à l'Energie Atomique;

-the guidance of the school board;

-the typing of the manuscripts and help in the edition by Lauris Balian;

-the role played by Nicole Coiffier and Annie Battendier in the preparation and the administration of the session;

-the help of Henri Coiffier and the whole housing and cooking staff for looking after our material needs;

-the cooperation of all the participants who contributed greatly to the lectures by their lively questions and comments.

Finally, we wish to thank again the lecturers for the many hours of preparation which went into their lectures and for the quality of their manuscripts, which we hope will make the present volume a useful instrument for the scientific community.

Roger Balian
Marc Chabre
Philippe F. Devaux

CONTENTS

Course 5. (Part I). Basic elements of immunology, by Michel Fougereau *293*

Course 5. (Part II). T lymphocytes in immunity, by Jacques F. A. P. Miller *325*

INTRODUCTORY COURSE

THE CELL MEMBRANE

S. Jonathan SINGER

Department of Biology B022
University of California, San Diego
La Jolla, CA 92093
U.S.A.

Contents

R. Balian et al., eds.
Les Houches, Session XXXIII, 1979 – Membranes et Communication Intercellulaire / Membranes and Intercellular Communication

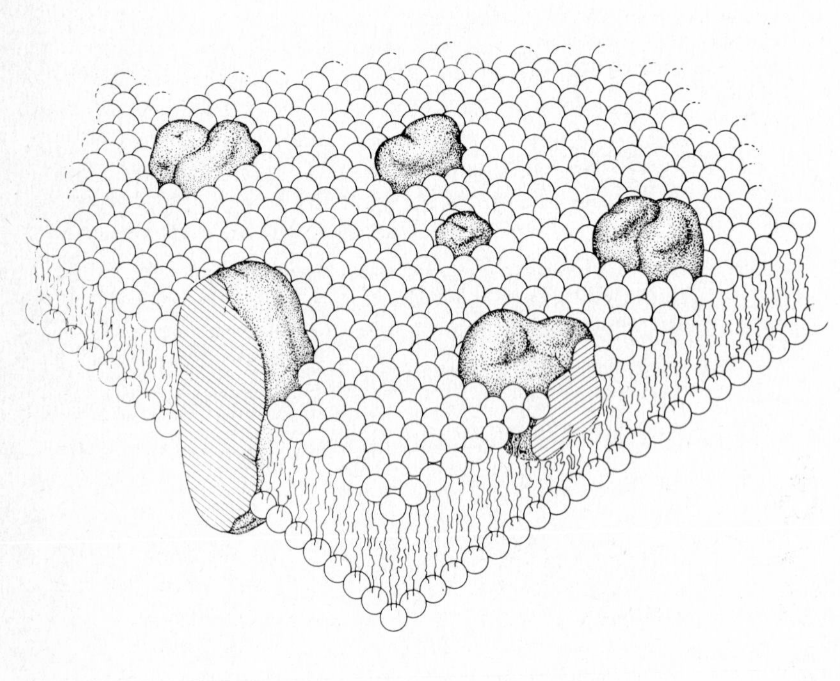

1. The composition of membranes

1.1. Lipids

1.1.1. Polar lipids

Polar lipids such as phospholipids and glycolipids: these constitute the bilayer matrix of membranes. In most real membranes, they may show enormous structural heterogeneity of their polar head groups, lengths, and degrees of unsaturation of their fatty acyl chains, chemical linkage of fatty chains to glycerol skeleton (acyl, ether), etc. It has been estimated that there are approximately 240 different molecular species of phospholipids in the human erythrocyte membrane. This gross heterogeneity is often ignored, but it must have some functional significance. First of all, it raises questions about the relevance of studies of one or two component lipid bilayer systems to real membranes. But, second, it raises the as-yet unanswered question, why? Why all this heterogeneity of phospholipids?

1.1.2. Non-polar lipids

Non-polar lipids, such as cholesterol, in contrast to the polar lipids, are not universal constituents of membranes. They are present in animal cell plasma membranes, but not intracellular membranes such as the endoplasmic reticulum. They are also absent from prokaryotic cell membranes. Therefore, they are not essential for the acquisition of membrane structure or function. They appear to play a role in "stiffening" membranes making them less fluid than they would otherwise be.

1.2. Proteins

Generally, the lipids are chemically inert and form an impermeable barrier to the flow of hydrophilic small molecules and ions. Proteins of membranes subserve most of the chemical functions of membranes, such as enzymatic (especially oxidation-reduction coupled to phosphorylation) activities, transport of ions, etc., and reception of signals such as hormonal and mitogenic stimuli. Two general classes of proteins associated with membranes can be distinguished.

1.2.1. Integral proteins

Operationally, these are recognized by their hydrophobic properties, i.e. the requirement for a detergent to solubilize them out of the membrane and their insolubility in aqueous buffers in the absence of detergent. Most membrane-bound enzymes, transport proteins, and hormone receptors are integral proteins.

1.2.2. Peripheral proteins

These are more readily removed from membranes by mild treatments, and when removed are often soluble and molecularly dispersed in aqueous buffers. A classic example is cytochrome C of the mitochondrial inner membrane. However, in addition, there are many "cytoskeletal" proteins, such as actin, myosin, and α-actinin, which in part exist inside eukaryotic cells peripherally associated with the cytoplasmic face of the plasma membrane. In erythroid cells, the protein spectrin is thus located. There are also "exoskeletal" proteins on some cells, including fibronectin and collagen on fibroblasts and some other cells.

1.3. Carbohydrate

This component of membranes exists covalently bound to one of the other two. It is attached in certain characteristic oligosaccharide chains to most if not all of the integral proteins (forming glycoproteins) that protrude from the outer surface of animal cell membranes and from prokaryotic and plant cell membranes. In the latter two cases the carbohydrate can define a relatively rigid outer casing for the cell (cellulose in the case of plant cells). With animal cells the oligosaccharides attached to glycoproteins do not form a rigid matrix, but, together with the other form of covalently-bound carbohydrates, the complex glycolipids, they undoubtedly play an important role in the "social behavior" of cells, their interactions with one another, organization into tissues, etc. The sialic acid residues on the glycoproteins of animal cells are largely responsible for their net negative surface charge density.

2. Thermodynamics and membrane structure

Considerations of equilibrium thermodynamics have been central to the development of current models of the molecular organization of membranes. Within this article, this topic will not be elaborated on any further; for a more extensive discussion see references [1, 2].

2.1. Interactions of primary importance

For our purposes, there are four kinds of interactions: hydrophobic, hydrophilic, hydrogen-bonding, and electrostatic.

2.1.1. Hydrophobic

These are responsible for the sequestering of non-polar groups away from contact with water. The free energy required, for example, to transfer a mole of methane from benzene to water solution is +2.6 kcal/mole at 25° C. Terms of this magnitude, summed over all the methylene groups of the fatty acid chains of the polar lipids, must play an important role in determining the bilayer structure adopted by the polar lipids in water. They play a similarly important role in determining protein conformation.

2.1.2. Hydrophilic

These determine the tendency for ionic and highly polar groups (such as saccharide residues) to remain in contact with water if offered a choice between an aqueous and a non-polar environment. An estimate given for the free energy required, for example, to transfer an ion-pair from water to benzene, is more than 50 kcal/mole [2].

2.1.3. Hydrogen bonding

This is of particular importance in connection with the integral proteins of membranes, because hydrogen bonding is maximized within a non-polar medium.

2.1.4. *Electrostatic*

These may be particularly important at the surface of a bilayer, where the zwitterionic polar head groups of the phospholipids are brought into proximity to one another.

2.2. *Structure of polar lipids*

This is discussed in greater detail by other speakers. Only two points are raised here. First, the bilayer lipid structure is clearly the result of maximizing both hydrophobic and hydrophilic interactions. Second, within this gross structural arrangement, more subtle thermodynamic factors operate, including an entropy that is associated with segmental flexing and rotational motions of the fatty acid chains of the polar lipids.

2.3. *Structure of integral proteins*

2.3.1. *Amphipathy*

In order to maximize hydrophobic and hydrophilic interactions, it was suggested that integral proteins adopt equilibrium conformations within the membrane that are amphipathic, exhibiting regions of different surface polarity on the same molecule, with hydrophilic surface(s) protruding from the membrane into the aqueous medium, and the hydrophobic surface buried within the bilayer. This suggestion has been supported by many recent structural studies of membrane proteins; examples are discussed, see ref. [2].

2.3.2. *Subunit aggregates and channels*

A thermodynamically satisfactory way, that has precedence in the structure of soluble proteins, to construct aqueous "pores" or channels across membranes is to form aggregates of two or more identical or different polypeptide chains, such that ionic and polar amino acid residues can line the aqueous channel. It is suggested that most transport proteins of membranes form such subunit aggregates.

2.3.3. α-helicity in integral proteins

The thermodynamic necessity to maximize hydrogen bonding in a non-polar environment imparts extensive α-helical conformation to the portions of integral protein molecules that are within the interior of membranes.

2.3.4. Oligosaccharides of integral glycoproteins

Hydrophilic interactions dictate that the saccharide residues attached to glycoproteins be exclusively located on those portions of the amphipathic molecules of the integral proteins that protrude into the aqueous medium. In addition, however, it turns out that these oligosaccharides are confined to the exterior surface of the plasma membrane (see subsection 2.5 on Membrane Asymmetry).

2.4. Structure of peripheral proteins

These structures are assumed to be no different in kind from those of ordinary soluble proteins. Their association with membranes is generally thought to be due to a specific affinity of a particular peripheral protein molecule for a site on the protruding portion of a particular integral protein molecule of the membrane.

2.5. Membrane asymmetry

The polar lipids of real membranes are generally asymmetrically distributed between the two halves of the bilayer, and the molecules of each integral protein are all oriented in a particular direction perpendicular to the plane of the membrane [3]. Two questions arise: how is such asymmetry achieved during the biosynthesis of a new membrane; and how is the asymmetry maintained against randomization by rotational diffusion? Only the latter question is considered at this juncture. Transmembrane rotations of the polar lipids and integral proteins of membranes are generally very slow although their lateral mobility in the same membranes can be very large (see next section). This is, almost certainly, in large part due to the hydrophilic interactions. The large free energy of activation that is required to move the polar portions of the polar lipids and integral proteins through the hydrophobic interior of the membrane to the other side greatly slows the rate of such motions.

3. Membranes as two-dimensional solutions

3.1. The fluid mosaic model

With no strong chemical forces acting between polypeptide chains and phospholipid molecules, the structure of membranes is a mosaic of globular integral protein molecules intercalated into a lipid bilayer. If the individual protein molecules exhibit a non-covalent directional bonding to one another, the resultant structure is a rigid, two dimensional lattice (such as exists in the bacteriorhodopsin purple membrane). In the absence of such protein–protein interactions, the membrane is a two-dimensional oriented solution of the integral proteins, randomly distributed in the bilayer lipid matrix. If the lipid matrix is fluid at the temperature of study, the result is a special kind of two-dimensional liquid solution [4].

3.2. The fluidity of membranes

By the early 1970s, it became clear that membrane proteins could move rapidly over long distances in the plane of a membrane. Two-dimensional diffusion constants have since obtained by various biophysical techniques and for several proteins which fall in the range of 10^{-9}–10^{-10} $cm^2\ s^{-1}$.

3.3. The regulation of membrane fluidity

In prokaryotes, it has been shown that perturbations of membrane fluidity (induced by temperature change or drugs) are rapidly restored by changes in the incorporation of fatty acyl groups of the membrane polar lipids. This indicates not only that there are membrane enzymes that sense such changes in membrane fluidity, but that the fluidity is regulated presumably because of its physiological importance [7, 8].

3.4. Lipid–protein interactions

It has recently been shown [9] that small molecule amphipathic compounds have a low solubility in real membranes but a high solubility in synthetic phospholipid bilayers. The compounds have included chlorpromazine (cationic), 2,4-dinitrophenol (anionic), and *n*-decanol (nonionic). This suggests that in many real membranes there exists a large internal pressure which excludes these amphipaths from the bilayer. The sources of this internal pressure are not yet all clear, but integral proteins appear to contribute to it as evidenced by reconstitution experiments. This is quite different from the "annulus" model of lipid–protein interactions, cf. [10], in which the immediate layer of phospholipid molecules surrounding an integral protein molecule is "bound", with the next layer essentially unperturbed. The low solubility of amphipaths in membranes suggests that the effects of protein on lipid structure may be fairly long range [11].

The two-dimensional solution appears, therefore, to be thermodynamically, highly non-ideal.

4. Transmembrane interactions

It should not come as a great surprise that the plasma membrane of a cell is not simply a semipermeable isolated sheath around a cell, but is in a state of dynamic interaction with cytoplasmic molecules and organelles. Many kinds of perturbations of membranes rapidly lead to changes in the interactions of membrane components with, in particular, cytoskeletal proteins.

4.1. The capping phenomenon

When antibodies, specific for a particular cell surface component, are bound to cells and are observed with fluorescently-labeled anti-antibodies in the light microscope, it is often found that the antibodies have collected to one region of the cell surface (a "cap") after about 20–30 min at 37° C. This process is inhibited by low temperatures or by inhibitors of energy metabolism. There is now substantial evidence to suggest that the cross-linking of surface components by their antibodies leads to an association (by mechanisms unknown) of such clusters with actin/myosin/α-actinin underneath the membrane, and that by an analogue of the muscle sliding filament mechanism, the clusters of surface components are then collected, in an energy-requiring process, into the cap [12].

4.2. Capping and endocytosis

The capping of a specific surface component by its antibodies is often accompanied by the endocytosis of that surface component into intracellular vesicles. The mechanisms involved are not clear, but the prior trans-membrane association of the clusters with the proteins actin/ myosin/α-actinin may be required for endocytosis to occur.

4.3. Cell–cell interactions as a mutual capping phenomenon

The physiological importance of capping phenomena may be in connection with specific cell–cell interactions, where a recognition molecule on the surface of one cell binds to a receptor molecule on the other. Under the proper circumstances these molecules may cap each other into the region of cell–cell contact; these intercellular bonds may indeed define the region of cell–cell contact.

4.4. The immobilization of surface components on flat cells

It has long been observed that, in contrast to the capping phenomenon that occurs with round cells such as lymphocytes, surface components on flat cells such as fibroblasts appear to be immobile. That is, the binding of antibodies to a specific surface component on such cells does not lead to a long-range redistribution of the antibodies into a cap. We have shown [12] that this is due to antibody-induced clusters of a surface component becoming linked across the membrane to actin/ myosin/α-actinin-containing fibers underneath the cell membrane. These so-called stress fibers often stretch the length of the flat cell. When clusters of a surface component undergo transmembrane linkage to the stress fibers, they thereupon become "immobilized".

The presumption is that the transmembrane linkage of clusters of surface components to actin/myosin/α-actinin occurs by the same (unknown) mechanism on both round and flat cells, but that the structural state of the actin/myosin/α-actinin is very different in the two types of cells, and this difference permits capping in the case of the round cell and immobilization in the case of the flat cell.

These observations can explain the observations that surface components appear to be more mobile in virally-transformed fibroblasts than in normal fibroblasts. Upon transformation of fibroblasts, their stress fibers undergo disaggregation, and this could lead to a change in apparent mobility of surface components [12].

4.5. The induction of polarity in cells

Many cells show distinct polarity, that is, specific structures are segregated to different ends of a single cell in a tissue, and other structures are organized at cell–cell contact regions. An example is the columnar epithelial cell, with its microvilli and brush border at one end of the cell facing the lumen of the tissue and the basal lamina facing opposite, cf. [13]. Cell–cell contacts are of several kinds in the brush border region, in the following sequence: tight junctions, belt desmosomes, and spot desmosomes. Each of these structures shows a highly characteristic and reproducible ultrastructure, both inside and outside the cell boundary. If we start with a cell exhibiting a fluid mosaic membrane which has no polarity, how is such polarity and organization produced? At present, the molecular basis for such ultrastructural organization is completely unknown. The likelihood is that interactions between cell membrane components and intracellular components (trans-membrane interactions) play important roles in these phenomena, but we have yet to define the components involved.

5. Biosynthesis of membranes

It is generally thought that new membrane synthesis does not occur *de novo*, but uses pre-existing membranes as templates. In gram-negative bacteria, possessing only a single membrane, it has been shown [3] that new phospholipid synthesis occurs exclusively on the cytoplasmic face of the membrane, and is then rapidly transferred to the opposite face. Apparently in a non-growing state such transfer is negligible (see subsection 2.5). The mechanism for such transfer during growth is not known.

Amphipathic molecules of integral proteins are not simply inserted into membranes. One mechanism of attachment appears to involve a signal sequence of some 20 or so largely hydrophobic amino acids on the *N*-terminal end of the polypeptide chain, which it is thought is involved in the initiation of oriented membrane insertion of the molecule [3]. Subsequent to insertion, the signal peptide is removed by proteolysis.

The asymmetry of membranes is achieved by these and other poorly understood mechanisms of biosynthesis and incorporation of lipid and protein constituents.

6. Conclusions

We are still in a primitive stage of understanding the molecular mechanisms that involve membranes in a whole range of phenomena of great physiological importance. However, we are beginning to understand: how membranes are organized, and how their components are synthesized and/or inserted into membranes; the dynamic properties of membrane components, and the role they play in cellular physiology and cell–cell interactions; the trans-membrane interactions that can be induced between membrane components and cytoskeletal proteins, and how these may be involved in the determination of cell polarity and intercellular connections.

References

[1] S. J. Singer, in: Structure and Function of Biological Membranes, ed. L. I. Rothfield (Academic Press, New York, 1971) ch. 4, pp. 145–222.
[2] S. J. Singer, in: Structure of Biological Membranes, eds. S. Abrahamsson and I. Pascher (Plenum Publ. Co., 1976) pp. 443–461.
[3] J. Rothman and J. Lenard, Science 195 (1977) 743.
[4] S. J. Singer and G. L. Nicolson, Science 175 (1972) 720.
[5] L. D. Frye and M. Edidin, J. Cell Sci. 7 (1970) 319.
[6] M. Edidin. Ann. Rev. Biophys. Bioeng. 3 (1974) 179.
[7] M. Sinensky, J. Bacteriol. 106 (1971) 449.
[8] L. O. Ingram, J. Bacteriol. 125 (1976) 670.
[9] M. Conrad and S. J. Singer, Proc. Nat. Acad. Sci. USA, 76 (1979) 5202.
[10] R. B. Gennis and A. Jonas, Ann. Rev. Biophys. Bioeng. 6 (1977) 195.
[11] S. Marcelja, Biochim. Biophys. Acta 455 (1976) 1.
[12] S. J. Singer, J. F. Ash, L. Y. W. Bourguignon, M. H. Heggeness and D. Louvard, J. Supramol. Struct. 9 (1978) 373.
[13] B. E. Hull and L. A. Staehelin, J. Cell Biol. 81 (1979) 67.

COURSE 1

PHYSICAL PROPERTIES OF MODEL MEMBRANES AND BIOLOGICAL MEMBRANES

Joachim SEELIG

Biozentrum der Universität Basel,
Klingelbergstrasse 70, CH4056 Basel, Switzerland

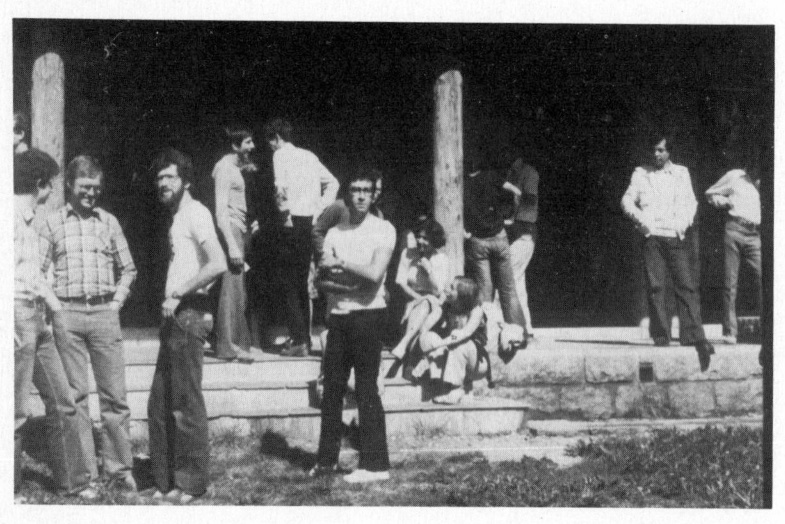

Contents

R. Balian et al., eds.
Les Houches, Session XXXIII, 1979 – Membranes et Communication Intercellulaire / Membranes and Intercellular Communication

1. Lipid monolayers

1.1. Surface pressure

An extensive literature exists on the formation and physical properties of monomolecular films (cf. Adamson 1976, Aveyard and Haydon 1973, Phillips 1972, Gaines 1966). A lipid monolayer can be produced by dissolving the lipid in an organic solvent such as hexane or chloroform and spreading a droplet of this solution on a water surface. The solvent then evaporates and a monomolecular lipid layer is formed. Since the lipids are amphiphilic molecules, the hydrophilic groups will tend to be in contact with water while the hydrophobic fatty acyl chains stick up in the air.

The conventional experimental arrangement to study monolayers is the Langmuir surface balance as shown schematically in fig. 1.1. The Langmuir trough is filled with water and a known amount of lipid is spread on the surface. The resulting monomolecular film is confined between a movable barrier and a float, the latter being connected to a torsion device. As the barrier is moved across the water surface the space occupied by the lipids is reduced and the film exerts a force on the float which can be measured by the torsion device. From the total area of the film and the known number of lipid molecules in the surface, the area-per-molecule, A, can be calculated. The measured force divided by the length of the float yields the surface pressure π. The results of monolayer studies are therefore represented as area–pressure (A–π) diagrams. (A = surface area-per-molecule in Å^2; π = surface pressure in dynes/cm.)

An alternative method for measuring the surface pressure follows from a consideration of the surface tension γ. If γ_0 is the surface tension of pure water and γ that of water covered by a monolayer then the surface pressure π is given by

$$\pi = \gamma_0 - \gamma. \tag{1.1}$$

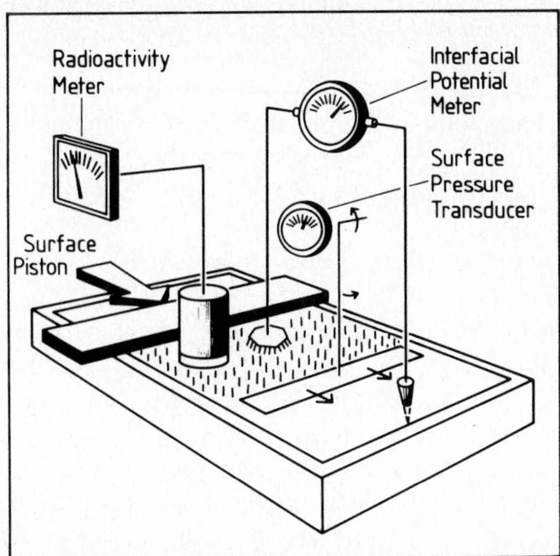

Fig. 1.1. Monolayer membrane model is formed by floating lipid molecules that have an affinity for water in a "trough". Movable piston and pressure transducer measure strength of attractive and repulsive forces between membrane's molecules; potentiometer connected to top of membrane and water beneath it measures electrical forces across it. [After A. D. Bangham, Hospital Practice (March 1973) p.79].

A particularly useful method to determine surface tensions is the Wilhelmy plate method (fig. 1.2). If a thin plate of glass or platinum is partially immersed in a liquid it will support a meniscus whose weight is

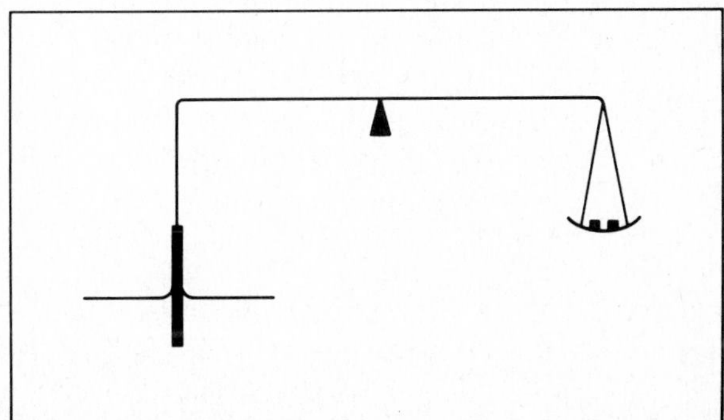

Fig. 1.2. Schematic diagram of the Wilhelmy plate method. [After Aveyard and Haydon (1973).]

given very accurately by the equation

$$W_{\text{total}} = W_{\text{plate}} + \gamma p, \tag{1.2}$$

where p is the perimeter of the plate. The various methods of measuring surface tension and surface pressure have been reviewed in detail by Gaines (1966) and by Adamson (1976).

1.2. Physical states of monomolecular films

Figure 1.3 shows an experimental area–pressure curve for the diester $C_2H_5OOC(CH_2)_{11}COOC_2H_5$ (cf. Aveyard and Haydon, 1973, pp. 94–96). At low pressure, the surface area-per-molecule is large compared to the molecular dimensions and the lipid molecules are thought to lie flat on the surface with both their polar groups in the water. In this very dilute state the lipid molecules appear to behave like a two-dimensional gas. The equation of state for a perfect two-dimensional gas is given by

$$\pi A = kT, \tag{1.3}$$

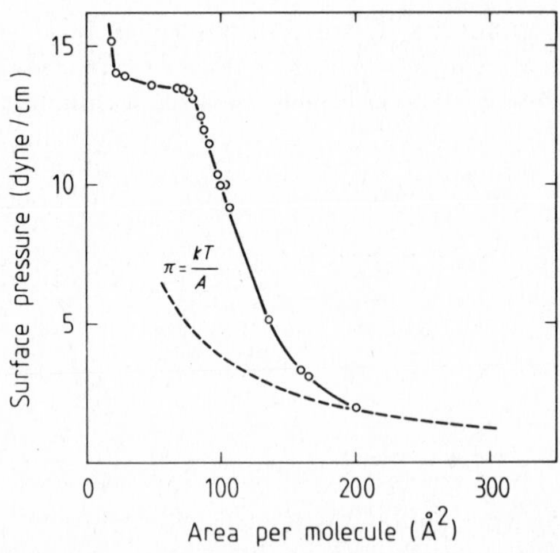

Fig. 1.3. The surface pressure as a function of area-per-molecule for the diester $C_2H_5OOC.(CH_2)_{11}.COOC_2H_5$ at the air–water interface at 1° C. The dashed curve is for an ideal two-dimensional gas. [After Aveyard and Haydon (1973).]

(k = Boltzmann constant, T = absolute temperature) and the system of fig. 1.3 obeys this equation (dashed line in fig. 1.3) at very low pressures and large areas. As the area is reduced, cohesive and repulsive interactions between the lipid molecules come into play and eq. (1.3) must be replaced by a van der Waals type of relation

$$\left(\pi + \frac{a_s}{A^2}\right)(A - A_0) = kT \tag{1.4}$$

where A_0 and a_s are constants. When the area-per-molecule is even further reduced (to less than about 80 Å^2 for the system of fig. 1.3), a condensation occurs (equivalent to the condensation of real gas). In this region the area–pressure isotherm is horizontal and a reduction of the surface area is not accompanied by an increase in the surface pressure. When the condensation is finished the area-per-molecule is about 25 Å^2. A further reduction of the surface area causes a dramatic pressure increase which very soon leads to a collapse of the monolayer. The limiting surface area of ~20 Å^2 suggests that at high surface pressures the diester is oriented vertically with only one polar group in water, since a limiting area of ~20 Å^2 is also typical for monocarboxylic acids and for fatty acyl chains attached at phospholipids.

The results of fig. 1.3 fall into the more general scheme summarized in table 1.1 and in fig. 1.4 (Gershfeld 1970, Gershfeld and Pagano 1972). The area–pressure diagram of fig. 1.4 is divided into a gaseous film, a transition region, and a condensed film, each of which can be further subdivided. (1) For areas larger than A_i (i = ideal) the monolayer behaves like a two-dimensional perfect gas. A_i is generally of the order of 50 000 Å^2/molecule. (2) At areas between A_v (v = van der Waals), typically 1 000–5 000 Å^2/molecule, and A_i the film behaves like a van-der-Waals gas. (3) Between A_v and A_c (c = condensed) the surface pressure is independent of the molecular area. In this region there exist two discrete surface phases in equilibrium, a condensed film and its two-dimensional vapor. The corresponding pressure π_v may thus be called surface vapor pressure. (4) At areas less than A_c, the monolayer exists as a single homogeneous condensed phase. In the condensed state the monolayer may form at least 3 different types of films, namely a liquid-expanded film (A_c~40–50 Å^2 for a normal aliphatic chain), a liquid-condensed film (A_c~25 Å^2), or a solid film (A_c~20 Å^2). Experimentally, the three types of films may be differentiated by their compressibility κ

$$\kappa = -\frac{1}{A}\left(\frac{\mathrm{d}A}{\mathrm{d}\pi}\right)_T \tag{1.5}$$

with κ being largest for the liquid-expanded film and smallest for the tightly-packed solid film (cf. Adamson 1976, pp. 129–133). In the solid film the molecules are probably in a well-aligned conformation, but the molecular arrangement in liquid-expanded and liquid-condensed films is still controversial. No spectroscopic probes are available to investigate the chain conformation of lipids at the air–water interface.

Monolayers of pure phospholipids have been studied extensively and excellent review articles are available (Cadenhead 1970, Phillips 1972). Generally these studies have been confined to the condensed film region of the area–pressure isotherm. As a representative example fig. 1.5 depicts the area–pressure curves for the homologous series of saturated 3-*sn*-phosphatidylcholines at the air–water interface (Phillips and Chapman 1968). At room temperature (22° C) the two 3-*sn*-phosphatidylcholines having short chains (C_{10}, C_{14}) form a liquid-expanded film, the two long-chain homologues (C_{18}, C_{22}) form a liquid-condensed film, while the lipid having C_{16} chains exhibits a well-defined transition point from a liquid-expanded to a liquid-condensed film. From such studies it can be concluded that at a given temperature and surface pressure the phospholipid packing is densest when both fatty acyl chains of the lipid are long and fully saturated; a looser configuration is obtained when

Table 1.1

State of the monolayer		Area/molecule[a] (normal aliphatic chain)
Gaseous film		
Ideal	$\pi A = kT$	$A_i \gtrsim 50\,000$ Å^2
van der Waals	$\left(\pi + \frac{a_s}{A^2}\right)(A - A_0) = kT$	$A_v \gtrsim 1\,000$–$5\,000$ Å^2
Transition region (Coexistence of two phases)		
Condensed film		
Liquid-expanded		$A_c \sim 40$–50 Å^2
Liquid-condensed		$A_c \sim 25$ Å^2
Solid		$A_c \sim 20$ Å^2

[a]According to Gershfeld and Pagano (1972).

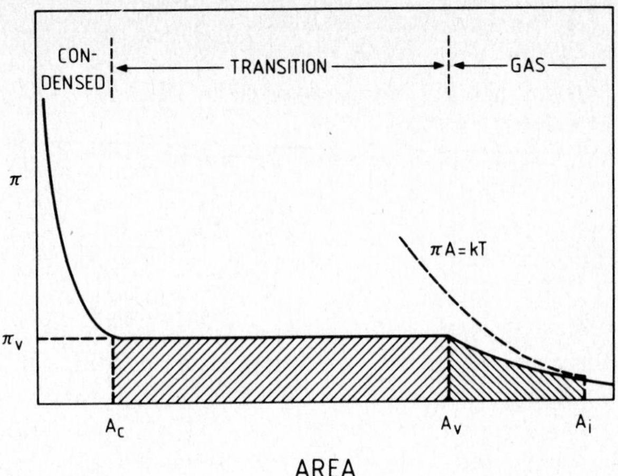

Fig. 1.4. Schematic representation of π-A isotherm in the transition region between a condensed state, area A_c and a gas, area A_v. The surface vapor pressure π_v is the value of the horizontal line in the diagram. See text for discussion. [After Gershfeld (1970).]

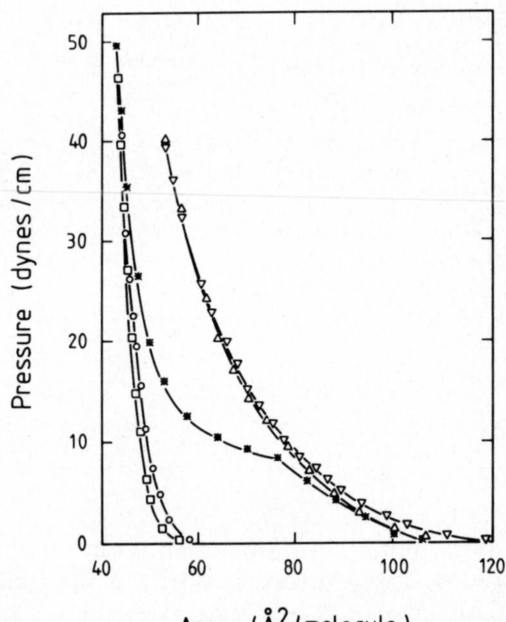

Fig. 1.5. Pressure-area curves for saturated 1,2-diacyl-L-phosphatidylcholines at the air-0.1 M NaCl interface at 22° C. (□) Dibehenoyl lecithin (C_{22}); (O) distearoyl lecithin (C_{18}); (X) dipalmitoyllecithin (C_{16}); (△) dimyristoyl lecithin (C_{14}); (▽) dicapryl lecithin (C_{10}). [After Phillips and Chapman (1968).]

one chain is either shorter or unsaturated (cf. Phillips 1972, Stoffel and Pruss 1969, Demel et al. 1967).

Another important factor in area–pressure diagrams is the temperature. This is illustrated in fig. 1.6 for monolayers of 1,2-dipalmitoyl-*sn*-glycero-3-phosphocholine. At 6.2° C the monolayer is almost totally condensed and the limiting area-per-phospholipid molecule is about 42 $Å^2$, i.e. 21 $Å^2$ per fatty acyl chain. As the temperature is raised an expanded region appears at low pressures. The 16.8 and 21.1° C-isotherms furthermore reveal well-defined transition points at which the expanded monolayer begins to condense. This transition disappears completely at temperatures larger than 41° C. Qualitatively, the area–pressure diagrams of lipid monolayers bear a close resemblance with the p-V diagram of a van der Waals gas.

1.3. Molecular packing characteristics of phospholipid–cholesterol films

Many cellular membranes such as liver plasma membranes or erythrocytes contain high levels of cholesterol in the molar ratio cholesterol : phospholipid of almost 1 : 1. Because of the importance of sterol molecules as building blocks of biological membranes, an extensive amount of work has been undertaken to understand the physical interactions of cholesterol with phospholipids (for reviews cf. Phillips 1972, Demel and de Kruijff 1976). Very early in these investigations it was observed that cholesterol exerts a condensing effect on the phospholipid molecules. For ideal mixing, a two-component monolayer would obey the equation

$$A_{\text{mix}} = nA_1 + (1-n)A_2 \tag{1.6}$$

where A_{mix} is the average molecular area, A_1 and A_2 are the molecular areas of the two single component films at the same surface pressure, and n is the mole fraction of component 1. However, experimentally it is found that mixtures of cholesterol and phospholipids deviate from ideal behavior by exhibiting smaller areas than predicted by equation (1.6). This is illustrated in fig. 1.7. Cholesterol alone forms a liquid-condensed monolayer with very little compressibility. The molecular area is 38 $Å^2$/ cholesterol molecule (Cadenhead and Phillips 1968). The molecules are oriented perpendicular to the interface at all pressures and it may safely be assumed that each molecule occupies essentially the same area in both pure and mixed films. The phospholipid used in the experiment depicted in fig. 1.7 is 1-stearoyl-2-oleoyl-*sn*-glycero-3-phos-

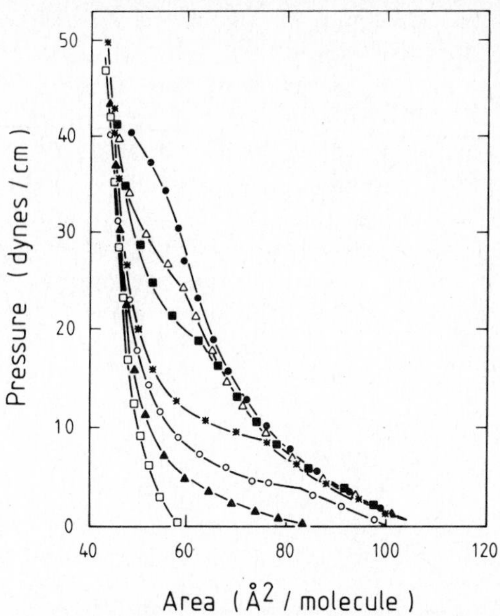

Fig. 1.6. Pressure-area curves 1,2-dipalmitoyl-L-phosphatidylcholine at the air-0.1 M NaCl interface at various temperatures: (●) 34.6° C; (△) 29.5° C; (■) 26.0° C; (X) 21.1° C; (O) 16.8° C; (▲) 12.4° C; (□) 6.2° C. [After Phillips and Chapman (1968).]

phocholine. While the fully saturated analogue 1, 2-distearoyl-*sn*-glycero-3-phosphocholine forms a liquid-condensed monolayer with a limiting area of 41 $Å^2$/ molecule, the introduction of a *cis* double bond increases the area-per-molecule drastically to 63 $Å^2$/ molecule. The dashed curve in fig. 1.7 then represents the proportionate average of the curves of the pure components and is found to be larger than the experimentally determined area of the mixture. The condensing effect of cholesterol is mainly a hydrophobic effect as evidenced by its dependence on the fatty acyl chain length and on the degree of unsaturation of the fatty acid constituents. No conclusive evidence exists that the phospholipid polar groups are also involved in this interaction (Demel and de Kruijff 1976, Müller-Landau and Cadenhead 1979). During the long history of studies on phospholipid–cholesterol systems a number of models have been suggested for the cholesterol–phospholipid interactions, in particular several authors have postulated phospholipid–cholesterol complexes of well-defined stoichiometry. Nevertheless, the subject has remained controversial. A thorough reinvestigation of this

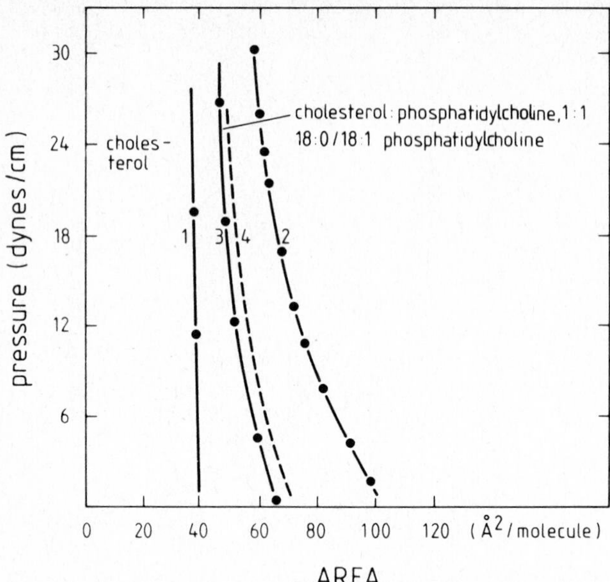

Fig. 1.7. Pressure vs area characteristics of monolayers of cholesterol, stearoyloleoylphosphatidylcholine and an equimolar mixture of the two lipids. 1 = cholesterol; 2 = stearoyloleoylphosphatidylcholine; 3 = equimolar mixture of cholesterol and stearoyloleoylphosphatidylcholine; 4 = proportionate average of the curves for the two pure lipids. [After Demel and de Kruijff (1976).]

problem has recently been undertaken for films composed of cholesterol and 1,2-dipalmitoyl-*sn*-glycero-3-phosphocholine (DPPC), providing many fresh data over a large concentration range (Müller-Landau and Cadenhead 1979). Figure 1.8 summarizes mean molecular area plots as a function of the cholesterol/DPPC film composition at various pressures. As a main conclusion it follows from these studies that, in contrast to earlier results, cholesterol and DPPC are miscible in all proportions. In a thermodynamic sense the monomolecular film is a homogeneous phase over the whole concentration range. On the molecular level, the hydrocarbon chains can, however, be divided into three groups based on their packing abilities: nearest neighbors with strong interaction, next nearest neighbors with weak interactions, and chains which are essentially unaffected. Maximal condensation is found to occur at approximately a molar ratio of 3 : 1 acyl chains/cholesterol (41.4 mole % cholesterol). These monolayer results are in excellent

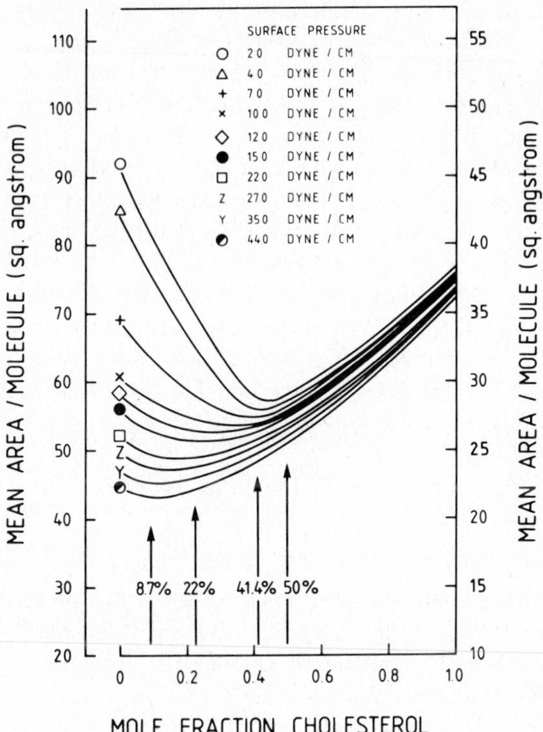

Fig. 1.8. Mean molecular area plots [DPPC, left-hand ordinate; cholesterol, right-hand ordinate] as a function of the cholesterol/DPPC film composition at indicated pressures. [After Müller and Cadenhead (1979).]

agreement with those obtained for lipid bilayers using deuterium magnetic resonance as a probing technique.

1.4. Enzyme reactions in lipid monolayers

Monolayers have been shown to be a useful tool in the study of interfacial properties of phospholipids and of spatial requirements for phospholipid–protein interaction. This will be illustrated as follows for a few selected examples.

The first system to be discussed is an enzyme complex in the inner membrane of *Salmonella typhimurium*. Gram-negative bacteria are generally surrounded by an inner and an outer membrane. The inner membrane corresponds to the plasma membrane of eukaryotic cells and carries out many different functions. The outer membrane has a different chemical composition and fewer functions have been identified so far. From the inner membrane of *Salmonella typhimurium*, two gylcosyl-transferase enzymes have been isolated and purified, catalyzing the sequential incorporation of glucose and galactose into a lipopolysaccharide (Rothfield and Pearlman 1965, Rothfield and Romeo 1971, Rothfield 1971). The lipopolysaccharide (LPS) is a glycolipid consisting of a lipid portion covalently linked to a complex phosphorylated polysaccharide. Most of the LPS is in the outer membrane, but some may be present in the inner membrane. The LPS is responsible for the endotoxin activity of *Salmonella typhimurium*. The reactions catalyzed by the glycosyltransferases in the synthesis of LPS are

$$\mathrm{UDP-Glc+LPS}\xrightarrow{\text{Enz. 1}}\mathrm{Glc-LPS+UDP}$$

$$\mathrm{UDP-Gal+Glc-LPS}\xrightarrow{\text{Enz. 2}}\mathrm{Gal-Glc-LPS+UDP.}$$

In order to activate these enzymes *in vitro* the presence of phosphatidylethanolamine, the major membrane phospholipid of this organism, is required. Reassembly of the active enzyme–lipid complex takes place in a stepwise fashion: (1) a monomolecular film of phosphatidylethanolamine is formed in a Langmuir trough. (2) LPS is injected into the aqueous subphase and penetration of LPS molecules into the monolayer is indicated by an increase in the surface pressure of the film (fig. 1.9). (3) the enzyme (I or II) is then injected into the subphase below the LPS-phosphatidylethanolamine monolayer. The incorporation of the enzyme into the monolayer is revealed by an additional increase in the surface pressure; and (4) in the final step the activated sugar is added to the subphase. After a suitable incubation period, the monolayer is removed and the incorporation of radioactively labeled sugar into LPS is determined demonstrating that the enzyme reaction has taken place within the monomolecular film. In contrast to this successful reconstitution a simple mixing of the components does not lead to any sugar incorporation into LPS. This indicates that the LPS molecule, the phosphatidylethanolamine and the glycosyltransferases must be organized in a particular spatial arrangement in order to become fully active.

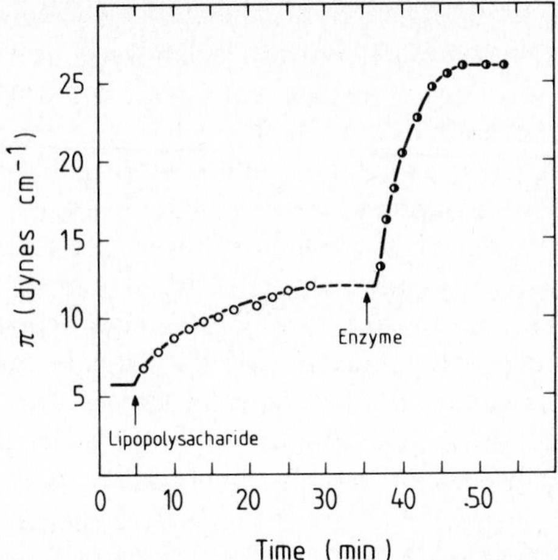

Fig. 1.9. Interaction of enzyme with a lipopolysaccharide-phosphatidylethanolamine monolayer. A film of *A. agilis* phosphatidylethanolamine was formed on the surface of the first compartment of the multi–compartment trough at a surface pressure of 6 dynes cm^{-1} (5.1 n moles). Lipopolysaccharide (200 μg/ml) was injected into the subsolution and after a further increase in surface pressure of 5.5 dynes cm^{-1} the film was moved onto the surface of the third compartment. The movement required 3 to 4 min, as indicated by the interrupted line in the graph. A solution of 1 M $MgCl_2$ was then injected under the binary film to a final concentration of 6 mM and transferase enzyme (in 5 mM phosphate buffer, pH 6,8, containing 20% glycerol) was injected into the subsolution to a concentration of 7μg/ml. In a parallel experiment, injection of the same amount of glycerol in phosphate buffer did not affect the surface pressure. –O–O– surface pressure after injection of lipopolysaccharide; –◑–◑– after injection of enzyme. [After Romeo et al. (1970).]

The physical state of the membrane phospholipids has also been found to be an important factor in regulating membrane properties. Overath et al. (1970) have demonstrated elegantly for *Escherichia coli* that changes in the temperature characteristic of *in vivo* parameters can be related to physical properties of isolated phospholipids in monolayers at an air–water interface. To this purpose Overath and colleagues employed an *E. coli* double mutant which was unable to synthesize or degrade unsaturated fatty acids, but incorporated exogenous fatty acids into the membrane phospholipids. By supplying fatty acids with various hydrocarbon chain structures (*trans* or *cis* double bond; various numbers of *cis* double bonds) to the growth medium, it was possible to modulate the physical properties of the *E. coli* membranes within certain limits. This was reflected most dramatically in the transport properties of the cells. Measuring the rate of efflux of thiomethyl-β-

galactoside gave well-defined breaks in the temperature characteristics (fig. 1.10). The break points were shifted towards lower temperatures with increasing extent of *cis*-unsaturation. This behavior was compared with the physical properties of monolayers formed from the extracted *E. coli* lipids. It was found that all lipids gave phase transitions from a liquid-expanded to a liquid-condensed state. The occurrence of this transition was dependent on the temperature (cf. also fig. 1.6); above a critical temperature only liquid-expanded films were observed. Table 1.2 then compares the temperature at which the liquid-condensed film first appears with the break point in thiomethyl-β-galactoside efflux. The good correlation between the two types of measurements indicates that the physical state of the lipids in the membrane influences the function of the membrane-bound transport system (cf. also Overath et al. 1971).

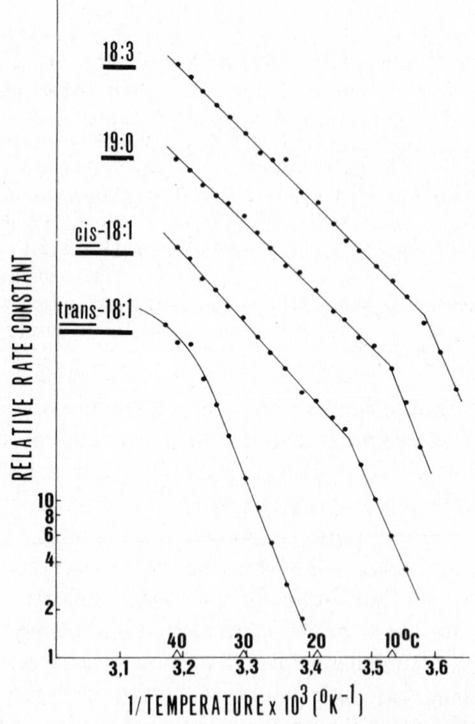

Fig. 1.10. Arrhenius plot of relative rate constants of [^{14}C] TMG efflux. The figure gives rate constants normalized to a temperature of 40° C. The rate constants in min $^{-1}$ at this temperature are: *cis*-18 : 1, 1.35; 18 : 3, 1.47; *trans*-18 : 1, 1.65; 19 : 0, 1.0. [After Overath et al., (1970).]

Table 1.2

Correlation of *in vivo* and *in vitro* phase transitions of membrane lipids in *Escherichia coli*[a]

	Fatty acid incorporated in phospholipid[b]			
	18 : 3	19 : 0	*trans*-18 : 1	*cis*-18 : 1
Efflux of thiomethyl-β-galactoside	6° C	10° C	38° C	15° C
Appearance of phase transition in monolayers	4° C	10° C	41° C	15° C

[a]According to Overath et al. (1970).

[b]18 : 3 *cis, cis, cis*-$\Delta^{9,12,15}$-octadecatrienoic acid; 19 : 0 DL-*cis*-9, 10-methylene-octadecanoic acid; and *trans*-18 : 1 *trans*-Δ^{9}-octadecenoic acid *cis* 18 : 1 *cis*-Δ^{9}-octadecenoic acid.

1.5. Monolayers and the lipid bilayer concept of biological membranes

The idea of a lipid bilayer as the basic building block of biological membranes goes back to early monolayer experiments of Gorter and Grendel (1925) who extracted the lipids from a defined number of erythrocytes, spread the lipids in a Langmuir trough and compared the area of the erythrocytes. Since the ratio of the areas was 2 : 1 Gorter and Grendel concluded that the amount of lipid in the erythrocyte would be sufficient to form a bimolecular leaflet of lipids in the cell membrane.

The original experiments of Gorter and Grendel contained a number of experimental weaknesses (cf. Branton and Deamer 1972, pp. 14 – 17, Zwaal et al. 1976). First the lipids were extracted with acetone and we now know that not all lipids can be removed by this treatment. Second, the red cell surface area was underestimated by about 30%. Third, and most important, Gorter and Grendel measured the monolayer area at an arbitrary, very low surface pressure (~9 dynes/cm). Since the surface area occupied by a phospholipid molecule critically depends on the applied surface pressure, the question arises which surface pressure best represents the situation in an intact biological membrane.

One approach to this problem is the use of phospholipases (Zwaal et al. 1975, Demel et al. 1975, Zwaal et al. 1976). The action of phospholipases purified from various sources on intact erythrocytes has been investigated in detail and two groups of phospholipases can be differentiated. One group of enzymes cannot hydrolyze the phospholipids of intact erythrocyte membranes, whereas the other group of phospholipases can attack red cells under the same circumstances (cf. table 1.3).

Table 1.3

Comparison of the effects of different phospholipases on erythrocyte membranes and monomolecular films[a)]

Phospholipases	Erythrocytes	Monolayers[b)] (dynes/cm)
Phospholipase		
A_2(pig pancreas)	−	16.5
D (cabbage)	−	20.5
A_2(*Cr. adamanteus*)	−	23.0
C(*B. cereus*)	−	31.0
A_2(*N. naja*)	+	34.8
A_2(*bee venom*)	+	35.3
Sphingomyelinase (*S. aureus*)	+	40.0
Phospholipase C (*C. welchii*)	+	40.0

[a)]According to Demel et al. (1975).
[b)]Maximal surface pressure at which these phospholipases can hydrolyze monomolecular films.

This behavior may be compared with the action of the same phospholipases on monomolecular films of various surface pressures as shown in fig. 1.11. Here a ^{14}C-labeled methyl group was introduced in the choline moiety of the lipid molecule and the enzymatic degradation by phospholipase C was followed by measuring the surface radioactivity. In fig. 1.11a, the surface pressure is ~29 dynes/cm. After a short lag period a rapid release of the phosphate–choline moiety is indicated by the decrease in radioactivity. The simultaneous decrease of the surface pressure can be explained by a rearrangement of the lipid molecules and a change in the packing density due to the formation of diacylglycerol. If the same experiment is performed at an initial surface pressure of 34.8 dynes/cm (fig. 1.11b), no degradation occurs. The detailed surface pressure dependence (fig. 1.11c) shows a rapid hydrolysis of phosphatidylcholine at pressures below 30 dynes/cm, whereas at higher pressures the hydrolysis stops completely. All phospholipases which were unable to attack red cells were also unable to degrade monomolecular phospholipid films at an initial surface pressure above 31 dynes/cm. On the other hand, those phospholipases which did attack intact erythrocytes were also able to degrade monomolecular films at all surface pressures. From these investigations which are summarized in table 1.3 it is safe to conclude that the lipid packing in the erythrocyte membrane is comparable with a lateral surface pressure between 31 and 34.8 dynes/cm. At this pressure the molecular area for an unsaturated

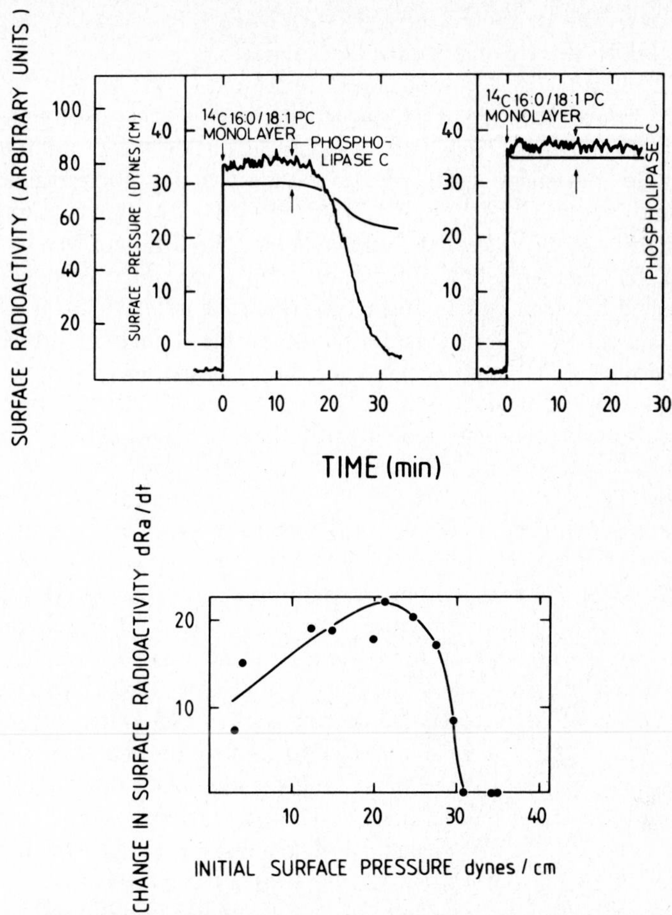

Fig. 1.11. (a) left and (b) right. Change in surface radioactivity (Ra) and surface pressure of ^{14}C-labelled palmitoyl-oleoyl phosphatidylcholine monolayers upon hydrolysis by phospholipase C from *B. cereus* (0.16 I.U.). The subsolution consists of 10^{-2} M tris pH 7.4 at 37° C. (c) Relation between the change in surface radioactivity and the initial surface pressure of ^{14}C-labelled palmitoyloleoyl phosphatidylcholine monolayers upon hydrolyses by phospholipase C from *B. cereus* (0.16 I.U.). [After Demel et al. (1975).]

phospholipid such as 1-palmitoyl-2-oleoyl-*sn*-glycero-3-phosphocholine is 58–59 Å^2/mol. Assuming a constant area of 38 Å^2/mol for cholesterol, a surface pressure of ~32 dynes/cm would lead to a monolayer area–erythrocyte surface area ratio of 1.5. This implies that the number of lipid molecules-per-red cell is not sufficient to form a bilayer covering the total red cell surface. On the basis of the present result only 75% of the erythrocyte surface can be made up by a lipid bilayer while the remainder must be occupied by proteins.

An interesting new development providing direct insight into the bilayer surface pressure is based on the observation that unilamellar bilayer vesicles (liposomes) when spread at an air–water interface are not stable, but disintegrate into a monomolecular phospholipid film (Verger and Pattus 1975, Pattus et al. 1978a). A detailed quantitative examination of this effect shows that after a lipid monolayer has been formed by disintegration of vesicles a lipid exchange equilibrium is established between vesicle and monolayer (Schindler 1979).

The results of a simple experiment in the Langmuir trough are depicted in fig. 1.12. A beaker containing a solution of unilamellar vesicles of well-defined size and chemical composition (1,2-dioleoyl-*sn*-glycero-3-phosphocholine; vesicle radius 350 Å) is placed in a Langmuir trough with the rim of the beaker remaining 1 mm below the water surface. The movable barrier of the Langmuir trough is fixed (constant surface area) and the increase in the surface pressure π is monitored as a function of time. The time course of π strongly depends on the vesicle concentration. At high vesicle concentrations a steady-state value of 24.5 ± 1.0 dynes/cm is reached and the data in fig. 1.12 suggest that this steady-state value should be approached independent of the initial vesicle concentration. By a number of different experiments and a thorough quantitative analysis of the problem, Schindler was able to demonstrate that a surface pressure of 24.5 dynes/cm is indeed the equilibrium surface pressure for the bilayer–monolayer transition in the above defined experimental system. The equilibrium pressure is dependent on the size of the vesicles and increases with increasing vesicle radius. The molecular picture which emerges from these studies can be summarized as follows. If a solution of unilamellar phospholipid vesicles is brought into contact with an air–water interface some of the vesicles disintegrate forming a monolayer. A layer of vesicles now assembles in close association with the monolayer. The concentration of vesicles which interact with the monolayer is found to exceed that in the bulk solution by a factor of 75. Two exchange processes take place in the adsorbed vesicle layer, namely (1) an exchange of intact vesicles between the adsorbed vesicle layer and the bulk solution and (2) an exchange of lipid molecules between the monolayer and the outer lipid layer of the adsorbed vesicles (Schindler 1979).

A bilayer surface pressure of 24.5 dynes/cm for vesicles of 1,2-dioleoyl-*sn*-glycero-3-phosphocholine is close to the value of 31 dynes/cm

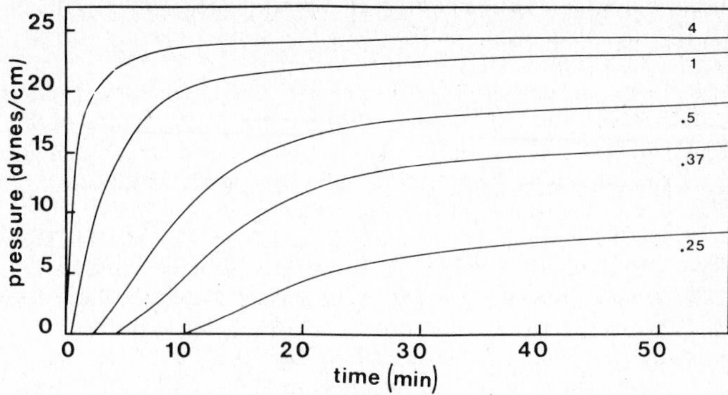

Fig. 1.12. Surface pressure rise at the interface of a vesicle containing aqueous solution as a function of vesicle concentration (labels in units of mg/ml). [After (Schindler 1979).]

as derived from phospholipase digestion experiments. The small but nevertheless significant difference may reflect the different chemical composition and size of the systems. More detailed results can be expected in the near future from monolayer studies of intact biological membranes, since it has been reported that even membranes like the inner and outer membrane of *E. coli* or intact erythrocytes can be spread at the air–water interface and form well-defined monomolecular films without loss or denaturation of membrane-bound protein (Pattus et al. 1978b).

References

Adamson, A. W. (1976) Physical Chemistry of Surfaces, 3rd ed. (Wiley, New York).

Aveyard, R. and D. A. Haydon (1973) An Introduction to the Principles of Surface Chemistry (University Press, Cambridge).

Branton, D. and D. N. Deamer (1972) Membrane Structure, (Springer Verlag, New York).

Cadenhead, D. A. (1970) in: Recent Progress in Surface Science, vol. 3, J. F. Danielli, A. C. Riddiford and M. D. Rosenberg, eds. (Academic Press, New York) pp. 169–192.

Cadenhead, D. A. and M. C. Phillips (1967) J. Coll. Interf. Sci. 24, 491.

Demel, R. A. and B. de Kruijff (1976) Biochim. Biophys. Acta 457, 109.

Demel, R. A., L. L. M. van Deenen and B. A. Pethica (1967) Biochim. Biophys. Acta 135, 11.

Demel, R. A., W. S. M. Geuris van Kessel, R. F. A. Zwaal, B. Roelofsen and L. L. M. van Deenen (1975) Biochim. Biophys. Acta 406, 97.

Gaines, G. L., Jr., 1966, Insoluble Monolayers at Liquid–Gas Interfaces, (Wiley Interscience, New York).

Gershfeld, N. L. (1970) J. Coll. Interf. Sci. 32, 167.

Gershfeld, N. L. and R. E. Pagano (1972) J. Phys. Chem. 76, 1231.

Gorter, E. and F. Grendel (1925) J. Exp. Med. 41, 439.

Müller-Landau, F. and D. A. Cadenhead (1979) Chem. Phys. Lip. 25, 315.
Overath, P., H. U. Schairer and W. Stoffel (1970) Proc. Natl. Acad. Sci. USA 67, 606.
Overath, P., H. U. Schairer, F. F. Hill and I. Lamnek-Hirsch (1971) Structure and Function of Hydrocarbon Chains in Bacterial Phospholipids, in: The Dynamic Structure of Cell Membranes, eds. D. F. H. Wallach and H. Fischer (Springer Verlag, Berlin) pp. 149–164.
Pattus, F., P. Desnuelle and R. Verger (1978) Biochim. Biophys. Acta 507, 62.
Phillips, M. C. and D. Chapman (1968) Biochim. Biophys. Acta 163, 301.
Phillips, M. C. (1972) The Physical State of Phospholipids and Cholesterol in Monolayers, Bilayers and Membranes, in: Progress in Surface and Membrane Science, vol. 5, eds. J. F. Danielli, M. D. Rosenberg and D. A. Cadenhead (Academic Press, New York) pp. 139–221.
Romeo, D., A. Hinckley and L. Rothfield (1970) J. Mol. Biol. 53, 491.
Rothfield, L. I. (1971) Some Aspects of the Structure and Assembly of Bacterial Membranes, in: The Dynamic Structure of Cell Membranes, eds. D. F. H. Wallach and H. Fischer (Springer Verlag, Berlin) pp. 165–179.
Rothfield, L. and M. Pearlman (1966) J. Biol. Chem. 241, 1386.
Rothfield, L. I. and D. Romeo (1971) in: Structure and Function of Biological Membranes, ed. L. I. Rothfield (Academic Press, New York) pp. 251–284.
Schindler, H. (1979) Biochim. Biophys. Acta 555, 316.
Stoffel, W and H. D. Pruss (1969) Hoppe-Seyler's Z. Physiol. Chem. 350, 1385.
Verger R. and F. Pattus, (1976) Chem. Phys. Lipids 16, 285.
Zwaal, R. F. A., R. A. Demel, B. Roelofsen and L. L. M. van Deenen (1976) TIBS 1, 112.
Zwaal R. F. A., B. Roelofsen, P. Comfurius and L. L. M. van Deenen (1975) Biochim. Biophys. Acta 406, 83.

2. Thermodynamics of phospholipid bilayers

2.1. Phase transitions in membranes

In the course of investigating the temperature behavior of biological membranes and also pure lipid-water systems it has frequently been observed that the experimental parameters do not vary smoothly with temperature but exhibit irregularities or discontinuities in one or more narrow temperature intervals. Some typical examples are:

(1) the enzymatic activity of membrane-bound proteins which shows distinct breaks at certain temperatures (Schairer and Overath 1969);

(2) changes in the fluorescence intensity and fluorescence anisotropy of fluorescent dyes (Overath and Träuble 1973);

(3) discontinuities in the excess specific heat of membranes and the protein-free lipids of *Acholeplasma laidlawii* (Steim et al. 1969, Melchior et al. 1970);

(4) temperature induced protein or lipid clustering as visualized by electron microscopy (Wunderlich et al. 1975).

This selection of techniques is by no means complete. Irregularities have also been detected with dilatometry, ^{1}H-, ^{2}H-, ^{13}C-, and ^{31}P-NMR, X-ray diffraction and epr-nitroxide spin labels. The observed changes are not due to the individual properties of a molecule but must be attributed to a large area of the membrane as a whole. Therefore, it is appropriate to denote these discontinuities or breaks in the experimentally observable parameters as phase changes or phase transition characterized by a transition temperature T_c.

Originally it was believed that the different experimental phenomena could be understood on the basis of just one molecular process, namely an order–disorder transition. The order–disorder transition is related to a melting of the hydrocarbon chains and can be described as a transition from a gel state to a liquid crystalline state. In the gel state the hydrocarbon chains are in the extended all-trans conformation, relatively rigid, and packed in a hexagonal lattice. The interchain separation is well-defined and gives rise to a sharp wide-angle X-ray reflex at $(4.2\ \text{Å})^{-1}$ corresponding to a chain–chain separation of 4.9 Å. Deuterium NMR data suggest that the chains are rotating around their long molecular axis (Davis 1979). In the liquid–crystalline state the segmental motions are drastically increased and the chains become disordered due to rapid trans–gauche isomerizations around carbon–carbon bonds. The chain–chain separation is a dynamic average of many different conformations and the sharp wide-angle reflex at $(4.2\ \text{Å})^{-1}$ is replaced by a diffuse reflex centered at $(4.6\ \text{Å})^{-1}$. Assuming again a hexagonal lattice, the average chain–chain separation in the liquid crystalline state is widened to 5.3 Å. The same diffuse $(4.6\ \text{Å})^{-1}$ reflex is also found in liquid hydrocarbons and this similarity was one of the earliest indications that the hydrocarbon chains in a lipid bilayer are disordered and liquid-like (Luzzati 1968).

An order–disorder transition is not the only mechanism capable of explaining the observed discontinuities in biomembranes. Another important type of structural reorganization are changes in the phase geometry. Phospholipid water mixtures form a variety of structurally different mesophases some of which are illustrated in fig. 2.1. By changing the water content, salt concentration, or temperature, transitions can be induced between the various mesophases which in turn would influence the biochemical parameters of the membrane.

Again a different kind of phase behavior is phase separations. Natural membranes generally contain mixtures of lipids which differ both in respect to their head groups and in their hydrocarbon chains.

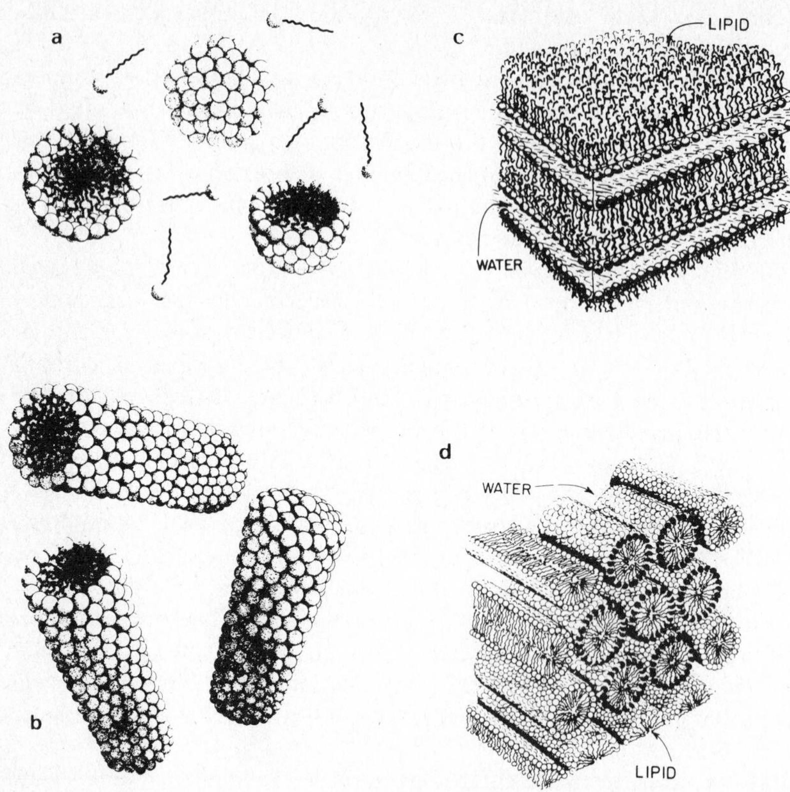

Fig. 2.1. Lyotropic liquid crystals. (a) Spherical micelles; (b) Rodlike micelles; (c) Bilayer (lyotropic smectic phase); and (d) Cylinders (lyotropic hexagonal phase). [From Rosevear (1968).]

The physical properties of such mixtures depend on the degree of similarity or dissimilarity of the lipid species. Lipids differing only by one or two carbon atoms in their fatty acyl chains can be expected to give ideal mixing in both the liquid crystalline and the gel phase whereas two dissimilar lipids will form a heterogeneous gel phase, i.e. in the extreme case the molecules will separate into two different regions corresponding to the pure compounds. Such a phase separation may not be limited to the gel state, but under certain conditions could also occur in the liquid–crystalline state.

2.2. *Thermodynamic definition of phase transitions*

A number of conditions can be specified if two phases are in thermodynamic equilibrium (Münster 1956, p. 220, Landau–Lifshitz 1958, pp. 253, 430). First of all, as for any bodies in thermal equilibrium, the temperatures T_1 and T_2 of the two phases must be equal

$$T_1 = T_2. \tag{2.1}$$

In addition, we must have the pressure of the two phases equal (if no external field is present) since the two phases must exert equal and opposite forces on each other over their surface contact

$$p_1 = p_2. \tag{2.2}$$

Lastly, we have the condition that the chemical potentials of the two phases must be equal

$$\mu_1(p, T) = \mu_2(p, T). \tag{2.3}$$

From the latter condition it follows

$$\begin{aligned} d\mu_1 &= d\mu_2 \\ d\bar{H}_1 - \bar{S}_1\, dT &= d\bar{H}_2 - \bar{S}_2\, dT \\ \bar{V}_1\, dp - \bar{S}_1\, dT &= \bar{V}_2\, dp - \bar{S}_2\, dT \\ \frac{dp}{dT} = \frac{\bar{S}_2 - \bar{S}_1}{\bar{V}_2 - \bar{V}_1} &= \frac{\Delta\bar{H}}{T\Delta\bar{V}} \end{aligned} \tag{2.4}$$

where the bars denote partial molar quantities (for pure compounds $\mu = G/n$, $\bar{S} = S/n$, etc.). This derivation shows that while the chemical potential μ is a continuous function of temperature, the volume V or the enthalpy H could be discontinuous. This is the basis for the thermodynamic definition of phase transitions according to Ehrenfest. A phase transition of nth order is characterized by the following properties. At the transition temperature the free Gibbs energy G and their derivatives up to the $n - 1$ order are continuous, the nth derivative is discontinuous and the $n+1$ derivative has a singularity. In particular, a first-order phase transition exhibits a discontinuity in the enthalpy H and a singularity in the specific heat C_p. This is illustrated schematically in fig. 2.2.

This short digression into thermodynamics shows that a rigorous and relatively simple thermodynamic classification of phase transitions exists. However, it also illustrates the difficulties in analyzing experimental

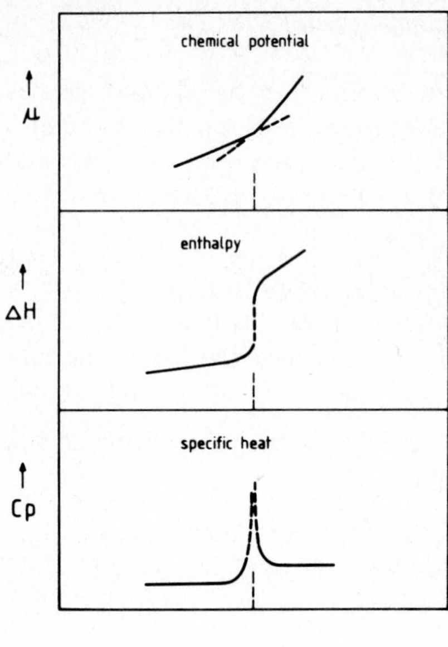

Fig. 2.2. Thermodynamic characteristics of a first-order phase transition.

results. If we want to determine the order of a particular phase transition unambiguously the only correct method is to follow the variation of the Gibbs free energy and its derivatives as a function of temperature. The closest we can get here for biomembranes is to measure the transition enthalpy and the excess specific heat in a calorimeter. On the other hand, many spectroscopic methods have been developed which also indicate phase changes. Here the spectroscopic probe detects molecular properties of the system and a discontinuity in a spectral parameter is not necessarily indicative of a change in the thermodynamic functions of state.

2.3. *Gel-to-liquid crystal phase transition of synthetic phospholipids*

All three processes, the melting of the hydrocarbon chains, the transition from one mesophase to the other, and the lateral phase separation are accompanied by changes in the heat content of the systems. Measurement of the excess specific heat and the transition enthalpy by means of differential scanning calorimetry (DSC), therefore, provides valuable insight into the energetic situation in lipid bilayers and other

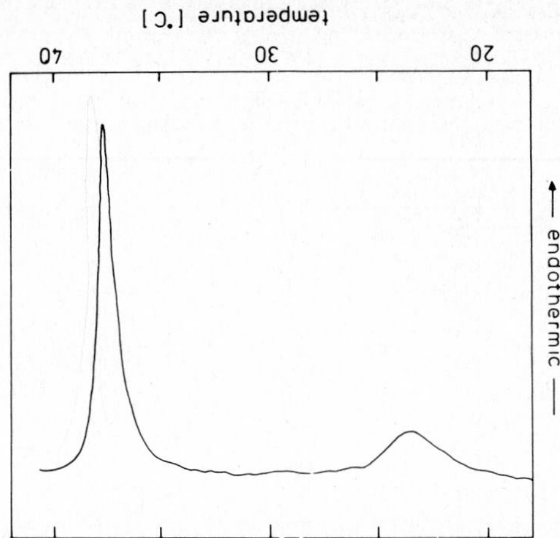

Fig. 2.3. Differential scanning calorimetric tracing of dispersions of 1,3-dipalmitoyl-*sn*-glycero-2-phosphocholine. 30 wt % lipid–70 wt % H_2O. The lipid exhibits a pretransition at around 23° C and a gel-to-liquid crystal transition at 35° C. [From Seelig, Dijkman, and de Haas (1979).]

mesophases. This approach has been pioneered mainly by the groups of Chapman (Chapman et al. 1967, Phillips et al. 1969, Chapman 1975, Chapman et al. 1977) and van Deenen (de Kruijff et al. 1972, 1973, van Dijck et al. 1975, 1976, 1978). A typical DSC scan for a synthetic phospholipid is reproduced in fig. 2.3. The excess specific heat C_p is experimentally accessible. Integration of the area underneath the C_p curve yields the transition enthalpy ΔH. At the phase transition, the gel phase and the liquid–crystalline phase are in equilibrium and the Gibbs free energy ΔG at the phase transition temperature T_c is therefore zero. The transition entropy ΔS can then be calculated according to

$$\Delta S = \Delta H / T_c. \tag{2.5}$$

In the following tables we have summarized calorimetric data for the most common classes of naturally occurring phospholipids, that is 3-*sn*-phosphatidylcholine (tables 2.1–2.3), 3-*sn*-phosphatidylethanolamine (table 2.4), 3-*sn*-phosphatidylglycerol (table 2.5), and 3-*sn*-phosphatidylserine (table 2.6). By far the most extensive literature exists for synthetic 3-*sn*-phosphatidylcholines, presumably because they are easy to prepare and to handle.

Table 2.1

Calorimetric data of the gel-to-liquid crystal phase transition of saturated 1,2-diacyl-*sn*-glycero-3-phosphocholines at maximum hydration[a]

Chain length	T_c (°C)	ΔH (kcal/mole)	ΔS (cal/mole deg.)	Refs.
12	−1.0	4.3	15.8	c)
	0[b]	4.3[b]	15.75[b]	d)
	−1.8	1.7	6.27	e)
13	13.7	4.8	16.6	f)
14	23.0	6.64	22.43	g)
	23.0[b]	6.8[b]	22.97[b]	d)
	23.9	5.4	18.19	e)
	23.7	6.26	21.10	h)
15	34.2	7.3	23.76	f)
16	41	8.66	27.58	g)
	41.5[b]	8.6[b]	27.34[b]	d)
	41.4	8.74	27.8	e)
	41.75	9.69	30.79	h)
	41.55	8.5	27.02	i)
	41	8.5	27.07	j)
	41.1	7.7	24.5	k)
	40.0	9.4	30.03	l)
17	48.6	9.8	30.5	f)
	47.8	9.2	28.7	m)
18	58	10.67	32.23	g)
	58.24	10.84	32.73	h)
	54.9	10.62	32.38	e)
	54	10.8	33.0	l)
22	75	14.88	42.76	g)

Regression analysis:

$$\Delta H = 0.58 \cdot 2n - 10.1 \text{ (kcal/mole)} \qquad R = 0.94$$
$$\Delta S = 1.54 \cdot 2n - 22.6 \text{ (cal/mole deg)} \qquad R = 0.90$$

a) The effect of ions on the phase transition of 3-*sn*-phosphocholines has been investigated by Simon et al. (1975) and by Chapman et al. (1977).

b) The data were derived from lipid dispersions in 50 vol % ethyleneglycol. The correlation coefficient R is generally improved if the statistical analysis is limited to the data of one particular group, indicating small systematic differences from group to group.

c) van Dijck et al. (1975), table I.

d) van Dijck et al. (1976).

e) Mabrey and Sturtevant (1976).

f) Seelig, unpublished results.

g) Phillips et al. (1969).

h) Hinz and Sturtevant (1972).

i) Albon and Sturtevant (1978).

j) Vaughan and Keough (1974).

k) Jacobson and Papahadjopoulos (1975).

l) van Dijck (1977).

m) Salvati et al. (1979).

Table 2.2

Thermodynamic data of the gel-to-liquid crystal phase transition of unsaturated 3-*sn*-phosphatidylcholines at maximum hydration

Chain composition	T_c (°C)	ΔH (kcal/mole)	ΔS (cal/mole deg)	Refs.
16 : 1 c/16 : 1 c dipalmitoleoyl	−36[a]	9.1[a]	38.3	b)
18 : 1 c/18 : 1 c	−14[a]	11.2[a]	43.2	b)
dioleoyl	−22	7.6	30.2	c)
	−21	7.7	30.6	d)
	−20	8.7	34.4	e)
18 : 1 tr/18 : 1 tr dielaidoyl	9.5[a]	7.3[a]	25.8	b)
18 : 0/18 : 1 c 1-stearoyl-2-oleoyl	3	5	18.1	f)
18 : 1 c/18 : 0 1-oleoyl-2-stearoyl	~15	6.7	23.2	g)
18 : 0/18 : 1 tr 1-stearoyl-2-elaidoyl	26	8.4	28.1	f)
16 : 0/18 : 1 c 1-palmitoyl-2-oleoyl	−5	8.0	29.8	h)
egg lecithin (~70 wt % 16 : 0/18 : 1)	−19	3.7		i)

a) The data were derived from lipid dispersions in 50 vol % ethyleneglycol.
b) van Dijck et al. (1976).
c) Phillips et al. (1969).
d) Barton and Gunstone (1975).
e) van Dijck (1977).
f) Phillips et al. (1972).
g) de Kruijff et al. (1972).
h) de Kruijff et al. (1973).
i) Blume (1976).

The following general conclusions can be deduced from these tables:

(i) Chain length dependence. For all four lipid classes the thermodynamic parameters ΔH, ΔS, and T_c increase with increasing chain length of the fatty acyl chains. In contrast to simple paraffins or pure fatty acids which exhibit an even–odd effect in the chain length dependence of their thermodynamic parameters (cf. Tanford 1973, table 6-2) no such effect has been found for the 3-*sn*-phosphatidylcholines (cf. table 2.1, also fig. 2.4).

(ii) Unsaturation. The incorporation of *cis* and *trans* double bonds lowers the transition temperature T_c. *Cis* double bonds are more efficient than *trans* double bonds in this respect. The downward shift of

Table 2.3

Thermodynamic data for fully hydrated 1,2-dioctadecenoyl-*sn*-glycero-3-phosphocholines as a function of the position of the *cis*-double bond[a)]

Position of *cis*-double bond	T_c (°C)	ΔH (kcal/mole)	ΔS (cal/mole deg)
2	+41	9.6	30.6
3	+35	8.7	28.2
4	+23	8.2	27.7
5	+11	7.8	27.4
6	+1	7.8	28.5
7	−8	7.6	28.6
8	−13	7.5	28.8
9	−21	7.7	30.2
10	−21	7.6	30.5
11	−19	7.8	30.7
12	−8	7.9	29.8
13	+1	8.2	29.9
14	+7	8.6	30.7
15	+24	8.9	29.9
16	+35	9.6	31.2
17	+45		

[a)]According to Barton and Gunstone (1975).

the phase transition depends also on the position of the double bond in the chain (cf. table 2.3). It is most pronounced if the double bond is located in the middle of the chain, i.e. the naturally occurring position, and becomes smaller as the double bond is moved to either end of the fatty acyl chains. Furthermore, a double bond in the *sn*-2 chain has a larger effect on the transition temperature than the same double bond in the *sn*-1 chain (table 2.2).

For unsaturated 3-*sn*-phosphatidylethanolamines not only the transition temperature T_c but also ΔH and ΔS are lowered compared to the saturated compounds. The same holds true for *trans*-unsaturated 3-*sn*-phosphatidylcholines whereas the situation in the *cis*-unsaturated analogues is more complex (cf. table 2.2).

(iii) Head group specificity. For lipids with two identical, saturated fatty acyl chains the transition temperature T_c depends on the type of polar group and increases in the order T_c (choline) = T_c (glycerol < T_c (serine) < T_c (ethanolamine). T_c (ethanolamine) is generally about 20° C higher than T_c (choline). For the dioleoyl-phospholipids this head group specificity of T_c appears to be smoothed out.

Table 2.4

Calorimetric data of the phase transition of saturated and unsaturated 1,2-diacyl-*sn*-glycero-3-phosphoethanolamines at maximum hydration

Saturated chains chain length n	T_c (°C)	ΔH (kcal/mole)	ΔS (cal/mole deg)	Refs.
12	29[a]	4.0[a]	13.2[a]	b)
	30	3.9	12.87	c)
	30.5	3.62	11.93	d)
14	47.5[a]	6.4[a]	19.96[a]	b)
	49.6	6.4	19.83	c)
	49.5	5.8	17.98	e)
	49	6.6	20.5	f)
16	60[a]	8.5[a]	25.53[a]	b)
	64.3	8.2	24.3	c)
	63.8	9.62	28.56	d)
	63.4	8.6	25.56	g)
18	71	10.9	31.69	c)
Unsaturated chains				
16 : 1 c/16 : 1 c 1, 2-dipalmitoleoyl	−33.5[a]	4.3[a]	17.9	b)
18 : 1 c/18 : 1 c 1, 2-dioleoyl	−16[a]	4.5[a]	17.5	b)
18 : 1 tr/18 ; 1 tr 1, 2-dielaidoyl	35(37)[a]	7.0[a]	22.7	b, h)

Regression analysis of saturated phosphatidylethanolamines

$\Delta H = 0.6 \cdot 2n - 10.5$ (kcal/mole) $R = 0.97$

$\Delta S = 1.62 \cdot 2n - 25.9$ (cal/mole deg) $R = 0.97$

a) The data were derived from lipid dispersions containing 50 vol % ethyleneglycol.
b) van Dijck et al. (1976).
c) Blume (1976).
d) Mabrey and Sturtevant (1977).
e) Mabrey and Sturtevant (1976).
f) Chapman et al. (1972) fig. 5.
g) Vaughan and Keough (1974).
h) Jackson and Sturtevant (1977).

Figure 2.4 provides a summary of the chain length dependence of ΔH and ΔS. Such a plot was first suggested by Phillips et al. (1969) for 3-*sn*-phosphatidylcholines and has been extended here to include the more recent data on 3-*sn*-phosphatidylethanolamine, 3-*sn*-phosphatidylglycerol, and 3-*sn*-phosphatidylserine. This figure illustrates that the transition enthalpies and entropies at a given chain length are almost independent of the polar groups.

Table 2.5

Thermodynamic data for the gel-to-liquid crystal phase transition of 1,2-diacyl-*sn*-glycero-3-phospho-*rac*-glycerol (sodium salt)[a]

Chain length	T_c (°C)	ΔH (kcal/mole)	ΔS (cal/mole deg)	pH/salt	Refs.
12	4	–	–	9.5 0.15 M NaCl	d)
	−4[b]	4.5[b]	16.7[b]	7.0 0.1 M NaCl	e, f)
14	23.7	6.94	23.4	9.5 0.15 M NaCl	d)
	23	6.8	23.0	7.0 0.12 M NaCl	g)
16	41.5	8.9	28.3	9.5 0.15 M NaCl	d)
	41.0	8.8	28.02	6.0 0.1 M NaCl	h)
	41.0	7.9	25.15	7.4 0.1 M NaCl	i)
	41.5[c]	8.9[c]	28.3[c]	7.0 0.1 M NaCl	j)
18	54.5	10.5	32.6	9.5 0.15 M NaCl	e)
18 : 1 c/18 : 1 c	−18	–		9.5 0.15 M NaCl	e)

Regression analysis

$$\Delta H = 0.5 \cdot 2n - 6.9 \text{ (kcal/mole)} \qquad R = 0.96$$
$$\Delta S = 1.27 \cdot 2n - 13.1 \qquad R = 0.95$$

a) Data on the influence of pH and Ca^{2+}/Mg^{2+} may be found in Findlay and Barton (1978) and van Dijck et al. (1978).
b) Optically pure 3-phosphatidyl-1′-glycerol.
c) Optically pure 3-phosphatidyl-3′-glycerol.
d) Findlay and Barton (1978).
e) Verkleij et al. (1974).
f) Ververgaert et al. (1975).
g) van Dijck et al. (1976).
h) van Dijck et al. (1978).
i) Jacobson and Papahadjopoulos (1975).
j) Wohlgemuth, R. et al. (1980).

Table 2.6

Calorimetric data of the phase transition of saturated and unsaturated 1,2-diacyl-*sn*-glycero-3-phospho-L-serine

Saturated chains chain length n	T_c (°C)	ΔH (kcal/mole)	ΔS (cal/mole deg)	Refs.
14	36.3	8.2	26.2	[a]
	38	8.35	26.8	[b]
	36.6	7.0 ± 0.5	22.6	[c]
16	53	9.0 ± 0.5	27.6	[c]
	53	3	9.2	[d]
Unsaturated chains				
18 : 1 c/18 : 1 c 1,2-dioleoyl	−11.6	8.8 ± 0.5	33.6	[c]

Regression analysis of ref. c:

$$\Delta H = 0.5 \cdot 2n - 7.0 \text{ (kcal/mole)}$$
$$\Delta S = 1.25 \cdot 2n - 12.4 \text{ (cal/deg mole)}$$

[a] van Dijck et al. (1978).
[b] Mombers et al. (1979).
[c] Browning and Seelig (1979).
[d] MacDonald et al. (1976).

Table 2.7

Summary of the regression analysis of tables 2.1 – 2.6

Compound	$\Delta H_{increment}$ (kcal/mole CH_2)	$\Delta S_{increment}$ (cal/deg mole CH_2)	H_0 (kcal/mole)	S_0 (cal/deg mole)
Hydrocarbons				
Odd numbers	0.85	1.77	−4.4	2.53
Even numbers	1.0	2.61	−3.2	2.08
Phospholipids				
1,2-diacyl-phosphatidyl-choline	0.58	1.54	−10.1	−22.6
1,2-diacyl-phosphatidyl-ethanolamine	0.6	1.62	−10.5	−25.9
1,2-diacyl-phosphatidyl-glycerol	0.5	1.27	−6.9	−13.1
1,2-diacyl-phosphatidyl-serine	0.5	1.25	−7.0	−12.4

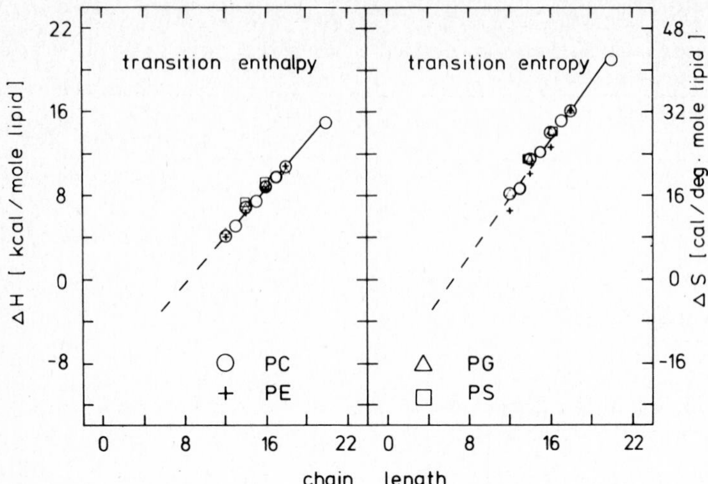

Fig. 2.4. Gel-to-liquid crystal phase transition. Chain length dependence of the transition enthalpy and the transition entropy of disaturated phospholipids.

For all four lipid classes a linear dependence of ΔH and ΔS on the chain length is observed which can be represented as

$$\Delta H = 2n\,\Delta H_{\text{increment}} + H_0 \tag{2.6}$$

$$\Delta S = 2n\,\Delta S_{\text{increment}} + S_0. \tag{2.7}$$

Here n is the number of chain segments per fatty acyl chain. The results of a linear regression analysis of the foregoing tables (2.1, 2.4–2.6) is given in table 2.7. Also included are the corresponding parameters for the melting of even- and odd-numbered paraffins (ΔH and ΔS values taken from Tanford 1973, table 6.2). Two conclusions are obvious: (i) $\Delta H_{\text{increment}}$ and $\Delta S_{\text{increment}}$ are very similar for the lipid classes investigated so far and (ii) $\Delta H_{\text{increment}}$ and $\Delta S_{\text{increment}}$ are clearly lower for phospholipids than for paraffins. Even though both systems are "fluid" above the transition temperature, as judged from the diffuse $(4.6\ \text{Å})^{-1}$ reflex, the hydrocarbon chains in a liquid-crystalline bilayer are still more restricted in their conformational freedom than in a true liquid paraffin (Phillips et al. 1969).

It is tempting to speculate for a moment on the H_0 and S_0 parameters. If a linear extrapolation were valid to zero chain length, then H_0 and S_0 should essentially represent the contribution of the head groups to the melting process. For alkanes both parameters roughly approach zero, since there is no head group. For phospholipids, however, one extrapolates a large negative S_0 value. Because the head groups become more flexible and mobile above the phase transition, as evidenced by NMR methods, this process alone can be expected to give a positive contribution to S_0. The large negative value would then suggest that upon melting a restructuring of the water molecules occurs resulting in a better ordered hydration layer.

The gel-to-liquid crystal transition of phospholipids is generally very sharp indicating that the phase transition is a highly cooperative process. The width of the transition is dependent on the prehistory of the sample and the purity of the lipid. Albon and Sturtevant (1978) prepared a highly purified 1,2-dipalmitoyl-*sn*-glycero-3-phosphocholine by zone refining the fatty acid and controlled crystallization of the lipid. The peak width at half-maximal excess specific heat was only 0.067° C and it seems safe to conclude from these measurements that the gel-to-liquid crystal transition closely approximates an isothermal first-order transition.

In order to obtain a feeling for the cooperativity of gel-to-liquid crystal transition, the melting process may be compared with a simple two-state equilibrium

$$A \rightleftharpoons B$$

without cooperativity (Träuble 1971, Mabrey and Sturtevant 1978). The degree of transition is defined as

$$\theta = (c_B / c_A + c_B) \tag{2.8}$$

where c_B and c_A denote the concentration of the molecules in states A and B, respectively. The temperature dependence of the equilibrium constant

$$K = \frac{c_B}{c_A} = \frac{\theta}{1-\theta}, \tag{2.9}$$

is given by the van't Hoff equation

$$\left(\frac{\partial \ln K}{\partial T}\right) = \frac{\Delta H_{\text{van't Hoff}}}{RT^2} = \frac{1}{\theta(1-\theta)} \frac{\partial \theta}{\partial T}. \tag{2.10}$$

At the midpoint of the transition ($T = T_c$, $\theta = \frac{1}{2}$) it follows

$$\Delta H_{\text{van't Hoff}} = 4RT_c^2 (\partial\theta / \partial T)_{T_c}. \tag{2.11}$$

$(\partial\theta/\partial T)_{T_c}$ is directly measurable from the steepness of the transition curve. For any strictly two-state process the ratio of ΔH_{cal} and $\Delta H_{\text{van't Hoff}}$ must be unity, whereas for cooperative processes $\Delta H_{\text{van't Hoff}}$ will be larger than ΔH_{cal}. Dividing $\Delta H_{\text{van't Hoff}}$ by ΔH_{cal} may thus yield the “cooperative unit”, i.e. an empirical parameter for the cooperative behavior of the system. However, even for comparative purposes the use of the “cooperative unit” remains unsatisfying since the steepness of the phase transition is extremely dependent on such uncontrollable factors as minor impurities or the prehistory of the lipid sample.

From a biological point of view the differences in the transition temperatures T_c of the various lipid classes are most intriguing and attempts have been made to provide qualitative or quantitative explanations of these differences. This is however a relatively difficult undertaking. Thermodynamically speaking, the transition temperature T_c is the ratio of ΔH and ΔS (cf. above),

$$T_c = \Delta H/\Delta S, \tag{2.12}$$

where T_c is the absolute temperature of the phase transition. A change in the transition temperature by 20–30° C is a small effect on the absolute temperature scale and even minor changes of ΔH and/or ΔS would be sufficient to induce the observed shifts in the transition temperature. A quantitative understanding of the variation of the transition temperature with the head group structure would therefore require a proper balancing of all the energies and entropies involved. So far the various attempts to emphasize the predominance of one specific molecular mechanism have not been very successful. It has been suggested, for example, that the 20–25° C lower transition temperatures of the saturated diacyl phosphatidylcholines compared to the corresponding phosphatidylethanolamines is a result of the crowding of the phosphatidylcholine head groups (Chapman et al. 1974, Vaughan and Keough 1974, Mabrey and Sturtevant 1977). However, neutron diffraction studies demonstrate that the determining factor in the packing of the phosphatidylcholines below and above the phase transition temperature is the space occupied by the fatty acyl chains and not that of the head groups (Büldt et al. 1978, 1979). The analysis of the neutron diffraction data leads to the conclusion that the orientation of the choline dipole is parallel to the membrane surface both below and above the gel-to-liquid crystal phase transition temperature. Model building of a phospholipid bilayer with the proper separation of the hydrocarbon chains shows that even in this parallel orientation the choline dipoles can easily be accommodated within the available bilayer surface (see fig. 2.5, Shepherd and Büldt 1978). The observed differences in the transition temperature of phosphatidylcholines and phosphatidylethanolamines are most probably not caused by steric repul-

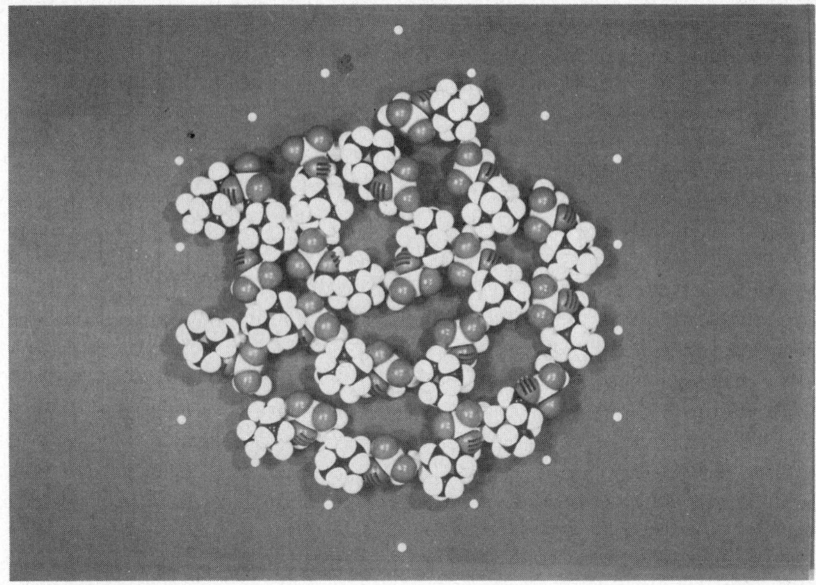

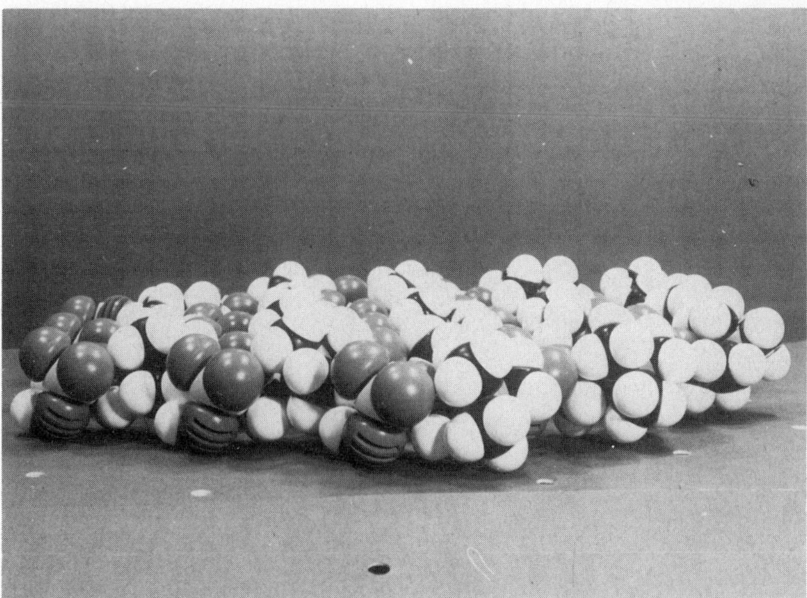

Fig. 2.5. Space filling models of the head-group region of bilayers composed of 1,2-dipalmitoyl-*sn*-glycero-3-phosphocholine. Top view and side view. The separations of the molecules were determined from neutron diffraction measurements. [From Shepherd and Büldt (1978).]

sion, but perhaps, by the different hydrogen bonding capacities of the choline and ethanolamine residues.

Träuble and Eibl have proposed that shifts in the phase transition temperatures may be connected with alterations in the electric charge density of the lipid bilayer (Träuble and Eibl 1974, 1975, Träuble et al. 1976). In this model the charges of the lipid bilayer are considered to be distributed evenly and the effect of the charge alteration at the phase transition is estimated using the Gouy–Chapman theory of the electric double layer. In brief, the model suggests that the electric charge density is reduced at the gel-to-liquid crystal transition due to lateral expansion of the membranes. The total change of the transition enthalpy, ΔH, therefore contains an electrostatic component, ΔH^{el}, in addition to a nonelectrostatic term, ΔH°. The transition temperature, T_{c}, may then be written as

$$T_{\mathrm{c}} = \frac{\Delta H}{\Delta S} = \frac{\Delta H^{\circ}}{\Delta S} + \frac{\Delta H^{\mathrm{el}}}{\Delta S} \qquad (2.13)$$

so that the electrostatic interaction changes the transition temperature according to

$$\Delta T_{\mathrm{c}} = \frac{\Delta H^{\mathrm{el}}}{\Delta S}. \qquad (2.14)$$

ΔH_{el} is calculated from the Gouy–Chapman theory leading to the final expression

$$\Delta T_{\mathrm{c}} = \frac{2RT}{\Delta S}\frac{\Delta f}{f}\sigma. \qquad (2.15)$$

In eq. (2.15) Δf is the increase in molecular area at the gel-to-liquid crystalline phase transition, f the area-per-lipid molecule, σ the number of elementary charges-per-lipid molecule, and RT the thermal energy. Equation (2.15) predicts that an increase in charge will reduce the transition temperature and vice versa. Qualitatively, this is in agreement with the experimental results obtained for charged lipids like methyl-phosphatidic acid (Träuble and Eibl 1974, 1975), phosphatidic acid (Träuble and Eibl 1974, Jacobson and Papahadjopoulos 1975), phosphatidylglycerol (Findlay and Barton 1978) and phosphatidylserine (MacDonald et al. 1976). Quantitatively the agreement between theory and experiment is less convincing (Jacobson and Papahadjopoulos 1975, Macdonald et al. 1976) and the available experimental evidence suggests that hydrogen bonding is at least equally important as the electrostatic effects.

References

Albon, N. and J. M. Sturtevant (1978) Proc. Nat. Acad. Sci. USA 75, 2258.
Barton, P.G. and F.D. Gunstone (1975) J. Biol. Chem. 250, 4470.
Blume, A. (1976) Ph.D. Thesis (Univ. of Freiburg, Germany).
Browning, J.L. and J. Seelig (1980) Biochemistry 19, 1262.
Büldt, G., H. U. Gally, A. Seelig, J. Seelig and G. Zaccai (1978) Nature 271, 182.
Büldt, G., H.U. Gally, J. Seelig and G. Zaccai (1979) J. Mol. Biol. 134, 673.
Chapman, D. (1975) Quart. Rev. Biophys. 8, 185.
Chapman, D., W.E. Peel, B. Kingston and T.H. Lilley (1977) Biochim. Biophys. Acta 464, 260.
Chapman, D., J. Urbino and K. M. Keough (1974) J. Biol. Chem. 249, 2512.
Chapman, D., R. M. Williams and B. D. Ladbrooke (1967) Chem. Phys. Lipids 1, 445.
Davis, J. H. (1979) Biophys. J., 27, 339.
de Kruijff, B., R. A. Demel and L. L. M. van Deenen (1972) Biochim. Biophys. Acta 255, 331.
de Kruijff, B., R. A., Demel, A. J. Slotboom, L. L. M. van Deenen and R. F. Rosenthal (1973) Biochim. Biophys. Acta 307, 1.
Findlay, E. J. and P. G. Barton (1978) Biochemistry 17, 2400.
Hinz, H. and J. M. Sturtevant (1972) J. Biol. Chem. 247, 6071.
Jackson, M. B. and J. M. Sturtevant (1977) J. Biol. Chem. 252, 4749.
Jacobson, K. and D. Papahadjopoulos (1975) Biochemistry 14, 152.
Landau, L. D. and E. M. Lifshitz (1958) Statistical Physics (Pergamon Press, London).
Luzzati, V. (1968) X-ray Diffraction Studies of Lipid–Water Systems, in: Biological Membranes, ed. D. Chapman, (Academic Press, New York) pp. 71–123.
Mabrey, S. and J. M. Sturtevant (1976) Proc. Nat. Acad. Sci. 73, 3862.
Mabrey, S. and J. M. Sturtevant (1977) Biochim. Biophys. Acta 486, 444.
Mabrey, S. and J. M. Sturtevant (1978) High Sensitivity Differential Scanning Calorimetry in the Study of Biomembranes and Related Model Systems, in: Methods in Membrane Biology, ed. E. Korn, vol. 9 (Plenum Press, New York) pp. 237–274.
MacDonald, R. C., S. A. Simon and E. Baer (1976) Biochemistry 15, 885.
Melchior, D. L. and J. M. Steim (1976) Ann. Rev. Biophys. Bioeng. 5, 205.
Mombers, C., A. J. Verkleij. J. de Gier and L. L. M. van Deenen (1979) Biochim. Biophys. Acta 551, 271.
Münster, A. (1956) Statistische Thermodynamik (Springer Verlag, Berlin).
Overath. P. and H. Träuble (1973) Biochemistry 12, 2625.
Phillips, M. C., H. Hauser and F. Paltauf (1972) Chem. Phys. Lipids 8, 127.
Phillips, M. C., R. M. Williams and D. Chapman (1969) Chem. Phys. Lipids 3, 234.
Rosevear, F. B. (1968) J. Soc. Cosmetic Chem. 19, 581.
Salvati, S., G. Serlupi-Crescenzi and J. De Gier (1979) Chem. Phys. Lipids 24, 85.
Schairer, H. U. and P. Overath (1969) J. Mol. Biol. 44, 209.
Seelig, J., R. Dijkman and G. de Haas (1980) Biochemistry 19, 2215.
Shepherd, J. C. W. and G. Büldt (1978) Biochim. Biophys. Acta 514, 83.
Simon, S. A., L. J. Lis, J. W. Kauffman and R. C. MacDonald (1975) Biochim. Biophys. Acta 375, 317.
Steim, J. M., M. E. Tourtellotte, J. C. Reinert, R. D. McElhaney and R. L. Rader (1969) Proc. Nat. Acad. Sci. USA 63, 104.
Tanford, C. H. (1973) The Hydrophobic Effect: Formation of Micelles and Biological Membranes (Wiley, New York).

Traüble, H. (1971) Naturwissenschaft. 58, 277.
Traüble, H. and H. Eibl (1974) Proc. Nat. Acad. Sci. USA 71, 214.
Traüble, H. and H. Eibl (1975) in: Functional Linkage in Biomolecular Systems, eds. F.O. Schmitt, D. M.Schneider and D. M.Crothers (Raven Press, New York) pp.59–90.
Traüble, H., M. Teubner, P. Woolley and H. Eibl (1976) Biophys. Chem. 4, 319.
van Dijck, P. W. M., P. H. J. Th. Ververgaert, A. J. Verkleij, L. L. M. van Deenen and J. de Gier (1975) Biochim. Biophys. Acta 406, 465.
van Dijck, P. W. M., B. de Kruijff, L. L. M. van Deenen, J. de Gier and R. A. Demel (1976) Biochim. Biophys. Acta 455, 576.
van Dijck, P. W. M., B. de Kruijff, A. J. Verkleij, L. L. M. van Deenen and J. de Gier (1978) Biochim. Biophys. Acta 512, 84.
Verkleij, A. J., B. de Kruijff, P. H. J. Th. Ververgaert, J. F. Tocanne, and L. L. M. van Deenen (1974) Biochim. Biophys. Acta 339, 432.
Ververgaert, P. H. J. Th., B. de Kruijff, A. J. Verkleij, J. F. Tocanne and L. L. M. van Deenen (1975) Chem. Phys. Lipids 14, 97.
Vaughan, D. J. and K. M. Keough (1974) FEBS Lett. 47, 158.
Wahlgemuth, R., N. Waespe-Šarčevič and J. Seelig (1980) Biochemistry, in press.
Wunderlich, F., A. Ronai, V. Speth, J. Seelig and A. Blume (1975) Biochemistry 14, 3730.

3. Molecular organization of phospholipid bilayers and biological membranes. Spectroscopic studies

3.1 Spectroscopic methods

3.1.1. Deuterium magnetic resonance (^{2}H-NMR)

Lipid bilayers are highly organized systems which are nevertheless fluid enough to allow considerable translational, rotational, and flexing movements of the constituent phospholipid molecules. The fluid (liquid crystalline) membranes behave like optically unaxial crystals with the optical axis being perpendicular to the surface of the membrane. This means that the rotational and flexing movements are characterized, on the average, by cylindrical symmetry, with the bilayer normal as the axis of motional averaging. Compared to an isotropic solution the movements of phospholipid molecules in membranes are thus anisotropic. Furthermore, the motional restrictions which are conveniently measured in terms of order parameters (Saupe 1968) vary with the position in the membrane, e.g. they are different for the hydrocarbon region than for the polar region. ^{2}H-NMR is ideally suited to quantitatively measure the motional restrictions and to provide a detailed picture of the phospholipid conformations in biomembranes. The principles of the method can be described as follows: by means of appropriate chemical synthesis some protons in a lipid molecule are replaced by deuterons. Since the van der Waals radii of the two isotopes are identical this substitution leaves the membrane virtually unchanged. Other methods like spin label electron spin resonance or fluorescence spectroscopy require the incorporation of bulky reporter groups into the membrane which leads to a distortion of the membrane. ^{2}H-NMR of selectively deuterated lipids thus offers the advantage of providing a non-perturbing probe technique. A second convenient feature of ^{2}H-NMR is the straightforward assignment of the signals. The natural abundance of deuterium in biological materials is negligibly low so that the ^{2}H-NMR signal of the selectively deuterated segment is the only resonance signal in the spectrum. This may be compared with proton and carbon-13 NMR of biomembranes and derived liposomes where a manifold of partially overlapping resonances is encountered. However, the most important advantage in the use of ^{2}H-NMR in the elucidation of membrane structures is the measurement of the segmental anisotropies which can be derived from the so-called deuterium quadrupole splittings (for a detailed review, cf. Seelig 1977). In brief, the deuteron has a nuclear spin $I=1$ which in an external magnetic field has three allowed orientations $m=+1, 0, -1$. The magnetic energy levels are equally spaced and, in the absence of quadrupole effects, the two allowed transitions $m=-1 \leftrightarrow m=0$ and $m=0 \leftrightarrow m=+1$ give rise to the same NMR signal. However, in addition to the magnetic moment the deuteron nucleus also possesses an electrical quadrupole moment as is indicated schematically in fig. 3.1. The interaction of the electric quadrupole with the electric field gradient of the surrounding bond electrons modifies the magnetic energy levels and removes the degeneracy of the two allowed quantum transitions. In particular, the $m=+1$ and $m=-1$ energy levels are shifted to exactly the same extent, while the $m=0$ level is affected differently. Consequently, the deuterium signal splits into two resonances since the two allowed transitions are now characterized by different energies (cf. fig. 3.1). The frequency separation between the two signals is the residual deuterium quadrupole splitting, $\Delta\nu_Q$. For a C-D bond in a perfectly ordered environment as, e.g. in a single crystal, the quadrupole splitting may reach a limiting value of 170 kHz (Burnett and Muller 1971), while in fluid membranes $|\Delta\nu_Q|$ is usually found to be in the range of $1 \text{ kHz} \leqslant |\Delta\nu_Q| \leqslant 60 \text{ kHz}$. It should be noted that in isotropic solution the quadrupolar effects are averaged out due to the rapid tumbling of the molecules through all angles of space so that the ^{2}H-NMR spectrum then consists of a single line. On the other hand,

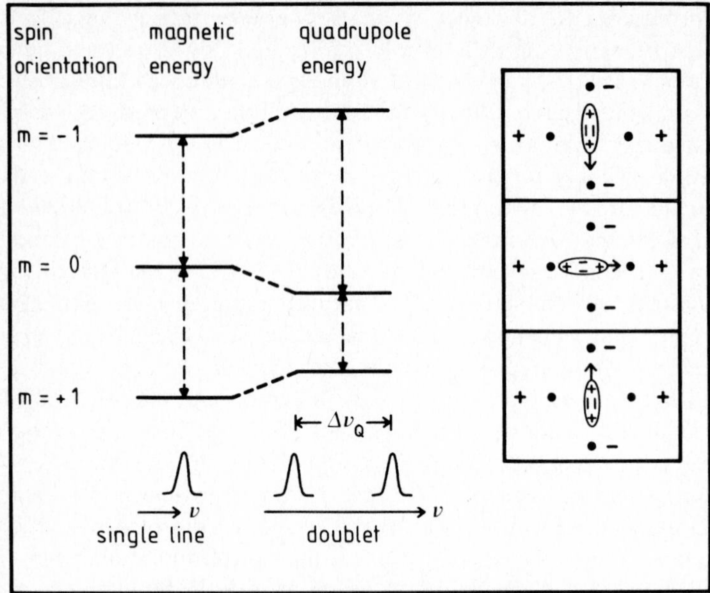

Fig. 3.1. The left part of the figure contains the energy levels for a spin $I=1$ system with and without quadrupole interactions. The insert describes schematically the interaction of an electric quadrupole with an array of four point charges. The orientation of the quadrupolar nucleus is determined by the orientation of its magnetic moment as indicated by the arrow. The figure illustrates that the orientations $m=+1$ and $m=-1$ experience identical electrical forces, while the interactions for $m=0$ are different. [From Seelig (1978b).]

the quadrupole separation is the larger, the more restricted the angular excursions of the labelled segment. A typical ^{2}H-NMR spectrum of a selectively deuterated lipid bilayer is reproduced in fig. 3.2 (Seelig and Niederberger 1974). The bilayer investigated in figure 3.2 is a lyotropic liquid crystal composed of a fatty acid, a deuterated long chain alcohol and water (phase composition: sodium octanoate 34 wt %, [1,1 $-{}^2$H] octanol 30 wt %, water 36 wt %). X-ray diffraction shows that in this ternary mixture the lipid molecules are arranged in bilayers which are separated from each other by layers of water. Both amphiphilic components, the fatty acid as well as the alcohol, are integral constituents of the lipid region. A macroscopic ordering of this phase can be induced by forcing it between two closely spaced, parallel glass surfaces. Shearing forces and the contact with the glass surfaces arrange the microdomains in parallel layers on the supporting plates. The axis of motional

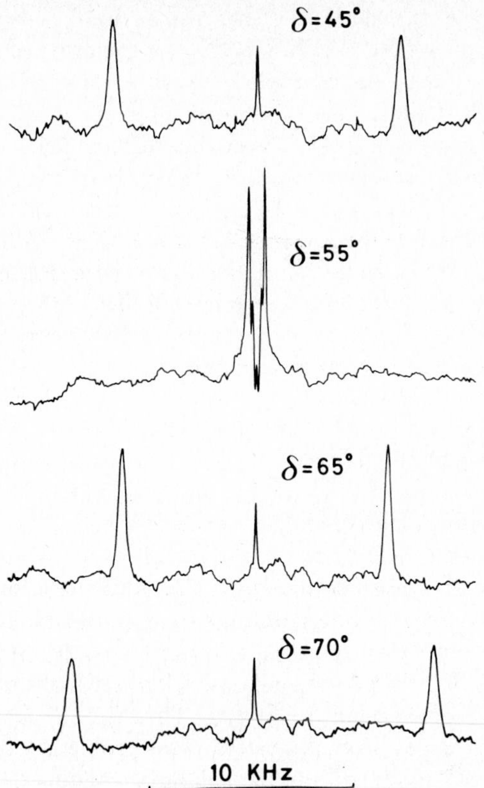

Fig. 3.2. Deuterium NMR spectra (13.8 MHz) of oriented bilayers. Phase composition: sodium octanoate 34 wt %, 1, 1-dideuteriooctanol 30 wt % and water 36 wt %. Approximately 20 mg liquid crystalline phase was sandwiched between a stack of 20 glass plates. δ denotes the angle between the magnetic field and the normal to the glass plates which is also the normal to the oriented bilayers. The sharp signal in the centre arises from isotropic motion of deuterium labelled molecules. During the preparation of the oriented sample a small fraction of an isotropic phase seems to form. A plot of the quadrupole splitting $\Delta\nu_Q$ against $(3\cos^2\delta - 1)/2$ yields a straight line with a maximum splitting of 57 kHz at $\delta = 0^0$. [From Seelig and Niederberger (1974).]

averaging (director axis z') is always perpendicular to the bilayer surface. For the macroscopically oriented sample the director axis is identical with the normal to the glass plates. The deuterium quadrupole splitting, $\Delta\nu_Q$, of a homogeneously oriented lipid bilayer obeys the relation (cf. Seelig 1977)

$$\Delta\nu_Q(\delta) = \tfrac{3}{2}(e^2qQ/h)S_{CD}\left(\tfrac{3}{2}\cos^2\delta - \tfrac{1}{2}\right) \tag{3.1}$$

where (e^2qQ/h) is the static deuterium quadrupole coupling constant (~170 kHz for paraffinic C-D bonds), S_{CD} is the order parameter of the C-D bond vector, and δ is the angle between the magnetic field and the bilayer normal. First, it may be seen that the residual deuterium quadrupole splitting of a lipid bilayer depends strongly on the orientation of the planar strata with respect to the external magnetic field. The quadrupole splitting will collapse if the membranes are oriented at the so-called "magic angle" with $\delta = 54.73°$, since $(3\cos^2 54.73 - 1) = 0$ for this orientation. On the other hand, the quadrupole splitting is largest if the bilayer normal is parallel to the magnetic field ($\delta = 0°$). Second, the quadrupole splitting depends on the molecular properties of the membrane as described by the order parameter $S_{CD} \cdot S_{CD}$ is defined according to

$$S_{CD} = \tfrac{1}{2}\left(3\,\overline{\cos^2\theta} - 1\right), \tag{3.2}$$

where θ is the instantaneous angle between the C-D bond vector and the bilayer normal, while the bar denotes a time-average over all motions which are fast compared to the static quadrupole splitting constant. The molecular interpretation of S_{CD} can be complicated at times since it is actually a tensorial average which depends on both the geometry of the deuterated molecule as well as on the statistical fluctuations of this molecule within the bilayer. The term "order parameter" is therefore misleading to a certain extent. This problem will be illustrated further below with more specific phospholipid examples.

The preparation of homogeneously oriented membranes is not easily achieved and remains the exception rather than the rule. Fortunately enough, ^{2}H-NMR is not limited to oriented samples but can be performed with 'powder-type' samples as well. The shape of the powder-type spectrum is then the average over the resonances of all possible bilayer orientations weighted by their corresponding geometric probability (cf. Seelig 1977). Figure 3.3 shows a typical ^{2}H-NMR spectrum at 41.5 MHz of a randomly dispersed bilayer system of similar chemical composition as defined above. For practical purposes the most important feature of fig. 3.3 is the frequency spacing of the two most intense peaks in the spectrum. These peaks arise from bilayer microdomains which are oriented perpendicular to the magnetic field ($\delta = 90°$) and the spacing of the two peaks therefore is

$$\Delta\nu_{powder} = \tfrac{3}{4}(e^2qQ/h)S_{CD}. \tag{3.3}$$

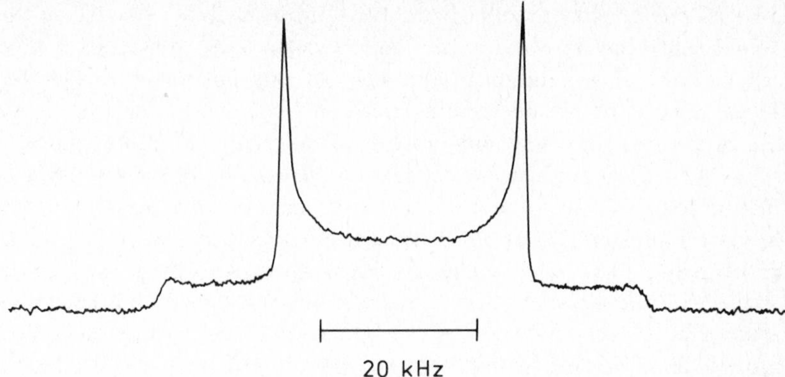

Fig. 3.3. ^{2}H-NMR spectrum (41.4 MHz) of a random distribution of liquid crystalline bilayers. Phase composition: [1,1-^{2}H] decanol 42 wt %, sodium decanoate 28 wt %, water 30 wt %. The separation of the intense inner peaks ($\delta = 90°$) corresponds to 30 kHz and that of the edges ($\delta = 0°$) to $\sim$60 kHz.

The edges of the spectrum correspond to orientations of the bilayer normal parallel to the magnetic field ($\delta = 0$) and the separation of the edges is therefore exactly twice as large as that of the inner peaks. The deuterium order parameter S_{CD} can therefore be easily determined from powder-type samples like, e.g. coarse dispersions of phospholipids in water. Figure 3.3 furthermore illustrates that the spectral intensity is much lower in the outer wings than at the $\delta = 90°$ orientations. Only recently has it been possible to actually measure the theoretically predicted line shape as shown in fig. 3.3, whereas in most earlier publications only the two most intense peaks could be detected. Obviously, this deficiency of the earlier spectra does not affect the evaluation of S_{CD}. On the other hand, it should be noted that S_{CD} cannot be evaluated from single-walled vesicles of small radius. For these systems the vesicle tumbling rate is fast compared to the residual quadrupole separation and the doublet will collapse into a singlet (cf. Stockton et al. 1976). Quadrupole effects are furthermore unique to nuclear spins with $I \geqslant 1$ and are not observed in more commonly employed NMR techniques like proton, carbon-13 or phosphorus-31 NMR since for these nuclei $I = \frac{1}{2}$.

3.1.2. Phosphorus-31 nuclear magnetic resonance (^{31}P-NMR)

The lipids in membranes are predominantly phospholipids and ^{31}P-NMR is thus an attractive tool to study the motion of the phosphate segment. The anisotropy of the phosphate movement is reflected in the chemical shielding anisotropy, $\Delta\sigma$, the physical basis of which may be explained as follows: the magnetic field experienced by the phosphorus nucleus is reduced by the bonding electrons (chemical shielding). Since the electron density is not isotropic but depends on the bonding pattern, the chemical shielding will be smallest (largest) along the molecular axis with the lowest (highest) electron density and the ^{31}P-NMR frequency will vary with the orientation of the phosphate segment with respect to the magnetic field. The chemical shielding anisotropy is most pronounced in the crystalline state where the resonance frequency for phospholipids may shift between -100 and $+100$ ppm (Kohler and Klein 1976, 1977; Griffin 1976; Herzfeld et al. 1978), while this effect is completely averaged out in isotropic solutions. Biomembranes represent an intermediate situation. The movements of the phosphate segment are neither completely free nor perfectly anisotropic with the result that the static chemical shielding anisotropy is only partially averaged out. This is demonstrated in fig. 3.4 which contains the rotation pattern for a planar oriented phospholipid bilayer (Seelig and Gally 1976). Depending on the orientation of the bilayer with respect to the magnetic field,

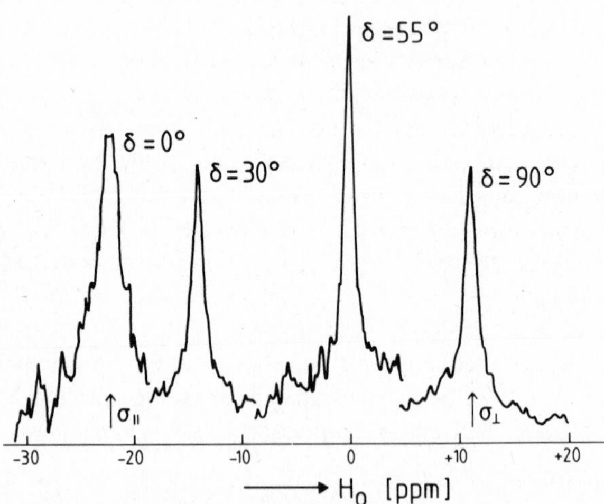

Fig. 3.4. Representative examples of proton-decoupled P-31 NMR spectra (36.5 MHz) obtained from planar oriented phospholipid multilayers (1,2-dipalmitoyl-*sn*-glycero-3-phosphoethanolamine). δ is the angle between the magnetic field and the normal to the plane of the membranes. Temperature 77° C and pH 5.5. The variation in linewidth could be caused by imperfect ordering of the multilayers. [From Seelig and Gally (1976).]

indicated by the rotation angle δ, the resonance frequency varies between -23 ppm for $\delta=0°$ (magnetic field parallel to the bilayer normal) and $+12$ ppm for $\delta=90°$ (magnetic field perpendicular to the bilayer normal). The chemical shielding anisotropy, $\Delta\sigma$, is defined as the difference between these two extreme values and amounts to -35 ppm. The chemical shielding anisotropy in ^{31}P-NMR is comparable to the deuterium quadrupole splitting in ^{2}H-NMR. However, the quantitative interpretation of $\Delta\sigma$ is more complicated than the corresponding analysis of the deuterium quadrupole splitting, $\Delta\nu_Q$, since $\Delta\sigma$ is determined by two independent order parameters compared to only one in the case of $\Delta\nu_Q$ (Niederberger and Seelig 1976, Seelig 1978a)

$$\Delta\sigma = S_{11}(\sigma_{11}-\sigma_{22}) + S_{33}(\sigma_{33}-\sigma_{22}). \tag{3.4}$$

Here the σ_{ii} are the principal elements of the static chemical shielding tensor whereas the S_{ii} are the order parameters of the corresponding

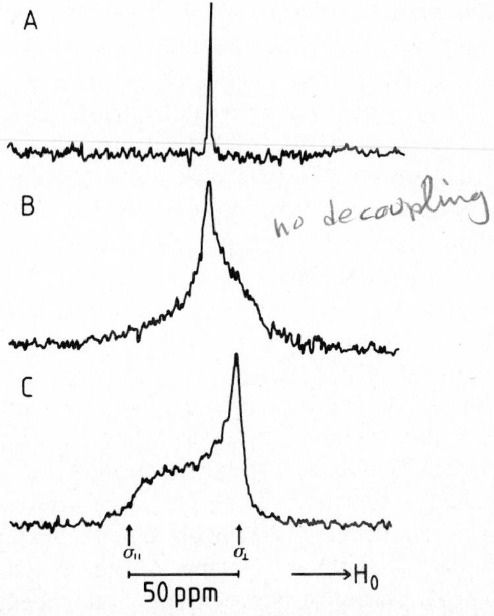

Fig. 3.5. P-31 NMR spectra (36. 5 MHz) of bilayers composed of 1,2-dipalmitoyl-*sn*-glycero-3-phosphocholine at 44° C. (a) Sonicated lipid dispersions (70 mg lipid/ml H_2O). (b) Non-sonicated phospholipid bilayers (50 wt % lipid; % H_2O) no proton decoupling. (c) The same as (b) but with proton decoupling. [From Gally et al. (1975).]

principal axes. The principal elements can easily be determined from measurements of crystalline samples (Kohler and Klein 1976, 1977; Griffin 1976; Herzfeld et al. 1978). However, a quantitative analysis of $\Delta\sigma$ is still not possible without additional assumptions since two independent order parameters should be evaluated from just one experimental result ($\Delta\sigma$). In spite of this theoretical difficulty the measurement of the chemical shielding anisotropy has been of central importance in the understanding of the headgroup structure of phospholipids in membranes. The pertinent literature has been reviewed recently (Seelig 1978a).

The measurement of $\Delta\sigma$ is not limited to planar oriented samples but $\Delta\sigma$ can also be obtained readily from random dispersions of phospholipid bilayers (Gally et al. 1975). A typical powder-type pattern of coarse liposomes is reproduced in fig. 3.5c. The important feature to note is that the edges of the powder-type spectrum correspond to $\sigma_{\perp}$ (high intensity shoulder, $\delta = 90°$) and $\sigma_{\parallel}$ (low intensity shoulder, $\delta = 0°$). Spectrum 3.5c was recorded under proton-decoupling conditions. Without proton decoupling the line-shape of the powder pattern is seriously distorted as is illustrated in fig. 3.5b. A reliable evaluation of $\Delta\sigma$ is not possible under these circumstances. Finally, in the case of small single-walled vesicles, produced by sonication of coarse lipid dispersions, rapid vesicle tumbling and lateral diffusion of lipid molecules within the plane of the membrane are effective mechanisms to average out the proton–phosphorus dipolar interactions and the phosphorus chemical shielding anisotropies. The P-31 NMR spectra of such vesicles exhibit therefore relatively sharp lines of about a few Hz linewidth as shown in fig. 3.5a.

3.1.3. Neutron diffraction

The principles of neutron diffraction are rather similar to those of X-ray diffraction but important differences exist due to the nature of the scattering centres. For X-rays, the scattering centres are the electrons of the atom, while for neutrons, the scattering centres are the nuclei. Each nucleus has a characteristic neutron coherent scattering amplitude which is different for different isotopes of the same element (Worcester 1976). The large difference between the coherent scattering length of hydrogen (−3.74 fermis) and deuterium (6.67 fermis) is particularly useful for the study of membranes. Using selectively deuterated lipids the deuterated membrane segments give rise to intense peaks in the neutron density profile (Worcester and Franks 1976, Büldt et al. 1978,

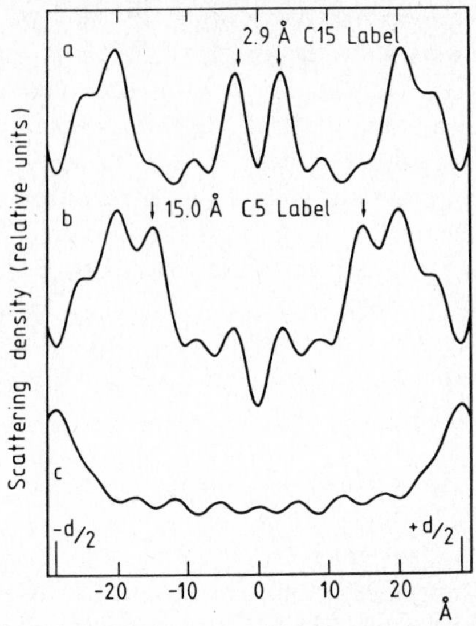

Fig. 3.6. Neutron diffraction profiles of 1,2-dipalmitoyl-*sn*-glycero-3-phosphocholine at low water content (5–6 wt %) and 20° C. (a) Deuterated at the C-15 position of both hydrocarbon chains. (b) At the C-5 position of both chains. (c) The water distribution as determined from a difference profile of C-5 deuterated lipid in D_2O and H_2O. The lamellar spacing was 57.4 Å [From Büldt et al. (1978).]

1979, Zaccai et al. 1979). This is illustrated in fig. 3.6 for bilayers of 1,2-dipalmitoyl-*sn*-glycero-3-phosphocholine (5–6 wt % H_2O, 20° C) with the deuterium label attached at the C-15 segment (fig. 3.6a) and at the C-5 position (fig. 3.6b). The position of the deuterated segment can thus be easily located within the membrane, with a precision of generally better than ± 1 Å.

3.2. The lipid–water interface

3.2.1. Water penetration

The polar head group region of a bilayer membrane constitutes the interface between the water-repellant hydrocarbon interior and the surrounding water. In addition to water it comprises the polar head group of the phospholipid [i.e. the zwitterionic or charged phosphoester groups; phosphocholine (PC), phosphoethanolamine (PE), etc.], the glycerol backbone, and the glycerol–fatty acid ester region. Neutron diffraction studies using the D_2O/H_2O exchange method reveal that the lipid–water boundary is diffuse and that water penetrates into the polar region up to a coordinate corresponding to the glycerol–fatty acid ester (Worcester and Franks 1976, Büldt et al. 1978). A water distribution profile obtained for bilayers of 1,2 -dipalmitoyl-*sn*-glycero-3-phosphocholine (DPPC) at low water content (5–6 wt %) is shown in fig. 3.6c, indicating a smooth decrease in the amount of water as one approaches the hydrocarbon layer. The penetration depth of water remains almost unchanged in a concentration range of 5–25 wt % H_2O. Furthermore, it has been demonstrated by means of ^{2}H-NMR that the aqueous layer is not homogeneous with respect to the physical state of the water molecules but that one must distinguish between bound, trapped and free water (Finer and Darke 1974). The site of attachment of the strongly bound water is not yet clear.

3.2.2. *Phospholipid conformation near the lipid–water interface*

Using acetic acid as a solvent it has been possible to crystallize rac-1,2-dilauroyl-glycero-phosphoethanolamine (DLPE) in bilayer form and to determine the conformation of the lipid molecule in the bilayer crystal (Hitchcock et al. 1974). This structure is shown in fig. 3.7. The polar head group, i.e. the phosphoethanolamine dipole, is aligned parallel to the surface of the membrane, whereas the glycerol backbone is orientated perpendicular to it. Furthermore, the beginnings of the two hydrocarbon chains have different orientations. The first two segments of the 2 chain (attached at the glycerol C-2 atom) are extended parallel to the bilayer plane while all following segments, starting with the C_{23} segment, are perpendicular to this plane. The 1 chain (attached at the glycerol C-1 atom) is at all positions extended perpendicular to the membrane surface.

A crystalline bilayer containing phospholipid molecules solvated by acetic acid is certainly different from a biomembrane surrounded by

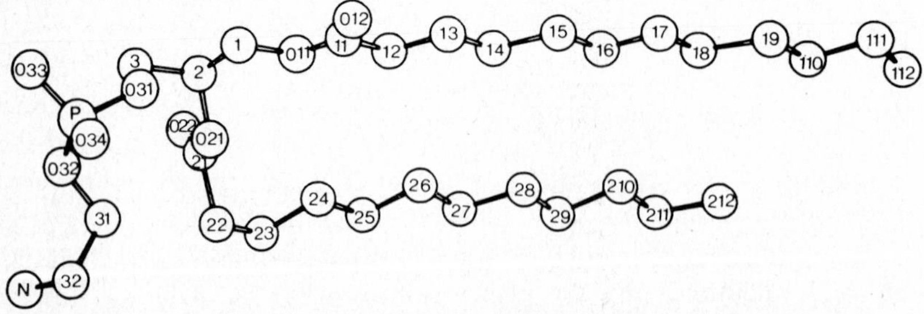

Fig. 3.7. The molecular conformation of rac-1,2-dilauroyl-glycero-3-phosphoethanolamine crystallized in bilayer form from acetic acid. [From Hitchcock et al. (1974).]

cellular fluids and the relevance of a phospholipid structure such as shown in fig. 3.7 for biomembranes seems rather questionable. However, recent ^{2}H-NMR and neutron diffraction studies of aqueous phospholipid dispersions strongly suggest that the principal features of fig. 3.7 are retained in biological membranes and that this conformation, with minor modifications, is characteristic of a wide variety of phospholipids. Let us briefly summarize the available evidence.

Neutron diffraction experiments of selectively deuterated 1,2-dipalmitoyl-*sn*-glycero-3-phosphocholine show that the three segments of the choline moiety are positioned at almost the same distance from the centre of the bilayer regardless of whether the bilayer is in the gel state (5–6 wt % H_2O; 20°C; average distance 24.8 Å) or in the liquid crystalline state (25 wt % H_2O; 50° C; average distance 21.2 Å) (Büldt et al. 1978, 1979). This constitutes a rather unambiguous proof for an orientation of the phosphocholine dipole parallel to the surface of the membrane. The same measurements also reveal that in the gel state the two hydrocarbon chains are out of step by about 1.5 carbon–carbon bonds. The C_{22} segment of the 2 chain is about 1.9 Å farther away from the centre of the bilayer than the corresponding C_{12} segment of the 1 chain, in agreement with fig 3.7. However, the displacement of the two fatty acyl chains with respect to each other is less pronounced in the gel state (~1.5 carbon–carbon bonds) than in the crystalline bilayer (~3 carbon–carbon bonds).

Distinct conformational differences between the beginnings of the two chains are also observed for fluid lipid bilayers and biomembranes above the phase transition temperature, using ^{2}H-NMR. This has first been shown for bilayers composed of 1,2-dipalmitoyl-*sn*-glycero-3-phosphocholine (Seelig and Seelig 1975) and the experimental spectra are reproduced in fig. 3.8. The quadrupole splitting of the deuterated C_12 segment (fig. 3.8B) is almost twice as large as that of the C_{22} segment (fig. 3.8C). This can again be explained by assuming a bent conformation of the 2 chain so that the average orientation of the C_{22} segment is parallel to the membrane surface while that of the C_{12} segment is perpendicular to it. The same spectral pattern has been observed since then for 1,2-dipalmitoyl-*sn*-glycero-3-phosphocholine in the presence of cholesterol (Haberkorn et al. 1977), for 1-palmitoyl-2-oleoyl-*sn*-glycero-3-phosphocholine (POPC) (Seelig and Seelig 1977, Seelig and Waespe-Sarcevic 1978), for 1,2-dipalmitoyl-*sn*-glycero-3-phosphoethanolamine (DPPE) and for 1,2-dipalmitoyl-*sn*-glycero-3-phosphoserine (DPPS) (Seelig and Browning 1978). For a quantitative comparison of the quadrupole splittings it is convenient to normalize the deuterium order

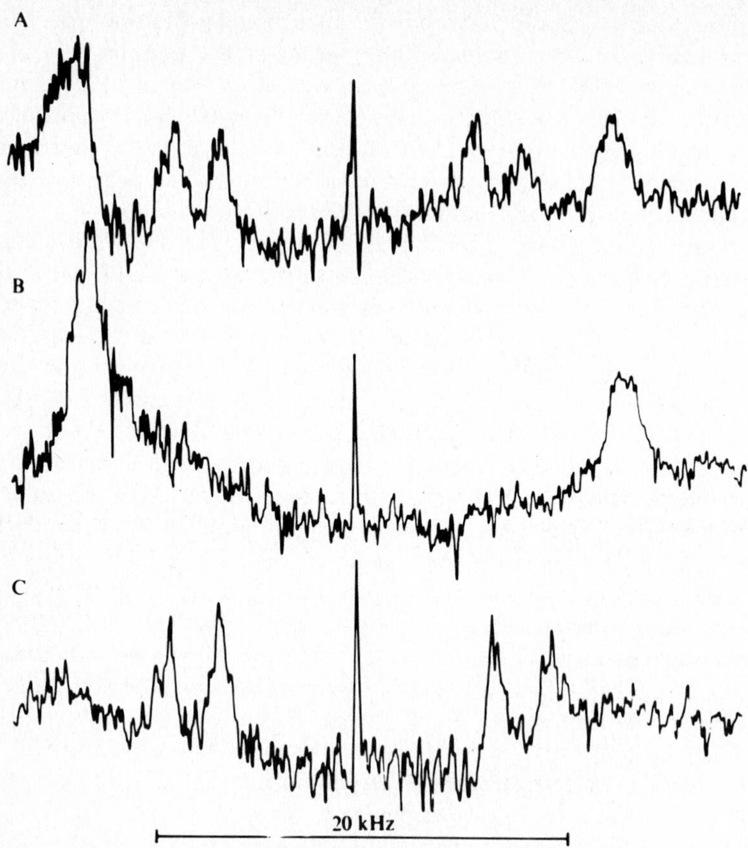

Fig. 3.8. Deuterium magnetic resonance spectra (13.4 MHz) of bilayers of 1, 2-dipalmitoyl-*sn*-glycero-3-phosphocholine at 50° C (50 wt % lipid, 50 wt % H_2O). (a) Both chains deuterated at the C-2′ segment (C_{12}, C_{22} in fig. 3.7). (b) *sn*-1 chain deuterated only (C_{12} segment in fig. 3.7). (c) *sn*-2 chain deuterated only (C_{22} segment in fig. 3.7). [From Seelig and Seelig (1975).]

profiles by referring them to a reduced temperature $\theta=(T-T_c)/T_c$(T = measuring temperature; T_c = gel-to-liquid crystal transition temperature; T, $T_c \hat{=}$ °K), the rationale being to eliminate all effects caused by differences in the gel-to-liquid crystal transition temperature which range from −5° C for POPC to 63° C for DPPE (DPPC, 41° C; DPPS, 51° C). The qualitative and quantitative similarity of the different lipid systems becomes obvious in fig. 3.9, where the C-2 segment deuterium order parameters of four synthetic lipids are

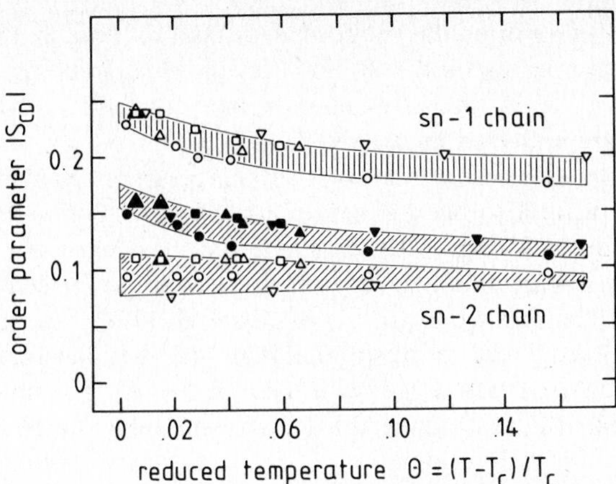

Fig. 3.9. Variation of the deuterium order parameter $|S_{CD}|$ of the C-2′ segments with reduced temperature. (▽), POPC; (○), DPPC; (□), DPPS; (△), DPPE. All lipids were dispersed in water 50 % lipid/50 % H_2O wt/wt) except DPPS which was prepared in buffer 0.5 M Na_2HPO_4, pH 7.2, 0.5 mM Na_2 EDTA at a phospholipid : H_2O ratio of 50 : 150 (wt/wt).

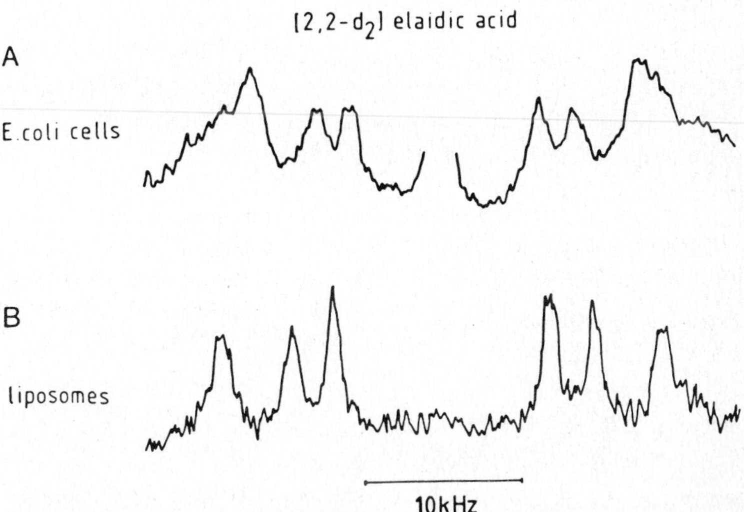

Fig. 3.10. ^2H-NMR spectra (61.4 MHz) of [2,2-$^2H_2$]-elaidate-enriched *E. coli* cells and derived liposomes. (a) Intact cells suspended in 0.1 M NaCl, 0.01 M $MgCl_2$, 0.01 M PIPES, pH 7.0, temperature 36° C. The central line arises from the natural abundance of deuterium in water. (b) Liposomes derived from elaidate-enriched cells in 0.1 M NaCl, 0.01 M $NaPO_4$, pH 7.0, 0.01 M EDTA 41° C. [From Gally et al. (1979).]

plotted as a function of the reduced temperature. Due to the different phase transition temperature of the various phospholipids, the actual temperature range in fig. 3.9 extends from −5 to 90° C. Nevertheless, all the data are collected in narrow bands, supporting the hypothesis of a similar physical state at a given θ temperature. Similar "spectral fingerprints" have also been observed for whole *E. coli* cells grown on [2, 2-^{2}H]-elaidic acid (fig. 3.10) suggesting that this particular feature of phospholipid conformation is unaltered even in the presence of more than 60 wt % membraneous protein (Gally et al. 1979).

The disposition and intrinsic flexibility of the phospholipid polar groups have been studied extensively by means of ^{2}H- and ^{31}P-NMR. Complete sets of data are available for phosphatidylcholine (Gally et al.

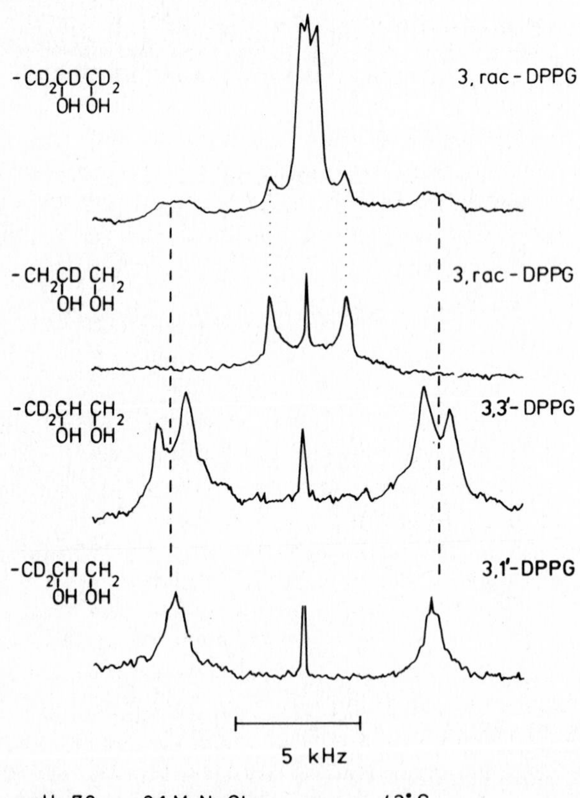

Fig. 3.11. ^{2}H-NMR spectra of 1,2-dipalmitoyl-*sn*-glycero-3-phosphoglycerol labelled at various head group segments. [From Wohlgemuth et al. (1980).]

1975), phosphatidyl-ethanolamine (Seelig and Gally 1976), phosphatidylglycerol (Wohlgemuth et al. 1979) and phosphatidylserine (Browning and Seelig 1979). The complexity of the results is illustrated in fig. 3.11 for bilayers composed of 1,2-dipalmitoyl-*sn*-glycero-3-phosphoglycerol (DPPG). In addition to the asymmetric carbon atom in the backbone, DPPG contains a second centre of optical activity at the C-2′ segment of the glycerol head group. Naturally occurring phosphatidylglycerol is characterized by an L-configuration of the glycerol backbone and a D-configuration of the glycerol head group which in the *sn* nomenclature (*sn* = *s*tereospecific *n*umbering) is denoted as 3,1′-phosphatidylglycerol. Figure 3.11 shows first a ^2H-NMR spectrum of DPPG with a perdeuterated glycerol head group (cf. formula below). The starting compound in the chemical synthesis was perdeuterated glycerol and since no optical resolution was attempted the final product contained a 1 : 1 mixture of the two diastereomers 3,3′-DPPG and 3,1′-DPPG. When dispersed in excess buffer the perdeuterated lipid exhibits a ^2H-NMR spectrum consisting of three quadrupole splittings with separations of about 10, 3.5, and 1 kHz at 45° C. The assignment of the splittings is achieved by synthesis of selectively labelled DPPG and some of the results are also summarized in fig. 3.11. In order to simplify the interpretation we denote the three glycerol head group segments with α, β, and γ, the α-segment being closest to the

$$\begin{array}{ccc} \alpha & \beta & \gamma \\ -CD_2 & CD & CD_2SB \\ & | & | \\ & OH & OH \end{array}$$

phosphate group. Figure 3.11 demonstrates that the largest quadrupole splitting comes from the α-CD_2 segment and the second largest from the β-CD segment. By exclusion the smallest splitting can thus be assigned to the γ-segment. α-deuterated 3,3′-DPPG shows an additional peculiarity in that the spectrum is composed of two overlapping powder patterns with slightly different quadrupole splittings. By stereospecific incorporation of just one deuteron into the α-segment (using anenzymatic method) it can be demonstrated that the two splittings in α-deuterated 3,3′-DPPG are due to the two deuterons of the α-CD_2 segment (Wohlgemuth et al. 1980) and not to a conformational equilibrium within the head group. Compared to 3,3′-DPPG the natural 3,1′-DPPG appears to be slightly more flexible since the α-CD_2 group gives rise to just one quadrupole splitting and its motional inequivalence is averaged out (cf. the two bottom spectra of fig. 3.11).

The phosphatidylglycerol head group data are well suited to illustrate two different aspects of ^{2}H-NMR. On the one hand, ^{2}H-NMR is an extremely sensitive technique which easily detects conformational and/or motional differences between the various lipid segments and even between the individual deuterons attached at the same methylene segment. This sensitivity can be exploited in a very fruitful but purely empirical manner to investigate such different effects as metal ion binding to polar groups (Brown and Seelig 1977, Akutsu and Seelig 1979), cholesterol–phospholipid head group interaction (Brown and Seelig 1978), or lipid–protein interaction (Gally et al. 1979). On the other hand, the detailed quantitative interpretation of the deuterium quadrupole splittings and derived $|S_{CD}|$ parameters [evaluated according to eq. (3.3)] is complicated and does not lead to unambiguous structural models for the polar groups. In fact, the deuterium order parameter is determined by (i) the number of conformations between which the head group may oscillate, (ii) the specific geometry of each allowed conformation, and (iii) any statistical fluctuations to which the phospholipid head group may be subjected, e.g. wobbling motions of the phospholipid molecule as a whole. Therefore, the analysis proceeds by conceiving physically reasonable statistical models for the head group structure and flexibility and by calculating the deuterium quadrupole splittings on the basis of this model. If the predicted quadrupole splittings deviate from the experimental results, the particular model is insufficient and must be rejected. If the theoretical data are consistent with the measurements, this will still not prove the model since it is easy to construct a more complicated model with a larger number of free parameters which will fit the data equally well. Several models have been investigated in detail for the phosphocholine (Gally et al. 1975, Seelig et al. 1977) and phosphoethanolamine head group (Seelig and Gally 1976). A completely rigid head group structure or a completely flexible head group with free rotation around the individual bonds are not in concord with the experimental observations and with certainty can be excluded. Both head groups are characterized by a restricted flexibility and the experimental data converge to a model in which the head groups execute jumps between two mirror-like conformations. The torsion angles of these conformations are furthermore very close to those derived by means of X-ray diffraction from phospholipid model compounds. This two-state model is probably the simplest model which at the present stage of our knowledge explains all the available experimental data. A more detailed discussion of this model may be found in the literature cited heretofore.

Addition of cholesterol induces only minor changes in the torsion angles of the phosphocholine and phosphoethanolamine head groups (Brown and Seelig 1978). The cholesterol molecule is embedded deeply in the hydrocarbon interior so that the cholesterol OH is hydrogen bonded to the glyceryl–fatty acid ester region and does not directly affect the zwitterionic head group region (Worcester and Franks 1976). On the other hand, binding of trivalent ions leads to distinct changes in the NMR parameters which must be attributed to specific ion-induced changes in the head group conformation (Brown and Seelig 1977).

As a general conclusion it follows from our measurements that the head groups probably fluctuate between only a few well-defined minima in the conformational energy profile. The energetically most favourable states seem to be almost independent of the state of the bilayer. The conformations characteristic of the crystalline state are carried over into the fluid bilayer where rapid transitions between the various conformations become possible. The phospholipid crystal structure shown in fig. 3.7, with appropriate dynamic modifications, seems also to be characteristic of biological membranes.

3.3 The structure of the hydrocarbon region

Synthetic phospholipids in excess water exhibit sharp phase transitions at a characteristic temperature T_c. In the gel state ($T<T_c$) the hydrocarbon chains are in an extended and highly ordered conformation. At temperatures $T \geqslant T_c$ the membranes become fluid and the hydrocarbon chains assume a disordered, liquid-like conformation. In order to obtain a more detailed insight into the chain configuration and chain packing in the "fluid" or disordered state of the membrane, we have selectively deuterated the various chain segments of phospholipid molecules and recorded the ^{2}H-NMR spectra of the corresponding bilayer phases above the phase transition temperature. The molecular interpretation of the deuterium quadrupole splittings and order parameters is simplified by the fact that the hydrocarbon chains are highly flexible and that the physical properties of the bilayer are characterized by axial symmetry with respect to the bilayer normal. It is then possible to relate the order parameter of the C-D bond, $|S_{CD}|$, to the order parameter of the long molecular axis, or to be precise, the average orientation of the chain segment to which the deuterium is attached (Seelig and Niederberger 1974). Let us define this segment direction as

given by the normal on the plane spanned by the two C-D bonds of a methylene group. With this definition the segmental orientations will coincide with the long molecular axis if the fatty acyl chain is frozen in the all-*trans* conformation. Since the segment direction is perpendicular to the C-D bond and, to a good approximation at least, also constitutes the rotation axis, the segmental order parameter S_{mol} can be derived for S_{CD} according to

$$S_{mol} = S_{CD}\left[(3\cos^2 90° - 1)/2\right]^{-1} = -2S_{CD}$$

In this model an order parameter $S_{mol} = 1$ corresponds to a completely

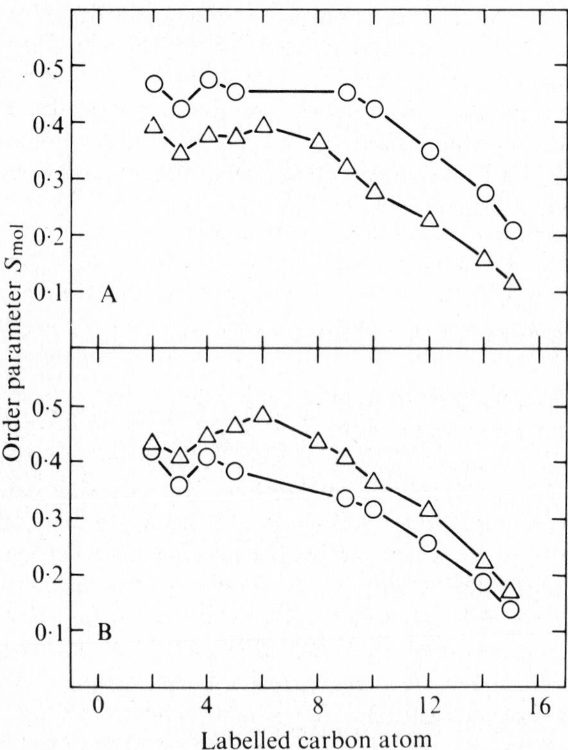

Fig. 3.12. Influence of *cis*-double bonds on the ordering of the hydrocarbon chains. Comparison of the deuterium order parameter S_{mol} for bilayers of 1,2-dipalmitoyl-*sn*-glycero-3-phosphocholine (○) and 1-palmitoyl-2-oleoyl-*sn*-glycero-3-phosphocholine (△) (phase composition 51.5 wt % H_2O/48.5 wt % lipid). (a) Both bilayers at identical temperatures 42° C. (b) Both bilayers at equal temperatures relative to the respective phase transition temperatures. △, POPC at 14° C = T_c + 19° C; O, DPPC at 60° C = T_c + 19° C. [From Seelig and Seelig (1977).]

ordered, all-*trans* conformation while $S_{mol}=0$ is characteristic of a completely disordered state of the hydrocarbon chains.

In fig. 3.12 the results obtained for a saturated bilayer, 1,2-dipalmitoyl-*sn*-glycero-3-phosphocholine (DPPC), are compared with those of an unsaturated phospholipid system, 1-palmitoyl-2-oleoyl-*sn*-glycero-3-phosphocholine (POPC) (Seelig and Seelig 1977). The gel-to-liquid crystal transition temperatures of DPPC and POPC in excess water are 41 and -5° C, respectively. To a first approximation the shape of the curves drawn through the order parameters are rather similar. The order profiles are characterized by a rather constant order parameter for the first 8 chain segments, followed by a gradual decrease of the chain order towards the methyl terminal. In the unsaturated lipid, POPC, the presence of the *cis*-double bond at the 9–10 position of the oleic acid chain introduces a rigid element into the otherwise flexible hydrocarbon chains. The *cis* conformation, furthermore, disturbs the parallel packing of the hydrocarbon chains and reduces the van der Waals interactions between adjacent hydrocarbon chains. This is reflected in the much lower transition temperature of POPC (−5° C) than that of DPPC (41° C) and also in the segmental order parameters. If compared at the same temperature (fig. 3.12a), the POPC bilayer is always found to be more disordered than the DPPC bilayer. It should be noted that the incorporation of a *cis*-double bond in a well-defined position in the hydrocarbon chain reduces the ordering in all parts of the hydrocarbon region. In fig. 3.12b the saturated and unsaturated bilayers are compared at equal temperatures relative to their respective phase transitions. The two order profiles are seen to run parallel and closely together in the first part of the chain until carbon atom 4 and then again for the terminal region starting from carbon atom 10. In the intermediate region the two curves depart from each other and it is now the unsaturated system which is the more ordered one. This increase in the order parameter can be interpreted as a local stiffening effect caused by the *cis*-double bond, which reduces the motional freedom of the adjacent chain segments.

A more extensive comparison of order profiles for various lipid systems is provided by fig 3.13. The order profiles of three synthetic lipids (POPC, DPPC, DPPS) are plotted at the same reduced temperature $\theta \approx 0.061$, corresponding to actual measuring temperatures of 11, 60, and 71° C (Seelig and Browning 1978). Also included in fig 3.13 is the order profile of the *Acholeplasma laidlawii* membrane measured at 42° C (Stockton et al. 1977). This natural membrane has no well-defined transition temperature, instead it shows a rather broad transition

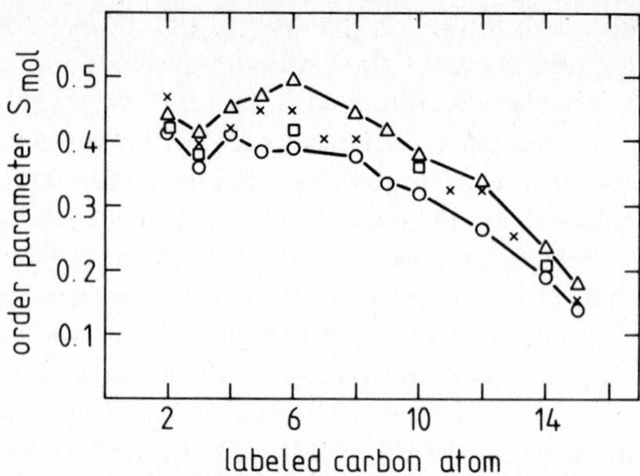

Fig. 3.13. Variation of the molecular order parameter, S_{mol}, with the segment position. (○) DPPC (Seelig and Seelig 1974), (△) POPC (Seelig and Seelig 1977); (□) DPPS (Seelig and Browning 1978); (X) *Acholeplasma laidlawii* (Stockton et al. 1977). The synthetic lipid membranes are measured at the same reduced temperature $\theta=(T-T_c)/T_c=0.0605$. [From Seelig and Browning (1978).]

around 25° C. Referred to this approximate phase transition temperature ($T_c \triangleq 298$ K), the measuring temperature of 42° C corresponds to $\theta=0.057$ which is tolerable for a comparison with the synthetic lipids measured at $\theta=0.061$. The figure 3.13 then shows that all the other profiles are relatively similar, in contrast to a comparison at the same temperature, e.g. 70° C. It is interesting to note that the extremes are defined by DPPC and POPC while DPPS and the *Acholeplasma laidlawii* membrane fall in between these boundaries. Thus the incorporation of a *cis*-double bond is seen to promote larger changes in the order profile than, for example, the introduction of a net negative charge in the polar head group (DPPC) or the incorporation of proteins into the membrane. The relatively small effect of proteins on the deuterium order has also been observed in recent reconstitution experiments with cytochrome oxidase containing bilayers (Seelig and Seelig 1978, Oldfield et al. 1978).

The average order parameter S_{mol} in figs. 3.12 and 3.13 is about 0.5 or less indicating a considerable chain flexibility. The molecular origin of this chain flexibility is rapid isomerizations between *trans* and *gauche* conformations of the carbon–carbon bonds. In solution, the average conformation of a hydrocarbon chain is essentially determined by intramolecular forces, i.e. the bond rotation potential for *trans*-*gauche* isomerizations and steric interactions between adjacent chain segments. The segment interactions are cooperative and are normally described in terms of a linear Ising model (Flory 1969). On the basis of this model the probabilities of *trans* and *gauche* states for a liquid polymethylene chain are found to be $p_t \approx 0.65$ and $p_g \approx 0.35$ at room temperature (cf. Flory 1969, p.82). In a bilayer the chain conformation is determined by intramolecular as well as intermolecular interactions. In this case the average chain conformation can be calculated on the basis of a model first proposed by Marčelja (1974). We have employed the Marčelja model to analyze the deuterium order parameters in the DPPC bilayer (Schindler and Seelig 1975). The probabilities of *trans* and *gauche* conformations were found to be $p_t = 0.69$ and $p_g = 0.31$ at 41° C, which is not significantly different from the corresponding probabilities for the liquid paraffin chain. Therefore, on the average, 9.5 bonds of a palmitic acyl chain are in the *trans* state while 4.5 are in the *gauche* state, regardless of whether the molecule is incorporated into a bilayer or is dissolved in a paraffinic liquid. However, the chain configurations in the systems are still not identical. In the liquid phase both ends of the chain are free to move, while in the bilayer one end is anchored in the lipid–water phase endowing the chain with a distinct polarity. Therefore, the probability of occurrence of *gauche* states becomes dependent on the position of the segment in the bilayer. Furthermore, coupled *gauche* rotations like kinks of jogs ($g^{\pm}tg^{\mp}$, $g^{\pm}tttg^{\mp}$) are favoured since they introduce a relatively small perturbation in the chain packing. Such conformational defects have been used to construct the disordered lipid bilayer model shown in fig. 3.14 (Seelig and Seelig 1974). The statistical–mechanical calculations show however that kink-like structures alone cannot account for the observed order profiles. Thus a pure kink model of lipid bilayers (cf. Träuble, 1971) is not in accordance with the physical reality of a fluid lipid bilayer.

Considering the specific effect of *cis*-unsaturation, this problem has been investigated extensively for bilayers composed of 1-palmitoyl-2-oleoyl-*sn*-glycero-3-phosphocholine. In one set of experiments the deuterium labels were attached to the palmitic acyl chain, and the influence of the double bond in the oleic acyl chain was probed indirectly by the neighbouring chain (cf. figs. 3.12 and 3.13). However, it is equally possible to selectively deuterate POPC in the *sn*-2 oleic acyl chain and fig 3.15 compares the $|S_{CD}|$-order profiles of the two chains (Seelig and Waespe-Šarčevič 1978). The *cis*-double bond appears as a pronounced discontinuity in the curve drawn through the order parameters. A quantitative analysis of the complete ordering tensor leads to the conclusion that the *cis*-double bond is not aligned exactly parallel to the bilayer normal but is tilted by a few degrees. After correcting for this

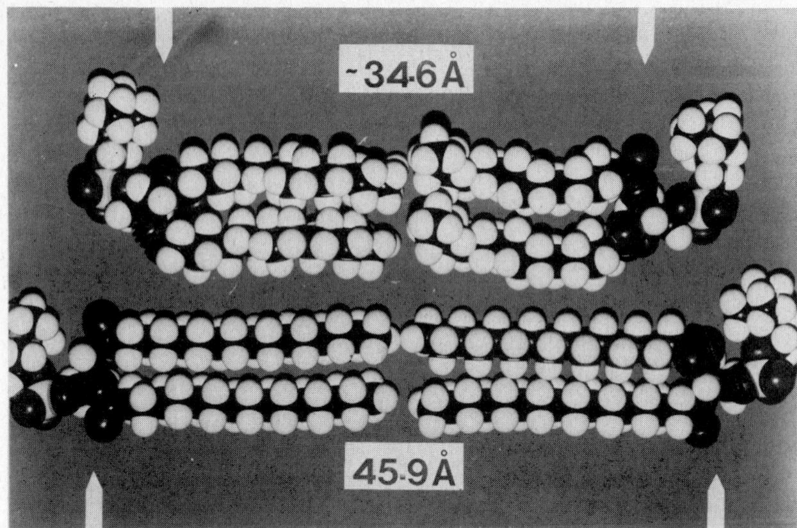

Fig. 3.14. Space filling models of lipid bilayers. The all-*trans* conformation of the fatty acyl chains in the gel state is compared with the disordered chain conformation in the fluid (liquid crystalline) state. [From Seelig and Seelig (1974).]

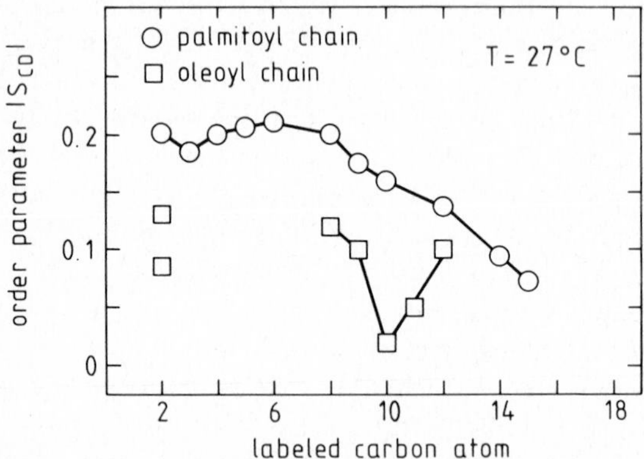

Fig. 3.15. Bilayers of 1-palmitoyl-2-oleoyl-*sn*-glycero-3-phosphocholine. Variation of the deuterium order parameter, S_{CD}, with segment position (○) *sn*-1 palmitic acyl chain; (□) *sn*-2 oleic acyl chain; (□) *sn*-2 oleic acyl chain. Measuring temperature 27° C. [From Seelig and Waespe-Šarčevič (1978).]

geometrical effect, the statistical fluctuations in the *sn*-1 and *sn*-2 chain are found to be identical. The segmental fluctuations in POPC bilayers are not dependent on the segment geometry but are determined by the distance from the lipid boundary.

Acknowledgements

This work was supported by the Swiss National Science Foundation Grant No. 3.409.78.

References

Akutsu, H. and J. Seelig (1980) manuscript in preparation.
Brown, M. F. and J. Seelig (1977) Nature 269, 721.
Brown, M. F. and J. Seelig (1978) Biochemistry 17, 381.
Browning, J. L. and J. Seelig (1980) Biochemistry 19, 1262.
Büldt, G., H. U. Gally, A. Seelig, J. Seelig and G. Zaccai (1978) Nature 271, 182.
Büldt. G., H. U. Gally, J. Seelig and G. Zaccai (1979) J. Mol. Biol. 134, 673.
Burnett, L. J. and B. H. Muller (1971) J. Chem. Phys. 55, 5829.
Finer, E. G. and A. Darke (1974) Chem. Phys. Lipids 12, 1.
Flory, P. J. (1969) Statistical Mechanics of Chain Molecules (Interscience-New York).
Gally, H. U., W. Niederberger and J. Seelig (1975) Biochemistry 14, 3647.
Gally, H. U., G. Pluschke, P. Overath and J. Seelig (1979) Biochemistry 18, 5605.
Griffin, R. G. (1976) J. Am. Chem. Soc. 98, 851.
Haberkorn, R. A., R. G. Griffin, M. D. Meadows and E. Oldfield (1977) J. Am. Chem. Soc. 99, 7353.
Herzfeld, J., R. G. Griffin and R. A. Haberkorn (1978) Biochemistry 17, 2711.
Hitchcock, P. B., R. Mason, K. M. Thomas and G. G. Shipley (1974) Proc. Nat. Acad. Sci. USA 71, 3036.
Kohler, S. J. and M. P. Klein (1976) Biochemistry 15, 967.
Kohler, S. J. and M. P. Klein (1977) Biochemistry 16, 519.
Marčelja, S. (1974) Biochim. Biophys. Acta 367, 165.
Niederberger, W. and J. Seelig (1976) J. Am. Chem. Soc. 98, 3704.
Oldfield, E., R. Gilmore, M. Glaser, H. S. Gutowsky, J. C. Hshung, S. Y. Kang, Tsoo E. King, M. Meadows and D. Rice (1978) Proc. Nat. Acad. Sci. USA 75, 4657.
Saupe, A. (1968) Angew. Chem. 80, 99.
Schindler, H. and J. Seelig (1975) Biochemistry 14, 2283.
Seelig, A. and J. Seelig (1974) Biochemistry 13, 4839.
Seelig, A. and J. Seelig (1975) Biochim. Biophys. Acta 406, 1.
Seelig, A. and J. Seelig (1977) Biochemistry 16, 45.
Seelig, A. and J. Seelig (1978) Hoppe-Seyler's Z. Physiol. Chem. 359, 1747.
Seelig, J. (1977) Quart. Rev. Biophys. 10, 353.
Seelig, J. (1978a) Biochim. Biophys. Acta 505, 105.
Seelig, J. (1978b) Progr. Coll. Polymer Sci. 65, 172.
Seelig, J. and J. L. Browning (1978) FEBS Lett. 92, 41.
Seelig, J. and H. Gally (1976) Biochemistry 15, 5199.
Seelig, J., H. Gally and R. Wohlegemuth (1977) Biochim. Biophys. Acta 467, 109.
Seelig, J. and W. Niederberger (1974) J. Am. Chem. Soc. 96, 2069.

Seelig, J. and N. Waespe-Šarčevič (1978) Biochemistry 17, 3310.
Stockton, G. W., C. F. Polnaszek, A. P. Tulloch, F. Hasan and I. C. P. Smith (1976) Biochemistry 15, 954.
Stockton, G. W., K. G. Johnson, K. Butler, A. P. Tulloch, Y. Boulanger, I. C. P. Smith, J. H. Davis and M. Bloom (1977) Nature 269, 267.
Träuble, H. (1971) J. Membr. Biol. 4, 193.
Wohlgemuth, R., N. Waespe-Šarčevič and J. Seelig (1980) Biochemistry, in press
Worcester, D. L. (1976) Neutron Beam Studies of Biological Membranes and Membrane Components, in: Biological Membranes, eds D. Chapman and D. F. H. Wallach, vol. 3 (Academic Press, London) pp. 1–44.
Worcester, D. L. and N. P. Franks (1976) J. Mol. Biol. 100, 359.
Zaccai, G., G. Büldt, A. Seelig and J. Seelig (1979) J. Mol. Biol. 134, 693.

SEMINAR

LIPID POLYMORPHISM AND THE OCCURRENCE OF NON-BILAYER PHASES IN MODEL AND BIOLOGICAL MEMBRANES*

B. de KRUIJFF, A. J. VERKLEIJ, J. LEUNISSEN-BIJVELT, C. J. A. van ECHTELD, W. J. GERRITSEN, C. MOMBERS, P. C. NOORDAM, J. de GIER and P. R. CULLIS**

Institute of Molecular Biology and Department of Biochemistry, State University of Utrecht, Padualaan 8, 3584 CH Utrecht, The Netherlands

1. Introduction

In the current models for biological membranes the lipids are organized in a continuous bilayer that forms the semipermeable barrier which selectively separates the cell content from its surroundings and which

*Lecture delivered at les Houches by B. de Kruijff.

**Department of Biochemistry, University of British Columbia, Vancouver, B.C. V6T 1W5.

R. Balian et al., eds.
Les Houches, Session XXXIII, 1979 – Membranes et Communication Intercellulaire / Membranes and Intercellular Communication

acts as a matrix for the more functional membrane proteins. However, these models do not account for two of the basic properties of the lipid part of biological membranes.

(a) The great variety of lipids found in a single membrane is not understood and only one lipid species like unsaturated phosphatidylcholine can satisfy the above requirements. Even more important is the observation that each membrane contains, next to bilayer-forming lipids, significant amounts of lipids that, in isolated form dispersed in buffer, do not adopt a bilayer configuration but organize themselves in different structures. Among those lipids are: unsaturated phosphatidylethanolamines [1–7], monoglucosyldiglycerides [8, 9], phosphatidic acid [10], and cardiolipin [11, 12] (in the presence of Ca^{2+}) which prefer the hexagonal H_{II} phase and phospholipid precursor molecules like lysophospholipids, fatty acids, and diglycerides which prefer micellar or other phases. The presence of these lipids can expect to actively mitigate against the bilayer structure of the membrane.

(b) Many different processes occur in biological membranes in which a part of the lipids has to temporarily leave the bilayer configuration. Clear examples are: membrane fusion (including endo-, exo-, and phagocytosis) and transbilayer movements of membrane lipids (flip-flop).

In this seminar we would like to develop the view that "non-bilayer" lipids are actively involved in these dynamic processes, a hypothesis that will first be tested in model membrane systems.

2. Model systems

The ability of hydrated membrane lipids to adopt a variety of phases in addition to the bilayer phase, has been demonstrated already some twenty years ago. The structural characteristics of these alternative phases have been solved by the extensive X-ray studies of Luzzati and co-workers [13–15]. The recent introduction of ^{31}P NMR in combination with freeze-fracture electron microscopy has made it possible to obtain detailed insight in the polymorphic phase behaviour of membrane lipids. This is illustrated in fig. 4.1 for an aqueous dispersion of phosphatidylethanolamine isolated from hen eggs. At low temperatures (below 25° C) this phospholipid organizes itself in extended bilayers as evidenced by the characteristic asymmetrical ^{31}P NMR spectrum with a high field peak and a low field shoulder [3, 4, 7, 16] and the smooth

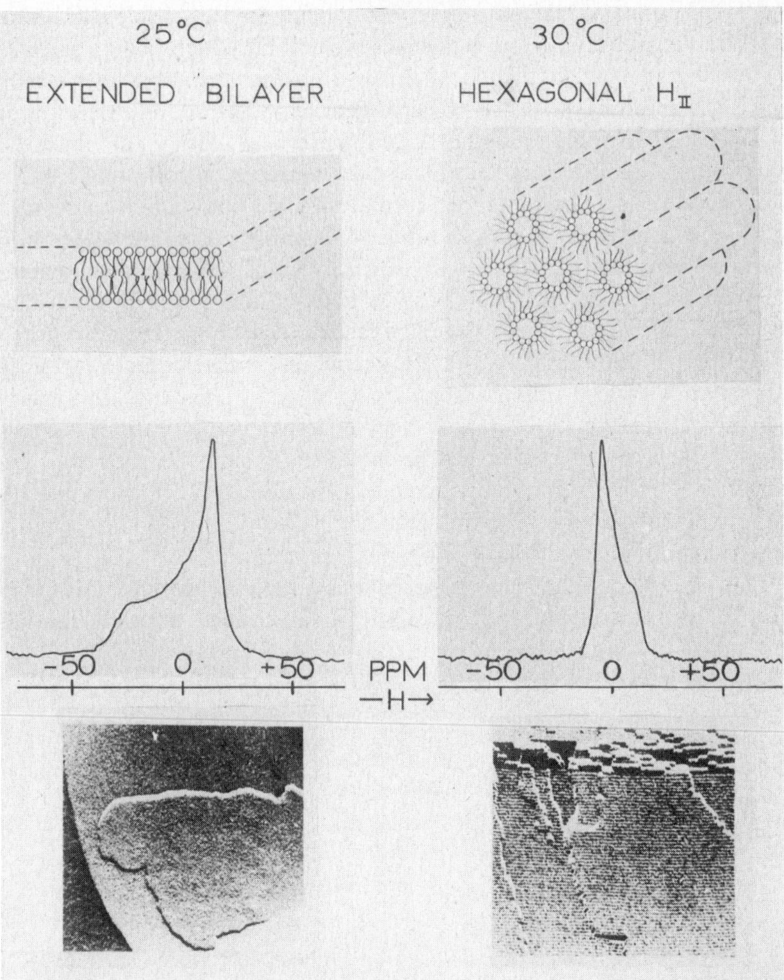

Fig. 4.1. ^{31}P NMR and freeze-fracture detection of bilayer (25° C) and hexagonal H_{II} phase (30° C) of an aqueous dispersion of egg phosphatidylethanolamine. Magnification of the micrographs about 100 000×.

fracture planes as observed by freeze-fracturing. In the temperature interval 25–30° C, a phase change occurs so that this lipid is now organized in the hexagonal H_{II} phase with the spectrum of half the spectral width and a reversed asymmetry [3, 4, 7, 16] and a freeze-fracture appearance of fracture planes being composed of long parallel lines [5]. The temperature of the bilayer-hexagonal transition is very sensitive to the degree of unsaturation of the acyl chains and is higher for more saturated species [7]. At the physiological temperature, naturally occurring phosphatidylethanolamines often prefer the hexagonal phase [7]. Other remarkable features of this transition are its sharpness and its low heat content. The complete transformation form bilayer to hexagonal or vice versa commonly occurs within a 5° C temperature interval for both synthetic and naturally occurring species (which have a heterogeneous fatty acid composition). The heat content of this phase change is an order of magnitude lower than the heat involved in the gel→ liquid crystalline phase transition as is illustrated in the thermogram of an egg phosphatidylethanolamine dispersion (fig. 4.2). The very low energy barrier between macroscopically very different configurations suggests that the acyl chain packing in both phases is similar which was also concluded from magnetic resonance experiments [17, 18] and has important consequences for the possible dynamic functional roles of non-bilayer lipid structures in biological membranes.

Phosphatidylcholines have a strong bilayer stabilizing effect on phosphatidylethanolamines [4, 6]. In contrast, cholesterol strongly destabi-

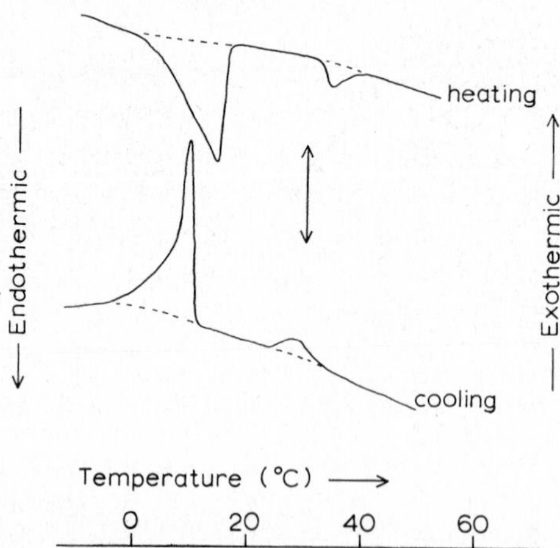

Fig. 4.2. Differential scanning calorimetry scans of an aqueous dispersion of egg phosphatidylethanolamine. The gel → liquid crystalline transition occurs from 0 –18° C. The arrow indicates the temperature of the bilayer → hexagonal transition as detected by ^{31}P NMR.

lizes the bilayer structure in unsaturated phosphatidylethanolamine containing systems [4, 6, 7]. The bilayer–hexagonal transition can also be isothermally induced by the addition of Ca^{2+}, both in pure systems like cardiolipin [11, 12] and phosphatidic acid [10], as well as in phosphatidylethanolamine–phosphatidylserine mixtures [19]. As a most interesting intermediate between the bilayer and hexagonal H_{II} phase a new phase is observed which is characteristic by a narrow symmetrical ^{31}P NMR resonance indicating isotropic motional averaging. This is illustrated in fig. 4.3 for a dioleoylphosphatidylethanolamine–dioleoylphosphatidylcholine–cholesterol (3: 1: 2) mixture in which, by a temperature increase, the isotropic phase was induced [9]. Freeze-fracturing of this sample shows the presence of numerous particles and pits of a uniform size of approximately 100 Å which are associated with the lipid bilayer [9]. ^{31}P NMR and freeze-fracturing evidence for lipidic particles was further obtained in phosphatidylcholine–cardiolipin (Ca^{2+}) and phosphatidylcholine–monoglucosyldiglyceride mixtures [9, 20]. As a tentative model for these lipidic particles we proposed [9, 20] the inverted micelle sandwiched between the monolayers of the lipid bilayer (see fig. 4.4d). Tumbling of the micelle and lateral diffusion of the lipids in the micelle will provide the isotropic motion detected in the ^{31}P NMR experiments. The additional possibility that rapid exchange may occur between the inverted micellar and surrounding bilayer lipids (fig. 4.4) adds a new dimension to the dynamics of lipids in membranes.

An important question in relation to the possible occurence of non-bilayer phases in biological membranes is whether such structures can be found in the hydrated total lipid extracts of these membranes. In the case of the human erythrocyte, the total lipids organize themselves in a bilayer at 37° C [21, 22] despite the presence of 30 mol % of phosphatidylethanolamine which, in isolated form above 10° C, adopts the hexagonal H_{II} phase [7] and therefore clearly demonstrates the bilayer's stabilizing capacity of the other membrane phospholipids. However, very recent work suggests that this situation is more exceptional than common. In fig. 4.5 the ^{31}P NMR and freeze-fracturing results of the total lipids of *E. coli* are presented at the growth temperature. It is now obvious that mainly the hexagonal H_{II} and an isotropic phases are observed. This latter phase might again be of an inverted micellar nature since particles and pits are found on the fracture planes. Very similar results are found for the total lipids of the photoreceptor [23] and the inner mitochondrial membrane [24].

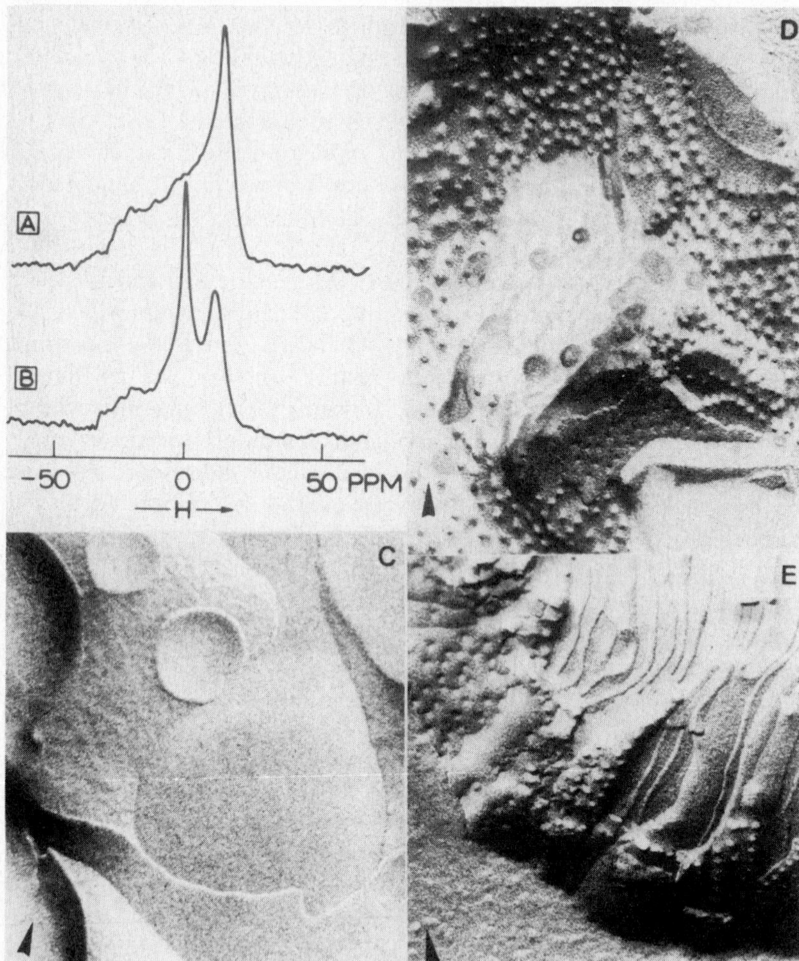

Fig. 4.3. ^{31}P NMR and freeze-fracturing of an aqueous dispersion of 18 : 1_c/18 : 1_c-phosphatidylethanolamine: 18 : 1_c/18 :1_c-phosphatidylcholine : cholesterol (3: 1: 2). (a) ^{31}P NMR and (c) freeze-fracturing of the sample at 10° C. (b) ^{31}P NMR and (d,e) freeze-fracturing of the sample at 10° C after being heated for 5 min at 60° C. Magnification of the micrographs about 1000 000×.

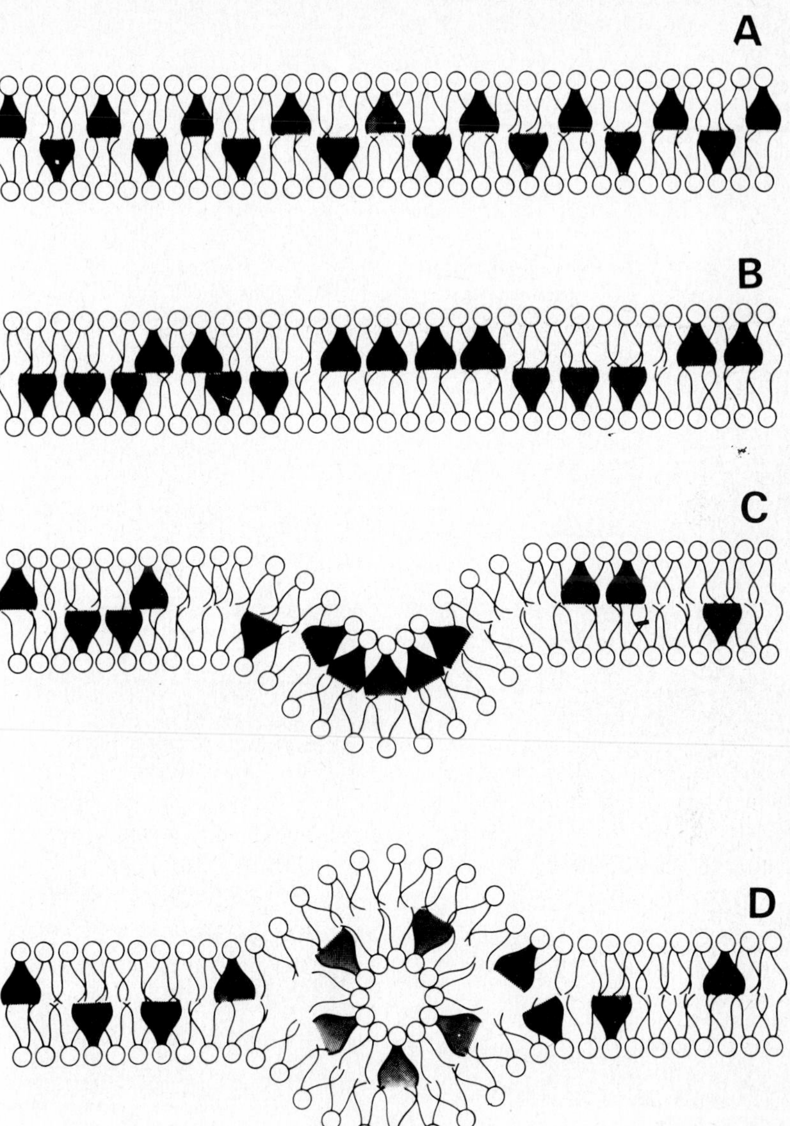

Fig. 4.4. Dynamic formation of inverted micelles in a lipid bilayer. In a lipid bilayer (a) composed of lipid molecules with an overall cylindrical shape (e.g. phosphatidylcholine) and molecules with a wedge shape (e.g. phosphatidylethanolamine indicated as dark molecules), statistically local high concentrations of these latter molecules (b) will cause an inward curvature of the lipid bilayer (c) reversibly leading to the formation of inverted micelles (d).

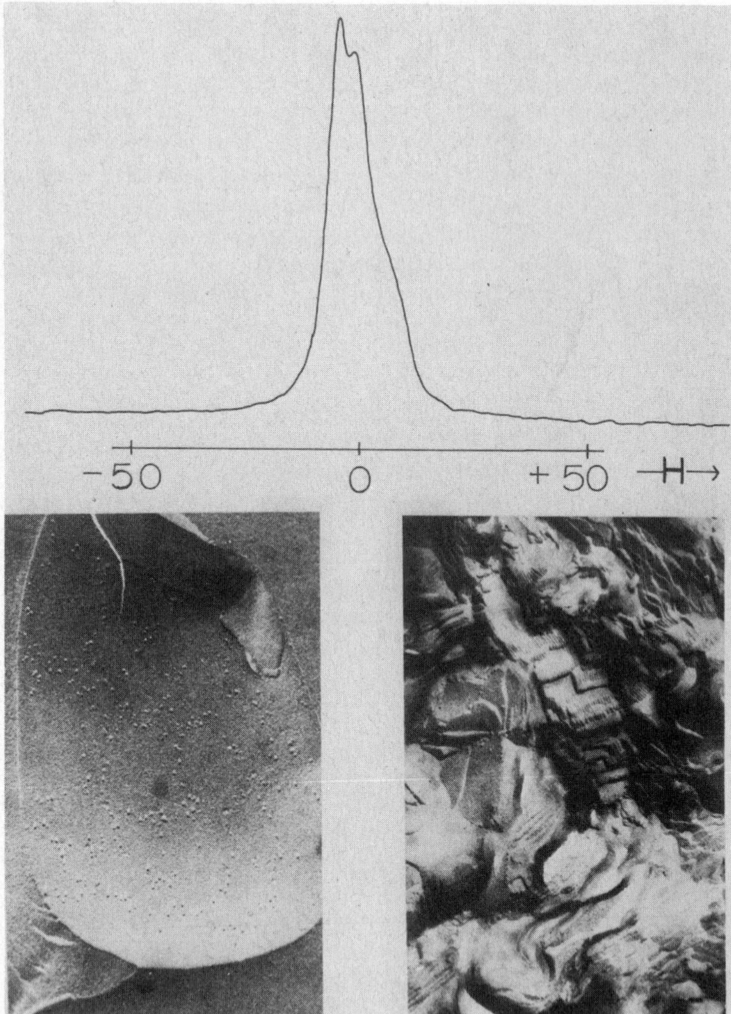

Fig. 4.5. ^{31}P NMR and freeze-fracturing of the total lipids of *E. coli* at 37° C. The micrographs (final magnification about 100 000×) show lipid bilayers associated with lipidic particles and the hexagonal H_{II} phase.

Since there is no evidence as yet for the existence of a hexagonal H_{II} phase lipid in biological membranes the "isotropic phase" is of particular interest, as experiments on different membranes do suggest lipid structures allowing such isotropic motion.

3. Biological membranes

One of the most closely characterized biological membranes is that of the human erythrocyte which exhibits ^{31}P NMR spectra (arising from at least 97% of the endogenous phospholipids [21, 22], which are fully consistent with virtually all the lipids being organized in a lipid bilayer (see fig. 4.6a). This bilayer is very stable and must, next to the membrane phospholipids, also be determined by cholesterol and/or membrane proteins because extensive phospholipid degradation by various phospholipases, producing high amounts of non-bilayer lipids like lysophospholipids, diglycerides, and ceramides, does not affect the bilayer structure [25]. This stability might be related to the low metabolic activity of the membrane, the long life span of the erythrocyte, and its exposure to large mechanical stresses during its passage through blood capillaries.

Support for the existence of non-bilayer lipid structures in intact biological membranes have recently been obtained for the metabolically very active endoplasmic reticulum membranes of rat, beef, and rabbit liver. Two laboratories [26, 27] have independently reported that the phospholipids in microsomes (isolated vesiculated fragments of the endoplasmic reticulum) give rise at 37° C to ^{31}P NMR line shapes (see fig. 4.6b) indicating isotropic motion of the lipids within the membrane. Most interestingly and in full agreement with the results on model membranes discussed in the previous section, at lower temperatures (below 30° C) an increasing fraction of the signal has the normal bilayer shape (fig. 4.6c). Strong ^{31}P NMR evidence has been obtained that this temperature-dependent phase change also occurs in the endoplasmic reticulum of intact rat liver [28]. These results would be consistent with the existence of inverted micellar or (short) cylindrical arrangements of lipid inside the bilayer. Furthermore, the results strongly indicate rapid exchange of bulk bilayer lipids with such structures. In addition it can be speculated that membrane proteins (possibly cytochrome P_{450} as suggested by Stier et al. [27]) actively encourage these manifestations of non-bilayer lipids as aqueous dispersions of the extracted lipids do show the normal "bilayer" spectra [26, 27].

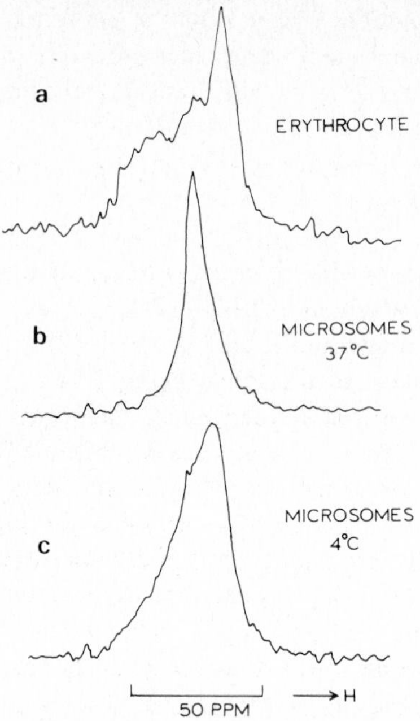

Fig. 4.6. ^{31}P NMR spectra of various biological membranes.

The sarcoplasmic reticulum membrane, although to a lesser extent than the endoplasmic reticulum membrane, also gives rise to ^{31}P NMR spectra indicating isotropic motion of (part) of the membrane phospholipids [29]. It is remarkable that similar findings were obtained already some eight years ago by Davis and Inesi [30], who concluded on the basis of ^{1}H NMR studies that some 20% of the endogenous sarcoplasmic reticulum lipid enjoyed isotropic motion on the NMR time scale.

There is also evidence that in the inner mitochondrial membrane a significant fraction of the phosphatidylcholine experiences isotropic motion possibly due to non-bilayer alternatives; this is implicit in the ^{2}H NMR results of Arvidson et al. [31]. These results are substantiated to some extent by recent ^{31}P NMR experiments [24] but must be treated with care in view of the observation that, for intact mitochondria at 37° C, changes in the functional state (P/O ratio) and the amount of "isotropic" ^{31}P NMR signal occurs within minutes of incubation at 37°

C [24]. For osmiophilic bodies from pig lung some 5% of the phospholipids undergo isotropic motion which was suggested to be due to apolar proteins [32].

4. Functional aspects of non-bilayer phases in membranes

Although the functional implications of the occurence of non-bilayer phases are obvious in many areas of membrane biology as discussed elsewhere [33], strong supportive evidence is only available in two cases, e.g. membrane fusion and lipid flip-flop.

Membrane fusion. Regardless of whether fusion is mediated by protein, lipid, or another agent, during some stage of the fusion process part of the lipids will have to leave the bilayer configuration. This was clearly demonstrated in the case of human erythrocyte ghosts where, upon treatment with fusogenic agents like fatty acids, the presence of the hexagonal H_{II} phase could be detected [34]. Furthermore, unilamellar phosphatidylcholine–cardiolipin (1:1) vesicles fuse upon the addition of Ca^{2+} in which the process is accompanied by the appearance of lipidic particles at the fusion interface [35].

Lipid flip-flop. It has been suggested that transient formation of intrabilayer inverted lipid-structures, like those shown in fig. 4.4, provide a mechanism for flip-flop processes resulting in redistribution of lipids across the bilayer [4]. Support for this hypothesis comes from measurements on microsomal membranes. At 37° C the phospholipids in these membranes undergo isotropic motion and have a fast flip-flop [36, 37]. At 4° C, mainly bilayer structure is observed, and the rate of phosphatidylcholine flip-flop appears to be drastically reduced [37]. In the sarcoplasmic membrane also isotropic motion of part of the phospholipids occurs and rapid transbilayer movements of lysophosphatidylcholine [29] and part of the phosphatidylcholine pool have been observed [38].

Other membrane systems in which rapid flip-flop occurs (e.g. certain bacterial membranes [39]) have lipid compositions which are also consistent with the occurence of non-bilayer structures. In fact, the data on the total lipids of *E. coli* (fig. 4.5) and the observation that in isolated *E. coli* inner membranes part of the phospholipids undergo isotropic motion [40] strongly support this hypothesis. However, it should be realized that alternative flip-flop mechanisms including protein mediated processes [41, 42] might be operating in membranes as well.

References

[1.] F. Reiss-Husson, J. Mol. Biol. 25 (1967) 363.
[2] R. P. Rand, D. O. Tinker and P. G. Fast, Chem. Phys. Lipids 6 (1971) 33.
[3] P. R. Cullis and B. de Kruijff, Biochim. Biophys. Acta 436 (1976) 523.
[4] P. R. Cullis and B. de Kruijff, Biochim. Biophys. Acta 507 (1978) 207.
[5] P. W. M. van Dijck, B. de Kruijff, L. L. M. van Deenen, J. de Gier and R. A. Demel, Biochim. Biophys. Acta 455 (1976) 576.
[6] P. R. Cullis, P. W. M. van Dijck, B. de Kruijff and J. de Gier, Biochim. Biophys. Acta 513 (1978) 21.
[7] P. R. Cullis, and B. de Kruijff, Biochim. Biophys. Acta 513 (1978) 31.
[8] Å. Wieslander, J. Ulmius, G. Lindblom and K. Fontell, Biochim. Biophys. Acta 512 (1978) 241.
[9] B. de Kruijff, A. J. Verkleij, C. J. A. van Echteld, W. J. Gerritsen, C. Mombers, P. C. Noordam and J. de Gier, Biochim. Biophys. Acta 555 (1979) 200.
[10] D. Papahadjopoulis, W. J. Vail, W. A. Pangborn and G. Poste, Biochim. Biophys. Acta 448 (1976) 265.
[11] R. P. Rand and S. Sengupta, Biochim. Biophys. Acta 513 (1972) 11.
[12] P. R. Cullis, A. J. Verkleij and P. H. J. Th. Ververgaert, Biochim. Biophys. Acta 513 (1978) 11.
[13] V. Luzzatti and F. Husson, J. Cell Biol. 12 (1962) 207.
[14] V. Luzzatti, T. Gulik-Krzywichi and A. Tardieu, Nature 218 (1968) 1031.
[15] V. Luzzatti and A. Tardieu, Ann. Rev. Phys. Chem. 25 (1974) 79.
[16] J. Seelig, Biochim. Biophys. Acta 515 (1978) 105.
[17] B. Mely, J. Charvolin and P. Keller, Chem. Phys. Lipids 15 (1975) 161.
[18] J. Seelig and H. Limacher, Mol. Cryst. Liq. Cryst. 25 (1974) 105.
[19] P. R. Cullis and A. J. Verkleij, Biochim. Biophys. Acta 552 (1979) 545.
[20] A. J. Verkleij, C. Mombers, J. Leunissen-Bijvelt and P. H. J. Th. Ververgaert, Nature 279 (1979) 162.
[21] P. R. Cullis, FEBS. Lett. 70 (1976) 223.
[22] P. R. Cullis and Ch. Grathwohl, Biochim. Biophys. Acta 471 (1977) 213.
[23] W. J. de Grip, E. H. S. Drenthe, C. J. A. van Echteld, B. de Kruijff and A. J. Verkleij, Biochim. Biophys. Acta 558 (1979) 330.
[24] Authors unpublished results.
[25] G. Vermeer, B. de Kruijff, J. Op den Kamp and L. L. M. van Deenen, Biochim. Biophys. Acta 596 (1980) 1.
[26] B. de Kruijff, A. M. H. P. van den Besselaar, P. R. Cullis, H. van den Bosch and L. L. M. van Deenen, Biochim. Biophys. Acta 514 (1978) 1.
[27] A. Stier, S. A. E. Finch and B. Bösterling, FEBS. Lett. 91 (1978) 109.
[28] B. de Kruijff and A. Rietveld, Biochim. Biophys. Acta (1979) submitted.
[29] A. M. H. P. van den Besselaar, B. de Kruijff, H. van den Bosch and L. L. M. van Deenen, Biochim. Biophys. Acta 555 (1979) 193.
[30] D. G. Davis and G. Inesi, Biochim. Biophys. Acta 241 (1971) 1.
[31] G. Arvidson, G. Lindblon and T. Drakenberg, FEBS. Lett. 54 (1975) 249.
[32] C. Grathwohl, G. E. Newman, P. I. R. Phizacherley and M. H. Town, Biochim. Biophys. Acta 552 (1979) 509.
[33] P. R. Cullis and B. de Kruijff, Biochim. Biophys. Acta 559 (1979) 399.
[34] P. R. Cullis and M. J. Hope, Nature 271 (1978) 672.

[35] A. J. Verkleij, C. Mombers, W. J. Gerritsen, J. Leunissen-Bijvelt and P. R. Cullis, Biochim. Biophys. Acta 555 (1979) 358.
[36] D. B. Zilversmit and M. E. Hughes, Biochim. Biophys. Acta 469 (1977) 99.
[37] A. M. H. P. van den Besselaar, B. de Kruijff, H. van den Bosch and L. L. M. van Deenen, Biochim. Biophys. Acta 510 (1978) 242.
[38] B. de Kruijff, A. M. H. P. van den Besselaar, H. van den Bosch and L. L. M. van Deenen, Biochim. Biophys. Acta 555 (1979) 181.
[39] J. E. Rothman and J. Lenard, Science 195 (1977) 743.
[40] E. Burnell, L. van Alphen, B. de Kruijff and A. J. Verkleij, Biochim. Biophys. Acta (1979) submitted.
[41] E. J. J. van Zoelen, L. L. M. van Deenen and B. de Kruijff, Biochim. Biophys. Acta 597 (1980) 492.
[42] B. de Kruijff, E. J. J. van Zoelen and L. L. M. van Deenen, Biochim. Biophys. Acta 509 (1978) 537.

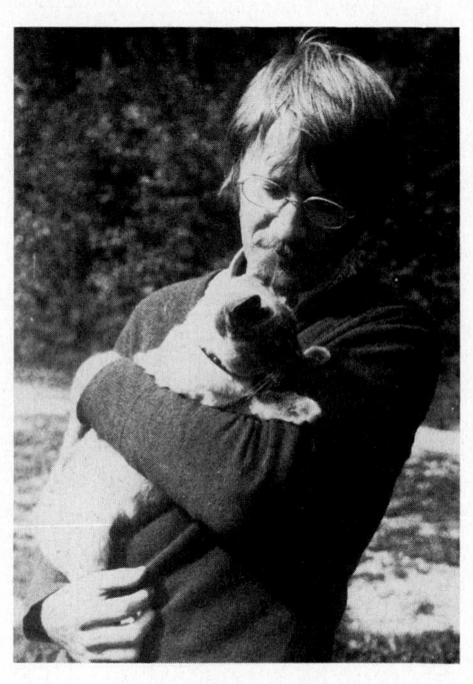

SEMINAR

SOLUBILITY OF INTRINSIC MEMBRANE PROTEINS IN PHOSPHOLIPID BILAYERS

Philippe F. DEVAUX

Institut de Biologie Physico-Chimique,
13 rue Pierre et Marie Curie,
75005 Paris,
France

1. Protein overall mobility and lipid–protein interaction in membranes

1.1. The paradox of the low lipid content of biological membranes

Intrinsic proteins are embedded in a phospholipid bilayer such that they form not a rigid structure but rather a dynamical association. There is increasing evidence that intrinsic proteins can experience a high degree of overall mobility. Both rotational and lateral diffusion of such proteins have been determined (see, in this book, the chapter by McConnell). However it has been found that the diffusion constant varies from one type of membrane to another in such a manner that differences in molecular weights do not fully explain the differences in mobility. For example, in the post-synaptic membrane of torpedo electric organ, the cholinergic receptor protein has a rotational correlation time larger than

R. Balian et al., eds.
Les Houches, Session XXXIII, 1979 – Membranes et Communication Intercellulaire / Membranes and Intercellular Communication

1 ms. Yet the molecular weight of the cholinergic receptor unit is about 40 000 Dalton, which is precisely the molecular weight of rhodopsin, a very mobile protein in the rod outer segment membranes ($\tau_c \simeq 10^{-5}$ s).

Therefore the following question is raised: what is responsible for the restriction in mobility of some membrane proteins? or alternatively how can a membrane optimize its protein mobility?

The simplest way to reduce protein mobility is to cross-link proteins together. Functional intrinsic proteins can be in oligomeric states. The acetylcholine receptor protein is certainly an oligomer. Ca^{2+} ATPase in the sarcoplasmic reticulum and glycophorin in red blood cell membranes are presumably in such a configuration. Intrinsic proteins can also be coupled to each other by electrostatic interactions via extrinsic proteins (actin). However, because intrinsic proteins by definition penetrate the phospholipid bilayer, their mobility depends largely on the lipid viscosity. Therefore, variations in the chemical composition of the lipids can influence protein mobility. Another very important parameter is the lipid to protein ratio. It influences not only the average viscosity of the lipid phase but also its ability to solubilize hydrophobic proteins, i.e. to disperse these proteins in the lipid matrix.

In most membranes, the ratio of phospholipids-to-proteins is one-to-one (in weight). The ratio is slightly lower in the case of complex membranes (such as mitochondria or *E. Coli* membranes) where numerous extrinsic proteins are present, but is slightly higher for specialized membranes containing almost one single type of intrinsic protein (discs, sarcoplasmic reticulum, myelin). One exception is stricking. It corresponds to the purple membrane (patches from halobacterium). There the proteins are in fact crystallized in a 2-dimensional array, and lipids obviously do not play the role of solvent but more likely are present only to assure the membrane impermeability. It can be calculated that in this latter system the ratio of phospholipids-to-proteins, in molar ratio, is ten-to-one. This is barely enough to form one single layer of phospholipids between each bacteriorhodopsin molecule.

It is possible to calculate such a molar ratio for the specialized systems containing a single major protein. For example in the disc membranes the ratio of phospholipids to proteins is 70 to 1; in the sarcoplasmic reticulum it is 100:1; in the Torpedo electroplax the number of phospholipids per acetylcholine receptor is about 130:1. These numbers are particularly striking if one realizes that a significant fraction of the total phospholipid pool is required to form just a single layer around each protein. Exact protein sizes would be helpful for these estimates. Unfortunately the tertiary structure of even the extensively studied rhodopsin or Ca^{2+} ATPase molecules are not available (nor is the 3-dimensional structure of any other membrane protein except bacteriorhodopsin). Combinations of various biophysical techniques however provide some information on the diameter of such proteins. Typically, rhodopsin is assumed to have a rod type shape with a diameter of about 30 Å (see the chapter by Chabre, in this book). Ca^{2+} ATPase has a much greater molecular weight than rhodopsin, but it has an asymmetrical shape with certainly a large hydrophilic fraction protruding out into the water. Therefore the hydrophobic core of a single Ca ATPase molecule is probably no more than 35–40 Å large. Using these rough numbers, plus an estimate of the average surface occupancy per phospholipid (about 64 Å^2), it can be found that about 20 phospholipids are required to surround rhodopsin with one double layer, and probably about 30 are needed to achieve the same result with Ca^{2+} ATPase. Consequently about one third of the total phospholipids are in direct contact with the proteins and only 3 or 4 phospholipid layers can be intercalated between two proteins.

Figure 1 represents the relative surface occupancy between lipids and proteins for the disc membranes. A random protein distribution is assumed. It is probably correct for rhodopsin but, as already pointed out, many other membrane proteins can form stable oligomers. In this case the number of lipid layers between groups of proteins can be slightly higher (see fig. 1b). Nevertheless these figures do not suggest an infinite dilution of solute in a solvent. For example, if the perturbation of a protein on the surrounding lipids extends beyond a single layer (say 2 or 3) then it extends practically to all lipids which means that all

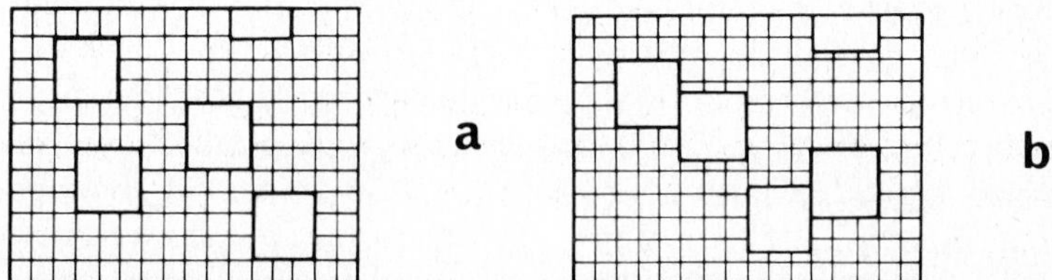

Fig. 1. (a) Schematic representation of the relative surface occupancy between phospholipids and proteins in a typical membrane such as the rod outer segment membranes (ratio of lipids-to-proteins 80 : 1). (b) The same membrane assuming proteins form oligomers. This does not seem to be the case for rhodopsin but is very likely for Ca^{2+} ATPase in the sarcoplasmic reticulum.

proteins interact with each other via the lipids. Eventually if this interaction produces an attraction, proteins will tend to aggregate.

The paradox is then the following: the function of many membrane proteins requires mobility, yet the actual amount of the two-dimensional solvent offered seems to be a minimum requisite for solubility.

Why don't biological systems synthesize larger amounts of lipids?

One explanation, proposed in the literature, is that a layer of tightly bound lipids would be enough to avoid protein aggregation. According to an alternative view, the whole lipid pool would be needed to achieve this function. In fact physical events taking place only at a certain level of lipids (such as protein overall mobility) could be a way to turn off lipid synthesis or trigger on lipid degradation. This latter model could explain the fixed ratio of lipid to protein in membranes.

1.2. Two different views of lipid–protein interactions in membranes

According to the model put forth by Griffith and coworkers in 1973 [1], intrinsic proteins are surrounded by a single layer of immobilized lipids. These lipids act as a molecular spacer preventing protein–protein aggregation. Although it was not ruled out that these lipids could exchange with the bulk lipids, like water molecules in a shell of hydration, it was originally proposed that the time scale of such exchange was several orders of magnitude lower than the exchange rate between 2 phospholipids in a bilayer. One concludes that proteins are accompanied in all their motions by this coat of lipids (see Metcalfe and Warren [2]).

A slightly different view corresponds to a picture whereby immobilized phospholipids are intercalated into the hydrophobic crevices of the protein. Such crevices exist perhaps between two parallel α-helices in the same protein. The lipids trapped can adapt to the protein shape and facilitate its solubility into a phospholipid bilayer.

However, the concept of stable immobilized lipids at the lipid–protein interface, is based on EPR experiments with purified proteins reassociated with low amounts of lipids in order to enhance lipid–protein interactions [1–3]. This makes some of the results questionable when they are extended to physiological conditions. Furthermore the two main proteins studied were cytochrome oxidase and Ca^{2+} ATPase. These two proteins were assumed to form free monomers. But there is now strong evidence against this in the literature. Therefore, immobilized lipids could in fact represent lipids trapped between adjacent proteins rather than in intrinsic surface defects of the proteins or in an immobilized boundary layer.

In the following, we shall present a different view of lipid–protein interactions. According to this model, intrinsic proteins are in fact dissolved in a rather homogeneous lipid solvent. But the solvent is near saturation under physiological conditions. Mild modifications such as the removal of small quantities of lipids, temperature variations or drug intercalation can result in important protein aggregations. We shall not speculate on how useful this mechanism could be for a cell, and why this may explain the regulation of lipid synthesis and breakdown. Rather we shall present experimental data taken essentially from EPR measurements and supporting this latter model. Particular attention will be given to rhodopsin, considered mainly as a model of intrinsic proteins. The results presented were obtained either in discs or in reconstituted systems and suggest that the immobilized lipids detected by EPR reflect the existence of hydrocarbon chains trapped between adjacent proteins rather than a specific halo of phospholipids surrounding rhodopsin molecules. Similar conclusions were brought about by Chapman et al. [4] from spin label experiments with gramicidin A, considered as a model for intrinsic proteins. The main emphasis of the discussion will not be the actual physical state of the lipids at the protein–lipid interface but rather the information gained by the spin label technique about lateral distribution and mobility of proteins. The real question about lipid–protein interactions is indeed to know to what extent lipids can control protein mobility or protein–protein interaction, and hence protein activity.

2. Techniques to determine protein solubility in lipids. Advantage of the spin label method

Biochemical assays have often been used as proof of protein reinsertion in lipids after purification, i.e. of protein solubility in given phospholipids. However it implies the a priori assumption that proteins partially immobilized are enzymatically inactive. This may not always be true.

Electron microscopy is a good technique to follow the lateral distribution of proteins and it should be used systematically as a control. But quantitative measurements by electron microscopy are very difficult. Furthermore a homogeneous distribution of particles does not exclude the possibility of cross linkage between particles.

For the previous reasons, a direct quantitative measurement of the proteins' rotational or lateral mobilities is necessary. This can be achieved in various ways, including photobleaching recovery (see in this book, the chapter by McConnell), transient dichroism and also EPR provided the proteins are labeled.

2.1. Measurement of the protein rotational correlation time τ_c by saturation transfer EPR

Proteins are covalently labeled with a derivative of *N*-ethyl maleimide corresponding to the following formula:

Spin label 1:

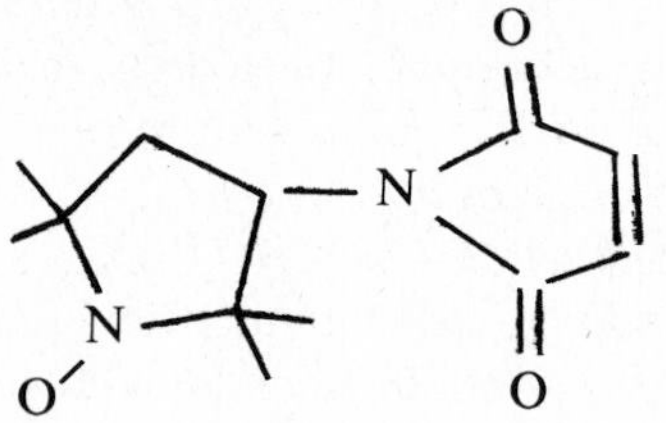

This molecule reacts readily with sulphydryl groups and is usually bound tightly enough to be an indicator of protein mobility. The technique to be used is the saturation transfer electron paramagnetic resonance, a new resonance technique introduced by Thomas et al. in 1976 [5, 6], applicable to rotational correlation times determination in the range 10^{-7} S $< \tau_c < 10^{-3}$ S.

At the present time, this method cannot provide accurate values of τ_c for membrane proteins because anisotropic motions have not been extensively studied by saturation transfer. Another limitation is that, in the case of heterogeneous samples, it is very difficult to sort out the various contributions from what looks like an average saturation transfer spectrum. It should be pointed out that the same problem is raised by most optical techniques particularly when looking at a decline in intensity due to a superposition of exponential terms.

2.2. Conventional EPR *with covalently bound long chain fatty acids as a means of detecting protein aggregation*

The spin labeling method can be employed in a more conventional way to determine the percentage of protein aggregation, provided a special class of amphiphilic spin labels are being used. The following molecules contain a reacting group (maleimide or isocynate) and a long chain spin labeled fatty acid.

Spin label 2: CH_3-CH_2-C-$(CH_2)_{14}$-COO$(CH_2)_2$- N (maleimide ring, O=, =O); O, NO (oxazolidine ring)

Spin label 3: CH_3-CH_2-C-$(CH_2)_{14}$-N = C = O; O, NO (oxazolidine ring)

Owing to the hydrophobic character of the alkyl chain, the reacting group on the spin label is positioned so as to react preferentially with a group on the protein (if available) that will allow the probe near the ω-2 methyl terminal to explore the protein's hydrophobic environment. That the nitroxides are not directly available from the aqueous phase and hence must be buried in the hydrophobic core of the membrane (see fig. 2) can be easily verified afterwards using either Ni^{++} or ascorbate as hydrophilic quenching agents. The full labeling procedure generally

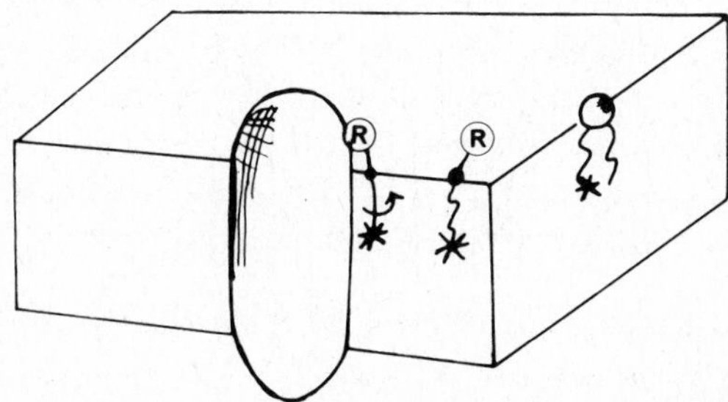

Fig. 2. Amphipatic spin labels are positioned in the membrane with the reacting group R pointing toward the aqueous phase, while the nitroxide (*) is buried in the hydrophobic phase.

requires the purification of the labeled proteins and delipidation followed by reinsertion (by dialysis) into defined lipids. By this procedure all unreacted spin labels are removed.

When spin labels 2 or 3 are used with rodopsin, and the protein reinserted into phosphatidylcholine vesicles, the EPR signal observed at high temperature (37° C) corresponds to a fast motion. This result indicates that the probe is immobilized neither in a hydrophobic cleft of the protein nor by an immobilized lipid annulus. On the contrary, the motion is typical of the motion expected in the bulk lipidic phase at 37° C. Similar probes have been attached to the ADP carrier in mitochondria and the cholinergic receptor protein and have lead to comparable results.

However if aggregation is provoked for example by crosslinking of the proteins by glutaraldehyde, a strong hindrance in the spin label's mobility is observed. Therefore these probes are capable of differentiating between state A (monomer) and state B (oligomer or aggregate) of fig. 3.

Because we are looking at the motion of the alkyl chains, situation A corresponds to a fast motion even in the conventional EPR time scale ($\tau_c \simeq 10^{-9}$ S), whereas situation B is associated with a "completely immobilized signal" ($\tau > 10^{-6}$ S). A typical spectrum corresponding to situation A is shown on fig. 4a, while spectrum c of figure 4 corresponds to the protein aggregate state. One can see that computer addition of the 2 spectra leads to a spectrum (b) revealing its heterogenous character and which cannot be confused with a state of intermediate viscosity. Provided one has an appropriate reference spectrum corresponding to

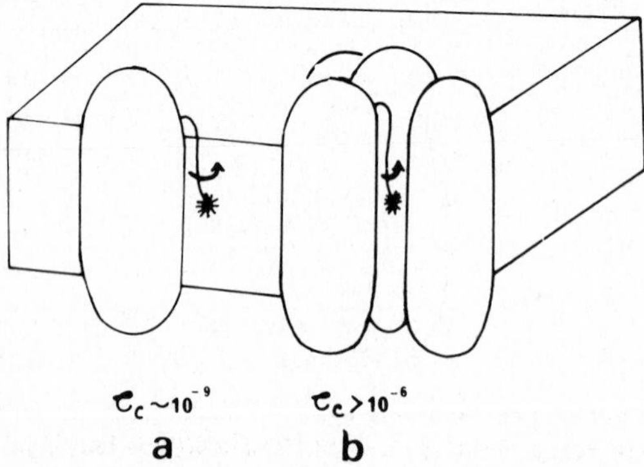

Fig. 3. Covalently bound fatty acid spin labels can differentiate between the monomeric state A and the oligomeric state B.

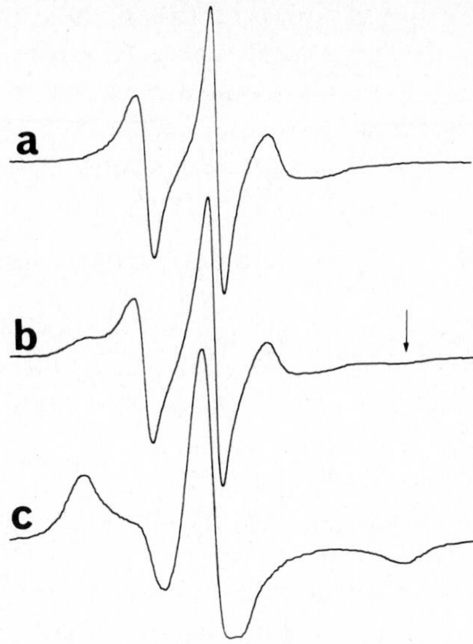

Fig. 4. Spectrum a and spectrum c are obtained respectively with a probe in a fluid environment and a probe strongly immobilized. The addition of a and c gives rise to spectrum b which shows unambiguously its heterogenous character. In spectrum b the immobilized signal represents 50% of the signal.

either the strongly immobilized spectrum or the pure mobile component, it becomes possible by computer subtraction and double intergrations to estimate the amount of label in the various states [7].

Therefore conventional EPR of long chain spin labels covalently bound to proteins provides a way to detect protein–protein contacts in membranes [8]. It does not tell the size of the aggregates but it enables one to estimate the fraction of proteins in such a configuration. On the other hand saturation transfer EPR with tightly bound spin labels gives the average rotational correlation time of the proteins and hence some indication of the size of the aggregates.

Finally if one tries to obtain detailed information on the motion and order parameter of lipid chains in contact with hydrophobic proteins, it is clear that NMR techniques and particularly ^{2}H NMR which provides a direct measure of the order parameters (see the chapter of this book by Seelig), are, in principle, much better techniques than EPR. No perturbing probes are necessary for ^{2}H NMR. However, the sensitivity of ^{2}H NMR is very small. At the present time it is not possible to bind a single deuterated chain to a protein and measure the order parameter of this chain in direct contact with a protein. Only average order parameters can be obtained. Therefore if the exchange rate between lipids is high, the information on the proteins is weak, much weaker than with EPR experiments, designed solely to detect protein–protein interactions, and for which the nitroxide cannot be considered as a perturbing agent.

3. Solubility of rhodopsin in various amphipatic environments

Rhodopsin from bovine retina was labeled with spin label 1, 2, or 3 and the protein's mobility as well as the viscosity of the direct hydrophobic environment was studied under different conditions. The investigated systems were: disc membrane fragments, partially delipidated discs membrane fragments, reconstituted rhodopsin, phosphatidylcholine complexes, and rhodopsin in detergent micelles (octyl-glucoside). These systems were studied at different temperatures and were also modified, either by the use of glutaraldehyde, as bifunctional reagent or by light driven aggregation. Freeze fracture electron microscopy was employed together with EPR in order to determine the state of aggregation.

Most of the results have been or will be published in more detail elsewhere [9–13]. We shall only summarize them here in order to be able to reach a general understanding of the system throughout these experiments.

3.1. Rhodopsin rotational diffusion in phospholipids

Cone was the first to show by means of optical techniques that rhodopsin has a very high rotational diffusion constant in the disc membrane [14]. By saturation transfer EPR with spin labeled rhodopsin, we were able to confirm Cone's results. A rotational correlation time of 20×10^{-6}s was obtained at 20° C in bovine retina. The activation energy is 9 Kcal/mole. It is not certain that this temperature dependence simply reflects the viscosity variation of the lipids. It has been demonstrated [15] that domains of rigid lipids appear below 20° C in bovine disc membranes. Therefore proteins could be partially segregated and protein–protein aggregation could be responsible for changes of τ_c. In fact as soon as lipids are removed from the discs (using phospholipase A_2 and bovine serum albumine), τ_c increases dramatically. This latter result is remarkable because it shows that all the endogenous lipids are required to assure protein mobility. If the system had, under physiological conditions, an excess of lipids, one would not expect to observe a change in protein mobility following the removal of only 20% of the lipids.

In order to reach a better understanding of the dependence of rhodopsin mobility on the temperature and lipid to protein ratio, we have reassociated purified rhodopsin with well-defined phospholipids. The protein's mobility in the recombinants was determined by saturation transfer EPR, while freeze fracture electron microscopy gave some indication of protein lateral distribution. Figure 5 shows the temperature dependence of rhodopsin rotational correlation time in different phosphatidylcholine environments (lipid-to-protein ratio 120:1, mol-to-mol). Note that dipalmitoylphosphatidylcholine (DPPC) undergoes a phase transition at 40° C, dimiristoylphosphatidylcholine (DMPC) at 23° C, while the transition temperature of dioleylphosphatidylcholine (DOPC) is below 0° C. As expected, in all cases τ_c decreases when temperature increases, but no obvious discontinuity appears at the phospholipid transition temperature. By contrast a spin labeled phospholipid gives rise to sharp spectral discontinuities at the phospholipid transition temperature when introduced in the same type of rhodopsin/rhodopsin/lipid recombinant. Thus the protein mobility does not solely reflect the phospholipid viscosity. Freeze-fracture electron micrographs of the samples helps explain the EPR results. Figure 6 shows that the particle distribution is quite different when the sample is quenched from above or below the phase transition temperature (T_c). This phenomenon is general with rhodopsin as demonstrated by Chen and Hubbell [16] who have studied by freeze fracture many rhodopsin–phospholipid recombinants: lipid crystallization creates protein depleted domains. Interestingly enough, these domains systematically appear above T_c, indicating that the phase separation starts before lipid

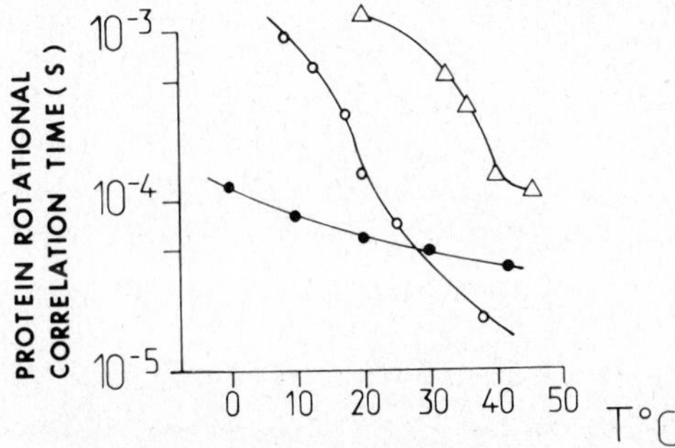

Fig. 5. Rotational correlation times for spin labeled rhodopsin incorporated into various phospholipid vesicles. The saturation transfer EPR technique is employed. Curves correspond respectively to (○) DMPC; (Δ) DPPC; (●) DOPC.

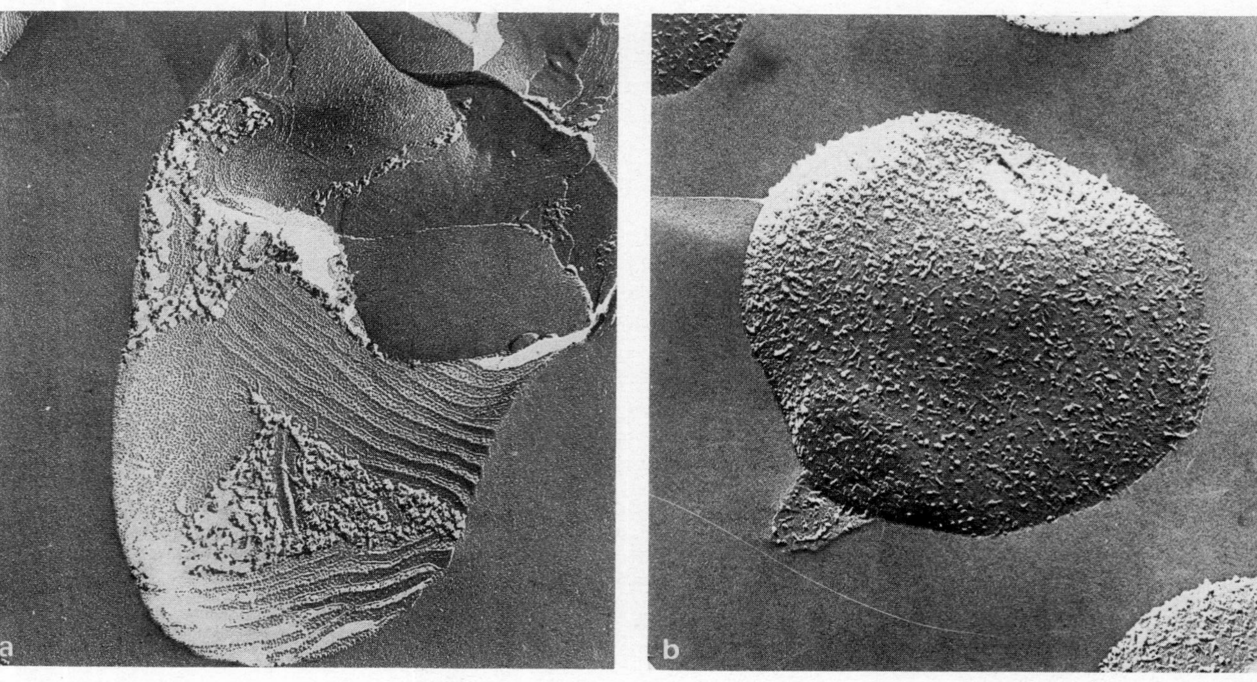

Fig. 6. Freeze-fracture electron micrographs of rhodopsin. DMPC recombinants: (a) frozen from 4° C in the dark and (b) frozen from 4° C after bleaching at 40° C. If the sample is frozen in the dark from 40° it resembles (b). Magnification respectively 35 000 and 41 000.

crystallization. Also the total protein depleted area is not at a maximum just below T_c but rather 10 or 15 degrees below T_c. A comparable phenomenon takes place in the case of a three-dimensional solvent-solute mixture, for example the solute precipitates usually before the freezing point of the solvent.

Finally, considering that aggregation must be a probable event in the protein-rich regions, we conclude that the temperature dependence of the rotational correlation time τ_c (fig. 5) must be interpreted as reflecting progressive protein segregation together with the lipid viscosity variation.

3.2. Viscosity of rhodopsin boundary layer

In the preceding subsection we have interpreted the results concerning rhodopsin's ability to rotate in terms of lipid–protein segregation. This interpretation is suggested by consideration of both freeze-fracture electron-micrographs and saturation transfer spectra. The use of long chain spin labeled fatty acid chains covalently bound to rhodopsin, together with conventional EPR, provides an independent way to quantitatively evaluate the fraction of aggregated proteins.

Figure 7 displays a typical set of spectra corresponding to spin label 2, covalently attached to rhodopsin in lecithin/rhodopsin vesicles (lipid-

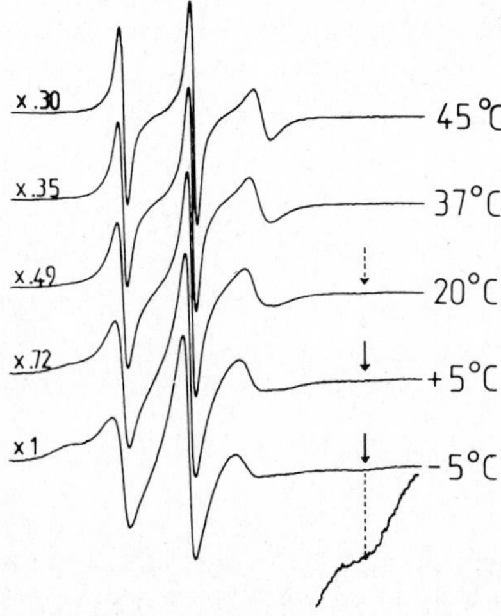

Fig. 7. EPR spectra of spin label 2 covalently bound to rhodopsin in rhodopsin-egg-lecithin vesicles. Lipid-to-protein ratio 500/1.

to-protein ratio: 500/1, mol-to-mol). The probe is buried in the hydrophobic core of the membrane but must be at the lipid–protein interface. The remarkable fact already mentioned in section 2, is that at 37° C (or above) the spectrum contains only 3 relatively narrow peaks which must be associated with a fast motion of the probe, in spite of its vicinity to the protein. Therefore this type of probe sees essentially a fluid environment at the boundary layer of rhodopsin under physiological conditions. This excludes the idea of a complete annulus of fluid lipids protecting rhodopsin molecules.

When the temperature is reduced the spectra obtained with spin label 2 show a second component corresponding to immobilized probes. At −5° C it represents about 50% of the signal. The spectral decomposition into two components (one "strongly immobilized" and one "weakly immobilized") was carried out from spectra obtained with different types of rhodopsin/lipid vesicles and under different physical conditions. Varying the lipid-protein ratio, the temperature and the chemical nature of the host lipids allowed us to draw diagrams corresponding to the fraction of immobilized signal detectable under the given conditions. Figure 8a shows the results gathered with rhodopsin-egg lecithin while fig. 8b corresponds to the data obtained with rhodopsin-DMPC. We have collected more data using DPPC or DOPC. The native disc membrane fragments and reconstituted systems with the endogeneous lipids have also been analyzed. Technical difficulties arise with the very unsaturated endrogeneous lipids, in particular spin reduction takes place. But the results compare with those obtained with egg lecithin or DOPC. Namely a substantial fraction of immobilized component exists at a low temperature (≃0° C), and disappears around 37° C.

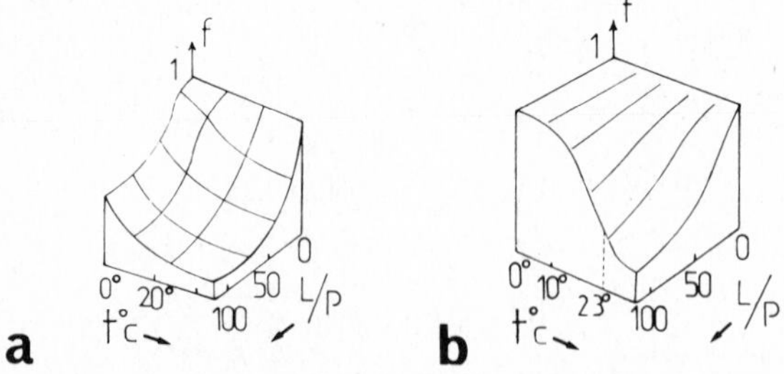

Fig. 8. These diagrams represent the fraction of immobilized signal detected near rhodopsin with covalently bound long chain spin labeled fatty acids. In fact they reveal the percentage of protein aggregation. Hence they correspond to solubility diagrams. In (a), host lipids are egg lecithin; in (b), DMPC.

In light of section 2's discussion, the simplest interpretation is to associate the immobilized signal with lipid chains trapped between adjacent proteins. Therefore fig. 8 diagrams would correspond to the fractions of aggregated proteins, i.e. fig. 8 represents solubility diagrams of rhodopsin in phosphatidylcholine.

3.3. Effect of light

In their 1973 article, Chen and Hubbell mentioned an interesting feature of the freeze-fracture micrographs obtained with rhodopsin DMPC recombinants. Namely if the samples are bleached at a temperature above T_c, and afterwards quenched from a low temperature ($T<T_c$), no protein segregation takes place. The electron micrographs are in fact identical to those obtained after glutaraldehyde fixation at a high temperature. As for the dynamical properties of rhodopsin observed by saturation transfer EPR with spin label 1, we have found that bleaching increases the rotational correlation time τ_c by about an order of magnitude. If a long chain spin label is being used (spin label 2 or 3), during the illumination a strongly immobilized component appears, which can represent up to 40 or 50% of the signal at 37° C (fig. 9). This strongly immobilized component is stable and cannot be reversed. Recording the EPR spectra at all temperatures after a prolonged

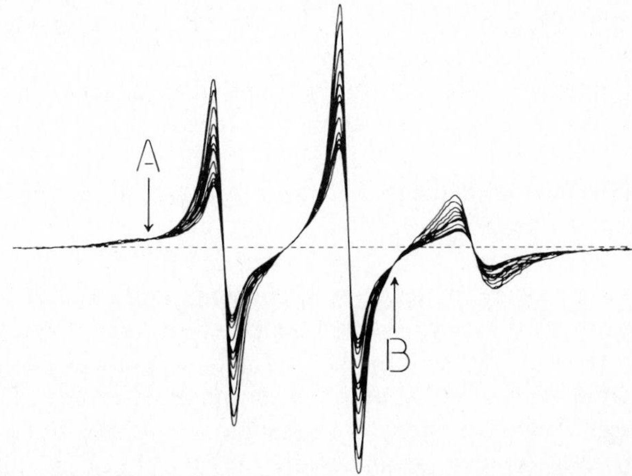

Fig. 9. Effect of light on the EPR spectrum of rhodopsin labeled with spin label 2, in rhodopsin-egg-lecithin vesicles. Temperature 37° C. Each scan represents 2 min. A and B are isosbestic points. Illumination produces an increase in the immobilized component.

illumination shows that a constant immobilized fraction is now superimposed to the temperature dependent immobilized signal.

The time scale at which the immobilization takes place after bleaching (about half an hour at 37° C) indicates that the observed phenomenon is probably not physiologically relevant. Nevertheless it is important to understand.

Our interpretation is that bleached rhodopsin molecules form oligomers stabilized by disulfide bridges. Indeed it is known that illumination of rhodopsin exposes new SH groups, furthermore, if the bleaching is carried out in the presence of dithiothreitol, which prevents disulfure bridges formation, protein depleted regions are still observed at low temperatures by freeze-fracture electron microscopy [16].

3.4. *Rhodopsin in detergent micelles*

When spin labeled rhodopsin molecules are in detergent micelles (octyl glucoside), no immobilized signal can be detected with spin label 2 (or 3) even at very low temperatures (0° C). If the immobilized signals seen in membranes were to be attributed to a conformational change of rhodopsin, one would expect to observe this phenomenon in a detergent which preserves the protein integrity. This negative result reinforces the idea that the immobilized component reflects rhodopsin solubility properties in phospholipids, which of course are not identical to the solubility properties in detergents. Finally, bleaching rhodopsin in detergents generates in a few minutes at 37° C an immobilized component, while aggregates of macroscopic size are progressively seen.

So, once more, with long chain spin labeled fatty acids the immobilized component is associated with protein–protein interactions.

3.5. *Conclusions on rhodopsin solubility properties in phospholipids and possible biological importance*

The previous observations lead us to conclude that, in the disc membranes, rhodopsin at a physiological temperature forms monomers free to diffuse without being surrounded by a halo of immobilized lipids. But if lipid to protein ratio, temperature or phospholipid composition (chain length, degree of unsaturation) are modified the probability of protein aggregation can increase dramatically or, to phrase it differently, rhodopsin solubility can decrease dramatically.

The general conclusion is that with unsaturated lipids forming bilayers of about 40 Å thickness, rhodopsin is totally solubilized around

37° C provided the ratio of lipid-to-proteins is about 80:1, (see fig. 8) which is precisely the physiological ratio of lipids-to-proteins in disc membranes.

Thus it is reasonable to conclude that the biological system is adapted in such a manner so as to permit the mobility of a maximum of proteins in a minimum of phospholipids. The biological function of rhodopsin is to be a light antenna which must carry its information rapidly to a different and extrinsic protein present in minute amounts in the discs (GTPase). This operation requires a high mobility which is favored by a high ratio of lipids to proteins. On the other hand, an excess of lipids would dilute the rhodopsin molecules and therefore decrease the efficiency of light capture. The system is probably optimized with all the lipids involved in the solubilizing function. The very fact that phospholipids extracted from bovine disc retina do not form bilayers at 37° C (but a hexagonal phase) shows the strength of the lipid–protein interaction, the function of which is to guarantee a fluid environment to the proteins rather than to form a protecting rigid annulus.

4. Other membrane proteins. The existence of oligomers. About the immobilized boundary layer

4.1. The ADP *carrier*

The direct lipid environment of other membrane proteins has been investigated with specific spin labels. For example in order to probe the hydrophobic environment of the ADP carrier in mitochondria, we have used long chain acyl CoA molecules [17] or long chain acyl atractylosides [18]. Those molecules have a high affinity towards the ADP carrier for which they function as specific inhibitors. In both instances we found that the probe, when near the ω-2 terminal of the alkyl chain, experiences a high mobility very close to – if not identical to – the mobility of a nitroxide bound to a phospholipid diffusing freely.

4.2. The acetylcholine receptor protein

It was found that a long chain spin labeled acyl choline [19]

spin label: 4 CH_3-CH_2-C-$(CH_2)_{14}$-COO$(CH)_2$+$(CH_3)_3$,
N

O N-O

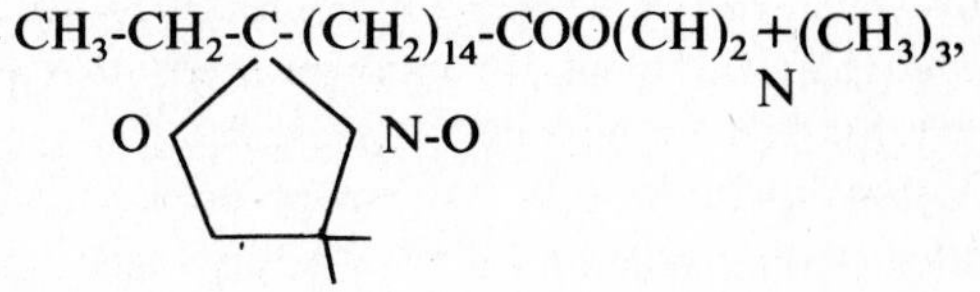

gives rise to a relatively mobile spectrum in Torpedo membrane fragments, although the molecule has a high affinity towards the cholinergic receptor protein. This shows that fluid lipids exist in the direct vicinity of this intrinsic protein, the particular property of which is to be completely immobilized at the time scale of saturation transfer [20]. This result suggests that in this particular case the proteins' immobilization is not due to a reduced lipid phase, generating protein aggregation, but more directly to protein–protein interactions. The mere addition of lipids to the cholinergic receptor membranes, for example by fusion, produces patches of lipids but no protein dilution nor any change in protein rotational correlation time. On the other hand, if lipid addition is preceded by a temporary pH increase, whose effect is to release a 43 000 Dalton extrinsic protein, the receptor protein becomes mobile as seen by saturation transfer [21]. At the same time electron microscopy indicates a more random protein distribution: the close packing is disrupted (fig. 10). This phenomenon is reversible. So protein–protein interactions are primarily responsible for post-synaptic stabilization.

Another interesting result on Torpedo membranes was pointed out first by Marsh and Barrantes [22]. They showed that a spin-labeled fatty acid gives rise to a spectrum containing an immobilized component, which seems to correspond to a constant fraction of labels, i.e. is temperature independent. However it was shown later [23] that a spin labeled phospholipid introcuded by means of a phosphatidyl choline exchange protein does not give rise to the same component, indicating that a specific binding of the fatty acid takes place. This is certainly correlated to the fact that spin labeled fatty acids behave as local anesthetics [24]. Thus one should be careful in concluding about boundary layer viscosity with probes that can be fixed in rather particular sites of a protein [25].

4.3. *Cytochrome oxidase*

An extensive work has been carried out by several groups mentioned before on cytochrome oxidase–lipid interactions using spin labeled fatty acids or phospholipids. However these authors did not verify the rotational mobility of cytochrome oxidase recombinants, i.e. its state of aggregation. Swanson et al. [26] have recently studied purified cytochrome oxidase in detergents or incorporated into liposomes. Spin label 2 was used to detect the lipid hydrocarbon region adjacent to the protein by conventional EPR. A strong immobilized component was found both in detergent micelles and in reconstituted membranes.

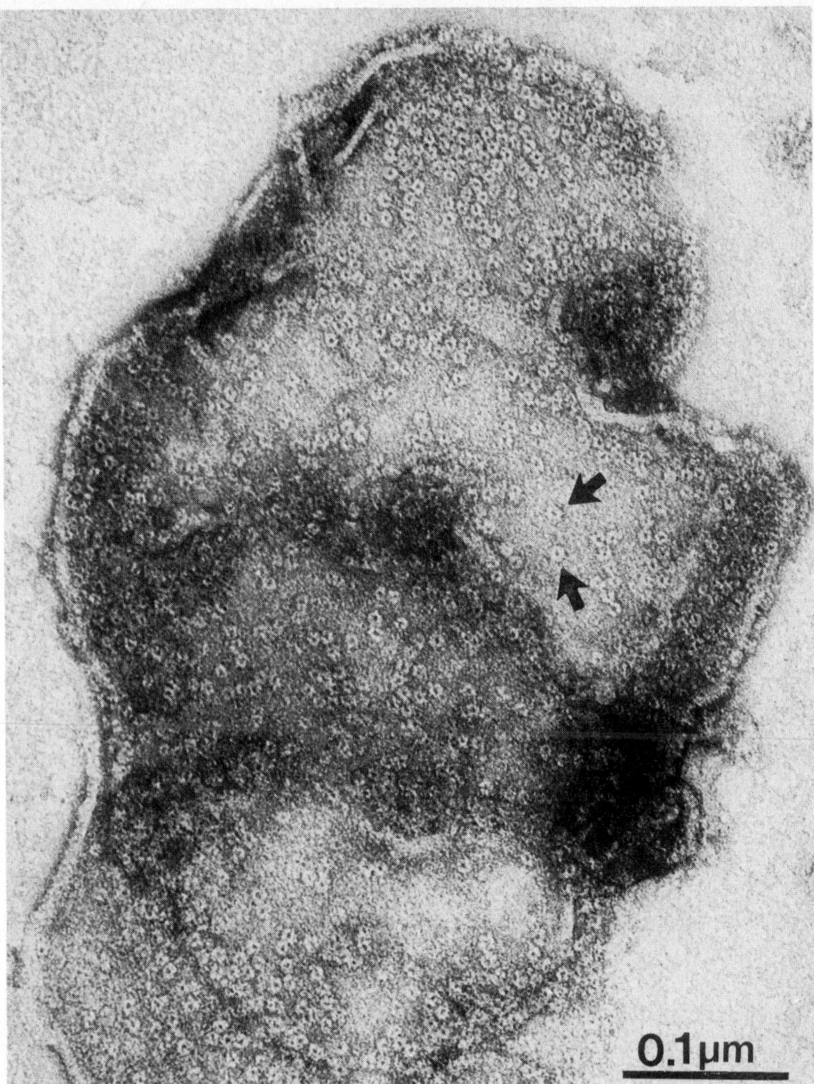

Fig. 10. Typical distribution of the cholinergic receptor proteins observed after treatment of the torpedo membrane at high pH, followed by fusion with lecithin. This figure is to be compared with the control electron micrographs of Torpedo membranes shown in the chapter by Popot in this book.

However, at the same time, saturation transfer with spin label 1 indicated the absence of protein-rotational mobility, suggesting an aggregated form. These authors then modified the cytochrome oxidase purification and reconstitution procedure and obtained spectacular modification both with spin label 1 and 2. Namely the overall protein's mobility and the boundary layer fluidity increased giving results very comparable to that of rhodopsin.

4.4. Ca^{2+} ATPase

In the case of Ca^{2+} ATPase there is evidence from fluorescence energy transfer measurements [27] that the protein also forms oligomers in reconstituted systems, and this could be the normal situation in the sarcoplasmic reticulum. Therefore spin labeled lipids could be trapped between 2 monomers. Recently in order to investigate sarcoplasmic reticulum we have used spin label 2 and the following nitrene derivative [28]

spin label 5: CH_3-CH_2-C-$(CH_2)_{14}$-COO$(CH_2)_2$-NH-$C_6H_3(NO_2)$-N_3 (oxazolidine ring O, N-O on the C)

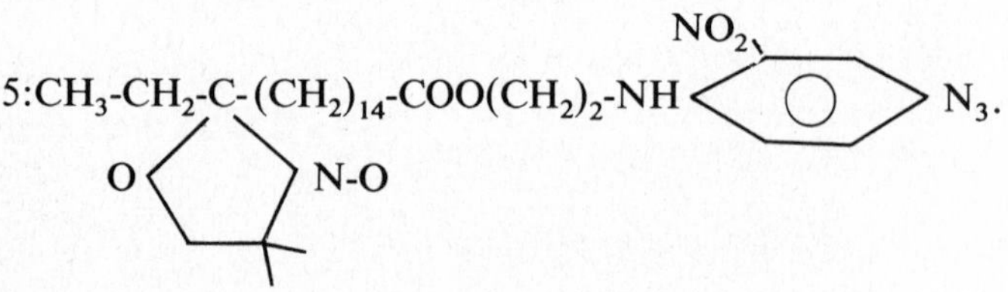

It is remarkable that both labels after incubation give rise at all temperatures to two components: an immobilized and a mobile component. However the immobilized component decreases if small amount of detergent is added. The most likely interpretation is that the immobilized component reflects the proteins oligomeric state that can be disrupted by detergent present at a non-solubilizing level.

4.5. About the "immobilized boundary layer" model

It appears that 5 different intrinsic proteins to which a spin labeled fatty acid is linked, can give rise to an EPR spectrum indicative of a high mobility. But all these proteins give rise, with the same spin labels, to an immobilized component under conditions where the probability of protein aggregation (or oligomerisation) is high, particularly at artificially low lipid to protein ratios. Thus we suggest that such proteins are not normally surrounded by an annulus of immobilized lipid chains.

The immobilized component whenever seen by EPR probably reveals protein-protein interactions, or, although this is presently unproven, the existence of specific hydrophobic crevices in the proteins.

Stable and functional oligomers may very well be rather common among membrane proteins, as they are among soluble proteins. Oligomers in solution, ribosomes for example, contain intercalated water molecules, similarly membrane proteins may contain a limited number of intercalated phospholipids, the dynamical properties of which must be very different from those of the lipids at the interface between intrinsic proteins and a bilayer.

Obviously the number of intercalated lipids must be smaller than the number of lipids required to surround the proteins. In the literature, the calculated fraction of immobilized lipids observed with cytochrome oxidase and Ca^{2+} ATPase accounts for a complete annulus. However, these estimates are based on the unverified assumption that a fatty acid (or phospholipid) spin label partitions equally well between the fluid membrane phase and what is assumed as an immobilized phase surrounding the proteins. Furthermore these calculations are usually extrapolated from observations made at low lipid concentration (i.e. under conditions of high probability of aggregation).

Finally ^2H NMR did not permit detection of a significant population of heterogenous lipids, when all phospholipids are deuterated, with either cytochrome oxidase [29, 30], Ca^{2+} ATPase [31], or rhodopsin [32]. Of course it can be argued that too rapid an exchange takes place for the time scale of NMR. But at least, it certainly does not reinforce the concept of an immobilized layer around intrinsic proteins.

So in conclusion, it appears that the model of an immobilized boundary layer surrounding intrinsic proteins, is far from being demonstrated.

5. General conclusion and prospective

As a general conclusion we think that lipid–protein interactions in membranes should be considered in terms of solvent–solute interactions. The biological systems seem to be optimized to provide solubility to monomers or limited oligomers with economy of lipids. This implies that all lipids are engaged in this task. Thus artificial modifications of temperature, lipid to protein ratio, lipid composition, ions, etc. can lead to spectacular modifications of the protein overall mobility and lateral distribution. As a working hypothesis it can be thought that these effects are means of physiological regulations in membranes. Similarly it is reasonable to assume that the complicated mixtures of phospholipids found in biological membranes are aimed at fulfiling maximum solubility of proteins with a minimum of solvent: mixtures of solvents are always more efficient in solubilizing any molecule in a three-dimensional milieu. This may mean that specific head groups are associated with specific proteins of regions of proteins. The important challenge is now to understand the role of specific head groups in given membranes.

Acknowledgements

The work discussed in this chapter is a collaborative work. J. Davoust is particularly responsible for most of the rhodopsin data. J. Olive and J. Cartaud did the electron microscopy. Other people whose work has been mentioned are J. Anderson, A. Baroin, A. Bienvenüe, E. Favre, P. Fellmann, A. Rousselet and B. Schoot. The author is also indebted to Drs. Swanson, Quintanilha, Thomas, Seelig and Bloom for making some data available before publication. This investigation was supported by research grants from the "Delegation à la Recherche Scientifique et Technique", the "Centre National de la Recherche Scientifique" and the "Université Paris VII".

References and notes

[1] P. C. Jost, O. H. Griffith, R. A. Capaldi and G. Van der Kooi, Proc. Natl. Acad. Sci. USA 70 (1973) 480.
[2] J. C. Metcalfe and G. B. Warren, in: Cell Biology, eds. Brinkley and K. Porter (The Rockefeller University Press, Boston, 1976) pp. 15–23.
[3] D. Marsh, A. Watts, W. Maschka and P. F. Knowles, Biochem. Biophys. Res. Comm. 81 (1978) 397.
[4] D. Chapman, B. A. Cornell, A. W. Eliasz and A. Perry, J. Mol. Biol. 113 (1977) 517.
[5] D. D. Thomas, L. R. Dalton and J. S. Hyde, J. Chem. Phys. 65 (1976) 3006.
[6] L. R. Dalton and J. S. Hyde, in: Spin Labeling, vol. II, ed. L. Berliner (Academic Press, 1979).
[7] It has been pointed out many times by P. Jost, see in Spin Labeling, vol. I, ed. L. Berliner (Academic Press, 1976) pp. 268, that the broad component is weak and often underestimated.
[8] This method is only applicable if one can show that the probe is not trapped in a crevice of a monomer.
[9] A. Baroin, A. Bienvenüe, and P. F. Devaux Biochemistry 18 (1979) 1151.
[10] E. Favre, A. Baroin, A. Bienvenüe and P. F. Devaux, Biochemistry 18 (1979) 1165.
[11] J. Davoust, B. Schoot and P. F. Devaux, Proc. Natl. Acad. Sci. (USA) 76 (1979) 2755.
[12] J. Davoust, A. Bienvenüe, P. Fellmann and P. F. Devaux, Biochem. Biophys. Acta 596 (1980) 28.
[13] J. Davoust, J. Olive, P. F. Devaux and A. Bienvenüe (1980) submitted.
[14] R. A. Cone, Nature 236 (1972) 39.
[15] M. Chabre, Biochem. Biophys. Acta 382 (1975) 322.
[16] Y. S. Chen and W. L. Hubbell, Exp. Eye Res. 17 (1973) 517.

[17] P. F. Devaux, A. Bienvenüe, G. Lauquin, A. Brisson, P. M. Vignais and P. V. Vignais, Biochemistry 14 (1975) 1272.
[18] G. J. Lauquin, P. F. Devaux, A. Bienvenüe, G. Villiers and P. V. Vignais, Biochemistry 16 (1977) 1202.
[19] A. Bienvenüe, A. Rousselet, G. Kato and P. F. Devaux, Biochemistry 16 (1977) 841.
[20] A. Rousselet and P. F. Devaux, Biochem. Biophys. Res. Comm. 78 (1977) 448.
[21] A. Rousselet, J. Cartaud and P. F. Devaux, C. R. Acad. Sci. Paris 289 (1979) 461.
[22] D. Marsh and F. J. Barrantes, Proc. Natl. Acad. Sci. (USA) 75 (1978) 4329.
[23] A. Rousselet, P. F. Devaux and K. W. Wirtz, Biochem. Biophys. Res. Comm. 90 (1979) 871.
[24] A. Brisson, P. F. Devaux and J. P. Changeux, C. R. Acad. Sci. Paris 280 (1975) 2153.
[25] This remark is valid for an EPR signal corresponding either to an immobilized or a mobile component. A mobile signal does not guarantee that the whole protein environment is fluid.
[26] M. Swanson, A. Quintanilha and D. D. Thomas, J. Biol. Chem. (1980) in press.
[27] J. M. Vanderkooi, A. Ierokomas, H. Nakamura and P. A. Martinosi, Biochemistry 16 (1977) 1262.
[28] P. Fellmann, J. Anderson, P. F. Devaux, M. le Maire and A. Bienvenüe, Biochem. Biophys. Res. Comm. (1980) in press.
[29] A. Seelig and J. Seelig, Hoppe Seyler's Z. Physiol. Chem. 359 (1978) 1747.
[30] E. Oldfield, R. Gilmore, M. Glaser, H. S. Gutowsky, J. C. Hshung, S. Y. Kung, E. King Tsoo, M. Meadows and D. Rice, Proc. Natl. Acad. Sci. USA 75 (1978) 4657.
[31] D. M. Rice, M. O. Meadows, A. O. Scheinmann, F. M. Goni, J. Gomez-Fernandez, M. A. Moscarello, D. Chapman and E. Oldfield, Biochemistry 18 (1979) 5893.
[32] A. Bienvenüe, M. Bloom, J. H. Davis and P. F. Devaux (1980) submitted.

COURSE 2

GLYCOPROTEINS IN MEMBRANES

Nathan SHARON

Department of Biophysics,
The Weizmann Institute of Science,
Rehovoth,
Israel

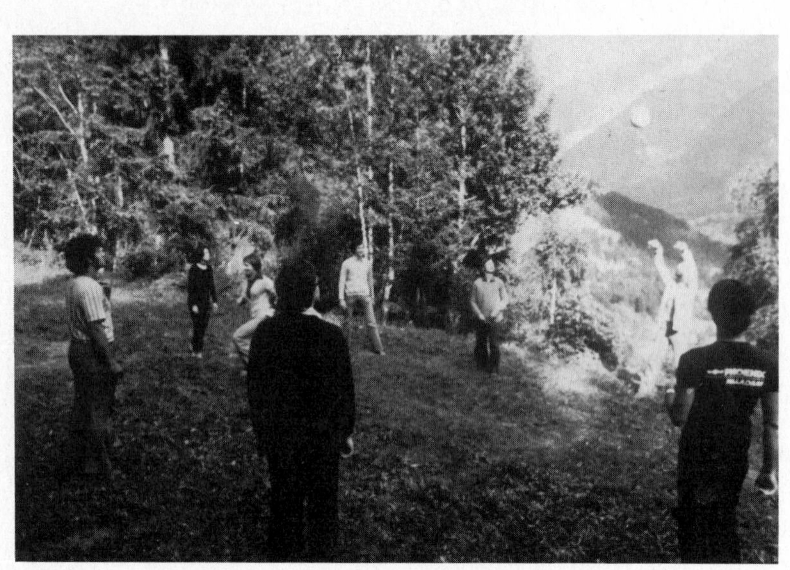

Contents

R. Balian et al., eds.
Les Houches, Session XXXIII, 1979 – Membranes et Communication Intercellulaire / Membranes and Intercellular Communication

1. Introduction

Understanding of cell membrane function requires a detailed knowledge of the biosynthesis, structure and organization of its individual constituents, as well as of the interactions between these constituents. In its simplest form a biological membrane can be viewed as a mosaic of integral membrane proteins and glycoproteins (as well as glycolipids) embedded in a fluid lipid bilayer, with peripheral loosely bound proteins attached at both the inner and outer membrane surfaces and with glycoproteins only at the latter (fig. 1). Quantitatively, proteins and lipids are the major constituents – at least 90% of the weight of most cell membranes. In the past, only these membrane constituents were believed to be of biological importance. However, with the increased awareness that carbohydrates play a crucial part in membrane function, the situation has changed markedly during the last decade. Carbohydrates comprise only a small portion by weight of the surface membrane of animal cells. For example, the human erythrocyte membrane, which is probably the best characterized cell membrane, contains 52% protein, 40% lipid, and just 8% carbohydrate. In this membrane, as in others investigated, all of the carbohydrate is attached either to proteins or lipids, forming glycoproteins and glycolipids respectively.

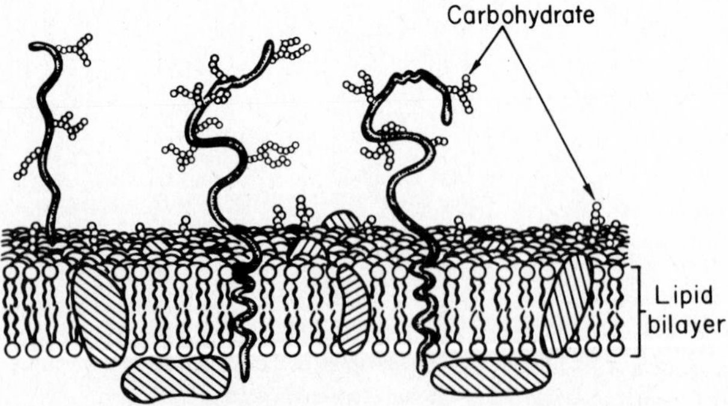

Fig. 1. Schematic representation of a cell surface membrane.

The oligosaccharide units of these glycoproteins and glycolipids are structurally diverse, and are asymmetrically distributed in the membrane, being found only on the outer surface of the cell.

It appears that virtually all cells come in a sugar coating, which imparts hydrophilic properties to the cells, since oligosaccharides are much less hydrophobic than lipids or proteins. Both their location and their structural diversity make the surface oligosaccharides admirably suited to act as specificity markers as well as sensitive antennae by which the cell may probe its environment to detect signals that may be transmitted to its interior.

Indeed, surface sugars have been shown to act as receptors for a variety of ligands, such as antibodies, hormones, toxins, lectins, and interferons. If one is allowed to generalize from the limited information thus far available, it would appear that most, and perhaps all, integral membrane glycoproteins span the entire width of the lipid bilayer. Thus, conformational changes in surface receptors or lateral interactions among them, caused by binding of ligands to the surface sugars, may create perturbations in the cell as a whole. Speaking metaphorically, shaking glycopeptide "trees" on the outer surface will also move their "roots", and thus be transmitted into the interior of the cell – to the cytoskeletal elements, the microtubules and microfilaments, to the cytoplasm and cell nucleus.

Cell surface sugars have been implicated in many other cell functions, such as intercellular communication, the control of cell growth, differentiation and malignancy, as well as in host-parasite relationship. It has also been suggested that cell surface sugars control the clearance of old erythrocytes from the circulatory system and the homing of lymphocytes to specific organs in the body.

There is some evidence for the presence of sugar in intracellular membranes such as those of the mitochondria and the nucleus, although in lower concentrations than in the plasma membrane. Studies of sugars in intracellular membranes have, however, been greatly hampered by cross contamination between different subcellular fractions.

Sugars are well suited to serve as specificity determinants, since a small number of monosaccharides can be linked in many combinations to form a large number of different oligosaccharides. A typical monosaccharide, such as glucose in its commonly occurring six membered pyranose ring form (fig. 2), has five hydroxyl groups, each of which can serve for the attachment of a second monosaccharide molecule. Moreover, the glycosidic linkage, at carbon-1, may be of different anomery,

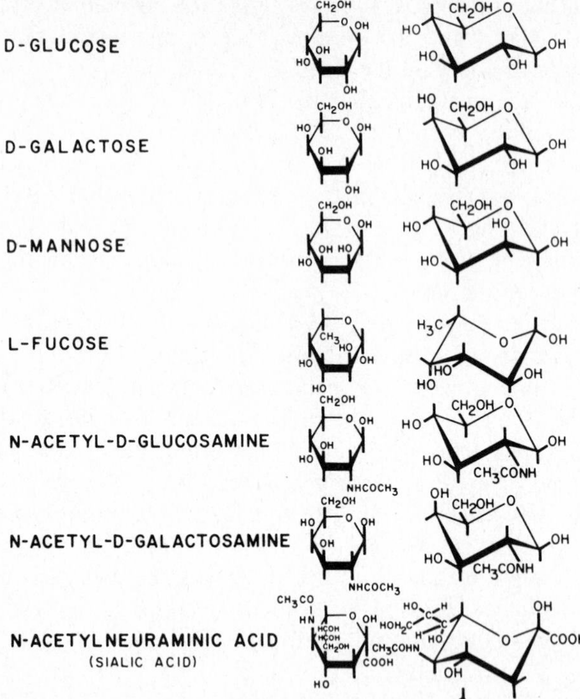

Fig. 2. Monosaccharide constituents of membrane glycoproteins and of intermediates of their biosynthesis. In the center column, the formulas of the sugars are drawn in their normal pyranose forms, according to the Haworth projection, and in the right column in their stable chair conformation.

either α or β (fig. 3). Two molecules of glucose or galactose can therefore form 11 disaccharides, and three of the same sugar – 176 trisaccharides. If the monosaccharides are of three kinds, e.g. glucose, galactose, and mannose, the number of isomeric trisaccharides that they can form is 1056. With longer oligosaccharides, not only linear structures can be formed, but also branched ones which greatly increase the potential number of isomers (fig. 3).

The information potential of sugars is thus much larger than that of amino acids, since three molecules of a neutral amino acid can form only one tripeptide, and three different amino acids – six tripeptides. As we shall see, the oligosaccharide units of membrane glycoproteins that have been characterized to date, contain between 4 and 15 sugar

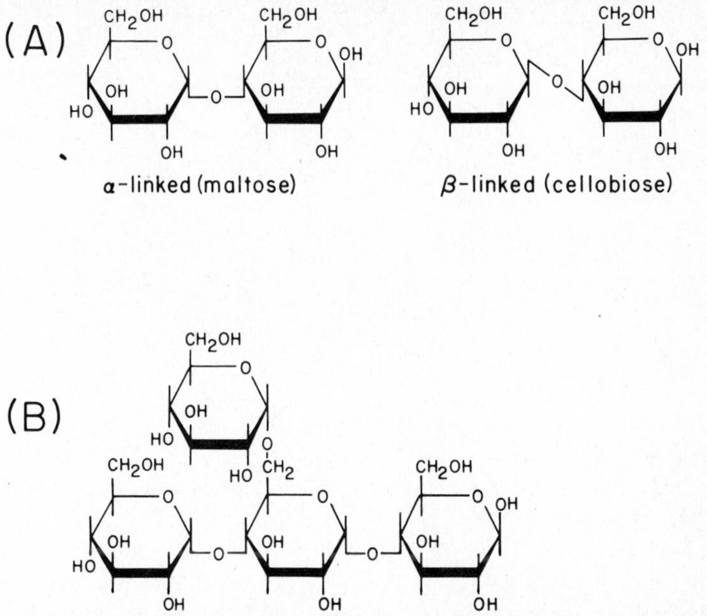

(A)

α-linked (maltose)

β-linked (cellobiose)

(B)

Fig. 3. Two ways of generating oligosaccharide diversity not available to proteins or nucleic acids. (A) α- or β-anomeric linkages; (B) branching. [Modified from Immunology, by L. E. Hood, I. L. Weissman and W. B. Wood, (Benjamin/Cummings Publishing Co., Calif., 1978) p. 314.]

residues, and are made up of only 3–5 different monosaccharide constituents. The number of arrangements possible of the larger oligosaccharides is astronomic indeed. Clamp, of the University of Bristol, has calculated the number of possible structures of an oligosaccharide with 12 residues consisting of 5 different monosaccharides. These 12 residues could, in theory, be linked together in more than 10^{24} different ways. However, the oligosaccharide structures encountered in glycoproteins, whether soluble or membrane bound, are known to be of restricted types. Consequently, the complete potential for structural diversity may not be utilized in nature, and it appears that there are certain limitations which drastically reduce the number of structures actually formed by living organisms.

These lectures will deal with membrane glycoproteins, with an emphasis on the structure, biosynthesis, and functions of their carbohydrate moieties. It is important to bear in mind that many of the

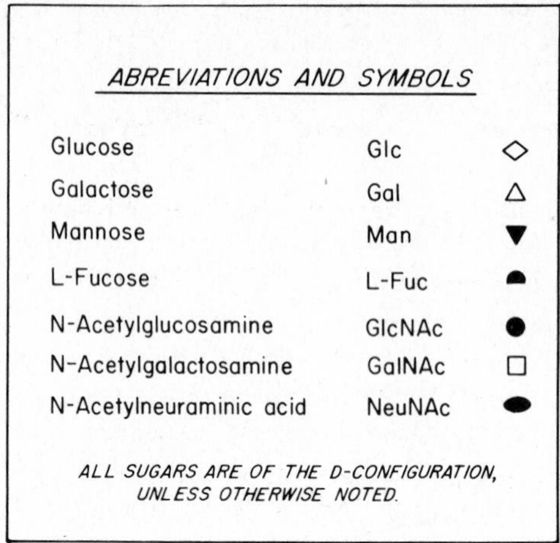

ABREVIATIONS AND SYMBOLS
Glucose
Glc
Galactose
Gal
Mannose
Man
L-Fucose
L-Fuc
N-Acetylglucosamine
GlcNAc
N-Acetylgalactosamine
GalNAc
N-Acetylneuraminic acid
NeuNAc
ALL SUGARS ARE OF THE D-CONFIGURATION,
UNLESS OTHERWISE NOTED.

Fig. 4. Common abbreviation used for denoting monosaccharides (center column) and symbols used in these lectures.

carbohydrate moieties of membrane glycolipids are structurally identical with those of membrane glycoproteins and that their biosynthesis may in part be carried out by the same enzymes. It seems likely, therefore, that their functions may occasionally be identical.

Proteoglycans (e.g. heparan sulfate, and the chondroitin sulfates that are prominent connective tissue constituents) are also ubiquitous, though minor, constituents of the cell coat of mammalian cells in culture. They are apparently not intrinsic membrane components, and will not be discussed here.

A list of abbreviations and symbols to be used is given in fig. 4.

1.1. What is a glycoprotein?

The covalent attachment of a carbohydrate to a polypeptide forms a glycoprotein. The number of attachment sites may vary between one, as found in glycoproteins such as chicken ovalbumin or bovine pancreatic ribonuclease, to over two hundred as in ovine submaxillary mucin. Oligosaccharides consisting of up to 20 monosaccharides, mostly in branched sequences, are common in glycoproteins. However, linear polysaccharide units of 50–100 sugar residues are found in the proteoglycans. Carbohydrates which crosslink polypeptide chains have not been encountered. The proportion of protein to carbohydrate in glycoproteins can vary widely, depending on the number and size of the oligosaccharides attached to the polypeptide chain. For example, collagen contains 1% carbohydrate by weight, glycophorin from the human erythrocyte membrane 60% carbohydrate, and the soluble blood group substances – 85%.

Glycoproteins are ubiquitous in nature as enzymes, hormones, lectins, immunoglobulins and structural elements. A particularly rich source of glycoproteins is human serum, where out of some 60 or 70 proteins that have been identified, there seem to be only two which do not contain sugar, i.e. albumin and prealbumin. Another rich source is hen egg-white, where apart from lysozyme probably all proteins are glycosylated. Although numerous glycoproteins have been detected in membranes, mostly from erythrocytes and lymphocytes of different animal species and from viral envelopes, only a handful of these have been purified and characterized (table 1). In fact, the first definitive structure of the carbohydrate units of a membrane glycoprotein, that of the vesicular stomatitis virus, was published only last year. This, and the few tentative structures available, e.g. for the oligosaccharides of glycophorin, support the general belief that the oligosaccharide moieties of membrane glycoproteins are largely identical to those present in many secretory glycoproteins.

The polypeptide chains of glycoproteins are synthesized in the same way as non-glycosylated proteins, on the ribosomes which use for this purpose information encoded in messenger RNA. The structure of the messenger RNA is determined by the genome, so that proteins are primary gene products. Ribosomal enzymes, though they play a role in

Table 1
Purified integral membrane glycoproteins

Glycoprotein	Source	Mol wt	Carbohydrate content (%)
Cytochrome b_5 reductase	Calf liver	33 000	
E_1 glycoprotein	Sindbis virus	50 000	10
Glycophorin	Human erythrocytes	31 000	60
G-protein	Vesicular stomatitis virus	70 000	9
Hemaglutinin	Influenza virus	210 000	25
Hepatic binding protein	Rabbit liver	{40 000, 48 000}	~10
Histocompatibility antigens	Mouse lymphocytes	45 000	10
Oligoaminopeptidase	Hog intestine	248 000	23
Polypeptide 3	Human erythrocytes	95 000	6–8
Rhodopsin	Bovine retina	40 000	~7

protein synthesis, have no influence on protein structure. In contrast, oligosaccharides and polysaccharides, whether free or attached to proteins, are not primary gene products. They are synthesized by enzymes known as glycosyltransferases, in the absence of any template. Oligosaccharide structure is thus determined by enzyme specificities and kinetic parameters, the latter dependent in part on local concentrations of substrate, enzyme, and product. This type of synthesis is much less accurate than RNA translation and results in an inherent heterogeneity in the carbohydrate portion of glycoproteins. Indeed, glycoproteins with identical protein sequences may have many different carbohydrate structures. For example, the single, carbohydrate unit of highly purified preparations of ovalbumin (mol wt 40 000 Daltons) has been shown to have 9 different structures attached to the same position of the polypeptide backbone. Similarly, α_1-acid glycoprotein from human serum (44 000 mol wt) has at least 23 carbohydrate structures at the five attachment points along its polypeptide chain. Such variation in the carbohydrate portion of glycoprotein is known as "microheterogeneity". Microheterogeneity poses special problems in purification and characterization of glycoproteins.

1.2. Monosaccharides

Although living organisms can form a large number of different monosaccharides – perhaps 200 or more – only six are found as constituents of membrane glycoproteins (fig. 2). Two of these, galactose and mannose, are simple hexoses ($C_6H_{12}O_6$), and are isomers of glucose; the latter, a sugar very widely occurring in nature appears to be absent from membrane glycoproteins, although it is present in intermediates of glycoprotein biosynthesis as well as in membrane glycolipids. L-fucose is related to these sugars, but it has a hydrogen atom in place of a hydroxyl at carbon-6, which makes it less hydrophilic. *N*-acetylglucosamine and *N*-acetylgalactosamine, as their names imply, are amino sugars derived from glucose and galactose, respectively, by substitution of the hydroxyl at carbon-2 with an aminoacetyl, or acetamido, group (CH_3CONH). *N*-acetylneuraminic acid, the most commonly occurring member of the sialic acid family, is the most complex of the membrane sugars. It is made up of a straight chain of nine carbon atoms, with a carboxyl group at carbon-1 and an acetamido group at carbon-5. Over twenty different sialic acids have been identified to date. They are formed by modifications of *N*-acetylneuraminic acid, e.g. by attachment of an additional acetyl group at carbon-4, carbon-9, or both, or the oxidation of the *N*-acetyl group to an *N*-glycolyl group ($CH_2OHCONH$) forming *N*-glycolylneuraminic acid. The carboxyl groups of sialic acids seem to be responsible for most of the negative charge on the surface of erythrocytes which, among other things, is believed to prevent the cells from agglutinating inside the blood vessels.

The chemistry of monosaccharides is highly complicated because their multiple hydroxyl groups have similar reactivities. Moreover, sugars have many different conformations. For example, although glucose is predominantly in one chair conformation (fig. 2), more than half a dozen unique ring forms of this sugar, in addition to the open chain molecule, are in equilibrium in water. The implications of these subtle conformational differences in biological systems is unknown.

2. Methodology

2.1. Isolation of membrane glycoproteins

The isolation and purification of membrane glycoproteins is hampered by microheterogeneity and by the scarcity of material. In addition, the hydrophobic nature of the transmembrane portion of the polypeptide often renders membrane glycoproteins insoluble in aqueous solutions, requiring the use of detergents. Characterization of the glycoproteins in the presence of lipids or detergents is difficult. Determining the location of a particular glycoprotein in the intact cell presents still another problem in distinguishing between cytoplasmic glycoproteins, those isolated from organelles, inner membranes, and the plasma membrane. Generally, two approaches have been employed: (i) selective prelabelling of the glycoproteins before isolation and (ii) the use of isolated membrane fractions as starting material for glycoprotein isolation.

Prelabelling has been useful in identifying glycoproteins on the outer cell surface. This technique provides direct evidence for the location of a particular glycoprotein, and is a useful handle for detecting the glycoproteins during the purification process. One type of prelabelling method employs the enzyme galactose oxidase. This enzyme oxidises preferentially the free hydroxyl group at carbon-6 of terminal non-reducing galactose (and *N*-acetylgalactosamine) residues in oligosaccharides and polysaccharides, converting this group to an aldehyde (fig. 5). This is followed by the addition of radioactive (^3H labelled) sodium borohydride, whereupon the aldehyde is immediately reduced

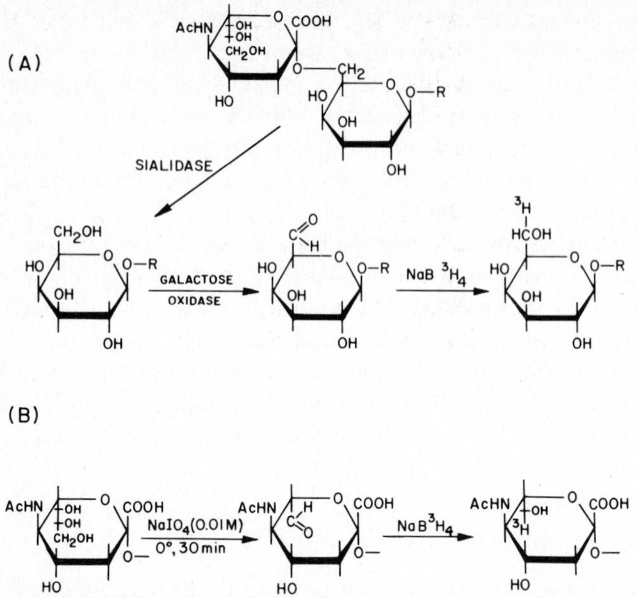

Fig. 5. Radioactive labelling of sugar residues in glycoproteins, glycolipids and on cell surfaces: (A) labeling of penultimate residues of galactose; (B) labelling of terminal nonreducing N-acetylneuraminic residues.

back to hydroxyl with the incorporation of a tritium in the galactose at carbon-6. Since galactose oxidase has a molecular weight of about 75 000 Daltons, it does not penetrate the cell membrane and only external galactose residues are labelled. Human erythrocyte membranes labelled by this method showed twenty radioactive bands on gel electrophoresis. Identical gels stained for sialic acid using the conventional periodic acid-Schiff (PAS) staining technique revealed only 5 bands. The potential problem of the sodium borohydride reacting with cell components other than the oxidized galactose can be avoided by pretreating the cell with the unlabelled reagent. A variation of the galactose oxidase–sodium borohydride technique is to first treat cells with the enzyme sialidase (known incorrectly as neuraminidase). The enzyme removes all terminal sialic acid residues from oligosaccharides exposing additional galactose residues which are then labelled as above.

Sialic acid residues on the outer cell surface can be labelled by another technique: mild treatment with sodium periodate cleaves the bond between the vicinal hydroxyl groups on carbon-7, carbon-8, and carbon-9 of sialic acid resulting in an aldehyde at carbon-7 which is subsequently reduced with radioactive sodium borohydride. The oxidation is done under conditions in which sodium periodate does not react with intracellular constituents. Other labelling techniques have also been employed but they are not specific for surface carbohydrates. For example, a radioactive sugar, such as [^{14}C] L-fucose is fed to cells and incorporated into glycoproteins biosynthetically.

The second general approach for membrane glycoprotein purification uses isolated membrane fractions as starting material. Current methods are based on breaking the cells by lysis or mechanically, followed by differential centrifugation to isolate the surface membrane fraction. Erythrocyte membranes were among the first to be isolated from cell

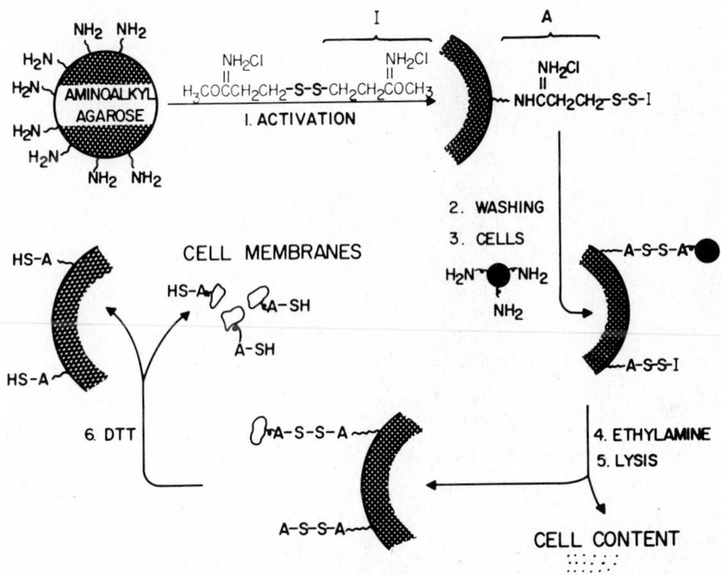

Fig. 6. Schematic illustration of cell membrane isolation by covalent fractionation on a solid support. Aminoalkyl agarose beads were activated (step 1) by reaction with imidoester groups (I) of the reversible crosslinking reagent 3,3′-dithiobispropionimidate, to form chemically stable amidine groups (A) which link dithioimidate groups to the beads. Following washing (step 2), the active beads were mixed with cells (step 3), leading to amidination of the beads' imidoesters by amino groups of cell surface components. The excess of imidoesters on the beads was deactivated by amidination with ethylamine (step 4), the covalently bound cells were lysed (step 5), and the cell content removed. Reduction by dithiothreitol (DTT) (step 6) of the disulfide bonds linking the resultant cell membranes and the beads, permitted the isolation of the cell membranes. [From Y. Eshdat and A. Prujansky-Jakobovits, FEBS Lett. 101 (1979) 43.]

lysates in the form of empty sacs or "ghosts". However, the isolation of plasma membranes from other cells poses many problems, most of which have not yet been overcome. Eshdat and Prujansky-Jakobovits in our department have recently developed a new technique for isolating cell membranes and their outer surface proteins (figs. 6 and 7). This technique is based on the covalent binding of cells to an insoluble matrix through a crosslinking agent with cleavable disulfide bonds. After attachment, the cells are lysed and washed; this is followed by reduction with dithiothreitol which detaches the membranes from the matrix.

Once the purified membrane fraction is obtained, the glycoproteins can be released by chaotropic agents or detergents. Conventional

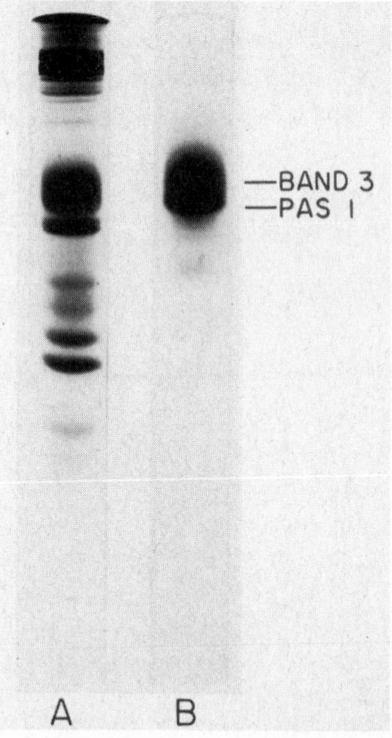

Fig. 7. Gel electrophoresis in sodium dodecylsulfate, detected by staining with Coomassie Brilliant Blue R-250: (A) ghosts obtained by covalent fractionation on solid support; (B) membrane proteins covalently bound to the solid support during attachment of the cells; the position of band 3 (polypeptide 3) and the major fraction of glycophorin (PAS 1) is indicated. Staining of the two gels with periodic-Schiff reagent resulted in patterns indicating the presence of glycophorin in both samples. (From Y. Eshdat and A. Prujansky-Jakobovits, loc. cit.)

methods such as gel filtration and ion exchange chromatography are employed to purify the glycoproteins. However, affinity chromatography on insolubilized lectins has recently become the method of choice for this purpose.

2.2. Lectins: reagents for glycoproteins

Lectins are cell agglutinating proteins of non-immune origin that are widely distributed in plants, but are also found in microorganisms and animals. They bind sugars with remarkable specificity (table 2). Many lectins combine preferentially with a single sugar structure, for example galactose or L-fucose, while some lectins exhibit a broader specificity and interact with several closely related sugars, e.g. mannose and glucose. Lectins such as phytohemagglutinin (PHA) interact only with complex carbohydrate structures like those that occur in glycoproteins, glycolipids, or on cell surfaces. To date over 50 lectins have been purified. They vary considerably in amino acid composition, sugar content, molecular weight, subunit structure, number of carbohydrate binding sites per molecule, and metal requirement. Many lectins contain covalently bound sugar and are themselves glycoproteins. However,

Table 2
Carbohydrate specificity of lectins

Sugar	Lectin: Name	Lectin: Abbreviation
Mannose, glucose	Concanavalin A,	Con A
	lentil lectin	LCA
Galactose	Soybean agglutinin,	SBA
	peanut agglutinin,	PNA
	Ricinus communis agglutinin	RCA
N-acetylglucosamine	Wheat germ agglutinin	WGA
N-acetylgalactosamine	Soybean agglutinin,	SBA
	Dolichos biflorus lectin,	
	helix pomatia agglutinin	HPA
L-fucose	*Lotus tetragonolobus* agglutinin	LTA
N-acetylneuraminic acid	Limulus (horseshoe crab) lectin,	LPL
	wheat germ agglutinin	WGA

concanavalin A, wheat germ agglutinin and peanut agglutinin, which are among the best characterized proteins of this class, are devoid of sugar.

Lectins can be used to determine the location and distribution of carbohydrates on cell surfaces. They are readily seen in the electron microscope if they are conjugated to ferritin, a protein with a very dense electron core. The ferritin conjugate of concanavalin A binds to the outer surface of the erythrocyte membrane and not to the inner cytoplasmic surface; ferritin–peanut agglutinin binds only to immature mouse thymocytes and not to the mature cells (fig. 8).

Affinity chromatography on lectins covalently attached to insoluble supports has been a valuable tool for purifying soluble glycoproteins. The finding that lectins retain their binding properties and specificity in the presence of moderate amounts of detergents has permitted their use for isolation of membrane glycoproteins by affinity chromatography.

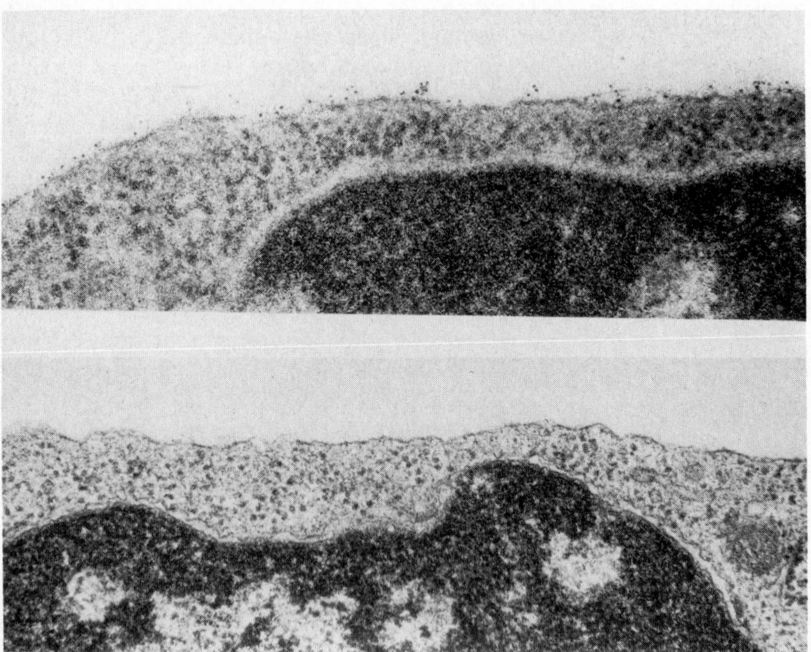

Fig. 8. Electron micrograph of immature mouse thymocyte labelled with ferritin-peanut agglutinin (top). For comparison, an electron micrograph of similarly treated mature mouse thymocyte that do not bind peanut agglutinin is also shown (bottom). (x 60 000, courtesy of E. Skutelsky.)

One advantage of this method is that preliminary structural information may be obtained during the purification process. The fact that a glycoprotein binds to a particular lectin is usually evidence that it contains certain carbohydrate structures for which the lectin is specific. The major drawback of affinity chromatography is that the membranes must be solubilized prior to glycoprotein isolation. Thus, the organization of receptor–ligand complexes cannot be studied. A new approach which conserves the membrane environment is by chemical crosslinking of ligands to receptors on membranes. This approach involves the use of reversible, photosensitive, heterobifunctional crosslinking reagents. Ligands are activated by attaching the crosslinking reagent via one of the reactive functional groups of the latter. After binding to the cell surface, irradiation leads to crosslinking of the activated ligands to the receptors (fig. 9). Jaffe in our Department has used this technique to study the binding of peanut agglutinin to human erythrocytes from which the sialic acid had been removed by enzymatic digestion. He developed a new and improved crosslinking agent, an *N*-hydroxysuccinimide ester

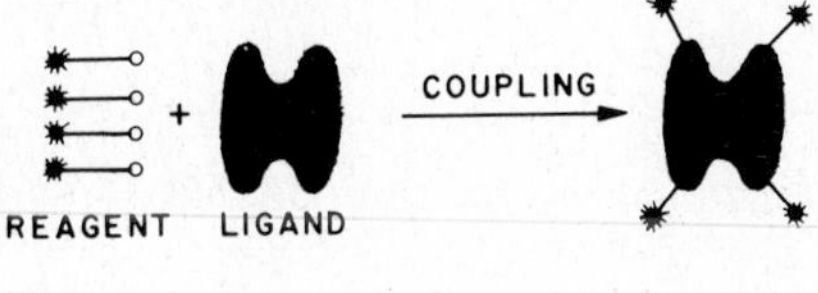

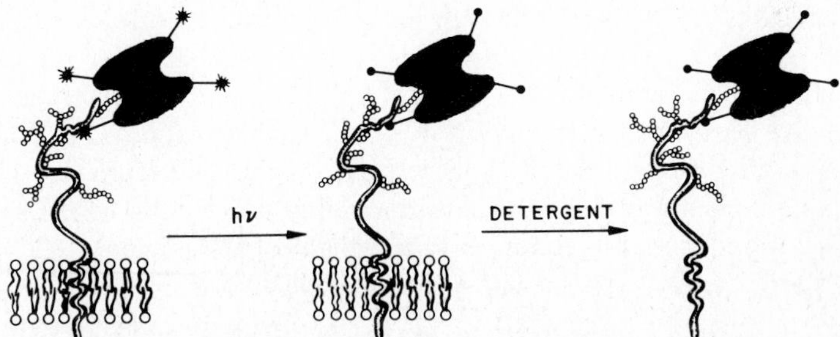

Fig. 9. Photoaffinity crosslinking (or macromolecular affinity labeling). A lectin, or another macromolecular ligand is activated by attaching to it a photosensitive heterobifunctional reagent. After binding of the modified lectin to surface receptors on cells, crosslinking is achieved by irradiation. The cells or membranes are then solubilized in a detergent (usually sodium dodecylsulfate) for analysis. [Modified from T. H. Ji, Biochim. Biophys. Acta 559 (1979) 39.]

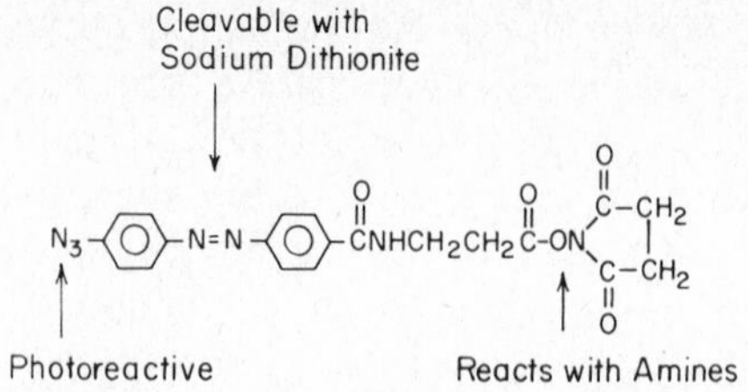

Cleavable with Sodium Dithionite

$N_3-C_6H_4-N{=}N-C_6H_4-\overset{O}{\overset{\|}{C}}NHCH_2CH_2\overset{O}{\overset{\|}{C}}-ON(COCH_2)_2$

Photoreactive   Reacts with Amines

Fig. 10. A new heterobifunctional and cleavable photosensitive crosslinking reagent [from C. L. Jaffe, H. Lis and N. Sharon, Biochem. Biophys. Res. Commun. 91 (1979) 402.]

derivative containing a photoreactive azide and a diazo group cleavable by sodium dithionite (fig. 10). The lectin was derivatized by attaching the reagent to the protein amino groups via the *N*-hydroxysuccinimide ester group of the reagent. After incubation with the modified lectin in the dark and removal of the unbound lectin by washing the cells, the latter were irradiated to photolyse the azide into a nitrene which formed a covalent linkage with the receptor. Analysis of the membranes of the treated cells revealed that peanut agglutinin bound mainly to asialoglycophorin (glycophorin lacking sialic acid residues). This method may be applicable to the study of a wide range of receptor–ligand (e.g. antibody, hormone or toxin) interactions.

2.3. *Physicochemical characterization of glycoproteins*

An important step in the characterization of any macromolecule is to determine its molecular weight. In the case of proteins, this task has been facilitated by the technique of sodium dodecylsulfate polyacrylamide gel electrophoresis, known in brief as SDS-gel electrophoresis. The method is based on the assumption that the ionic detergent SDS binds to denatured proteins in a fixed weight ratio, and that the protein-SDS complex has a rigid rod-like shape. Therefore, the charge on this complex and hence the distance migrated by the protein in the gel, are proportional to the molecular weight of the protein.

Glycoproteins pose special problems since the presence of large amounts of carbohydrate affects both detergent binding and the hydrodynamic behaviour of detergent–glycoprotein complexes. Carbohydrate heterogeneity in glycoproteins has also been shown to complicate SDS-gel electrophoresis. Thus, on polyacrylamide gel electrophoresis in SDS, glycophorin migrates as proteins with a molecular weight in the range of 39 000 to about 90 000, depending upon the experimental conditions. Its true molecular weight, estimated from compositional analysis and peptide sequencing, and by ultracentrifugation in the presence of SDS, is about 30 000. Enzymatic removal of sialic acid from glycophorin which causes a decrease of about 20% in the mass of the molecule, results in an increase in the apparent molecular weight, and this further points out the problems associated with the determination of the molecular weight of glycoproteins by SDS-gel electrophoresis.

Polypeptide 3 (also known as Band III) from the human erythrocyte membrane is an example of a glycoprotein that gives a broad band on SDS-gel electrophoresis, and there is increasing evidence that this diffuseness is due to heterogeneity of its oligosaccharide moieties. The leading and trailing edges of the band differ in reactivity towards galactose oxidase and in their ability to bind concanavalin A. Proteolytic removal of the most heavily glycosylated region of polypeptide 3 yields a large protein fragment that migrates with a much sharper band on SDS-gel electrophoresis, while a carboxy terminal fragment of the glycoprotein, which contains the glycosylated region, yields a more diffuse band than the intact glycoprotein; the components in this fragment vary in their binding of different lectins (concanavalin A, PHA and *Ricinus communis* agglutinin).

There are also great difficulties in establishing the molecular weight of glycoproteins by gel filtration since in this technique too proteins containing a substantial amount of carbohydrate behave in an anomalous manner. While a linear relationship exists for most globular proteins between their elution volumes on Sephadex gel columns and the logarithm of their molecular weights, glycoproteins such as fetuin, ovomucoid and thyroglobulin do not conform to the above relationship. This appears to be due to a greater hydration in solution brought about by the carbohydrate units, resulting in a more expanded structure for glycoproteins than that for proteins not containing carbohydrate. The use of gel filtration for the purpose of molecular weight determination of glycoproteins is therefore precluded, or at most, may be employed with great caution.

Another difficulty in estimating the molecular weight of carbohydrate-rich glycoproteins is the occurrence of non-covalent interactions that may lead to the formation of intermolecular complexes, as clearly demonstrated with ovine submaxillary mucin. This glycoprotein, containing about 63% sugar, forms large aggregates with molecular weight ranging from $0.5–1.0 \times 10^6$ Daltons, that can be dissociated at high salt concentrations but not by urea, guanidine hydrochloride or SDS at concentrations that normally dissociate proteins into subunits.

Values reported in the literature of molecular weights of glycoproteins determined by ultracentrifugation are frequently incorrect, not only because association has not been eliminated, but also because the partial specific volumes on which the molecular weight calculations are based have not been experimentally measured and the calculated values are incorrect. With glycoproteins that can be dissociated into monomers or subunits in SDS, accurate subunit molecular weight values can be obtained by sedimentation analysis, provided that the amount of detergent bound is experimentally evaluated. Using this technique, it has been conclusively shown that glycophorin has a molecular weight of 29 000, a value in agreement with that calculated from its composition and the sequence analysis of its polypeptide moiety.

Accurate values for the molecular weight of glycoproteins can also be obtained indirectly, by measuring the molecular weight of the protein moiety (sometimes designated as apoprotein) after removal of the carbohydrate. This approach has only recently become feasible with the availability of highly purified glycosidases that act on glycoproteins. The most promising enzymes for this purpose are the endoglycosidases, such as endo-β-N-acetylglucosaminidase. Yeast invertase treated with endo-β-N-acetylglucosaminidase to remove its carbohydrate units almost completely, gave discrete protein bands on SDS-acrylamide gel electrophoresis, from the migration of which it was concluded that the carbohydrate-free enzyme is composed of two 60 000 Dalton subunits. The molecular weight of ovine submaxillary mucin was estimated accurately for the first time with the aid of two exoglycosidases – sialidase and α-N-acetylgalactosidase – that removed sequentially the sugar

Table 3

Molecular weights of mucin, asialomucin and apomucin in 0.5 M sodium chloride[a)]

	Mol wt	
Preparation	Experimental	Calculated
Mucin	559 000–640 000	154 150
Asialomucin	224 300	108 000
Apomucin	58 300	

[a)]From H. D. Hill, Jr., J. A. Reynolds and R. L. Hill, J. Biol. Chem. 252 (1977) 3791–3798.

constituents of the disaccharide units attached on the average to every third amino acid residue (serine or threonine) of this glycoprotein (table 3). It was concluded that ovine submaxillary mucin consists of molecules of 154 000 Daltons, that associate via carbohydrate–protein and/or carbohydrate–carbohydrate interactions, into high molecular weight aggregates.

2.4. Structural studies of the carbohydrate units

Structural characterization of glycoproteins requires examination of the polypeptide backbone, the carbohydrate units, and the carbohydrate–peptide linkage(s). Analysis of the peptide moiety is carried out using methods developed for the determination of protein structure, whereas special techniques are required for studies of the carbohydrate and its linkage to the protein. Elucidation of the structure of the carbohydrate units is rarely done on the intact molecule. This is both because most glycoproteins contain several different carbohydrate units, and due to the microheterogeneity of the oligosaccharides. As a rule, it is necessary first to isolate the carbohydrate units, either as glycopeptides after exhaustive proteolytic digestion of the glycoproteins, e.g. by pronase, or in the form of carbohydrate chains devoid of amino acids, by the use of endoglycosidases or by chemical cleavage of the carbohydrate–peptide linkages. Since only minute quantities of material are usually available, especially when the starting materials are membrane glycoproteins, it is advisable to radioactively label the glycopeptides and oligosaccharides to facilitate their detection and analysis. The carbohydrate chains, either with or without amino acids attached, are isolated and purified by gel filtration, ion-exchange chromatography, fractionation on immobilized lectins and preparative paper electrophoresis. Careful application of these methods permits the resolution of mixtures containing closely related carbohydrate chains into strictly homogenous products. An impressive illustration of the resolving power of ion-exchange chromatography in combination with paper electrophoresis is the isolation of nine homogenous asparaginyl-oligosaccharides from a pronase digest of crystalline ovalbumin. Incidentally, it also serves as a clear example of the microheterogeneity of glycoproteins, mentioned earlier.

In order to characterize an oligosaccharide unit completely, the following information must be obtained: (i) carbohydrate composition; (ii) molecular weight; (iii) sequence of sugar residues; (iv) position of linkages; (v) anomeric configuration; and (vi) the nature of carbohydrate–peptide linkage. Although by no means a routine task, the

Table 4
Structural analysis of glycopeptides

Information	Method
Composition	GLC of alditol acetates in acid hydrolysate
Mol wt	Gel filtration
Sequence of sugar residues	Digestion by glycosidases
Anomeric configuration of linkages	Digestion by glycosidases, nuclear magnetic resonance
Position of linkages	Methylation analysis, periodate oxidation, nuclear magnetic resonance
Structure of carbohydrate–peptide linkage	Examination of acid and alkali lability, β-elimination reaction

refinement of old carbohydrate methodology and the development of new techniques (primarily NMR analysis) (table 4), have made it possible to obtain all this information on as little as 0.5–1.0 mg of material.

Compositional analysis of oligosaccharides and glycopeptides still depends to a considerable extent on old time colorimetric and paper chromatographic techniques carried out on either the intact or acid hydrolysed material. However, gas-liquid chromatography of acid hydrolysed or methanolysed samples is becoming the method of choice, since it permits the separation and estimation in a single run of all the monosaccharides that commonly occur in glycoproteins. Other procedures in use are automated ion exchange chromatography and quantitative paper electrophoresis.

Molecular weight estimations of glycopeptides are done by gel filtration on columns calibrated with oligosaccharides of known molecular weight, e.g. homologous cellodextrins or more recently asparaginyl-oligosaccharides isolated from ovalbumin.

Methylation analysis, introduced in the thirties, is still the most important method for structural studies of complex carbohydrates, including glycoproteins. It involves methylation of all free hydroxyl groups of the compound examined, followed by acid hydrolysis. During this hydrolysis the glycosidic linkages are cleaved but the methyl-ether linkages are stable. The product is a mixture of partially methylated sugars and the free hydroxyls in these mark the positions to which the sugars are linked in the starting material. A qualitative and quantitative analysis of this mixture is best carried out after conversion of the sugars to suitable derivatives such as alditol acetates, and is done by combined gas liquid chromatography and mass spectrometry (GLC–MS). The results obtained provide complete information on the linkage positions in the starting material.

Another chemical approach is Smith degradation, a sequential application of periodate oxidation, borohydride reduction, and mild acid hydrolysis. Periodate oxidizes vicinal unsubstituted hydroxyl groups to produce characteristic degradation products which are stabilized by reduction. From the analysis of the acid hydrolysate of the oxidized-reduced glycopeptide (or oligosaccharide) it is possible to make deductions about the structure of the starting material. In addition to the chemical techniques, various exoglycosidases (sialidase, β-galactosidase, β-*N*-acetylglucosaminidase, and α-mannosidase, etc.) have been used to degrade sugar chains from their non-reducing ends. Sequential digestion with very pure enzymes will reveal not only the sequence of sugars but also their anomeric configuration based on the specificity of the glycosidases for α- or β-linkages. The recently isolated endoglycosidases have proven to be of enormous aid in glycoprotein research. Of particular use are the endo-β-*N*-acetylglucosaminidases because of their specificity in cleaving *N*-acetylglucosamine linkages within the core of glycosidic units. The endo-β-*N*-acetylglucosaminidase H isolated from cultures of *Streptomyces griseus* can remove carbohydrate side chains composed of *N*-acetylglucosamine and mannose from either glycopeptides or intact glycoproteins. Another enzyme, endo-β-*N*-acetylglucosaminidase D, also splits the core di-*N*-acetylglucosamine (GlcNAcβ1→4GlcNAc) but displays a different specificity for the type of oligosaccharide chains that may be attached to the disaccharide. Since these different endoglycosidases attack glycopeptides with different branch patterns, they offer a very powerful potential for elucidation of glycoprotein structure. Other useful glycosidases are the endo-α-*N*-acetylgalactosaminidase that removes galactosyl-β1→3-*N*-acetylgalactosamine disaccharides attached to glycoproteins and the endo-β-galactosidase capable of cleaving the internal galactosyl linkages in the repeating sequence ... Galβ1→4-GlcNAcβ1→3Galβ1→4 . . . .

Considerable structural information can also be obtained by nuclear magnetic resonance, which is discussed elsewhere in this book (Dorland and Vliegenthart's chapter). Other useful techniques are partial chemical degradation, e.g. by acid, acetolysis, or hydrazinolysis, and the use of anticarbohydrate antibodies or lectins.

Identification of the carbohydrate–peptide linkages is carried out either on the intact glycoprotein or on the isolated glycopeptides. Preliminary information can be obtained from analytical studies. Thus, the presence of mannose in a glycoprotein is suggestive of an *N*-acetylglucosaminyl–asparagine linkage, while the presence of *N*-acetylgalactosamine is indicative of an *N*-acetylgalactosaminyl–serine (or threonine) linkage. Hydroxylysine, a characteristic constituent of the collagens, suggests the presence of the galactosyl–hydroxylysine linkage. These and other commonly occurring carbohydrate–pyridine linkages are listed in table 5. Only the first two types of linkage have been found to date in membrane glycoproteins and they will be discussed in more detail.

The *N*-glycosidic linkage is relatively stable to mild acids and is only partially hydrolysed under conditions that lead to cleavage of *O*-glycosidic linkages in oligosaccharides. Indeed, the first isolation of *N*-acetylglucosaminyl-asparagine, in the early 1960s, was from an incomplete acid hydrolysate of the asparaginyl–carbohydrate obtained from an exhaustive proteolytic digest of ovalbumin. The linkage is also relatively stable under mild alkaline conditions. Alkaline cleavage under drastic conditions liberates the carbohydrate unit, and when the reaction is carried out in the presence of $NaBH_4$, the terminal reducing *N*-acetylglucosamine residue is converted into *N*-acetylglucosaminitol.

The most characteristic feature of the *O*-glycosidic linkage to serine and threonine is its extreme lability to alkali, as it is split at a measurable rate in most cases by 0.1 M alkali at room temperature. This cleavage is not hydrolysis in the usual sense, but β-elimination, the mechanism of which is shown in fig. 11. The product of the reaction is an unsaturated amino acid which breaks down to give pyruvic acid or α-ketobutyric acid from serine or threonine, respectively. If a reducing agent such as sodium borohydride is added together with the alkali, and the reaction mixture hydrolysed in acid, the corresponding saturated amino acid, alanine or α-aminobutyric acid, is obtained together with a sugar alcohol, galactosaminitol. Although the β-elimination reaction is rarely quantitative, analysis (e.g. on the amino acid analyser) of the loss of serine and threonine, the increase of alanine and the amount of α-aminobutyric acid and galactosaminitol formed in the presence of sodium borohydride, provide information not only on the nature of the carbohydrate–peptide linkage, but also on the approximate number of *O*-glycosidically linked serine and threonine residues in the glycoprotein.

Table 5
Carbohydrate–peptide linking groups

Compound	Occurrence	
	Soluble glycoproteins	Membrane glycoproteins
N-GLYCOSIDIC		
β-*N*-acetylglucosaminyl-asparagine 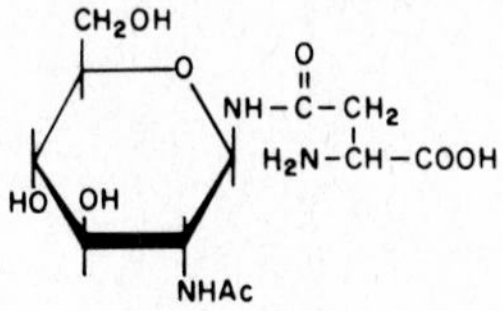	Widely distributed	+
O-GLYCOSIDIC		
α-*N*-acetylgalactosaminyl-serine (R = H) or threonine ($R = CH_3$) 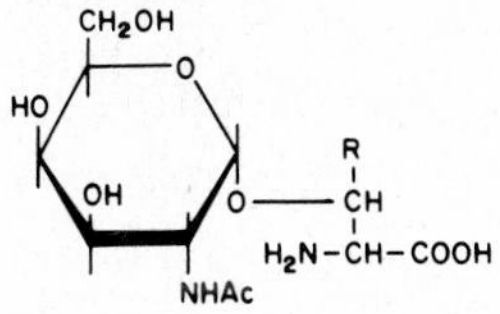	Animal glycoproteins	+
Xylosyl-serine 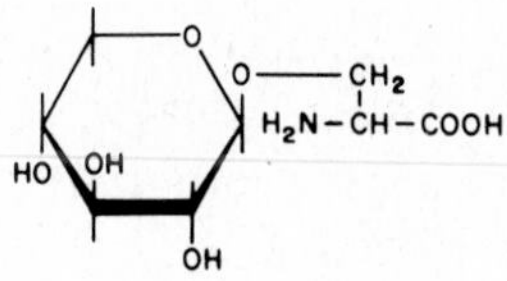	Proteoglycans	–
Galactosyl-hydroxylysine 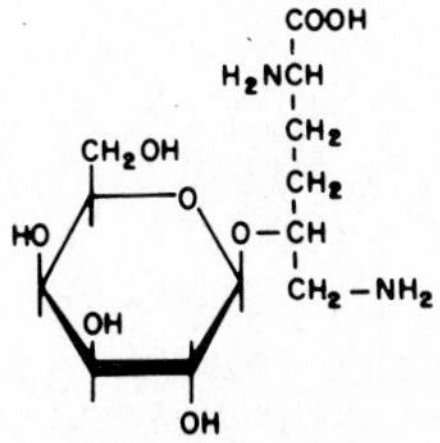	Collagens	–
L-arabinosyl-hydroxyproline 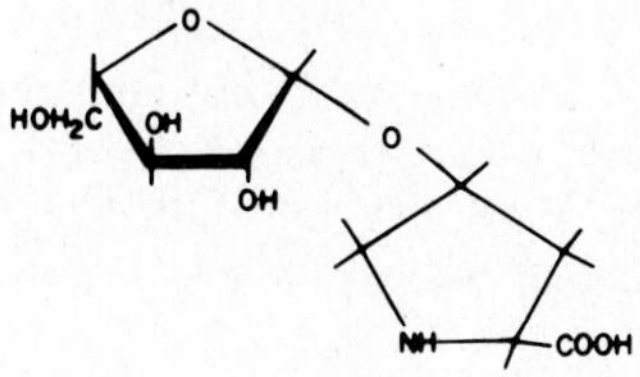	Plant glycoproteins	–

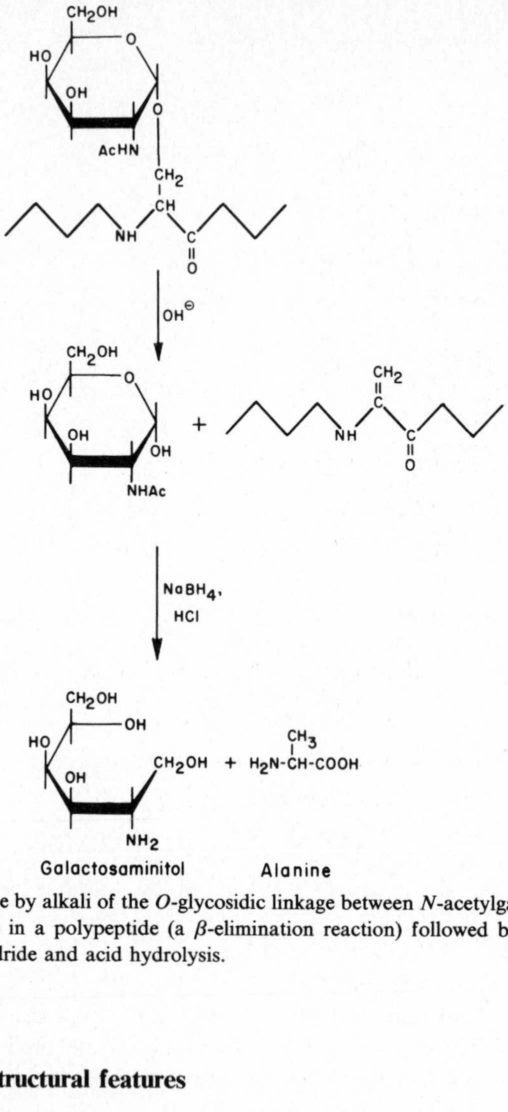

Fig. 11. Cleavage by alkali of the *O*-glycosidic linkage between *N*-acetylgalactosamine and a serine residue in a polypeptide (a β-elimination reaction) followed by reduction with sodium borohydride and acid hydrolysis.

3. General structural features

The great improvements in methodology and the increased interest in glycoproteins, have resulted during the past decade in rapid progress in the structural elucidation of the carbohydrate units of glycoproteins, primarily of soluble glycoproteins. Some typical examples of such structures are given in fig. 12.

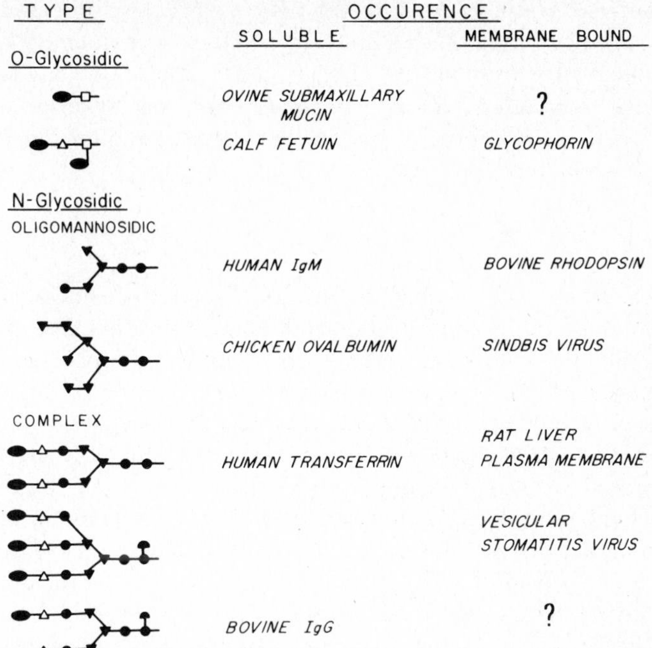

Fig. 12. Structures of carbohydrate units found in soluble and membrane bound glycoproteins.

3.1. O-glycosidic units

Few, if any, generalizations can be made about the *O*-glycosidically linked units. The sugar structures vary from a single galactose residue, as found in collagen, to branched oligosaccharides ("megalosaccharide") of 16 to 18 monosaccharide residues found in the soluble blood group substances, to the much longer linear polysaccharides of the proteoglycans. Perhaps the only common feature which emerges is the presence of the disaccharide galactosyl $\beta 1 \rightarrow 3 N$-acetylgalactosamine linked to serine or threonine in many glycoproteins. In its unsubstituted form, this disaccharide is found in certain immunoglobulins, in the antifreeze glycoproteins of antarctic fish as well as in certain membranes, e.g. those of pig lymphocytes. More frequently, the disaccharide occurs in a substituted form. Thus current evidence, though not yet complete, shows that each of the 15 *O*-glycosidic units of glycophorin consists of the disaccharide to which 2 *N*-acetylneuraminic acid residues are linked, $\alpha 2 \to 6$ and $\alpha 2 \to 3$, to the *N*-acetylgalactosamine and galactose, respectively (fig. 12). Such structures have been found in soluble glycoproteins, for example fetuin and human chorionic gonadotropin. The Gal$\beta 1 \to 3$GalNAc in a substituted form occurs also in other glycoproteins, such as porcine submaxillary mucins and the blood group substances mentioned above.

3.2. N-glycosidic units

N-glycosidically linked oligosaccharides contain considerably more common features than the *O*-glycosidic ones. It appears that in all the *N*-glycosidic units the inner core, which comprises the residues next to the linkage with the peptide, has an identical structure. It consists of a pentasaccharide, $Man_3(GlcNAc)_2$, in which the two *N*-acetylglucosamine residues are at the terminal reducing end of the molecule and are $\beta 1 \to 4$ linked. One of the mannose residues is attached to this disaccharide by a $\beta 1 \to 4$ linkage; it is flanked by the two remaining mannose residues linked $\alpha 1 \to 3$ and $\alpha 1 \to 6$, thus forming a branched structure (fig. 13).

The core oligosaccharide is attached to the polypeptide through a glycosidic linkage to the amide group of asparagine residues. Its peripheral mannose residues are almost always substituted and here too certain regularities can be discerned: either the substitution is by additional mannose residues, in the form of short or long oligosaccharides, that are usually branched, or by the disaccharide *N*-acetylglucosaminyl$\beta 1 \to 4$galactose (GlcNAc$\beta 1 \to 4$Gal), known also as *N*-acetyllactosamine, to which sialic acid is often attached (fig. 12). There are thus two main types of *N*-glycosidic units—the simple, mannose-rich or oligomannosidic and the complex, *N*-acetyllactosamine. *N*-glycosidic units of both types have been found in numerous animal glycoproteins. However, in plant and yeast glycoproteins, only oligomannosidic units seem to be present.

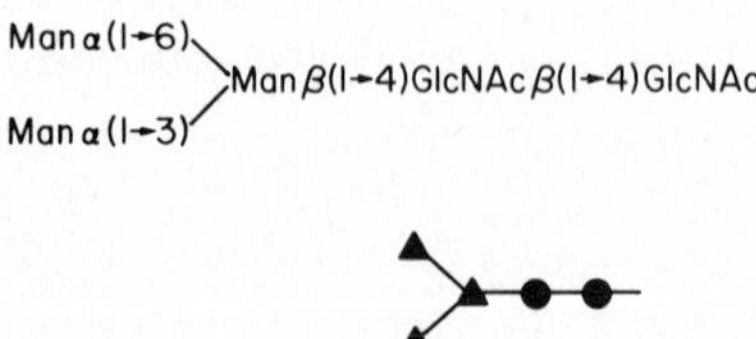

Fig. 13. Structure of the *N*-glycosidic core pentasaccharide.

Several membrane glycoproteins have also been shown to contain such units. The best characterized of these is the oligosaccharide of the *G*-protein from the outer membrane of vesicular stomatitis virus, in which the pentasaccharide core is substituted by three chains of NeuNAcα2→3Galβ1→4GlcNAc and by an L-fucose residue which is attached to the asparagine-linked *N*-acetylglucosamine residue (fig. 12). Two such carbohydrate units are present in the *G*-protein, at approximately asparagine residues 150 and 400.

The outer chains of the vesicular stomatitis virus oligosaccharide are identical to those in fetuin, transferrin, α_1-acid glycoprotein, thyroglobulin and chorionic gonadotropin, except for the linkage of sialic acid to galactose which may be different (2→6 instead of 2→3 in the *G*-protein). It may be safely assumed that the single *N*-glycosidic unit of glycophorin, for which only tentative structures are available, will prove to be very similar too. The fucose in the vesicular stomatitis virus glycoprotein core is attached in the same position as that reported for different immunoglobulins, mouse histocompatibility-2 alloantigen and glycopeptide S1 of glycoprotein E2 of Sindbis virus. A similar structure with two outer chains has been reported for a Sindbis virus glycopeptide, whereas structures with four outer chains have been found in α_1-acid glycoprotein (in addition to structures with two and three outer chains).

Structural variants of the outer chains have, however, been encountered, such as the sequence Galβ1→3Galβ1→4GlcNAc in a glycoprotein from calf thymocyte membranes. In influenza virus glycoproteins, sulfate groups are attached to *N*-glycosidic units. Mannose residues which are phosphorylated at the 6-position are found in lysosomal enzymes (e.g. β-*N*-acetylhexosaminidase and β-glucuronidase) that are glycoproteins: they seem to play an important functional role in the uptake of these enzymes by fibroblasts. People who lack the kinase necessary to phosphorylate mannose suffer from I-cell disease.

Attempts have been made to predict protein glycosylation sites according to amino acid sequences. The sequence Asn-X-Ser/Thr appears to be necessary, but is not sufficient for glycosylation of the asparaginyl residue since not all polypeptides containing this sequence have glycosylated asparaginyl residues. One model which tries to account for the observation that the sequence Asn-X-Ser/Thr is required for *N*-glycosylation assumes that the asparagine carbonyl group can form a hydrogen bond with the serine (or threonine) hydroxyl group and thus enhance the amide reactivity. For this hydrogen bonding to occur, a cyclic structure has to be formed embracing 13 atoms which is the same number as that occurring in the α-helix of a polypeptide chain. However, most glycosylated sites are probably in β-bend (or β-turn) regions. Thus, from X-ray crystallographic studies of bovine ribonuclease A, which is identical to the glycosylated ribonuclease B, it was concluded that in the latter protein the *N*-glycosidic Asn-34 is in a β-bend. Furthermore, in immunoglobulin IgG, the only glycoprotein for which a three dimensional structure is known (fig. 14), the carbohydrate is also attached at a β-bend. Unfortunately, X-ray diffraction studies of other glycoproteins have been hampered by a lack of adequate crystals.

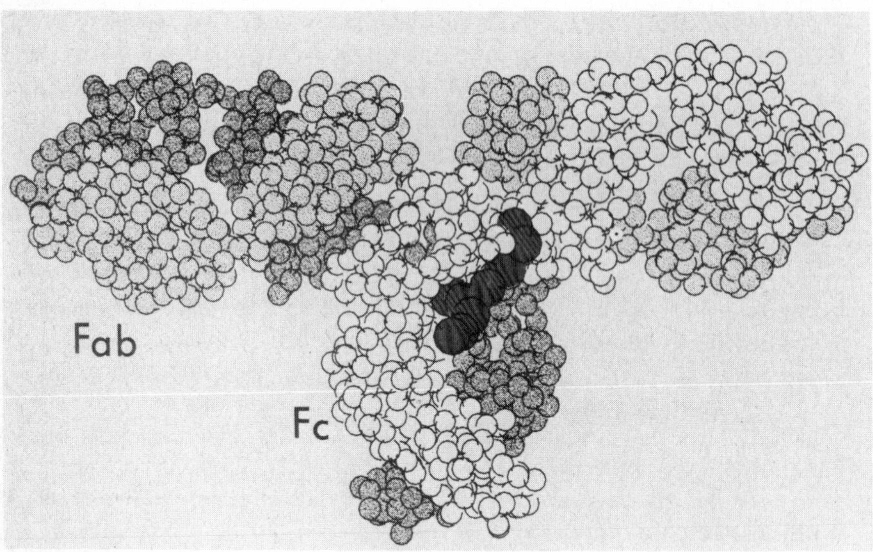

Fig. 14. Space-filling view of a human immunoglobulin, the Dob Ig molecule. One complete heavy chain is in white and the other is dark gray; the two light chains are lightly shaded. The large black spheres represent the individual hexose units of the complex carbohydrate. In this view, the 2-fold axis of symmetry is vertical. A crevasse is seen between the C_H2 of the white heavy chain and the C_L domain of the Fab on the left. [From E. W. Silverton, M. A. Navia and D. R. Davis, Proc. Natl. Acad. Sci. USA 74 (1977) 5140.]

4. Biosynthesis

The polypeptide chains of glycoproteins are synthesized by the same machinery that produces non-glycosylated proteins. Sugar addition to proteins leading to their conversion into glycoproteins occurs either directly from sugar nucleotides (figs. 15 and 16) or indirectly through sugar-linked lipid intermediates (fig. 15). The structure of the carbohydrate units is determined primarily by the specificity of glycosyltransferases which add with great precision monosaccharides or oligosaccharides from the donors to suitable acceptors. As mentioned in the introduction, genetic control of the oligosaccharide sequence of glycoproteins is achieved without the direct participation of DNA or

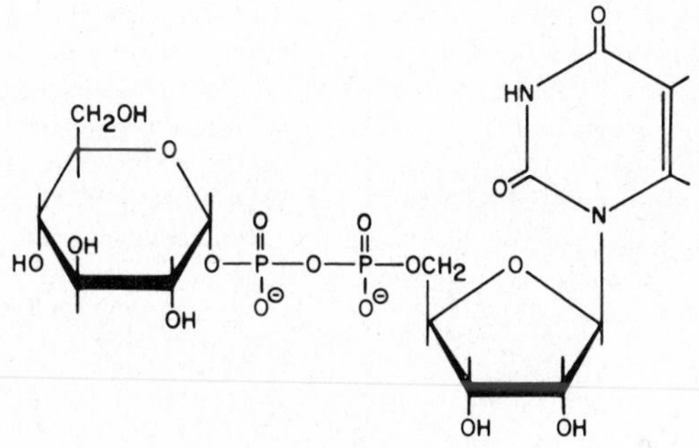

Uridine diphosphate glucose (UDP-Glc)

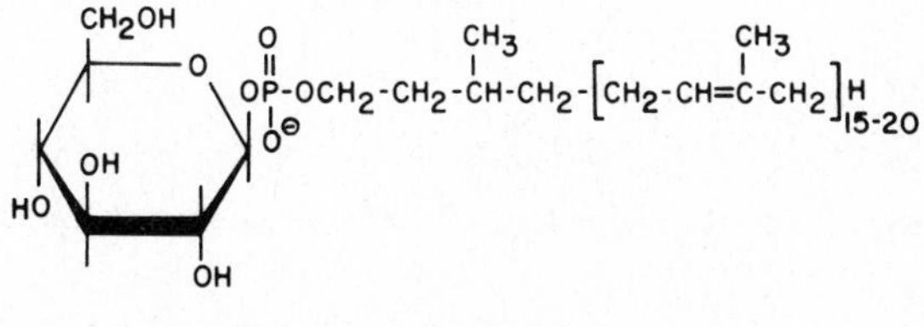

Dolichyl monophosphate glucose (Dol-P-Glc or Glc-P-Dol)

Fig. 15. Two types of activated monosaccharides which serve as donors in transglycosylation reactions. Note that in uridine diphosphate glucose the anomeric configuration of the glucose is α, whereas in dolichyl monophosphate glucose it is β.

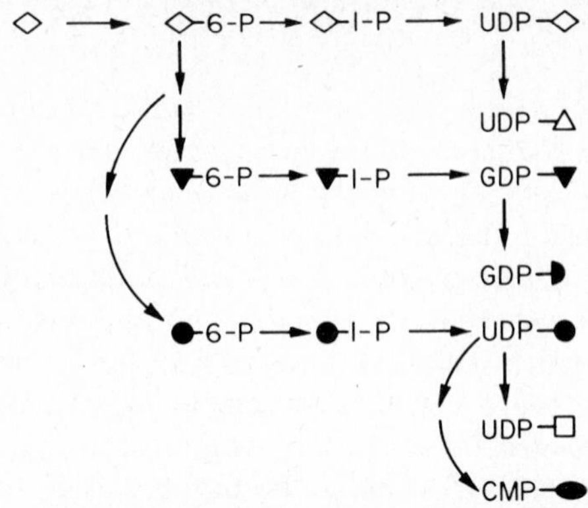

Fig. 16. Formation of sugar nucleotides. All activated sugars can be considered as derived from glucose. Glucose-6-phosphate obtained by phosphorylation of glucose, is converted into the corresponding derivatives of mannose and *N*-acetylglucosamine. The 6-phosphates are then modified into the corresponding sugar 1-phosphates, which by reacting with uridine triphosphate UTP (for glucose 1-phosphate and *N*-acetylglucosamine 1-phosphate) or guanosine triphosphate GTP (for mannose 1-phosphate) yield the corresponding sugar nucleotides UDP-Glc, UDP-GlcNAc, and GDP-Man. The first two of these serve as direct precursors of UDP-Gal and UDP-GalNAc, respectively, and the third of GDP-L-Fuc. In addition, UDP-GlcNAc is converted by a complex sequence of reactions into *N*-acetylneuraminic acid, which by reacting with cytidine triphosphate (CTP) affords CMP-NeuNAc.

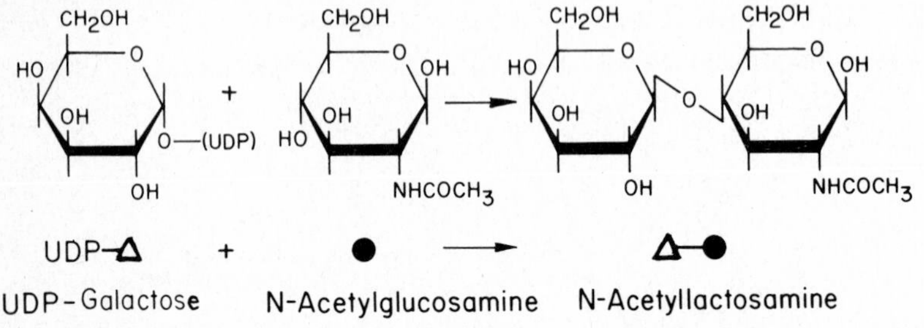

CH$_2$OH, HO, OH, O—(UDP), OH + CH$_2$OH, OH, HO, NHCOCH$_3$ → CH$_2$OH, HO, OH, O, OH + CH$_2$OH, OH, OH, NHCOCH$_3$

UDP-Galactose + N-Acetylglucosamine → N-Acetyllactosamine

Fig. 17. Synthesis of *N*-acetyllactosamine catalysed by a galactosyltransferase: an example of a transglycosylation reaction.

RNA, but rather indirectly by controlling the properties of the glycosyltransferases, which are the primary gene products.

The glycosyltransferases are classified according to the sugar transferred, e.g. sialyltransferases, galactosyltransferases (fig. 17), etc. While some of the enzymes act on both low and high molecular weight acceptors, others have a preference for the larger acceptors. Glycosyltransferases act in sequence, the product of one enzyme serving as the substrate of the next one.

4.1. O-glycosidic units

Biosynthesis of *O*-glycosidically linked units appears to be a simpler process than that of the *N*-glycosidic units, since it occurs by the direct and sequential addition of one monosaccharide at a time to the growing polypeptide, without the apparent participation of any lipid-linked intermediates (fig. 17).

Most of our knowledge in this area comes from studies of ovine and porcine submaxillary mucins, each of which carries numerous small carbohydrate units, that are *O*-glycosidically linked. The first step in the formation of these units is the transfer of *N*-acetylgalactosamine, from UDP-*N*-acetylgalactosamine to an hydroxyamino acid in the polypeptide backbone. The specificity requirements of the *N*-acetylgalactosaminyltransferase that catalyses this reaction are not known. In the synthesis of ovine submaxillary mucin, the next step is the attachment of sialic acid to the protein-linked *N*-acetylgalactosamine residues; the donor for this reaction is cytidine monophosphosialic acid (CMP-NeuNAc), and the enzyme is a specific sialyltransferase which forms the NeuNAcα2$\rightarrow$6GalNAc disaccharide units of the glycoprotein. Since no further attachment of sugar residues is possible after this step, addition of sialic acid can be considered as a termination signal. If, however, galactose is attached to form the Galβ1$\rightarrow$3GalNAc disaccharide, the different oligosaccharides present in bovine submaxillary mucin are synthesized (fig. 18). The relative proportions of the sialyltransferases and galactosyltransferases control this branch point. A similar sequence of reactions may be responsible for the formation of other *O*-glycosidic units, e.g. of the type found in glycophorin.

The sialyltransferase mentioned above, that catalyses the attachment of sialic acid in α2$\rightarrow$6 linkage to mucins, is different from the sialyltransferase involved in the elongation of *N*-glycosidic units to be discussed later. The enzyme can transfer *N*-acetyl, *N*-glycolyl, *N*-acetyl-7(or 9)-*O*-acetyl, and *N*-acetyl-4-*O*-acetylneuraminic acids from their respective CMP derivatives to endogenous acceptors at similar rates; it is thus not specific for the acyl groups attached to neuraminic acid. The different ratios of the various sialic acids found in salivary mucus glycoproteins from different species apparently do not depend

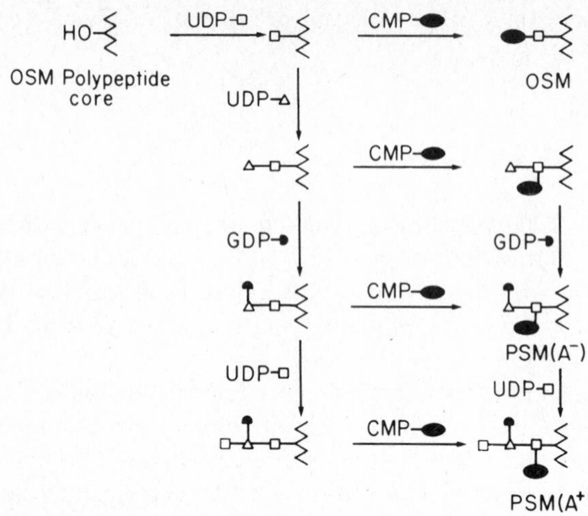

Fig. 18. Biosynthesis of ovine submaxillary mucin (OSM) and porcine submaxillary mucin (PSM) blood groups A^- and A^+. [Modified from H. Schachter, in: The Glycoconjugates, eds. M. I. Horowitz and W. Pigman vol. II (Acad. Press 1978) pp. 87–181.]

on the sialyltransferases but on the activities of the oxidoreductases and acetyltransferases which modify *N*-acetylneuraminic acid.

Another well studied group of glycoproteins containing the GalNAc-Ser/Thr linkage are the blood group substances. Gastric mucosa and submaxillary glands from humans of blood type A, B, or O, contain an *N*-acetylgalactosaminyltransferase which incorporates *N*-acetylgalactosamine into human blood group glycoproteins rendered carbohydrate-poor by mild acid hydrolysis followed by treatment with α-*N*-acetylgalactosaminidase. A similar *N*-acetylgalactosaminyltransferase is found in human sera from individuals of blood types A, B, and O.

The blood group substances provide the best example of genetic control of carbohydrate structure by the synthesis of specific glycosyltransferases (fig. 19). Four independent gene systems – ABO, Hh, Lele, and Sese – control the assembly of the non-reducing oligosaccharide termini of the blood group substances responsible for the immunological activities of these macromolecules. The ABO gene locus is responsible for two enzymes: an *N*-acetylgalactosaminyltransferase specified by the A gene and a galactosyltransferase specified by the B gene. Both enzymes attach the appropriate sugar by α1→3 linkage to galactose substituted on its C-2 by an α-L-fucosyl moiety. The third

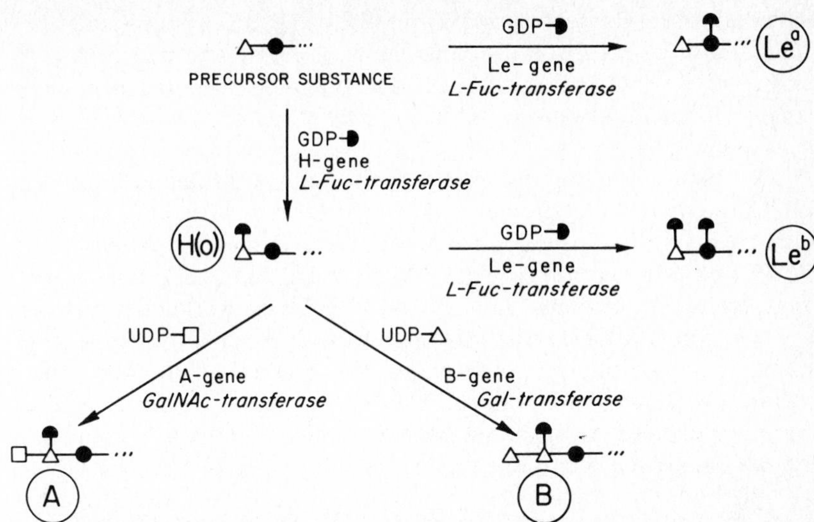

Fig. 19. Simplified scheme describing the genetic control of the biochemical pathways of the biosynthesis of the A, B, H(O) and Lewis (Le[a] and Le[b]) human blood group determinants.

gene at the ABO locus, the O gene, is inactive and does not produce a functional glycosyltransferase. The Lele locus produces one enzyme, a fucosyltransferase specified by the Le gene, that attaches L-fucose in an $\alpha 1 \rightarrow 4$ linkage to a subterminal *N*-acetylglucosamine residue; the Le gene is apparently inactive. At the Hh locus, the H gene controls a second fucosyltransferase that transfers L-fucose to the terminal β-galactose to form $\alpha 1 \rightarrow 2$ linkages; the h gene is apparently inactive.

The Sese locus does not specify an enzyme but in some unknown way controls the expression of the H gene. The absence of the Se gene results in suppression of the H-dependent fucosyltransferase in some secretory tissues (but not in other tissues, such as those responsible for the synthesis of the antigen on the red blood cell surface). Therefore, individuals lacking either the H gene (genotype hh) or the Se gene (genotype Sese) do not secrete blood group substances with H, A, or B antigenic activities, even if they possess the A or B genes.

The A gene specified α-*N*-acetylgalactosaminyltransferase has been found in a wide variety of species and tissues, but usually occurs in only a limited number of individuals within a species.

The enzymes show a high degree of acceptor specificity; all acceptors contain a terminal β-galactose residue substituted with an $\alpha 1 \rightarrow 2$ linked

L-fucose. Human and porcine gastric mucosa *N*-acetylgalactosaminyltransferase from individuals with the A gene can convert high molecular weight H(O) substance to immunologically active A substance and transform human red blood cells of types O and B into types A and AB, respectively.

The action of the four enzymes described above is summarized in fig. 19. The carbohydrate structures that they form are depicted, together with their associated serologic activity. Clearly, these determinants of blood type are secondary gene products, in that the primary gene products are the enzymes and it is these enzymes, working in concert, that determine which structures are formed. Such a mechanism of synthesis has an important biological consequence: it provides a biochemical explanation for antigens, whether membrane bound or soluble, that are produced by "gene interaction", namely antigens present in a hybrid that are not found in either parent. The Le^b is one of these. Thus, a child born to parents one of whom is $Le^+H^+Se^-$ and the other Le^-Se^+ would synthesize an oligosaccharide that neither parent could make alone.

4.2. N-glycosidic units

Research carried out during the last decade in many laboratories has demonstrated that unlike the *O*-linked oligosaccharides, the *N*-glycosidic ones are first assembled on a lipid carrier. The carrier is dolichol phosphate, a phosphorylated polyprenol containing between 17 and 21 isoprene units (fig. 15). Retinol, or vitamin A, may also serve as a carrier of sugars in some mammalian glycosylation reactions. Lipid linked intermediates were originally shown to participate in the biosynthesis of complex bacterial polysaccharides such as peptidoglycans or the lipopolysaccharides of Gram negative bacteria. Although the exact role of the lipid-linked saccharides is not known, it appears that they serve to transport the hydrophilic sugars into or through the hydrophobic membrane environment to the location where polymerization (in bacteria) or attachment to polypeptide chains (in eukaryotic cells) occurs.

It appears that an identical lipid linked oligosaccharide or "G-oligosaccharide" precursor is formed in animals, plants, and yeast, consisting of two residues of *N*-acetylglucosamine and, most likely, nine of mannose. Quite surprisingly, the G-oligosaccharide contains also two or three residues of glucose, a sugar not found in *N*-glycosidic units of glycoproteins. The structure of the G-oligosaccharide is given in fig. 20.

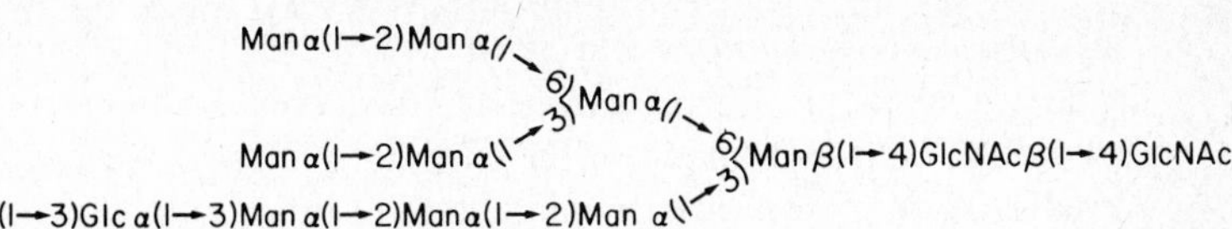

Fig. 20. Structure of the glucose-containing oligosaccharide intermediate of *N*-glycosidic units (G-oligosaccharide).

Notable is the presence of the $Man_3(GlcNAc)_2$ pentasaccharide core which, as emphasized earlier, seems to be a constant part of all *N*-glycosidic units. The sequence of reactions by which the G-oligosaccharide is formed is known as the "dolichol phosphate cycle" and is summarized in fig. 21. It is based on experiments with preparations from higher animals, plants, yeasts, and in virus infected cells, although usually only a few of the reactions of the cycle have been demonstrated in a single system. Certain reactions such as the removal of one phosphate from dolichol pyrophosphate (reaction 7 in fig. 21), are strictly speculative. Moreover, little is known about the enzymes involved in the other reactions and none of them have been purified.

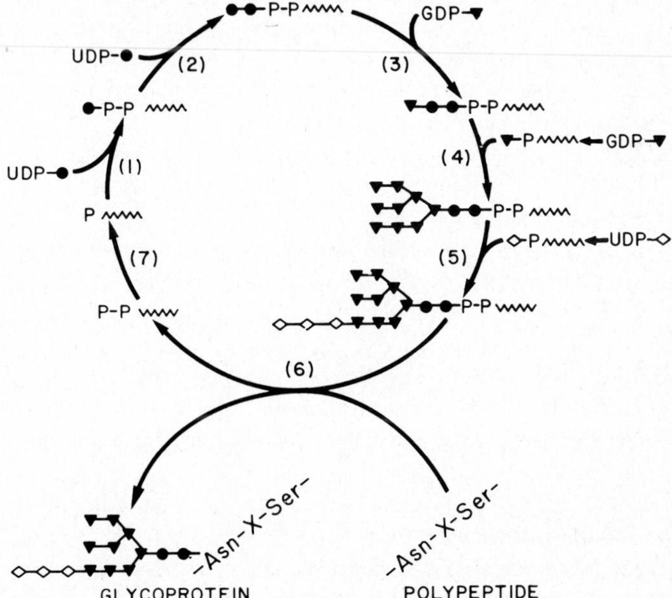

Fig. 21. The dolichol phosphate cycle of protein glycosylation (P/\/\/\dolichyl phosphate).

All the glycosylation reactions of the dolichol phosphate cycle proceed with inversion of configuration. Thus, whereas mannose is α-linked in GDP-Man, it is β-linked in the Man-P-lipid and α-linked again when transferred from this intermediate to the lipid-bound oligosaccharide. On the other hand, the innermost β-linked mannose arises through a direct transfer from the nucleotide donor. In a similar manner, the outer β-linked *N*-acetylglucosamine residue of the GlcNAcβ1→4GlcNAc unit is transferred directly from UDP-GlcNAc, where it is α-linked (reaction 2, fig. 21). The only apparent exception to the rule is the formation of GlcNAc-P-P-lipid (reaction 1, fig. 21) in which the sugar remains α-linked. However, in contrast to the other transfer reactions, this step does not involve the rupture of a sugar 1-phosphate bond. Inversion of configuration of the bond linking the preformed G-oligosaccharide to the P-P-lipid most likely occurs upon the transfer of this unit to the protein acceptor, to form the GlcNAc-β-Asn linkage (reaction 6, fig. 21).

Evidence for the participation of the dolichol phosphate cycle in *N*-glycosylation has been obtained by studies with inhibitors. The most specific of these is tunicamycin, an antibiotic from *Streptomyces lysosuperificus*, that inhibits selectively the transfer of *N*-acetylglucosamine 1-phosphate to dolichol phosphate (reaction 1, fig. 21). Other less specific inhibitors of *N*-glycosylation, such as the antibiotics bacitracin or amphomycin and the mannose analogs 2-deoxyglucose of 2-fluoromannose, also block the formation of the G-oligosaccharide.

Once the G-oligosaccharide is assembled, it is transferred en bloc to the amide of an asparaginyl residue which is part of a sequence Asn-X-Ser/Thr in a growing polypeptide chain (reaction 6, fig. 21). The transfer reaction to protein also seems to be of general occurrence and has been found in a variety of tissues and cells. The requirement of the Asn-X-Ser/Thr sequence for glycosylation implies that the enzyme involved in the formation of the *N*-acetylglucosaminyl–asparaginyl linkage has the same specificity, regardless of the enzyme source, be it hen oviduct, liver plasma cell, thyroid, or even plant or yeast cells. It is also possible that one or more amino acid residues on either side of the Asn-X-Ser/Thr sequence is partly contained in the combining site of the putative transferase, and that the precise nature of these other residues may affect the binding of the enzyme to its substrate.

Most of the information about the transfer of the G-oligosaccharide to protein has been obtained from studies in animals, primarily in cells infected with certain viruses. Such cells serve as excellent material not only for the study of glycoprotein synthesis, but also for membrane assembly and biogenesis. Extremely valuable information has been obtained in experiments with vesicular stomatitis virus and Sindbis virus, which are of the RNA type and have a coat containing only one and two glycoproteins, respectively. As previously mentioned, the vesicular stomatis virus G-protein contains two identical oligosaccharide units of the complex type, whereas in Sindbis virus each of the two glycoproteins carries one complex and one mannose rich oligosaccharide (fig. 12). On infection, protein synthesis of the host cell is suppressed and replaced by that of viral proteins. The biosynthesis of the oligosaccharide moiety is carried out by the glycosyltransferases of the host, since the virus is too small to possess the large amount of genetic information necessary for coding for the many enzymes required in oligosaccharide biosynthesis. However, different viruses growing in the same cells may possess different oligosaccharides. It must therefore be assumed that the structure of the viral carbohydrate is somehow specified by the primary sequence of its polypeptide. In other words, the polypeptide contains information which determines whether it will have at a certain position in the chain a complex oligosaccharide, a mannose-rich one, or none. It is further clear that the same lipid intermediate is the precursor for the biosynthesis of both the oligomannosidic and the complex chains, so that a mechanism must exist for the removal or "trimming" of the glucose and excess mannose residues before attachment of the sugars of the NeuNAc-Gal-GlcNAc to the chains is possible.

Experiments using chick cells infected with vesicular stomatitis virus have shown that the transfer of the G-oligosaccharide to protein is very rapid and can be readily detected within 3–5 min. The presence of two (or three) glucose residues in the preformed lipid linked oligosaccharide is required for efficient transfer of the latter to proteins. Within 3–5 min after transfer, processing of the oligosaccharide begins and by 30 min the three glucose residues have been excised. This is followed by rapid removal of four mannose residues resulting in the formation of a heptasaccharide $Man_5(GlcNAc)_2$ linked to protein (fig. 22). Similar reactions have been observed in other systems, e.g. in Chinese hamster ovary cells infected with vesicular stomatitis virus, in influenza infected cells, as well as in mouse plasmacytoma cells and thyroid slices.

The enzymes involved in the trimming process are under active investigation. The glucose residues of the G-oligosaccharide are hardly affected by the commonly available glucosidases but are removed by a

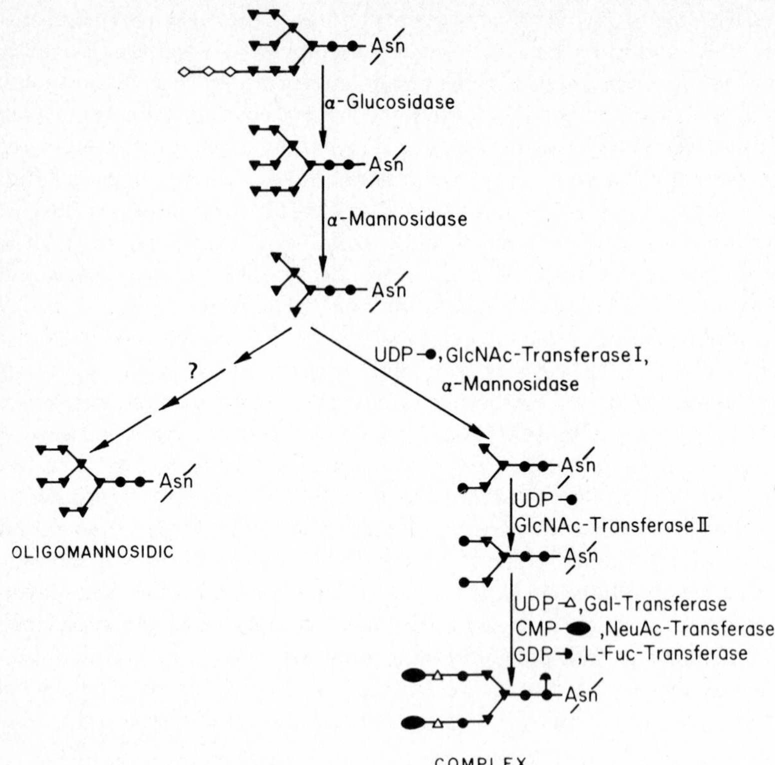

Fig. 22. Trimming and elongation of protein-linked *N*-glycosidic units.

microsomal enzyme. On the other hand, an α-mannosidase active in processing is found in the Golgi fraction.

Conversion of the $Man_5(GlcNAc)_2$ heptasaccharide into the common core pentasaccharide requires the attachment of one of the *N*-acetylglucosamine residues present in the branches of the complex oligosaccharide units. This residue is attached by *N*-acetylglucosaminyltransferase I to the Manα1→3 moiety of the protein linked $Man_5(GlcNAc)_2$. The addition of the first *N*-acetylglucosamine residue controls the entire elongation process. The removal of the two peripheral mannose residues attached to Manα1→6, addition of the second *N*-acetylglucosamine residue to the latter mannose, and of L-fucose, all depend on the action of this enzyme, as does the subsequent addition of galactose and sialic acid to form the completed complex units.

The enzyme which adds the galactose in $\beta 1 \rightarrow 4$ linkage to the peripheral *N*-acetylglucosamine residues attached to the core oligosaccharide is probably the best characterized glycosyltransferase. This galactosyltransferase (fig. 16) is widely distributed in mammalian tissues, and is believed to be related, if not identical, to the A protein of milk lactose synthetase, an enzyme confined to the lactating glands.

Elongation of the *N*-acetyllactosamine units is completed by the addition of sialic acid residues in $\alpha 2 \rightarrow 3$ or $\alpha 2 \rightarrow 6$ linkages to the galactose residues or, occasionally, of L-fucose in $\alpha 2 \rightarrow 3$ linkage to the *N*-acetylglucosamine. The action of the sialyltransferase and L-fucosyltransferase in certain tissues appears to be mutually exclusive (fig. 23).

A recently purified sialyltransferase specific for the formation of $2 \rightarrow 6$ linkages incorporates sialic acid only into acceptors containing the Gal$\beta 1 \rightarrow 4$GlcNAc sequence, and there is evidence that optimal transfer occurs when the *N*-acetylglucosamine residue is in $\alpha 1 \rightarrow 2$ linkage to mannose. Very little is known about the glycosyltransferase that attaches sialic acid to *N*-glycosidic units by the $\alpha 2 \rightarrow 3$ linkage. As mentioned earlier, a transferase has been isolated that incorporates sialic acid into an $\alpha 2 \rightarrow 3$ linkage with galactose in the sequence Gal$\beta 1 \rightarrow 3$-GalNAc (present in *O*-glycosidic units).

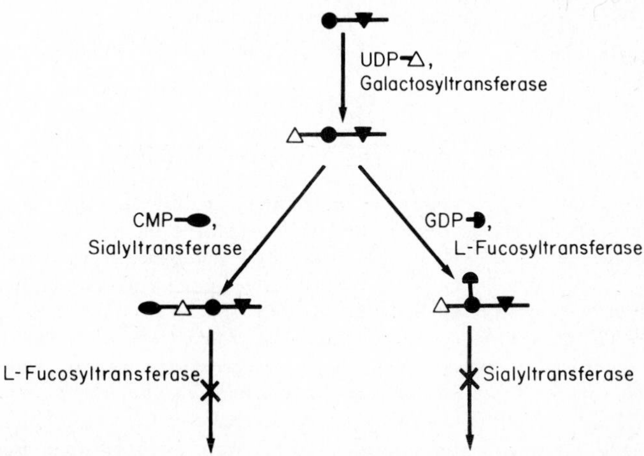

Fig. 23. Mutually exclusive action of sialyltransferase and fucosyltransferase in the biosynthesis of *N*-acetyllactosamine type *N*-glycosidic units [from J. C. Paulson, J. -P. Prieels, L. R. Glasgow and R. L. Hill, J. Biol. Chem. 253 (1978) 5617.]

Glycoproteins may undergo additional modification reactions. These include attachment of phosphate or sulfate residues to the carbohydrate as well as conversion of *N*-acetylneuraminic acid to its various derivatives, e.g. *N*-glycolyl or *N*-acetyl-4-*O*-acetylneuraminic acid.

The extensive studies of Schachter and his coworkers have shown that the *N*-acetylglucosaminyltransferase, L-fucosyltransferase, galactosyltransferase and sialyltransferase described above are highly enriched in the Golgi apparatus of a variety of tissues, and that this subcellular organelle is the major site of elongation. Supportive evidence comes from work in which intact cells were pulsed with radioactive sugars, and the cells were examined by autoradiography or measurements were

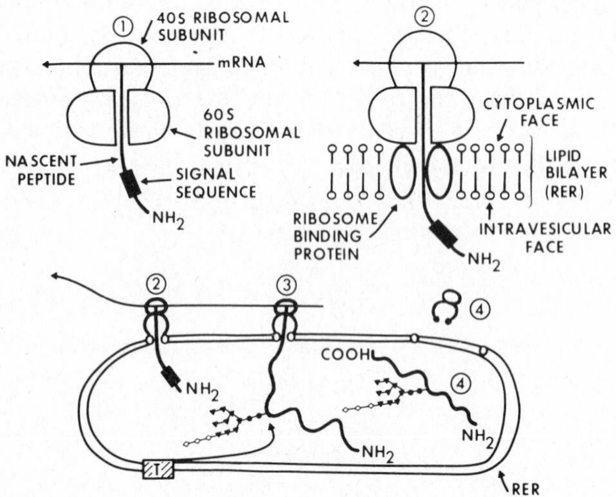

Fig. 24. Schematic representation of biosynthesis and secretion of *N*-glycosylated glycoproteins. (1) Translation begins on free ribosomes with the formation of the signal sequence which serves to direct the free ribosome to the endoplasmic reticulum membrane. (2) The ribosome becomes attached to the rough endoplasmic reticulum (RER) membrane via a putative ribosome-binding protein, which assists in the passage of the nascent peptide through the membrane into the intravesicular space. (3) As the ribosome moves along the mRNA, translation continues and more of the nascent peptide enters the intravesicular space. The signal sequence is probably cleaved off at some stage in assembly. (4) The preformed G-oligosaccharide is transferred from its dolichol carrier to the growing peptide chain. After completion of the latter, the ribosome is released from the endoplasmic reticulum membrane. Trimming (or processing) of the G-oligosaccharide starts with the removal of three glucose and four mannose residues.

made of incorporation of radioactivity into glycoproteins in different subcellular fractions.

Once elongation and sugar modifications are completed within the Golgi apparatus, the finished glycoprotein migrates towards the plasma membrane within a transport vesicle. The vesicle membrane fuses with the plasma membrane. At this stage secretory glycoproteins are extruded from the cell whereas membrane glycoproteins probably become part of the plasma membrane by a lateral diffusion process.

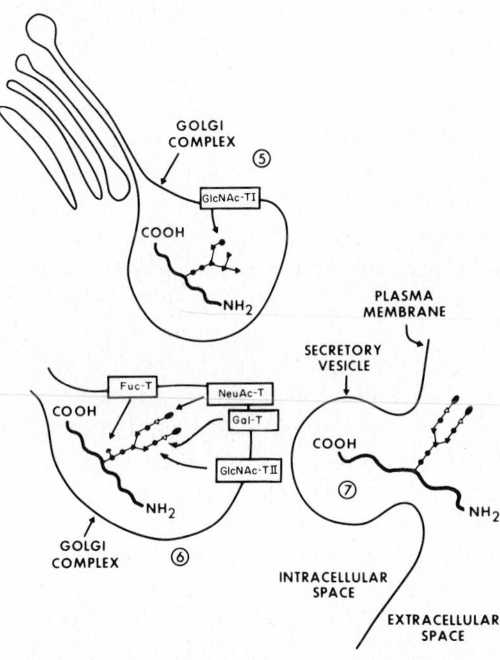

Fig. 24 continued (5) The glycoprotein migrates to the Golgi apparatus, where an *N*-acetylglucosamine residue is attached to the $\alpha 1 \rightarrow 3$ linked mannose by *N*-acetylglucosaminyltransferase I. (6) The two mannose residues attached to the $\alpha 1 \rightarrow 6$ linked mannose are removed and elongation is completed by the action of *N*-acetylglucosaminyltransferase II, galactosyltransferase, sialyltransferase, and L-fucosyltransferase. (7) The mature glycoprotein is carried in a secretary vesicle to the plasma membrane, where fusion of the vesicle with the latter occurs. The glycoprotein is either inserted into the membrane by lateral migration or secreted to the extracellular space. [Modified from H. Schachter, S. Narasimhan and J. R. Wilson, Am. Chem. Soc. Symp. Ser. 80 (1978) 21.]

4.3. Cellular location

Studies of cells infected with vesicular stomatitis virus have provided insight into the temporal and topological relationship between the biosynthesis of the polypeptide chain and the transfer of the G-oligosaccharide from dolichol pyrophosphate to specific asparagine residues. In a cell-free system consisting of the viral mRNA, wheat germ ribosomes, and microsomal membranes from dog pancreas, an intermediate form of the vesicular stomatitis virus glycoprotein (*G*-protein) has been identified. It differs from the mature, completed glycoprotein in that its carbohydrate units are chiefly of the oligomannosidic, instead of the *N*-acetyllactosamine type present in the mature glycoprotein. A similar intermediate has been detected in cells infected with the virus.

Synthesis of the viral protein occurs on polyribosomes (polysomes), although it is apparently initiated on free ribosomes (fig. 24). The attachment of the free ribosomes to the membrane of the endoplasmic reticulum is mediated by a signal sequence which resides within the first thirty *N*-terminal amino acids of the nascent peptide chain. Concomitant with the formation of the polysomes, passage of the peptide begins through the membrane bilayer into the intravesicular space of endoplasmic reticulum. As the ribosome moves along the messenger RNA, translation occurs and more of the nascent peptide enters the intravesicular space. Transfer of preformed oligosaccharide units from the lipid intermediate to the asparagine residues occurs probably very soon after the latter emerge on the lumen side of the endoplasmic reticulum. Sometime during the synthesis the signal sequence may be cleaved by a peptidase designated as "signalase".

In the absence of endoplasmic reticulum membranes, translation of the viral messenger RNA is completed but the resulting protein has no carbohydrate and the signal sequence is retained. The completed glycoprotein is synthesized only if endoplasmic reticulum membrane is added before the first 70 amino acids have been polymerized. It has been suggested that at a later stage of synthesis part of the polypeptide chain will already have folded in the cytoplasm and will be unable to interact with the endoplasmic reticulum membrane or to cross the permeability barrier of the lipid bilayer. If the endoplasmic reticulum membrane is disrupted by detergents after 150 amino acid residues, but before all 500 have been polymerized, the resulting protein is an intermediate form never observed in nature, with just one carbohydrate chain. The formation of the novel intermediate provides strong evidence that the carbohydrate units of the glycoprotein are added in sequence, as the polypeptide passes through the endoplasmic reticulum (fig. 24).

In vivo, the glycoprotein then migrates to the Golgi apparatus where trimming and elongation reactions (discussed earlier) are taking place, and then to the plasma membrane.

Studies of the biosynthesis of glycophorin A in a continuous leukemic cell line have indicated a pathway resembling that described above for the biosynthesis of viral membrane glycoproteins. Using antibodies specific for glycophorin A, an incompletely glycosylated precursor, with an apparent molecular weight close to that of the completed glycophorin, was detected in a microsomal fraction, indicating that in this system, too, glycosylation starts in the endoplasmic reticulum when the polypeptide is still ribosome-bound. The precursor bound to immobilized lentil lectin (specific for mannose and glucose) but not to *Ricinus communis* lectins (specific for galactose), and did not contain sialic acid, from which it was concluded that the precursor already contains a part of the *N*-glycosidic chain located at the asparagine in position 26 of the peptide backbone. Comparison of the apparent molecular weights (as estimated by SDS-gel electrophoresis) of the precursor, of asialoglycophorin and of glycophorin suggested that the precursor contains the *O*-glycosidically linked *N*-acetylgalactosamine residues as well, which is in agreement with the finding that initial *O*-glycosylation of a rat epithelial mucin also occurs at the ribosomal level. Whether the glycophorin precursor contains an additional NH_2-terminal signal sequence which is found in most glycoprotein precursors is not known.

Soluble glycoproteins, both secretory and cytoplasmic, are probably synthesized like membrane glycoproteins, *N*-glycosylation occurring cotranslationally on nascent chains.

5. Organization

Generalizations about the structure of membrane glycoproteins and their organization in the membrane bilayer (fig. 1) are based on limited data, primarily studies of the human erythrocyte, of enveloped viruses and to some extent also of lymphocytes. Integral membrane glycoproteins, such as glycophorin and the histocompatibility antigens (as well as non-glycosylated membrane proteins) are amphiphatic molecules, containing a hydrophobic sequence which interacts strongly with the lipid bilayer. The carbohydrate units are often clustered near one end of the molecule, and this hydrophilic portion is exposed on the external side of the plasma membrane (or at the inner face, opposite the cytoplasmic face, of intracellular membranes). Thus, carbohydrates show an asymmetrical distribution across the membrane bilayer, as do the lipid constituents of the two halves of the bilayer. Indeed, asymmetry is one of the key features of membranes.

At least some of the intrinsic glycoproteins pass all the way through the bilayer, i.e. they span the membrane, so that they are exposed to both the external and internal environment. The internal segments of such intrinsic glycoproteins (and proteins) may be closely associated with some of the extrinsic proteins at the cytoplasmic face of the membrane. The transmembrane glycoproteins may thus provide a means of communication across the bilayer, either for the transport of solutes and water, or for the transmission of signals in response to external stimuli, such as hormones, antibodies, or other cells.

5.1. Human erythrocyte membrane

The asymmetry of distribution of the carbohydrate units is particularly striking in glycophorin which comprises between 5–10% of the weight of the human erythrocyte membrane, each cell having about 500 000 molecules of the glycoprotein.

Glycophorin (fig. 25), extensively investigated by Marchesi and his coworkers, consists of a polypeptide chain of 131 amino acids, which comprises about 40% of the mass of the molecule. Sixteen carbohydrate units are attached to the polypeptide. Fifteen of the units are *O*-glycosidically linked to serine or threonine residues, and one is *N*-glycosidic. All the carbohydrate is found in the first 50 residues of the *N*-terminal portion of the glycoprotein; the carbohydrate distribution is especially dense at the extreme *N*-terminus, where each of the residues from 2 to 4 and 10 to 15 carries one *O*-glycosidic unit.

Another striking feature of the glycophorin molecule is the high concentration of non-polar amino acids located roughly midway between the amino terminal third of the polypeptide chain and the carboxy-terminal third. On the basis of a variety of labelling studies, it has been suggested that the amino acids extending from residue 71 to residue 90 may be the segment of glycophorin buried within the lipid bilayer of the membrane. This peptide, which can be produced by tryptic digestion of the soluble glycophorin, is insoluble in aqueous buffers but can be solubilized in both non-ionic and ionic detergents.

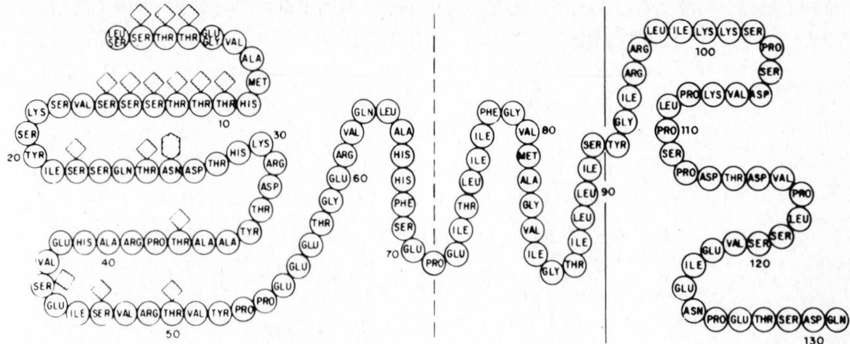

Fig. 25. The amino acids of glycophorin arranged to simulate, in a very general way, the positions they might have if the glycophorin molecule were arranged perpendicularly to the lipid bilayer of the membrane. Limits of the bilayer are defined by the two vertical lines; the solid vertical line, which passes between residues 92 and 93, should be the approximate location of the polar groups of the inner half of the phospholipid bilayer. [From V. T. Marchesi, Seminars in Hematology 16 (1979) 3.]

Under the latter conditions the peptide has an α-helical conformation. Indeed, this segment of the glycophorin polypeptide contains almost all of the α-helical content of the intact glycophorin. It is therefore likely that this hydrophobic portion may be in an α-helical conformation when the glycophorin molecules are embedded within the intact membrane of the human erythrocyte. There is a considerable amount of experimental data in support of the idea that glycophorin is a transmembrane glycoprotein (fig. 26). Thus, incubation of erythrocytes with trypsin removes from their surface the first 30–40 residues of glycophorin, together with the bulk of the carbohydrate. Lectins, such as wheat germ agglutinin (which probably interacts with the sialic acid residues of glycophorin), bind only to the outer surface of the human erythrocyte membranes. Also, glycophorin is radioactively labelled in intact erythrocytes by periodate-NaB^3H_4 or after removal of its sialic acid residues by galactose oxidase-NaB^3H_4; no increase in labelling is observed upon similar treatment of erythrocyte ghosts (or inside-out membranes) which are permeable to these reagents. Experiments with non-permeating protein labelling reagents, such as ^{35}S-formylmethionylsulfate, methyl phosphate, or lactoperoxidase catalysed iodination, have shown that in intact cells only the *N*-terminal part of the glycophorin is labeled, whereas when the cells are made permeable to these reagents, the C-terminal end is also labelled.

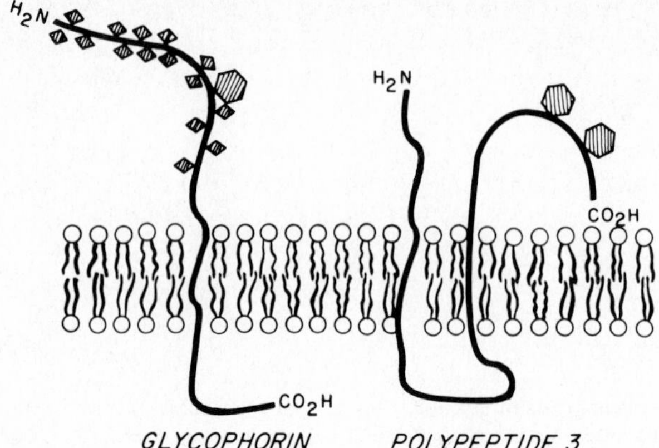

Fig. 26. A schematic representation of the arrangement of glycophorin and polypeptide 3 in the membrane of the human erythrocyte, according to V. T. Marchesi and M. J. A. Tanner, respectively. ◇ - *O*-glycosidic units; ⬡ - *N*-glycosidic units.

The application of immunocytochemical techniques has provided conclusive evidence for the transmembrane orientation of glycophorin. These experiments employed antibodies against a peptide fragment consisting of 17 amino acids from the C-terminal end of the glycophorin molecule (residues 102–118). Ferritin conjugates of the antibodies bound exclusively to sites distributed uniformly along the inner surfaces of frozen sections of intact erythrocyte membranes.

Another erythrocyte membrane glycoprotein which is under active investigation is polypeptide 3 (Band III), which mediates anion movements across the membrane. This glycoprotein appears as a diffuse band on SDS-gel electrophoresis and migrates as if it had a molecular weight of approximately 90 000. There are reasons to believe that the diffuse electrophoretic mobility of polypeptide 3 may be due at least in part to carbohydrate heterogeneity (see earlier discussion).

Polypeptide 3 has been isolated and purified in several laboratories and found to contain approximately 5–8% carbohydrate on a weight basis. The carbohydrate is composed of mannose, galactose, and *N*-acetylglucosamine in the approximate ratios of 1:2:2; in addition, traces of fucose and glucose are frequently found. This composition suggests that the oligosaccharides attached to polypeptide 3 contain *N*-glycosidic units of the complex type.

The primary structure of polypeptide 3 is not known, and there is still some question as to whether it is composed of one or several polypeptide chains. The protein is comprised of three distinct molecular domains, which include an external segment of approximately 35 000 Daltons, and a cytoplasmic segment of approximately 40 000 Daltons. This general picture has been developed as a result of an elegant series of experiments employing differential enzymatic digestions and radiolabelling of various red cell membrane preparations, principally by Steck and his coworkers. These investigators showed that incubation of intact red cells with chymotrypsin results in the production of a 38 000 Dalton peptide that seems to be exposed on the external surface of the lipid bilayer and a 55 000 Dalton fragment that remains embedded in the membrane. The 55 000 Dalton piece can be further degraded into 41 000 Dalton and 23 000 Dalton peptide by mild tryptic digestion and specific chemical cleavage, respectively. It has also been found that the 23 000 Dalton peptide is derived from the *N*-terminal end of polypeptide 3. The latter finding indicates that polypeptide 3 has a transmembrane orientation essentially opposite to that of glycophorin in that glycophorin has its *N*-terminal end external to the lipid bilayer while polypeptide 3 appears to have its *N*-terminus on the cytoplasmic side of the membrane. Polypeptide 3 also has a considerably larger amount of its polypeptide segment situated on the cytoplasmic side of the cell membrane. This view is, however, at variance with that of Tanner and his coworkers. According to the latter, polypeptide 3 spans the membrane at least twice, so that both its termini are on the outer surface of the cell (fig. 26).

5.2. *Viral envelopes*

Apart from the human erythrocyte, little is known about the structure and organization of glycoproteins in surface membranes of most other cells. Considerable information has, however, accumulated on the structure of viral envelopes, that share many properties with other biological membranes. Because of their structural simplicity, such envelopes are very suitable models for membrane research. All these viruses (e.g. influenza virus, vesicular stomatitis virus and Semliki Forest virus) have a lipid bilayer membrane with glycoprotein projections (or spikes) that envelope their internal nucleocapsid, in which the viral nucleic acid is located.

A well studied example is the Semliki Forest virus. This virus is a spherical particle with a diameter of about 65 nm; it contains about 240 spike-like glycoprotein projections on its membrane. Each spike is 7–10 nm long and is composed of three glycopolypeptides: E1 (mol wt

49 000), E2 (mol wt 52 000), and E3 (mol wt 10 000). The viral nucleocapsid consists of one RNA molecule (mol wt 4.5×10^6), which is complexed with about 240 copies of a basic protein (mol wt 30 000).

The location of the viral glycoproteins in the lipid bilayer has been studied by digesting the external portions of the glycoproteins with a protease and then analysing their membrane-bound fragments. SDS-acrylamide electrophoresis showed that three fragments with molecular weights ranging from 9 000 to 5 000 remained in the membrane of protease-treated Semliki Forest virus. With virus in which the polypeptides had been labeled with a gradient of radioactivity increasing towards their C-termini, it was possible to ascribe two of the fragments to the C-terminal portion of the E2 glycoprotein and one to the C-terminus of the E1 glycoprotein. Amino acid analyses of these fragments showed that they contained a high proportion of non-polar amino acids. Thus, the C-termini of both E1 and E2 glycoproteins have a hydrophobic nature and they attach the glycoproteins to the lipid bilayer of the virus. The third glycoprotein, E3, does not interact with the viral lipid bilayer, and appears to be attached to the outer region of the E1 and/or the E2 glycoprotein (fig. 27).

The C-terminus of the E2 glycoprotein spans the lipid bilayer of the virus, and a small segment of it, approximately 30 amino acids, is located on the internal side of the membrane. This has been shown in several ways. Firstly, it is possible to covalently link the major part of the glycoprotein to the underlying nucleocapsid by treating virus particles with protein–protein crosslinking reagents such as dimethyl suberimidate of dithiobispropionimidate. Since these reagents can link proteins within a range of only about 10 Å (which corresponds to one-quarter of the bilayer thickness), the spanning parts of the membrane glycoprotein must be crosslinked to the nucleocapsid. Secondly, if the viral membranes are lysed with small amounts of the non-ionic detergent Triton X-100, parts of the E2 glycoprotein can be detected on the internal side of the viral envelope by surface-labelling techniques. Thirdly, it is possible to solubilize all lipids from the virus particles without removing the glycoprotein spikes by using the anionic detergent octylglycoside.

6. Function

Since biologically-active glycoproteins are so widely distributed in nature, and all cells come in a sugar coating, it is pertinent to ask what are the functions of sugars in glycoproteins and on cell surfaces. The search

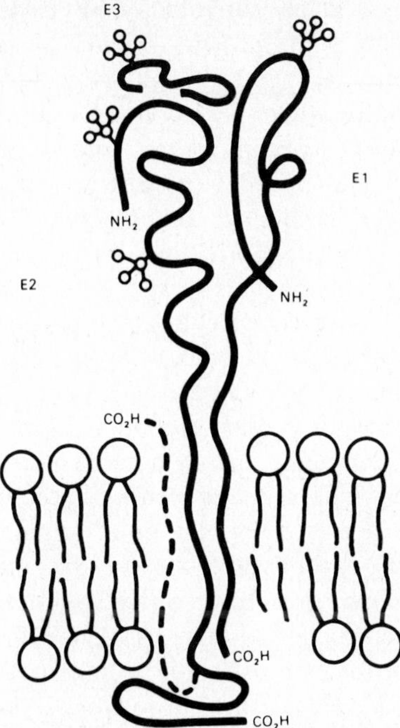

Fig. 27. Topography of glycoproteins in the membrane of Semliki Forest virus. The C-termini of the E1 and the E2 glycoproteins attach these proteins to the lipid bilayer. The E2 protein spans the membrane. The dashed line indicates that the C-terminus of E2 may loop back to the external membrane surface. The E3 glycoprotein is not attached to the lipid bilayer. The three glycoproteins form E1-E2-E3 complexes in the viral membrane. Two carbohydrate units are attached to the E2 polypeptide and one of each of the E1 and E3 polypeptides. [From H. Garoff, Biochem. Soc. Trans. 7 (1979) 301.]

for an answer to this intriguing question is further motivated by the belief that every structure in nature must have a function, otherwise it would not have persisted throughout evolution. In this context, it is important to bear in mind that glycosylation of proteins is an expensive operation for an organism to carry out, since it requires a large amount of genetic information and the production of many enzymes, cofactors and intermediates.

6.1. Soluble glycoproteins

Carbohydrates in soluble glycoproteins appear to act in a variety of ways. In particular, they may modify the physicochemical properties of proteins by changing their hydrophobicity, electrical charge, mass, and size. The conformation of the protein is generally not affected, as long as the carbohydrate content is not high. However, carbohydrate rich glycoproteins, especially when they contain considerable amounts of sialic acid, may acquire special conformations. Salivary mucins, for example, have an extended rod like structure, by virtue of the high density of negatively charged sialic acid residues. Similarly, the first 15 *N*-terminal residues of glycophorin that carry 9 sialic acid-containing oligosaccharides (fig. 25) may also exist in a rod-like structure. The carbohydrate, however, rarely affects the biological activities of proteins, whether as catalysts, hormones, carriers, lectins, interferons, etc. Furthermore, contrary to an earlier suggestion, glycosylation is not generally a prerequisite for protein secretion. In most glycoproteins the carbohydrate is not immunogenic; a notable exception are the blood group substances, in which sugar sequences at the non-reducing end of carbohydrate chains act as determinants of immunological specificity. Last, but not least, carbohydrates serve as important recognition markers on glycoproteins in solution as well as on cell surfaces.

Recently it has been suggested that the carbohydrate may function in directing the protein to its most stable conformation. Yeast invertase from which more than 90% of the carbohydrate has been removed by endo-β-*N*-acetylglucosaminidase regained its activity at a markedly slower rate after denaturation in guanidine hydrochloride than the fully glycosylated enzyme. Moreover, fluorescence as well as circular dichroism measurements of the two forms of the enzyme after renaturation revealed differences in their conformations.

It has been known for a long time that glycoproteins, particularly if they are sugar rich, are more resistant to proteolysis *in vitro* than non-glycosylated proteins. Recent studies of the effect of tunicamycin on glycoprotein synthesis have led to the conclusion that the carbohydrate protects proteins also against proteolysis *in vivo*, in the course of their biosynthesis. Non-glycosylated fibronectin synthesized in chick embryo fibroblasts in the presence of tunicamycin was degraded intracellularly at a much faster rate than the glycosylated protein. Inhibition of the formation of mature Semliki Forest and fowl plague viruses in the presence of the antibiotic was ascribed to proteolysis of the non-glycosylated precursor proteins, since at least one of these (the sugar-free precursor of fowl plague virus hemagglutinin) was detected in the tunicamycin treated cells when a specific trypsin inhibitor was included in the growth medium.

A mutant (Orsay) of vesicular stomatitis virus has been described in which assembly of non-glycosylated enveloped protein occurs at 30° but not at 38°. It has been suggested that the non-glycosylated protein retains its conformation only at the lower temperatures, whereas at the high temperature glycosylation is required to stabilize the molecule. On the other hand, non-glycosylated forms of vesicular stomatitis virus and of Sindbis virus proteins synthesized in the presence of tunicamycin were metabolically stable. However, the proteins could not be detected on the host cell surface at any stage during the process of infection.

It has indeed been reported that inhibition of glycosylation prevented the migration of viral glycoproteins from the rough endoplasmic reticulum to the smooth intracellular membranes and their insertion into the outer membrane of the infected cell. Strong inhibition of immunoglobulin secretion was also observed in certain cells. This, however, is not a general phenomenon, as in many other cells there was no inhibition of protein secretion in the absence of glycosylation.

The role of carbohydrate as recognition markers has been best demonstrated in the control of the lifetime of serum glycoproteins in the circulatory system and their uptake into liver cells, as well as for the uptake of lysosomal enzymes by fibroblasts.

The classical work of Ashwell and Morell has demonstrated that removal of sialic acid from circulating glycoproteins by sialidase leads to a dramatic enhancement in the rate of their clearance from the circulatory system of rabbits (fig. 28), rats , and mice. The removal of as

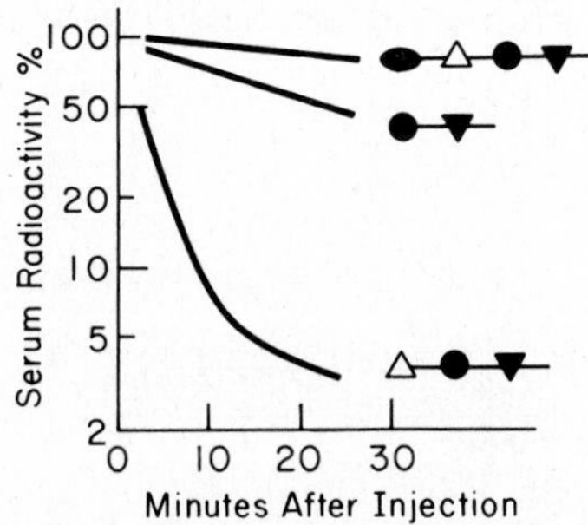

Fig. 28. Disappearance from rabbit serum of radioactively labelled ceruloplasmin (top curve), asialoceruloplasmin (bottom) and asialoagalactoceruloplasmin (middle). The symbols denote the structure of the terminal nonreducing part of the native and modified glycoprotein. [Redrawn from data of G. Ashwell and A. G. Morell, Adv. Enzymol. 41 (1974) 99.]

few as two sialic acid residues per molecule of ceruloplasmin (out of a total of about ten) is sufficient to reduce the halflife of the glycoprotein in circulation from 54 h to 3–5 min. The asialoglycoproteins are rapidly taken up and catabolized by the liver. Uptake depends on the recognition by the liver cells of exposed galactose residues on the glycoprotein. Treatment of the desialylated glycoproteins with β-galactosidase or galactose oxidase abolishes this recognition and considerably extends the time they remain in the circulatory system, as does replacement of the missing sialic acid with the aid of sialyltransferase. A glycoprotein that binds specifically asialoglycoproteins has been isolated from rat liver membranes and has been designated as the hepatic (carbohydrate-) binding protein. It exhibits lectin activity in that it agglutinates human and rabbit erythrocytes and acts as a mitogen on sialidase-treated lymphocytes; both activities are inhibited by galactose and its derivatives. Binding of asialoglycoproteins, agglutination of erythrocytes and mitogenic stimulation of lymphocytes, appear to involve interaction with the same combining sites of the hepatic binding protein.

Clearance systems in which sugars other than galactose serve as determinants have also been identified and in some cases the specific carbohydrate binding proteins have been isolated (table 6).

A different system in which carbohydrates on soluble glycoproteins serve as determinants of recognition is that responsible for the intercellular segregation and selective pinocytosis of certain lysosomal glycosidases by fibroblasts. Such pinocytosis was initially observed in studies of the uptake of "corrective factors" by enzyme-deficient human fibroblasts taken from patients with different mucopolysaccharidoses (e.g. the Hurler and Hunter syndromes); the "corrective factors" were

Table 6

Clearance of glycoproteins from the circulatory system into the liver of different animals

Marker	Animal	Lectin isolated
Galactose	Rabbit	+
	Rat	+
Mannose/*N*-acetyl-glucosamine	Chicken	+
	Rabbit	+
	Rat	+
L-fucose	Mouse	–

later identified as the hydrolases missing in the deficient cells. The kinetics of uptake of the different lysosomal hydrolases display saturability and selectivity expected of a receptor-mediated process. For example, selectivity for β-glucuronidase uptake was evident from the fact that only certain relatively acidic forms of the enzyme, called "high-uptake" forms, were taken up by rates that greatly exceeded the rate of non-specific endocytosis. Direct proof of binding of a lysosomal enzyme, α-L-iduronidase, to receptors on cultured fibroblasts has recently been obtained.

Several hydrolases, all glycoproteins, that are not pinocytosed selectively are secreted by fibroblasts from patients with the I-cell disease, that are homzygous for a single gene mutation. To explain the molecular basis of this defect, it was proposed by Neufeld that the normal lysosomal hydrolases have a common recognition marker which is essential for their uptake by fibroblasts and that the marker is absent or cryptic in I-cell disease patients. Since periodate treatment destroyed the capacity of the normal enzymes to be taken up by the cells (without affecting their catalytic activity) it was further postulated that the recognition marker is a carbohydrate. The marker has now been identified as mannose-6-phosphate. This was first suggested on the basis of studies with β-glucuronidase, in which it was demonstrated that the uptake of this enzyme was competitively inhibited by low concentrations of mannose-6-phosphate, as well as by yeast mannans containing this sugar. In addition, treatment of the enzyme with alkaline phosphatase decreased its uptake while its catalytic activity remained unimpaired. Similar results were obtained for the uptake of several other lysosomal hydrolases, such as β-*N*-acetylglucosaminidase and α-L-iduronidase.

Recent work has shown that β-*N*-acetylglucosaminidase produced by normal fibroblasts is phosphorylated, whereas the same enzyme synthesized by I-cells is not, and that the mannose-6-phosphate residues of α-*N*-acetylglucosaminidase and of β-glucuronidase are present in *N*-glycosidic side chains of the high-mannose type. Moreover, the rate of uptake of the various forms of the latter enzyme that were separated by ion exchange chromatography, varied directly with their content of mannose-6-phosphate. Mannose-6-phosphate has also been found in a bovine testicular glycoprotein that is a powerful inhibitor of β-galactosidase uptake by I-cell disease skin fibroblasts.

The biological role of the mannose-6-phosphate specific system has not yet been ascertained. It was believed for some time that the system functions in directing the migration of lysosomal enzymes from their synthetic sites in the endoplasmic reticulum to the outside of the cell and their re-entry by uptake by specific pinocytosis, either into the same cell or into neighbouring cells. It now appears that this secretion-recapture pathway is only of minor importance in the life cycle of lysosomal enzymes. Thus, attempts to interfere with this putative pathway by, for example, the addition to normal cultured fibroblasts of mannose-6-phosphate or of antibodies to α-L-iduronidase failed to deplete the cells of their lysosomal enzymes nor did it lead to extracellular accumulation of the latter. It seems, therefore, more likely that the recognition marker functions mainly as an intracellular traffic signal to prevent enzyme secretion and to direct the acid hydrolases to lysosomes (fig. 29).

It has been further suggested that the recognition marker also affects processing of oligosaccharide chains on acid hydrolases, since most

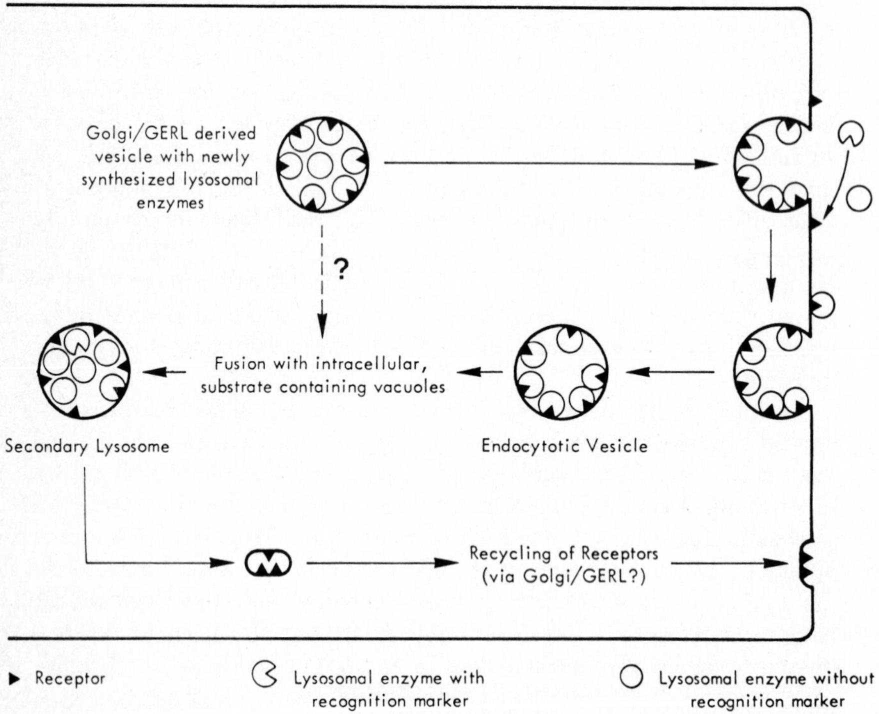

Fig. 29. Life cycle of a lysosomal enzyme (GERL = Golgi endoplasmic reticulum). (Courtesy of K. von Figura.)

enzymes secreted by I-cells contain *N*-glycosidic units of the *N*-acetyllactosamine type, in contrast to the normal enzymes that are rich in oligomannosidic chains. In its absence, as in I-cell disease, the enzymes remain soluble, are processed in the Golgi complex (where *N*-acetyllactosamine-type chains are synthesized) and secreted.

6.2. Cell surface carbohydrates

A variety of approaches are being employed to investigate the role of cell surface sugars in recognition phenomena, either in cell–molecule, cell–virus, or cell–cell interactions (tables 7, 8). Most of these cannot, however, distinguish between cell surface oligosaccharides that are part of glycoproteins, and those that are attached to lipids. This is one of the main reasons why there is hardly any single biological activity or function of cell surface sugars that can at present be ascribed to a specific membrane glycoprotein.

The finding, some 30 years ago, that agglutination of human erythrocytes by influenza virus is abolished by treatment of the cells with sialidase was the first demonstration that cell surface sugars may serve as attachment sites for viruses. This conclusion was strengthened when it was found that agglutination is inhibited by very low concentrations of sialoglycoproteins and that the latter lose their inhibitory activity upon desialylation. Final proof was obtained very recently by

Table 7
Methods for studying biological roles of cell surface sugars

Method	Systems investigated
Hapten inhibition	Lectin-cell Bacteria-epithelial cell
Modification of cell surface sugars	Blood group determinants Virus-cell Lymphocyte stimulation by periodate, galactose oxidase
Interaction with membrane constituents	Toxin-cell Hormone-cell Interferon-cell
Biological changes in cell surface sugars or lectins	Slime mold aggregation
Inhibitors of *N*-glycosylation	Embryonal development

Table 8
Recognition of cell surface sugars by biologically active agents

Agent	Sugar determinant
Fibronectin	NeuNAc-Gal-GlcNAc-Gal
Lectins	
Concanavalin A, lentil lectin	Man, Glc
Peanut agglutinin	Galβ1$\rightarrow$3GalNAc
Lima bean and soybean agglutinins	GalNAc
Limulin, wheat germ agglutinin	NeuNAc
Potato and wheat germ agglutinins	$(GlcNAc)_{1-3}$
Lymphokines	
Interferon	NeuNAc-Gal-GalNAc
Leukocyte inhibitory factor	GlcNAc
Migration inhibitory factor	L-Fuc
Toxins	
Abrin, ricin	Gal
Botulinus, cholera, tetanus	$(NeuNAc)_{0,1}$-Gal-GalNAc
Viruses	
Influenza, Sendai	NeuNAc

the demonstration that enzymatic attachment of sialic acid to asialoerythrocytes restores their ability to be agglutinated by the virus.

Several lines of evidence, including the use of lectins, glycosidases, and glycosyltransferases have proven beyond doubt that sugars are the immunodeterminants of the blood type specific ABH antigens on human erythrocytes (table 9). As early as 1953, it was shown, by Morgan and Watkins, that *N*-acetylgalactosamine specifically inhibited type A specific lectins from *Vicia cracca* and lima bean; they concluded that this sugar serves as a determinant of human blood group A specificity. Similarly, the agglutination of group O cells by the type H(O)-specific lectins from eel serum and the seeds of *Lotus tetragonolobus*, was best inhibited by methyl α-L-fucoside, indicating that the α-L-fucosyl residue is a determinant of H(O) specificity. These conclusions have been fully substantiated in subsequent studies both of the soluble blood group substances (see earlier section) and of erythrocytes. For example, treatment of blood type B erythrocytes with α-galactosidase leads to a loss of the B activity, which can be restored by enzymatic reattachment of the α-galactosyl residues. Furthermore, if instead of α-galactosyl residues, α-*N*-acetylgalactosamine residues are attached to the α-galactosidase treated cells, blood type A activity appears. Other blood group determinants, such as those belonging to the P and I/i type are also specified by sugars (table 9).

The ABH activity is present both in glycolipids, primarily of high molecular weight (macro- or megalolipids) and in polypeptide 3, but contrary to earlier claims not in glycophorin. It is likely that the same, or closely related, glycolipids and glycoproteins also carry the blood type I/i activity.

The contribution of sugars to human blood type M and N specificities is apparently less direct. The action of sialidase on blood type M or N erythrocytes leads to the loss of this blood type specificity, and reattachment of sialic acid by sialyltransferase results in regeneration of the original activity. In this system, however, it seems impossible to convert type M erythrocytes into N erythrocytes, or vice versa. Since glycophorin carries the M and N determinants and glycophorins from M and N individuals differ in the amino acids present in positions 1 and 5 of their sequence, the suggestion was made that the M and N specificities are determined by the structure of both the carbohydrate and the polypeptide of glycophorin. It should be noted, however, that the physiological role of the various blood group substances, either in soluble form or on erythrocytes, is completely obscure. They are certainly not required for the well-being of humans, since individuals lacking the ABO or MN blood types are known.

Inhibition by low concentrations of specific monosaccharides of the various effects of lectins on cells (primarily agglutination and lymphocyte stimulation) provides the best evidence that cell surface sugars serve as receptors for lectins (table 8). This is further supported by the

Table 9

Blood group determinants on human erythrocytes specified by sugars

Blood group	Sugar immunodeterminant
A	GalNAcα1→3
B	Galα1→3
H	Fucα1→2
Le^a	Fucα1→4
Le^b	Fucα1→2, Fucα1→4
P_1	Galα1→4
i	. . . Galβ1→4GlcNAc . . .
I	GlcNAcβ1→6 \| . . . Galβ1→4GlcNAc . . .
MN	NeuNAcα2→3, 6

demonstration that treatment of lymphocytes by sialidase, β-galactosidase, and galactose oxidase affects their response to specific lectins (table 10). The receptors for lectins may also be either glycoproteins or glycolipids, or both. Thus, glycophorin is a receptor for some lectins (e.g. wheat germ agglutinin, phytohemagglutinin, and *Ricinus communis* agglutinin) and asialoglycophorin is a receptor for peanut agglutinin; moreover, partial proteolysis of the human erythrocyte cell surface markedly diminishes its interaction with some of these lectins. On the other hand, exhaustively proteolysed human erythrocytes bind other lectins (e.g. soybean agglutinin), as do liposomes containing membrane glycolipids. Whether glycoproteins or glycolipids are the predominant receptor depends both on the lectin and on the cells. An interesting case is that of cold agglutinin MKV, an immunoglobulin with lectin-like properties, which is specific for sialic acid. Based on the finding that both human and dog erythrocytes are agglutinated by the cold agglutinin MKV, but only the agglutination of the former is diminished by treatment of the cells with ficin, it was suggested that the receptors for the agglutinin on human cells are sialoglycoproteins whereas on dog cells they are sialoglycolipids.

The specific inhibition of the action of toxic lectins and of lymphokines by simple sugars and of the action of bacterial toxins by gangliosides has led to the conclusion that binding to cell surface sugars is the initial event in this action. The effects of glycoprotein hormones, too, are inhibited by gangliosides, albeit only at high concentrations and

Table 10

Effects of enzymatic modification of lymphocyte surface sugars on their response to mitogens

	Mitogen			
Surface carbohydrate	SBA, PNA	Periodate	Galactose oxidase	Con A
●—△—●—▼	−	+	−	+
↓ Sialidase				
△—●—▼	+	−	+	+
↓ β-Galactosidase				
●—▼	−	−	−	+

under unphysiological conditions, casting some doubt on the proposal that cell surface sugars are receptors for these ligands.

In analogy to the role of carbohydrates on the survival of glycoproteins in the circulating system, sugars on cell surfaces may be important in determining the life span of circulating cells and their distribution in specific organs in the body. This was first demonstrated with rat lymphocytes treated with a glycosidase preparation from *Clostridium perfringens*. While untreated cells homed to the spleen, enzyme treated lymphocytes upon reinjection migrated to the liver instead.

The correlation between decreased sialic acid content, electrophoretic mobility, and the age of erythrocytes in circulation has given rise to the hypothesis that the decrease in sialic acid is correlated with the physiological mechanism of erythrocyte senescence and thereby is the signal responsible for the removal of the older erythrocytes from circulation. This hypothesis seemed to be further substantiated by the finding that enzymatic removal *in vitro* of sialic acid from erythrocytes resulted in a drastic shortening of their life span upon reinjection into circulation, as well as in an enhancement of erythrocyte phagocytosis by peritoneal macrophages *in vitro*. Thus, human erythrocytes which normally persist in the circulatory system for 120 days, are absorbed within hours and phagocytosed by liver Kupffer cells and by spleen macrophages after treatment with sialidase.

Upon ageing, however, there is a gradual loss not only of sialic acid but of equimolar amounts of other carbohydrates as well, indicating that whole carbohydrate chains are eliminated, rather than sialic acid alone. Moreover, treatment of desialylated erythrocytes with galactose oxidase did not increase their life span in the circulatory system. Also, peanut agglutinin, a lectin that interacts with desialylated human erythrocytes, did not bind to old erythrocytes. It seems therefore unlikely that exposure of subterminal galactosyl residues alone, is the physiological factor responsible for the removal of senescent erythrocytes from the circulatory system. Rather, it is possible that sialic acid protects the erythrocytes from clearance and sequestration not by covering an internal galactose marker, but by preventing the binding of immunoglobulins and the subsequent uptake into macrophages mediated by the Fc receptor.

Intercellular adhesion, whether homotypic or heterotypic, is a crucial step in key processes such as fertilization, cellular differentiation and organogenesis on the one hand and host-parasite relationships on the other. There are ample indications for the role of cell surface sugars in such adhesion (table 11). Most of the evidence for this concept is, however, circumstantial, despite the voluminous literature on the subject.

It is well established that there are pronounced changes in cell surface sugars during cell growth, differentiation and oncogenesis, as demonstrated chiefly by studies with lectins and glycosidases. For example, many but not all transformed cell lines are agglutinated by much lower concentrations of lectins than the parental normal cell lines, although the number of lectin receptors remains essentially unchanged. On the other hand, changes in the number of lectin receptors, in particular for peanut agglutinin, have been found during lymphocyte maturation in mouse and man (fig. 30). The functions of these and most other sugar markers of lymphocyte subpopulations are not known. One attractive possibility is that the specific acquisition of components at the cell surface occurring during differentiation affects cell location by providing surface receptors for interaction with certain tissues, for example in the thymus cortex. Other surface sugars may be required for cell activation or cooperation in the immune system.

Attempts have been made to assess the role of cell surface sugars in embryonal development by examining the effect of tunicamycin on this process. It was found that tunicamycin at concentrations that completely block *N*-glycosylation prevented sea urchin embryogenesis and gastrulation, as well as several other stages of development. Tunicamycin also caused dramatic and specific changes in the morphology of

Table 11

Cell surface sugars in intercellular adhesion and recognition

Cells	System	Sugar	Lectin
Bacteria	Adhesion to animal cells	Man, L-Fuc	+
Brown algae	Fertilization	Man, L-Fuc	
Sea urchin	Fertilization		+
Sea urchin, embryo	Aggregation	Gal	
Slime molds	Cohesive aggregation	Gal, GalNAc	+
Sponge	Aggregation	GlcUA[a]	+
Teratocarcinoma	Intercellular adhesion	$(Man)_n$	
Yeast	Mating	Man?	

[A]GlcUA = glucuronic acid.

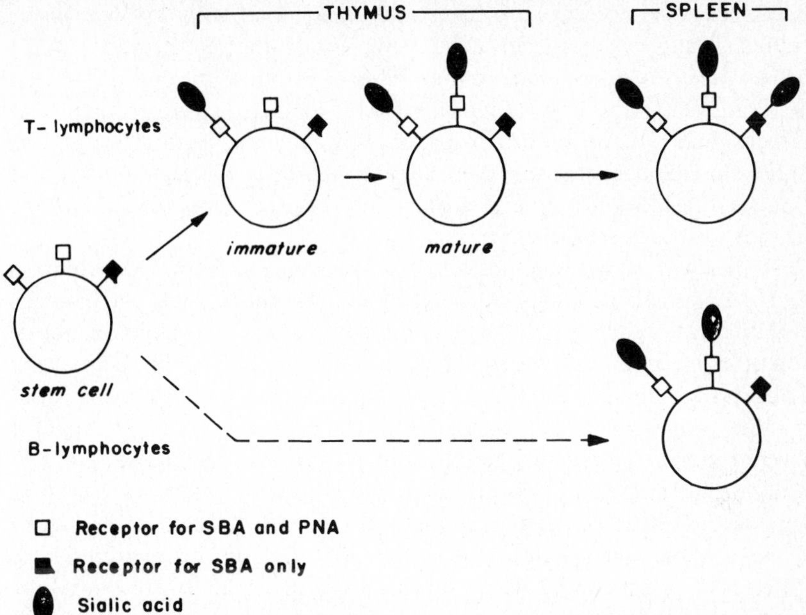

Fig. 30. Model for changes in lectin receptors on lymphocyte surfaces during differentiation and maturation. [From N. Sharon and Y. Reisner, in: Molecular Mechanisms of Biological Recognition, ed. M. Balaban (Elsevier, Amsterdam, 1979) pp. 95–106.]

mouse embryos grown in tissue culture. These alterations were noted only when the embryos were treated with the antibiotic while in the blastocyst stage or later in development. The data, while showing that *N*-glycosylation is essential for normal embryonic development, do not provide proof that the morphological changes induced by tunicamycin are a direct outcome of the lack of glycosylation of surface proteins.

A well-studied system of cell–cell recognition is that involved in the sexual mating of compatible yeasts. Opposite types (type 5 and 21) of haploid cells of *Hansenula wingeii* are coated by substances that cause their immediate aggregation upon mixing. These substances are released from the cell surface by proteolysis. Type 5 factor, a glycoprotein consisting of 85% mannose, 10% protein, and 5% phosphorus, contains specific binding sites for the type 21 factor. The latter is a small acidic glycoprotein that contains 5% carbohydrate with a core structure typical of *N*-glycosidic oligosaccharide chains.

Participation of cell surface sugars in gamete recognition has been examined by testing the ability of plant lectins to inhibit fertilization in mammals, sea urchins, protozoa and algae, but with no conclusive results. Using another approach, it was found that fertilization of the brown alga, *Fucus serratus*, was inhibited by binding of polysaccharides containing mannosyl or L-fucosyl residues to sperm or by pretreatment of eggs with α-mannosidase or α-L-fucosidase. Thus, fertilization in this organism is apparently based on the association between mannosyl and L-fucosyl residues on the egg surface and specific carbohydrate binding ligands on the sperm surface.

Studies with slime molds have further provided support for the notion that cellular association may be mediated by the interaction between carbohydrate binding proteins on one cell and specific oligosaccharide receptors on an apposing cell. Thus, differentiation of slime molds from a vegetative (single cell) to a cohesive (aggregated) form is accompanied by the appearance of both cell surface lectins and of specific glycoproteins. Moreover, simple sugars such as galactose and *N*-acetylgalactosamine inhibit cell aggregation in this system. However, in view of the restricted sugar specificity of the lectins, which in all species of slime mold investigated is confined to the above saccharides, it is difficult to understand how they can control the highly species-specific aggregation process.

Evidence based chiefly on inhibition studies with simple sugars, has been accumulating that bacteria such as *Escherichia coli* and *Salmonella typhi* interact with animal cell surfaces via mannose residues on the latter (fig. 31). This carbohydrate specific interaction appears to be mediated by a mannose specific lectin present on the surface of the bacteria. Similarly, recognition of L-fucose by *Vibrio cholerae* may be responsible for the attachment of this bacterium to intestinal cells, which is probably mediated by a lectin specific for L-fucose on the bacterial surface. Such studies, in addition to providing insight into the mechanism of bacterial adherence and its role in infection, may also lead to the development of new methods for prevention of infection, by inhibitors of attachment. Indeed, it was found that methyl α-mannoside instilled into the bladder, prevented colonization of the urinary tract of mice infected with *Escherichia coli* (fig. 32).

Attempts have been made to study the role of carbohydrates in intercellular adhesion with the aid of sugar derivatized beads. Chicken hepatocytes bound specifically to polyacrylamide gels to which *N*-acetylglucosamine was chemically attached, while rat hepatocytes adhered specifically to galactoside beads. The cell ligands involved in these interactions are not known, but in the case of the chicken hepatocytes, they may be related or identical to the chicken liver

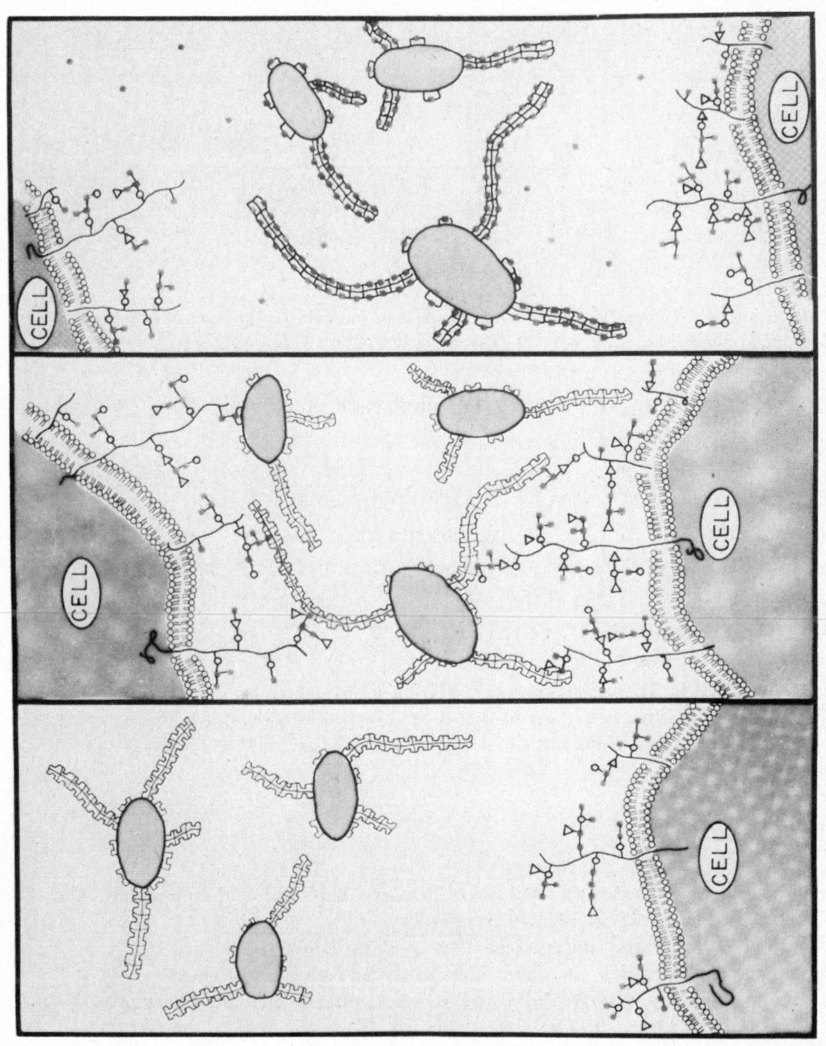

Fig. 31. Model depicting the binding of *Escherichia coli* to sugars on animal cell surface, via a bacterial lectin, and the inhibition of the binding by a specific sugar. (Courtesy of Y. Eshdat.)

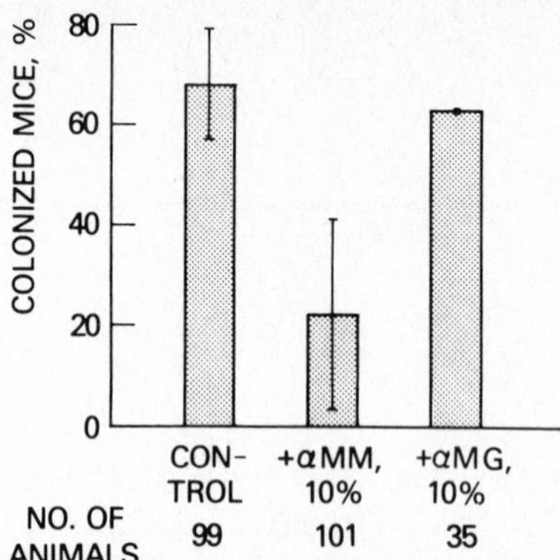

Fig. 32. Effect of methyl-α-mannoside (αMM) and of methyl-α-glucoside (αMG) on the colonization of the urinary tract of mice by *Escherichia coli*. [Data from M. Aronson, O. Medalia L. Schori, D. Mirelman, N. Sharon and I. Ofek, J. Infect. Dis. 139 (1979) 329.]

binding protein responsible for the clearance of glycoproteins from the circulating system.

It would thus appear that in many systems recognition is based on the interaction between cell surface carbohydrates and lectins on apposing syltransferases seems less likely, not the least because the evidence for the presence of these enzymes on cell surfaces is inconclusive.

Acknowledgements

Thanks are due to Thomas Sakmar and Helwig Reidl, whose notes, taken during the lectures in Les Houches, helped me in the preparation of this manuscript. Thanks are also due to Drs. Marc Chabre, Phillipe Devaux and Roger Balian for their hospitality and for organizing a marvellous summer course.

Further reading

N. Sharon, Complex Carbohydrates: Their Chemistry, Biosynthesis and Functions (Addison Wesley, Reading, MA, 1975) pp. 465.

R. C. Hughes, Membrane Glycoproteins (Butterworths, London, 1976) pp. 367.

Cell Surface Glycoproteins: Structure, Biosynthesis and Biological Functions, eds. R. L. Juliano and A. Rothstein, in: Current Topics in Membranes and Transport, vol. 11 (Academic Press, 1978) pp. 518.

H. Lis and N. Sharon, Lectins – Their Chemistry and Application to Immunology, ed. M. Sela, in: The Antigens, vol. 4 (Academic Press, 1977) pp. 429–529.

N. Sharon and H. Lis, Glycoproteins, eds. H. Neurath and R. L. Hill, in: "The Proteins" vol. 5 (Academic Press, 1980) in press.

SEMINAR

APPLICATION OF NMR TO THE STRUCTURAL ELUCIDATION OF COMPLEX CARBOHYDRATES*

L. DORLAND and J. F. G. VLIEGENTHART

Department Bio-Organic Chemistry, State University,
Croesestraat 79, 3522 AD Utrecht,
The Netherlands

The structural analysis of the carbohydrate chains of glycoproteins is usually carried out by a combination of chemical and enzymic methods. Some frequently used techniques are: periodate oxidation, Smith degradation, permethylation analysis, acetolysis, alkaline degradation (β-elimination), and sequential degradation with glycosidases. Despite the high degree of sophistication reached by these methods, it is evident that still quite a number of uncertainties remain even with regard to the monosaccharide composition. For example, it is sometimes difficult to estimate accurately the number of mannose and *N*-acetyl-hexosamine residues.

During the last few years high resolution ^{1}H-NMR spectroscopy has obtained a firm position among the techniques available for structural studies of biomolecules. In the structure elucidation of carbohydrates

*Lecture delivered at Les Houches by L. Dorland.

R. Balian et al., eds.
Les Houches, Session XXXIII, 1979 – Membranes et Communication Intercellulaire / Membranes and Intercellular Communication

high resolution ¹H-NMR spectra give valuable information about qualitative and quantitative aspects of the carbohydrate structure. For relatively large compounds the spectra are not completely interpretable. However, already a partial interpretation of the spectra can furnish relevant structural information. The structural reporter groups which are useful for this aim are those that comprise the signals of (a) the anomeric protons; (b) special non-anomeric protons, resonating outside of the poorly resolved bulk, e.g. the H-2 protons of mannose- and the H-3 protons of sialic acid residues; and (c) protons of substituents like *N*-acetyl, *N*-glycolyl and *O*-acetyl groups.

In the following, a few examples will be presented of what in principle can be done with 360 MHz ¹H-NMR spectroscopy.

Figure 1 gives the structure for the carbohydrate chain of human serotransferrin. Jamieson [1] proposed on the basis of periodate oxidation, partial acid hydrolysis, methylation analysis, and enzymic degradations the upper formula of fig. 1, whereas Spik [2] arrived at a more symmetric structure using essentially the same techniques. The principle differences are the following: Jamieson found 4 mannose residues and suggested GlcNAc→Asn to be directly attached to mannose; Spik found only 3 mannose residues and she proposed the occurrence of a *N*-acetylchitobiose unit linked to asparagine.

In fig. 2 the overall 360 MHz ¹H-NMR spectrum of the asialo serotransferrin glycopeptide [3] is given. Simple integration of the

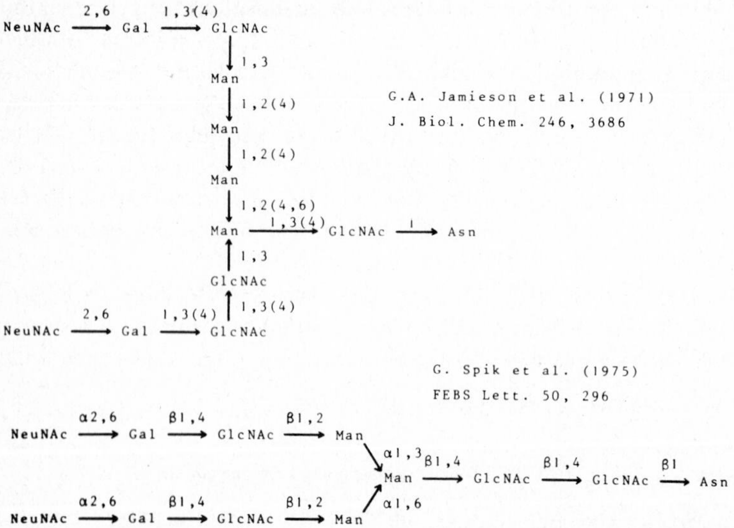

```
           2,6        1,3(4)
NeuNAc  ------> Gal ------> GlcNAc
                              | 1,3
                              v
                             Man
                              | 1,2(4)                G.A. Jamieson et al. (1971)
                              v                       J. Biol. Chem. 246, 3686
                             Man
                              | 1,2(4)
                              v
                             Man
                              | 1,2(4,6)
                              v     1,3(4)            1
                             Man ---------> GlcNAc ------> Asn
                              ^
                              | 1,3
                            GlcNAc
                              ^
           2,6        1,3(4)  | 1,3(4)
NeuNAc  ------> Gal ------> GlcNAc

                                                    G. Spik et al. (1975)
                                                    FEBS Lett. 50, 296

          α2,6        β1,4           β1,2
NeuNAc  ------> Gal ------> GlcNAc ------> Man
                                              \ α1,3  β1,4            β1,4           β1
                                               Man ------> GlcNAc ------> GlcNAc ------> Asn
          α2,6        β1,4           β1,2     / α1,6
NeuNAc  ------> Gal ------> GlcNAc ------> Man
```

Fig. 1. Proposed structures for the carbohydrate chain of human serotransferrin.

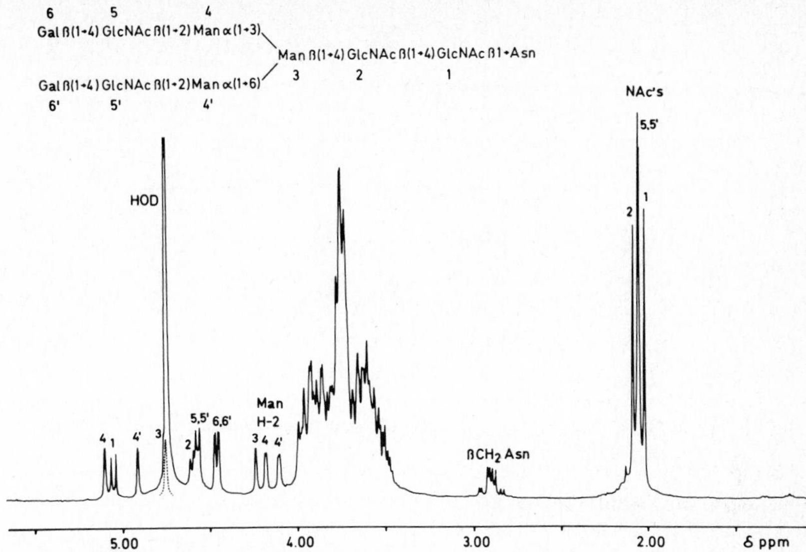

Fig. 2. 360 MHz ^{1}H-NMR spectrum of the asialo-serotransferrin glycopeptide in D_2O.

mannose H-2 and H-1 protons shows immediately that only 3 mannose residues are present in this structure, which excludes the structure given by Jamieson. In fact the proposal of Spik is correct, but before considering this in more detail, I want to mention that this report is limited to complex glyco-chains, coupled via an *N*-glycosidic linkage to asparagine in glycoproteins. According to the carbohydrate composition, these can be divided into two groups having in common a pentasaccharide core, which consists of a *N*-acetylchitobiose–Asn moiety, linked to a mannotriose branching unit. In the first family of the Asn glycans the pentasaccharide is substituted by one or more *N*-acetyl lactosamine units. These structures can be further extended by sialic acid and/or fucose residues in terminal positions. In the second family the pentasaccharide bears oligomannose chains. The total number of mannose residues in these type of compounds can vary considerably. Both groups of structures are presented in fig. 3.

In figs. 4–6 a few structures of the lactosamine type are presented to define the compounds which have been investigated. Figure 4 presents the extension of the pentasaccharide core with two *N*-acetyl lactosamine units. This is defined as the biantennary structure [4]. Figure 5 gives a further extension with a *N*-acetyl lactosamine moiety affording the triantennary structure, and fig. 6 shows the tetraantennary structure [4]. Compounds also occur which represent partial structures of the afore-

A
SA$_{n'}$
Fuc$_{n''}$
(Gal → GlcNAc)$_n$
Man
Man → GlcNAc → GlcNAc → Asn
Man
B
(Man)$_n$
Man
Man → GlcNAc → GlcNAc → Asn
Man

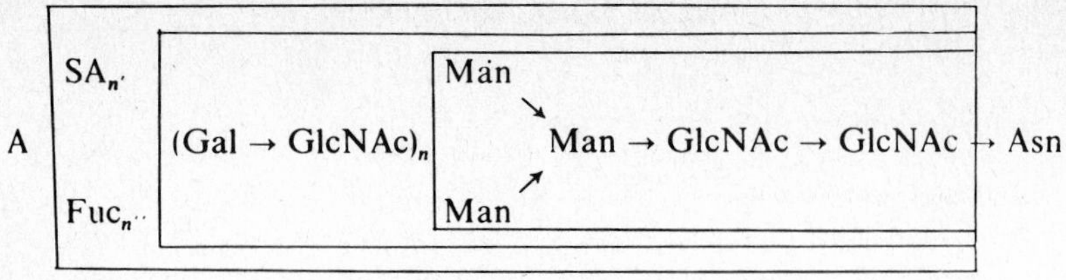

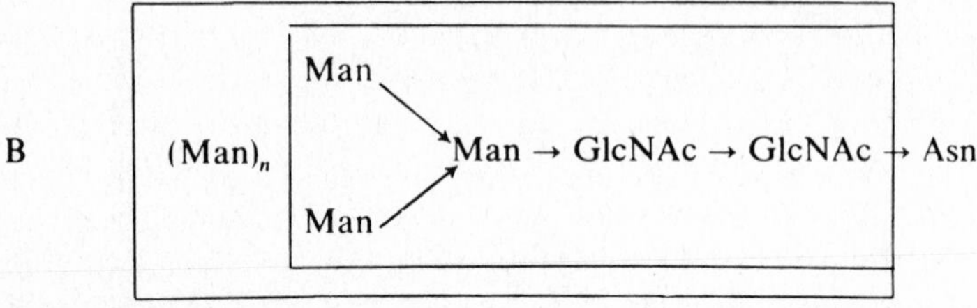

Fig. 3. Two types of *N*-glycosidic carbohydrate structures occurring in glycoproteins.

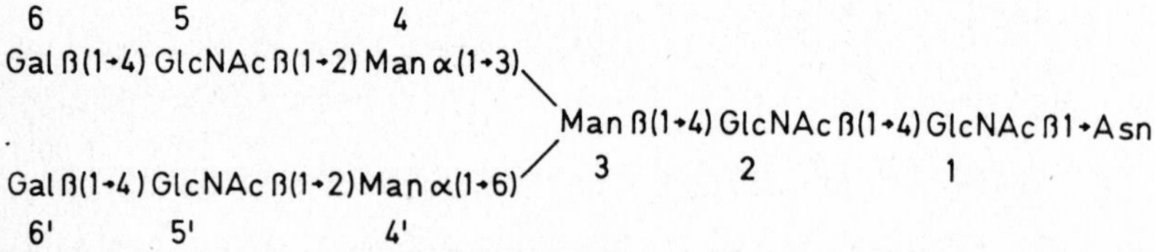

6 5 4
Gal β(1→4) GlcNAc β(1→2) Man α(1→3)
Man β(1→4) GlcNAc β(1→4) GlcNAc β1→Asn
3 2 1
Gal β(1→4) GlcNAc β(1→2) Man α(1→6)
6' 5' 4'

Fig. 4. Biantennary structure.

8 7
Gal β(1→4) GlcNAc β(1→4)
6 5 4
Gal β(1→4) GlcNAc β(1→2) Man α(1→3)
Man β(1→4) GlcNAc β(1→4) GlcNAc β1→Asn
3 2 1
Gal β(1→4) GlcNAc β(1→2) Man α(1→6)
6' 5' 4'

Fig. 5. Triantennary structure.

8 7
Gal β(1→4) GlcNAc β(1→4)
6 5 4
Gal β(1→4) GlcNAc β(1→2) Man α(1→3)
Man β(1→4) GlcNAc β(1→4) GlcNAc β1→Asn
3 2 1
Gal β(1→4) GlcNAc β(1→2) Man α(1→6)
6' 5' 4'
Gal β(1→4) GlcNAc β(1→6)
8' 7'

Fig. 6. Tetraantennary structure.

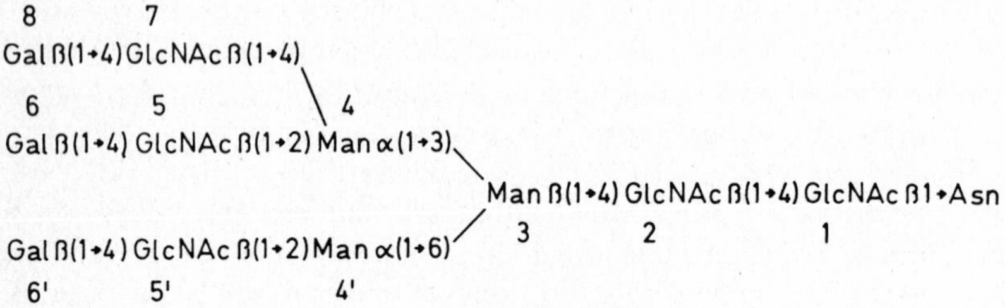

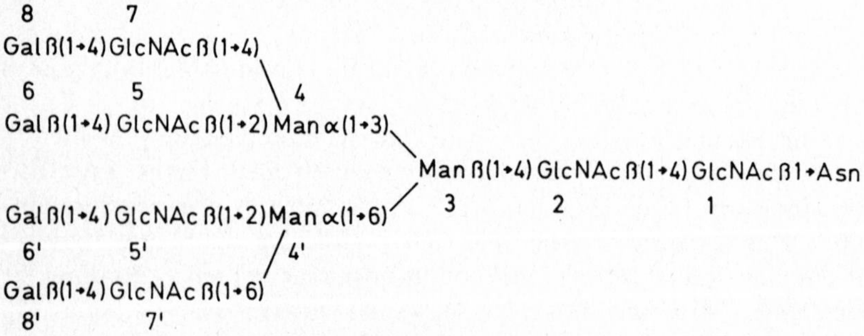

mentioned classes of carbohydrate chains. In particular from glycoproteins which have a large heterogeneity, these partial structures can be obtained.

The 360 MHz ^{1}H-NMR spectrum of the general structural element GlcNAcβ→1 Asn could completely be interpreted [5]. The coupling constant $J_{1,2}=9.8$ Hz is indicative of a β-glycosidic bond of the GlcNAc residue. The $^4C_1$ (D) chair conformation of the pyranosyl ring of the GlcNAc residue could be deduced from the vicinal coupling constants $J_{HH'}$ using an adapted Karplus equation. Another frequently occurring structural element in glycoproteins is Fucα(1→6)GlcNAcβ1 →Asn. The 360 MHz ^{1}H-NMR spectrum of this compound is also completely interpretable. Characteristic for the fucose residue are the resonances of the anomeric proton ($\delta=4.90$ ppm; $J_{1,2}=3.7$ Hz) and the protons of the CH_3 group ($\delta=1.21$ ppm; $J_{5,6}=6.6$ Hz). The coupling constant of 3.7 Hz is indicative of an α-glycosidic bond of the fucose residue. The ring conformations of both sugar residues were determined: for GlcNAc the $^4C_1$ (D) chair and for Fuc the $^1C_4$ (L) chair [5]. The attachment of fucose to position 6 of GlcNAc gives rise to changes in the chemical shifts for H-4, 5, and 6 of GlcNAc when compared with the data of GlcNAcβ1→Asn. Also the value of the geminal coupling constant $J_{6,6'}$ of GlcNAc is changed ($-12.7 \rightarrow -11.4$ Hz).

As soon as the number of monosaccharides increases the pattern of the non-anomeric protons becomes far too complex to be analysed in full detail.

An example of a complex Asn-glycopeptide is the asialo-glycopeptide obtained from human serotransferrin, which spectrum is given in fig. 2. The resonances of this glycopeptide can be divided into signals from the following groups of protons:

(a) Anomeric protons (9); at this temperature, one is hidden under the HOD line. This signal can be visualized by recording the spectrum at another temperature.
(b) The H-2 protons of mannose residues.
(c) The remaining non-anomeric protons.
(d) β-CH_2 protons of asparagine.
(e) CH_3 protons of the *N*-acetyl groups.

It is impossible to interpret the bulk of the non-anomeric protons. However, many structural details of this compound are reflected in the chemical shifts of the anomeric protons and the H-2 protons of the mannose residues. Integration showed that 9 anomeric protons are present, which is in accordance with the proposed number of monosaccharide units. An extra check for the number of amino sugar residues

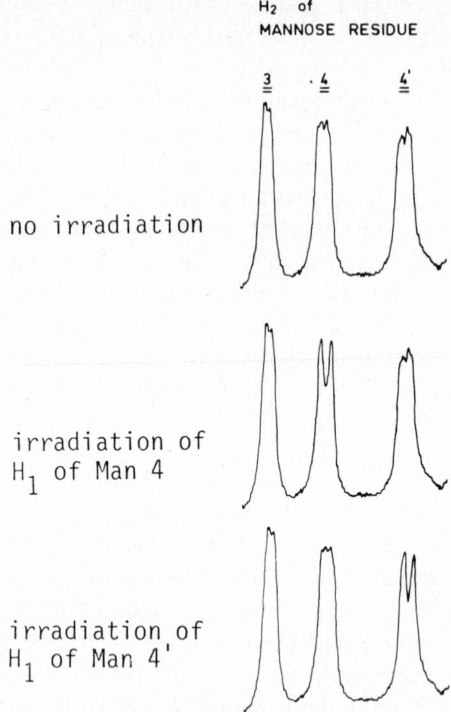

Fig. 7. Assignment of the mannose H-2 protons by selective irradiation.

can be obtained from integration of the *N*-acetyl signals. We arrived at this interpretation on the basis of a wide variety of partial structures, each containing a characteristic part of this molecule. The H-2 protons of the mannose residues could be assigned by selective irradiation of the H-1 protons of the mannose residues (fig. 7). From the NMR spectrum of this glycopeptide and the spectra of the various reference compounds some conclusions can be drawn:

(1) The chemical shifts of the various anomeric protons in the intact glycopeptide and the partial structures thereof occur at characteristic positions.

(2) The primary structure and the type of the glycosidic linkages are reflected by the chemical shifts and the coupling constants of the anomeric protons of the various monomers. The total NMR spectrum can be used as a fingerprint.

(3) The mannotriose branching core, surrounded by GlcNAc residues can be recognized on the basis of the pattern of the mannose H-2 proton resonances.

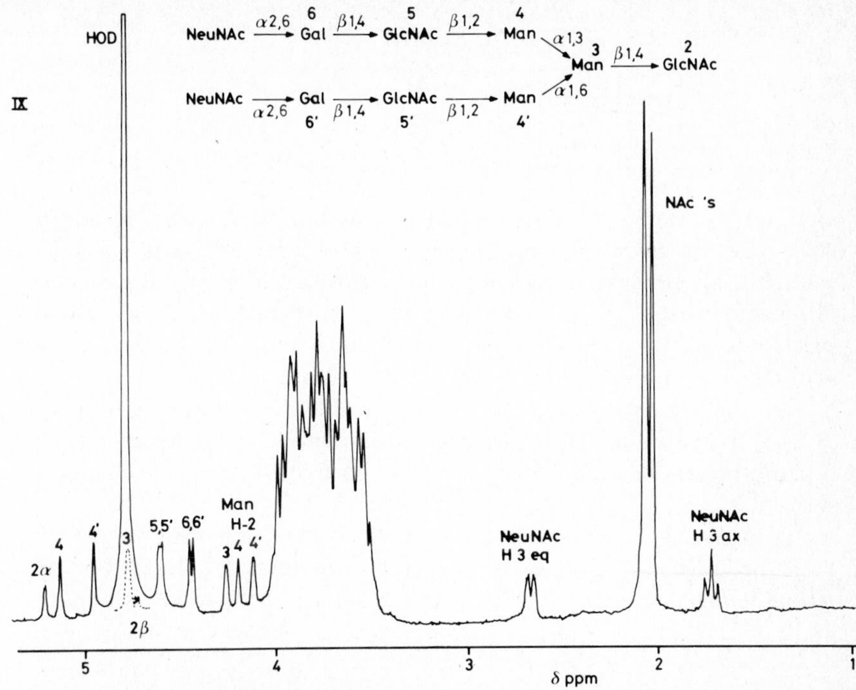

Fig. 8. 360 MHz ^{1}H-NMR spectrum of sialo-oligosaccharide IX in D_2O.

The occurrence of sialic acid at terminal positions of the biantennary structure has some remarkable influences on the spectrum, depending on the type of glycosidic linkage. First $\alpha(2{\rightarrow}6)$ linked sialic acid, as present in the oligosaccharide IX, isolated from urine of sialidosis patients [6]. Figure 8 gives the 360 MHz ^{1}H-NMR spectrum of this sialo-oligosaccharide and its structure. Additional signals in the spectrum of the sialo-compound are those of the H-3_{eg} and H-3_{ax} protons of sialic acid. The introduction of sialic acid at position 6 of the galactose residues gives rise to a few small but significant shift increments for some anomeric protons. There is a downfield shift of H-1 of Man 4 and 4′ and GlcNAc 5 and 5′, whereas an upfield shift is present for the anomeric protons of Gal 6 and 6′. When only one sialic acid residue occurs in $\alpha(2{\rightarrow}6)$ linkage to Gal, then its location in the biantenna can be inferred from the spectrum. For this purpose the chemical shifts of the anomeric protons of the mannose residues 4 and 4′ are used.

Sialic acid also occurs in $\alpha(2{\rightarrow}3)$ linkage to Gal. Such a sialic acid residue can easily be recognized from the chemical shifts of the H-3_{eq}

Table 1

Linkage	Chemical shift of H-3	
	Equatorial	Axial
NeuAcα(2→3)Gal	2.76	1.80
NeuAcα(2→6)Gal	2.67	1.72

and H-3_{ax} protons. These values together with those for α(2→6) linked sialic acid are given in table 1. The only H-1 that undergoes a significant shift on attachment of sialic acid to position 3 of galactose is that of galactose itself. In fig. 9, the spectrum is presented of a sialo-oligosaccharide having the biantennary structure with α(2→3) linked sialic acid residues in both branches. In contrast to α(2→6) linked sialic acid it is, in a monosialo biantenna, not possible to distinguish whether α(2→3)-linked sialic acid is attached to the upper or the lower branch because the anomeric protons of Gal 6 and 6′ have the same chemical shift.

An interesting glycoprotein is α_1-acid glycoprotein which shows a large heterogeneity in the carbohydrate structures [7]. Bi-, tri-, and tetraantennary structures occur in this protein. Furthermore, in the tri- and tetraantennary structures fucose can be present in an α(1→3)

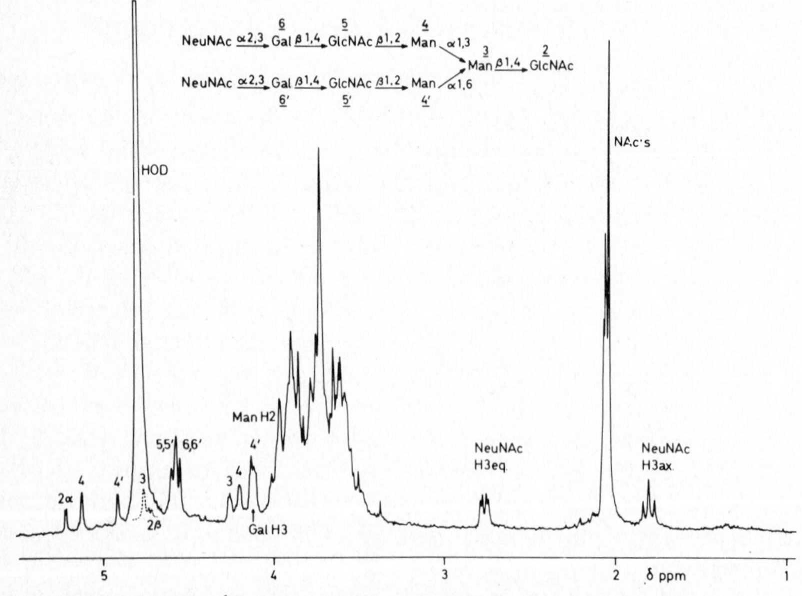

Fig. 9. 360 MHz ^{1}H-NMR spectrum of sialo-oligosaccharide VII in D_2O.

Table 2

	Chemical shift of					
	H-1 of mannose			H-2 of mannose		
Structure	3	4	4′	3	4	4′
Biantenna	4.764	5.121	4.928	4.247	4.189	4.110
Triantenna	4.757	5.119	4.924	4.215	4.215	4.109
Tetraantenna	4.754	5.127	4.866	4.215	4.215	4.092

linkage to GlcNAc. The determination of the antenna type can be carried out by high resolution proton NMR spectroscopy [8]. The substitution pattern of the mannotriose branching core is reflected in the chemical shifts of the H-1 and H-2 protons of the mannose residues as shown in table 2.

Another interesting glycoprotein is conalbumin or ovotransferrin [9]. The carbohydrate moiety differs in several respects from sero- and lactotransferrin. For example, it does not contain galactose and sialic acid. The 360 MHz ^{1}H-NMR spectrum and the carbohydrate structure are given in fig. 10.

The interpretation was made on guidance of some ^{1}H-NMR spectra of partial structures of this glycopeptide. On the basis of the spectral data of the partial structures we discovered that the shift increments

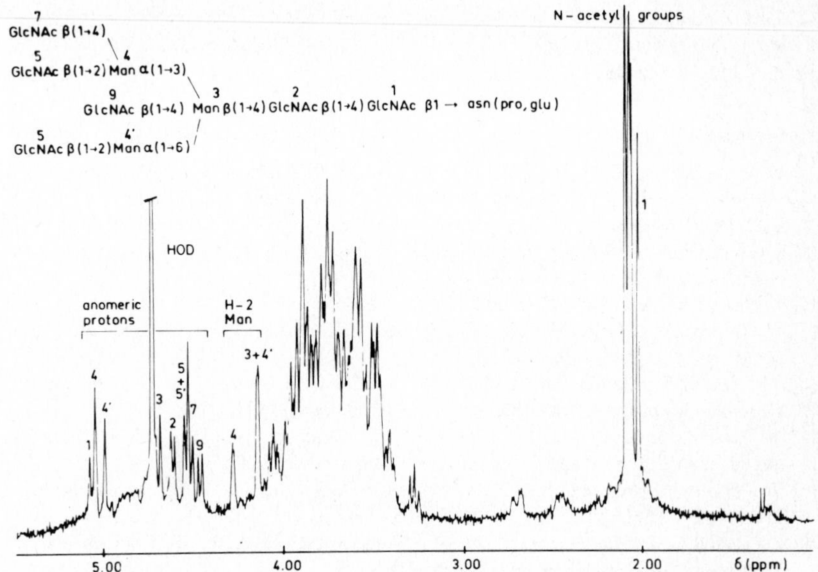

Fig. 10. 360 MHz ^{1}H-NMR spectrum of a glycopeptide from ovotransferrin.

	δ H_1 of residue									δ H_2 of residue		
	1	2	3	4	4'	5	5'	7	9	3	4	4'
predicted chemical shift	5.072	4.616	4.688	5.062	5.004	4.555	4.555	4.522	4.471	4.150	4.275	4.151
observed chemical shift	5.079	4.621	4.685	5.062	5.001	4.543	4.543	4.516	4.468	4.143	4.284	4.143

Fig. 11. Predicted and observed chemical shifts for the glycopeptide of ovotransferrin.

which result from making compounds more complex by the addition of a monosaccharide are, in general, additive. This opened the possibility to predict the spectra of compounds which are closely related to the set of reference compounds. In fig. 11 the comparison is shown of the predicted and observed values for the characteristic protons of this glycopeptide. The agreement is excellent.

To summarize: high resolution ^{1}H-NMR spectroscopy is a powerful technique for the structure determination of the carbohydrate chains of glycoproteins.

Acknowledgements

Thanks are due to Dr. J. Montreuil and co-workers, Lilly, France and to Dr. K. Schmid and co-workers, Boston, USA.

These investigations were supported by the Netherlands Foundation for Chemical Research (SON) with financial aid from the Netherlands Organization for the Advancement of Pure Research (ZWO).

References

[1] G. A. Jamieson, M. Jett and S. L. DeBernardo, J. Biol. Chem. 246 (1971) 3686.
[2] G. Spik, B. Bayard, B. Fournet, G. Strecker, S. Bouquelet and J. Montreuil, FEBS Lett. 50 (1975) 296.
[3] L. Dorland, J. Haverkamp, B. L. Schut, J. F. G. Vliegenthart, G. Spik, G. Strecker, B. Fournet and J. Montreuil, FEBS Lett. 77 (1977) 15.
[4] J. Montreuil, Pure Appl. Chem. 42 (1975) 431.
[5] L. Dorland, B. L. Schut, J. F. G. Vliegenthart, G. Strecker, B. Fournet, G. Spik and J. Montreuil, Eur. J. Biochem. 73 (1977) 93.
[6] L. Dorland, J. Haverkamp, J. F. G. Vliegenthart, G. Strecker, J.-C. Michalski, B. Fournet, G. Spik and J. Montreuil, Eur. J. Biochem. 87 (1978) 323.
[7] B. Fournet, J. Montreuil, G. Strecker, L. Dorland, J. Haverkamp, J. F. G. Vliegenthart, J. P. Binette and K. Schmid, Biochemistry 17 (1978) 5206.
[8] L. Dorland, J. Haverkamp, J. F. G. Vliegenthart, B. Fournet, G. Strecker, G. Spik, J. Montreuil, K. Schmid and J. P. Binette, FEBS Lett. 89 (1978) 149.
[9] L. Dorland, J. Haverkamp, J. F. G. Vliegenthart, G. Spik, B. Fournet and J. Montreuil, Eur. J. Biochem. 100 (1979) 569 .

COURSE 3
(PART I)

INTERNAL DYNAMICS OF PROTEINS

(Abstract)

Martin KARPLUS

Department of Chemistry, Harvard University, Cambridge, MA, U.S.A.

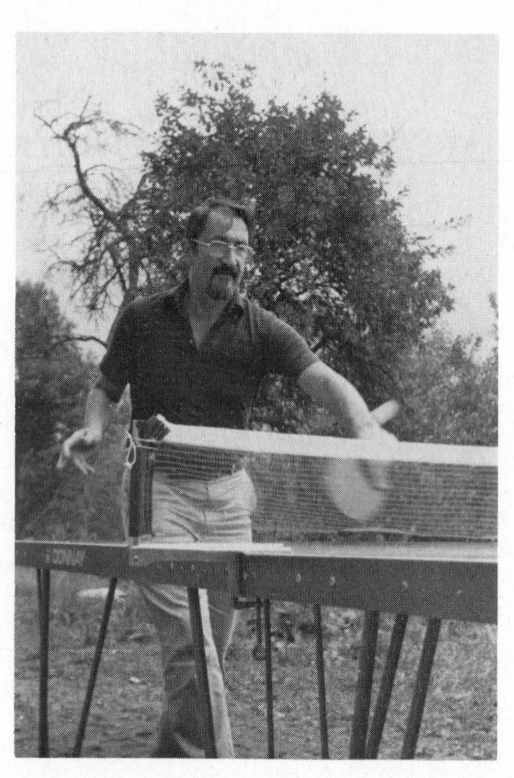

The topics which have been covered by professor M. Karplus in his series of lectures are essentially contained in a forthcoming review article (ref. [1]). A brief abstract is given here.

Since the internal dynamics of globular proteins play an essential role in their function, it is important to understand the origin and detailed nature of the motions that occur at the atomic level. A variety of experimental and theoretical methods are now being employed to probe these motions. In this review, we describe some of the methods and present their advantages and limitations. Particular emphasis is given to recent theoretical approaches, which have not been reviewed previously. An attempt is made to provide a coherent picture of the structure, flexibility, and dynamics of the interior of the protein molecule and to use this picture to outline the contributions of motional phenomena to protein function.

General references

M. Karplus and J. A. McCammon, Internal Dynamics of Proteins, in: CRC Reviews, to be published.

R. Balian et al., eds.
Les Houches, Session XXXIII, 1979 – Membranes et Communication Intercellulaire / Membranes and Intercellular Communication

SEMINAR

DYNAMIC ASPECTS OF THE STRUCTURE OF GLOBULAR PROTEINS BY HIGH RESOLUTION NMR SPECTROSCOPY

The fluid-like structure of the internal hydrophobic core of muscular parvalbumins*

Adrien CAVÉ and Joseph PARELLO

Equipe de Recherche de Biophysique, C. N. R. S.
Laboratoire de Chimie Structurale, U. S. T. L.,
34060 Montpellier,
France

"...la substance ne serait plus qu'un système multirésonnant, qu'un groupe de résonances, qu'une sorte d'amas de rythmes qui pourraient absorber et émettre certaines gammes de rayonnements. On peut prévoir, dans cette voie, une étude toute temporelle des substances qui serait le complément de l'étude structurale" [G. Bachelard, La Philosophie du Non (P.U.F., Paris, 1940).]

1. Introduction

Although it has been accepted for years that regulatory effects involving proteins are related to conformational adjustments brought about by external perturbations (binding of ligands, substrates, inhibitors), only

*Seminar delivered at Les Houches by J. Parello.

R. Balian et al., eds.
Les Houches, Session XXXIII, 1979 – Membranes et Communication Intercellulaire/Membranes and Intercellular Communication

more recently has it been recognized that dynamic properties of the protein molecule (conformational fluctuations) can play an important role in the ability of the proteins to undergo conformational transitions (for a comprehensive review see ref. [1]). Different types of internal motions have been detected with proteins in solution using varied spectroscopic techniques [1]. The movements can affect extended parts of the protein structure (flexible domains, local helix-coil transitions, backbone warps) and/or more localized atomic elements (rotations of side chains).

NMR (nuclear magnetic resonance) spectroscopy has played a major role in detecting the mobility of localized parts of a protein molecule. The first proton NMR spectrum of ribonuclease obtained at 40 MHz strongly suggested that a protein does not behave as a rigid assembly [2]. In a rigid structure, the broadening of the proton signals would be caused by the overall reorientation of the protein, and no high-resolution NMR spectrum could be obtained. For native proteins in solution, NMR studies indicate that side chains exhibit more sizable fluctuations than the polypeptide backbone. The most fully characterized motions revealed by NMR studies are the 180° rotations about the C^{β}-C^{1} bond of tyrosine and phenylalanine observed in the proton NMR of proteins at very high magnetic fields. Evidence from a number of proteins shows that tyrosine and phenylalanine rings commonly rotate with rates greater than 10^3 s^{-1}, even when these residues are buried in the protein interior: bovine pancreatic trypsin inhibitor or BPTI [3–5], cytochrome C [6], lysozyme [7], and muscular parvalbumins [8]. For general reviews, see refs. [9]–12]. There are a few cases where evidence for lower reorientation rates has been found [4, 13]. In some cases, it has been possible to extract definite rate constants and estimates of the enthalpy and entropy of activation for aromatic ring flipping [13, 14]. The enthalpies of activation range downward from 40 kcal/mol and the entropies of activation range downward from 70 e.u. The observed activation enthalpies are in reasonable agreement with theoretical calculations [15, 16].

A remarkable example of conformational mobility is provided by muscular parvalbumins. Optical studies (UV and CD) with parvalbumins suggested the existence of conformational mobility for the side chains of phenylalanyl residues due to rotational isomerism about the C^{α}-C^{β} and C^{β}-C^{1} bonds [17]. A ^{13}C NMR study of one parvalbumin from carp muscle provided more direct evidence that the aromatic rings of the phenyalanyl residues possess greater motion than the overall molecular rotation can provide [18, 19]. Proton NMR spectroscopy shows that all phenylalanyl residues, which belong to the central hydrophobic core of the tertiary structure (usually 8 residues), undergo rapid $\pm$ 180° rotations about the C^{β}-C^{1} bonds [8].

The present review gives a comprehensive discussion of the dynamic and conformational features of the muscular parvalbumins which have been established by ^{1}H NMR spectroscopy. The relevance of conformational mobility in proteins to evolutionary mechanisms, regulatory effects, and enzymic catalysis is discussed.

2. Rotational isomerism of the side-chains of phenylalanine and tyrosine residues

2.1 Conformational characteristics

The concept of conformational* variation of a molecule which results from rotation about single bonds has been discussed and documented since the thirties [20]. An energy description of a molecular system comprising a carbon-carbon single bond (butane-like system) requires the establishment of the dependence of the potential energy of the molecule on a single parameter χ, the angle of torsion around the bond (or dihedral angle between two planes, one defined by a designated C_1-R bond and the C_1-C_2 bond, and the other defined by the C_1-C_2 bond and a designated C_2-R′ bond). Among the great number of momentary arrangements of conformations about the C_1-C_2 bond, only three conformations (staggered) correspond to energy minima and are therefore stable. For a non-symmetrically substituted butane-like molecule, the staggered conformers do not possess the same energy.

Let us consider the conformational possibilities of the side-chains of phenylalanine and tyrosine residues due to rotational isomerism about the single bond C^{α}-C^{β} and C^{β}-C^{1} (C^{4}-O in the case of tyrosine).

*The term "conformation" is to be used to denote any one of the infinite number of momentary arrangements of the atoms in space that result from rotation about single bonds. For further information the reader is referred to the textbook "Stereochemistry of Carbon Componds" by E. L. Eliel (McGraw-Hill Book Co., Inc., New York, 1962).

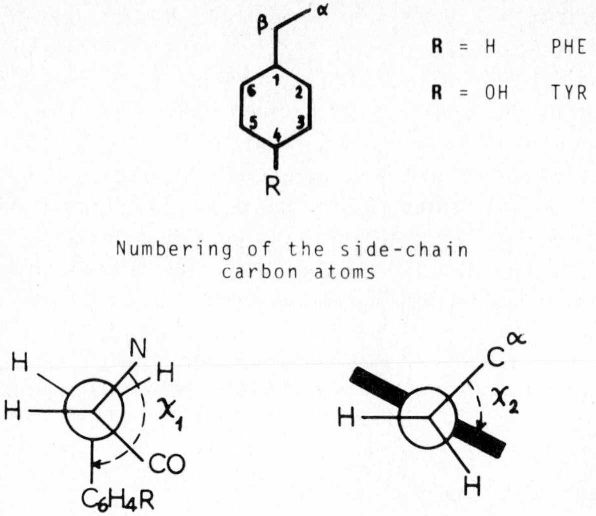

R = H PHE

R = OH TYR

Numbering of the side-chain carbon atoms

Newman projections

Left : about C^{α}-C^{β} Right : about C^{β}-C^{1}

Fig. 1. Rotational isomerism of the side-chains of phenylalanine and tyrosine.

Figure 1 shows the Newman projection formulae* of the side-chains of phenylalanine and tyrosine. Two angles of torsion χ_1 and χ_2 are sufficient to define the system. Conventions used to define the dihedral angles χ_1 and χ_2 are those in ref. [21].

*"In the Newman projection formula the molecule is viewed from front to back in the direction of the bond linking the two atoms of the single bond. These two atoms thus exactly eclipse each other and are represented by two superimposed circles (actually one circle only appears in the drawing). The bonds and groups attached to the central atoms are projected into a vertical plane; the bond thus appears as the spokes of a wheel at angles of 120° for each carbon, the spokes for the rear carbon being displaced by a given angle (dihedral angle) with respect to the bonds on the front carbon. In order to distinguish the two sets of bonds, the set from the front carbon is drawn to the center of the circle but that from the rear carbon ends at the periphery" [20]. Eclipsed conformations correspond to the superimposition of rear and front bonds. Staggered conformations correspond to a displacement of the rear bonds by an angle of 60° with respect to the front bonds (or vice versa). The term "rotamer" is also used to define varied rotameric conformations.

The staggered rotamers about the C^{α}-C^{β} bond of phenylalanine or tyrosine correspond to χ_1 values of 60°, 180°, and 300°. According to energy calculations the most stable conformers of phenylalanine and tyrosine are the six rotamers corresponding to $\chi_1 = 60°$ or 180° or 300° and $\chi_2 = 60°$ or 120°. The distribution of the conformational parameters χ_1 and χ_2 of the phenylalanine side-chains within the tertiary structure of a globular protein, given in fig. 2, is based on the results of an X-ray diffraction analysis of a parvalbumin from carp muscle in the crystalline state [22]. Three different sets of χ_1 values are observed: about 120° (eclipsed rotamer), about 210° (nearly staggered rotamers) and around 300° (fully staggered rotamers). χ_2 values are spread over an interval ranging from 40° to 150° comprising unstable local rotamers. However, it must be emphasized that these values are time-averaged over different types of conformational situations. Furthermore the accuracy of the crystallographic method must also be taken into account in defining the conformational parameters χ_1 and χ_2.

2.2. *Rotation about the C^{β}-C^{1} bond and* ^{1}H NMR *spectroscopy*

Let us consider the case of the aromatic ring of a phenylalanine residue with a rigid side-chain within the tertiary structure of a globular protein.

Consider the conformer I (or II) without any allowed rotation about the C^{β}-C^{1} bond (see fig. 3). The magnetic influence of the surrounding protein is usually different for each of the five aromatic protons (labelled 2 to 6) because of the very asymmetric arrangement of the polypeptide

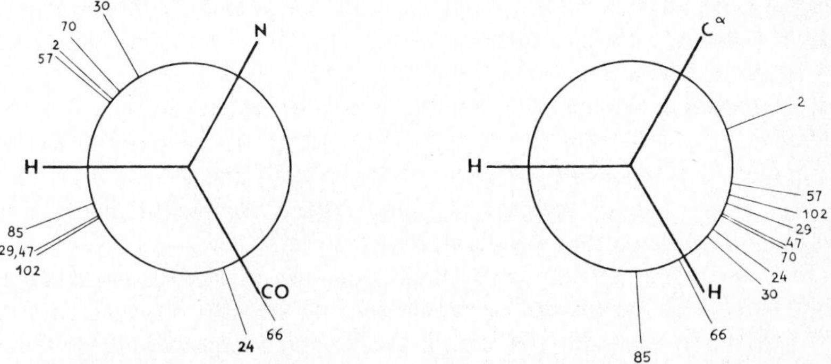

Fig. 2. Side-chain conformations of the 10 phenylalanine residues of carp parvalbumin (pI 4.25) in the crystalline state. Left: χ_1 angle. Right: χ_2 angle. Phenylalanine residues are numbered according to their position in the sequence.

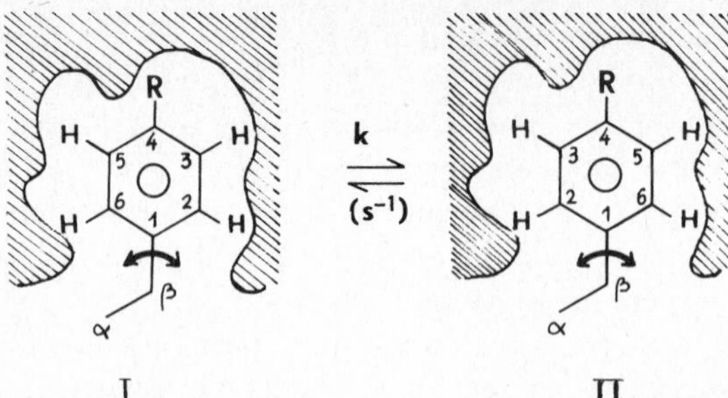

Fig. 3. Proton exchange by interconversion between the two identical conformers I and II ($\Delta\chi_2 = \pm 180°$) through rotation about the C^{β}-C^1 bond of phenylalanine (R=H) or tyrosine (R=OH). *Ortho* (2) ↔ *ortho* (6); *meta* (3) ↔ *meta* (5). *Para* (4) remains unperturbed. k is the first-order intramolecular rate of interconversion in s^{-1}.

backbone and the side-chains in the tertiary structure. Therefore the chemical shifts δ_2 to δ_6 (or resonance frequencies ν_2 to ν_6) of the phenylalanine aromatic protons must all be distinct on the basis of symmetry considerations (a deceptively simple spectrum might, however, originate due to casual equivalences: $\delta_2 \simeq \delta_6$ and/or $\delta_3 \simeq \delta_5$). Such a spin system of five non-equivalent aromatic protons can be labelled ABCDE according to the nomenclature used in NMR spectrum analysis [23]. However, a large number of small organic compounds, which contain a monosubstituted benzene ring, are characterized by NMR spectra which are much simpler than ABCDE spectra. The five spin system is usually observed as an AA′BB′C spectrum, for which the two *ortho* protons are equivalent ($\delta_2 = \delta_6$), as well as the two *meta* protons ($\delta_3 = \delta_5$). The *para* proton has a distinct chemical shift δ_4. The observation of an AA′BB′C system is due to the fact that a symmetrical situation is encountered with respect to the C^1-C^4 axis if the rate of interconversion (k in s^{-1}) between the two energetically identical rotamers ($\Delta\chi_2 = \pm 180°$ C) is sufficiently large in comparison to the frequency differences of the *ortho* protons $|\nu_2$-$\nu_6|$ and the *meta* protons $|\nu_3$-$\nu_5|$. This is usually the case for small organic compounds in solution within a large interval of temperature.

Time-averaging effects are well documented in NMR spectroscopy [24]. The NMR spectra can be dependent on a number of parameters of the system (temperature, pH, etc.) if the observed molecule takes part in various rate processes. Let us consider a molecular system in which a chemical exchange process occurs so that at different times a given proton will occupy either the chemical position I or the chemical position II. If this exchange is sufficiently rapid, a coalescence of some signals will be observed. This is a manifestation of the uncertainty principle which may be written in the form, $\tau . \Delta\nu \simeq \frac{1}{2}\pi$, where $\Delta\nu$ is the separation of the corresponding resonance lines I and II (under no-exchange conditions) and τ is the smallest time for which two separate states can be distinguished. When the exchange is sufficiently rapid, the lifetimes of the states will become less than this critical value and the signals cannot be separated. Under these conditions, the observed chemical shift of the single line is a mean value, $P_I\nu_I + P_{II}\nu_{II} = \nu_{obs}$, where P_I and P_{II} are the fractions in each state ($P_I + P_{II} = 1$).

If the tertiary structure of the globular protein was totally rigid, the proton NMR spectrum would in general include five distinct signals (each with an intensity of one proton) for the aromatic protons of each phenylalanine residue (see fig. 4A). However, if motion is allowed to occur about the C^{β}-C^1 bond, there is the possibility of two equally stable conformers I and II, which arise through ± 180° variations of χ_2 (flipping motion). If the rate of interconversion between I and II is much larger than the greatest frequency difference $|\nu_2$-$\nu_6|$ or $|\nu_3$-$\nu_4|$ (rapid rotation on the NMR time scale) both *ortho* signals will coalesce to yield a single signal with an intensity of two protons at equal distance from the signals 2 and 6. This is due to the fact that both interconverting conformers have the same potential energy so that the $P_I = P_{II} =$ 50%.

Similar behaviour is observed for the two *meta* protons H_3 and H_5. The chemical shift of proton H_4 is unaffected since the flipping motion is a rotation about the C^{β}-C^1 direction. The NMR spectrum under rapid rotation conditions is given in fig. 4B. A three signal NMR spectrum (with intensities 2-2-1) is observed for the five aromatic protons of a phenylalanine residue.

It therefore appears that the analysis of multiplicity of the aromatic region in the proton NMR spectrum of a protein will provide clear information regarding the dynamic state of the phenylalanine side-chains within the compact globular structure. Similar behaviour is expected for the aromatic protons of tyrosine. In this case the *para* position is substituted by a hydroxyl group (see fig. 1) so that only a system of four aromatic protons is to be considered. In the case of rigidity or slow rotation the NMR spectrum will show four distinct signals each with the intensity of one proton, while in the case of fast rotation only two signals with the intensity of two protons each will appear. The last case corresponds to an AA′BB′ system. For proteins, the observed spectrum

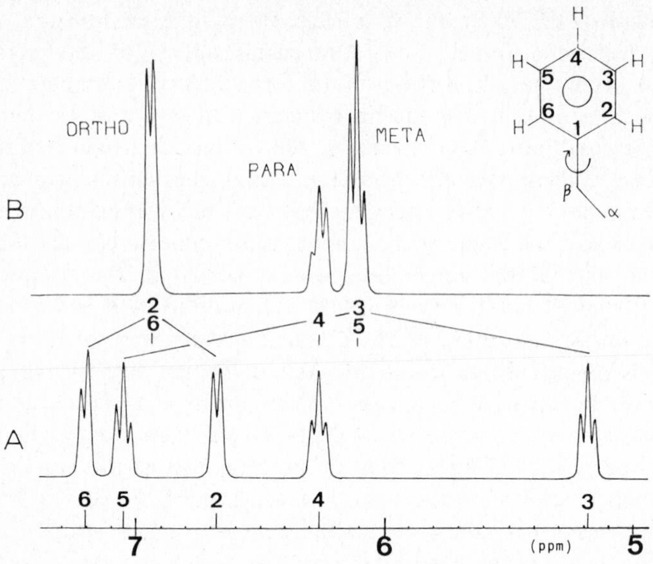

Fig. 4. Theoretical ^{1}H NMR spectrum of the aromatic counter-part of a phenylalanine residue. Calculations were carried out with the aid of a computer program (LAOCN 3 NMR program) adapted to the case of the aromatic five spin system of a phenylalanyl residue at the resonance frequency of 270 MHz using a standard coupling constant for an alkyl monosubstituted benzene ($J_{ortho}=J_{2,3}=J_{3,4}=J_{4,5}=J_{5,6}=8$ Hz; $J_{meta}=J_{2,4}=J_{3,5}=J_{4,6}=J_{2,6}=2$ Hz; and $J_{para}=J_{2,5}=J_{3,6}=0.5$ Hz) as well as a Lorentzian line-shape with 4 Hz in half-width (no spin–spin coupling with non-aromatic protons of the side-chain is considered). (A) Rigidity or slow rotation about the C^{β}-C^1 bond. The adopted chemical shifts for protons 2, 3, 4, 5, and 6 correspond to a given phenylalanine (Phe-29) within the tertiary structure of carp parvalbumin pI 4.25. Calculations which allow a prediction of chemical shifts for the 50 aromatic protons of this protein molecule were carried out according to theoretical predictions ([45]; see also fig. 13) and the atomic coordinates of the static model of carp parvalbumin established by X-ray crystallography [22]; ν_5-ν_3= 500 Hz and ν_6-ν_2= 140 Hz. The theoretical simulation involved the five spin system of the ABCDE-type (for nomenclature see ref.[23]). (B) Rapid rotation about the C^{β}-C^1 bond (i.e. interconversion rate k much higher than 500 s^{-1}). The theoretical simulation involves a five spin system of the AA′ BB′ C-type (for nomenclature see ref. [23]). Non-symmetrical multiplets (doublets, triplets) are observed in spectrum A (resonances 5 and 6) and in spectrum B (resonances 4,3–5). This is due to second-order effects which occur when the chemical shift difference (in frequency units) between two spin–spin coupled resonances is not sufficiently large in comparison to the spin–spin coupling constant(s). For further details on secondary order effects in high-resolution NMR spectra see ref. [23].

is constituted of two apparent doublets (*meta* protons at high field position) with a spacing of about 8 Hz (*ortho–meta* vicinal spin–spin coupling coupling constant) since the smaller coupling constants (through more than three bonds) are not usually resolved.

Varying the rate of interconversion between conformers I and II (fig. 3) will affect the positions as well as the shapes of the corresponding NMR signals. At intermediate rates close to the above-mentioned critical frequencies the resonance pattern of the aromatic protons of the Phe (or Tyr) will be complex (coalescence phenomenon). However, the actual line-shape can be analyzed theoretically and the rate constant k can be thus determined (see below).

Globular proteins usually contain several Phe and/or Tyr residues. Therefore the aromatic region of the proton NMR spectra, although usually the less complex part of the spectrum, contains a great number

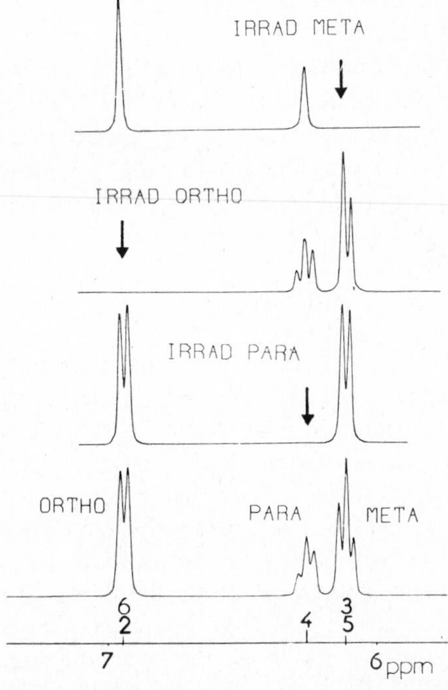

Fig. 5. Theoretical predictions under double resonance conditions for rapid rotation about the C^{β}-C^{1} bond (for calculation conditions see legend to fig. 4). Vertical arrows indicate the position of the saturating frequency.

of resonances which overlap at least partially even in conditions of very high-resolution. The different groups of aromatic resonances (*meta*, *ortho* and *para* protons) belonging to a given phenylalanine residue (or tyrosine residue) are to be identified. A method well adapted to identify a system of spin–spin coupled protons is the technique of multiple resonance (for a review see refs. [25, 26].) Decoupling can thus be achieved affording signals of lesser multiplicity. The most usual technical procedure is to introduce one saturating frequency. Figure 5 illustrates the expected effects of such a decoupling technique in the case of the five spin system of the aromatic protons of a phenylalanine residue under rapid rotation conditions. The use of two saturating frequencies is also very well adapted to the case of the aromatic signals of phenylalanine, since simultaneous irradiation of the *ortho* and *para* signals yield a singlet for the *meta* protons (see fig.12).

3. Dynamic studies with muscular parvalbumins by ^{1}H NMR spectroscopy

Muscular parvalbumins afford a striking example where multiple resonance techniques coupled to Fourier transform NMR spectroscopy and mathematical techniques to improve the resolution have been extensively used to analyze the aromatic patterns of the proton NMR spectra of these proteins which usually contain 10 phenylalanine residues, i.e. 50 aromatic protons [8, 27].

3.1. General properties of parvalbumins

Parvalbumins (Pa) form a class of homologous globular proteins of low-molecular weight (about 11 500 Daltons) which are present in the muscles of most vertebrates [28]. They are characterized by a high proportion of phenylalanine and alanine residues, an acidic isoelectric point (pI) and a high affinity for calcium ions. Several parvalbumin components can occur within the same species. These components are usually named by their isoelectric point following the proposal of Pechère [29]. The sequences of more than ten parvalbumins from different species are known [28, 30]. A phylogenetic classification into two main series α and β has been made on the basis of the known primary structures [28, 30].

The three-dimensional structure of parvalbumins can be inferred from the results obtained by X-ray crystallography with component pI

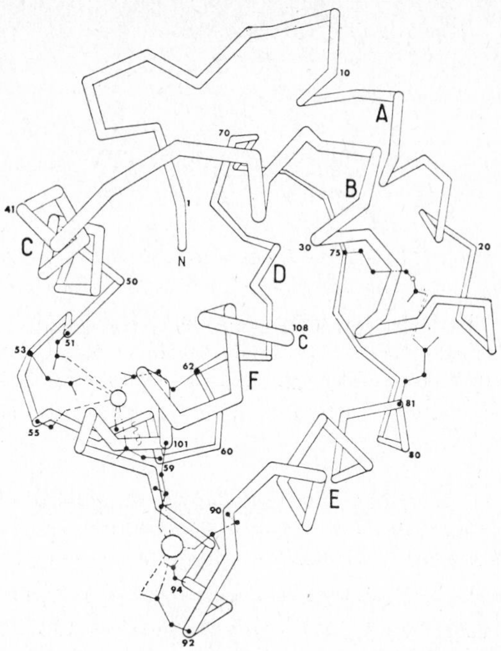

Fig. 6. Pictorial represesentation of the three-dimensional structure of the carp 4.25 parvalbumin. The course of the peptide backbone was drawn from a photograph of a model of the molecule built with Kendrew–Watson parts from the electron density maps. The small capital N and C letters designate the N- and C-terminus of the chain, respectively. The large capitals, A–F, refer to the six helical fragments in the molecule. The residues implicated in calcium binding are represented by thin lines, and the coordinating bonds by dashed lines. A similar symbolism applies to the Arg 75–Glu 81 salt bridge. The hydrogen bond connecting the two calcium binding regions is represented by an undulating stroke. (Courtesy of Dr. J. Demaille; reproducted from ref. [28].)

4.25 from carp muscle ([22, 31]; see fig. 6). The protein molecule has the approximate shape of a prolate ellipsoid of revolution (fig. 7). The polypeptide main chain is composed of six well-defined secondary structure domains (helices A, B, C, D, E, and F) separated by less-defined domains or loops (named by two letters: for instance the CD loop is that part of the sequence comprised between helix C and helix D). The protein has a well-defined internal core consisting of the side-chains of hydrophobic residues: 7 phenylalanine, 4 isoleucine, 5 leucine, and 3 valine residues plus half of the side-chains of Phe-47, Leu-86, and Leu-105 [22]. The main chain encloses this core but it does not pass through it. Each of the six loops, AB, . . . , CD, . . . , EF has one

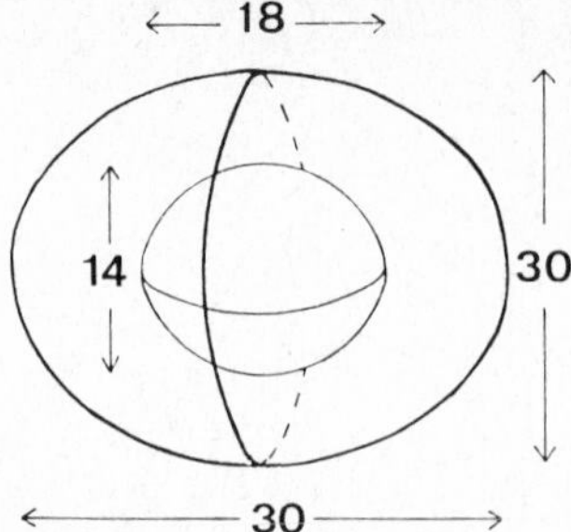

Fig. 7. The carp parvalbumin (pI 4.25) molecule has the general shape of a prolate ellipsoid of revolution. Volume of the entire molecule: 16 900 Å^3. The central oblate ellipsoid core (hydrophobic core) contains side-chains of phenylalanine, isoleucine, leucine, and valine residues (volume 2 400 Å^3). Drawing adapted from fig. 2 in ref. [22]. Dimensions in Å.

core group either at its beginning or its end. In general, at each turn of the six helices there are one or two groups that contribute to the core from the inner part of the helix. Parvalbumins are usually isolated with two calcium ions per protein molecule ($PaCa_2$) which are strongly bound to the polypeptide chain with an intrinsic binding constant of about 10^9 M^{-1} [32]. X-ray crystallography of carp parvalbumin pI 4.25 shows that the two Ca^{2+} ions occupy two specific sites at the CD and EF loops [22]. Competition experiments show that these cationic sites can accommodate a great variety of ions differing in their charges and dimensions [33]. Ca^{2+} has the highest affinity among the alkaline–earth cations. Mg^{2+} interacts with parvalbumins with an affinity constant of about 10^5 M^{-1} [34]. This is an important observation when considering the biological function of these proteins. *In vivo* parvalbumins are found in the presence of a relatively high concentration of Mg^{2+} ions (about 5 mM according to ref. [35]; parvalbumin concentration between 0.05 and 2 mM according to ref. [36]). A reversible exchange between Ca^{2+} and Mg^{2+} is likely to occur during muscle contraction [37]. In relation to this exchange a Ca–Mg secondary site (with similar affinities for both ions) has been inferred from NMR studies using ^{25}Mg resonance [38] and relaxation techniques in the presence of paramagnetic ions [33].

3.2. *Proton* NMR *studies at high field*

^{1}H NMR spectroscopy at high magnetic field is very well adapted to characterize the conformational features of parvalbumins in solution

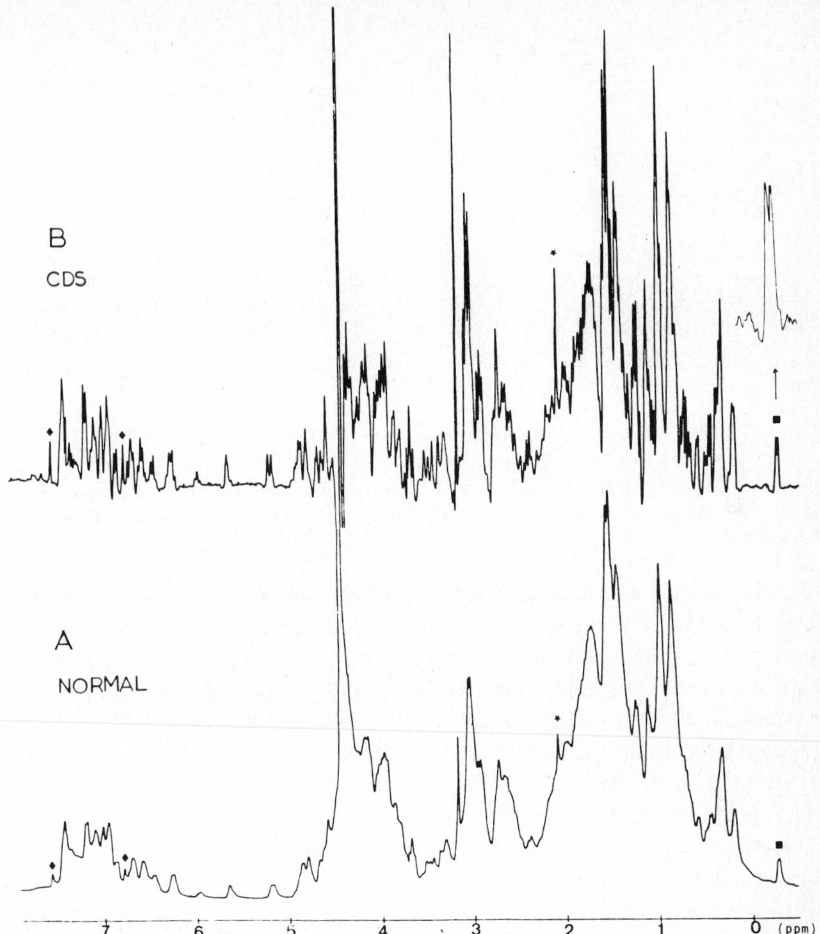

Fig. 8. ^1H NMR spectrum at 270 MHz of an 8 mM carp parvalbumin (component pI 4.25) solution in D_20 at pH 6.8 and 52° C (1024 transients, pulse length 16 μs, delay time 0.513 s and sweep-width 4000 Hz). (A) Normal Fourier transform spectrum. (B) Convolution difference spectrum (CDS) calculated from the same FID (free induction decay) as in (A), using $t_1 = 0.25$ s, $t_2 = 0.08$ s, and $K = 0.98$ [for definitions see R.A. Dwek, NMR in Biochemistry (Clarendon Press, Oxford, 1973) pp. 370–372]. All the labile protons have been previously exchanged by deuterons. (◆) imidazole protons of His-26; (★) *N*-terminal acetyl group; (■) aliphatic methyl group (CH-CH_3).

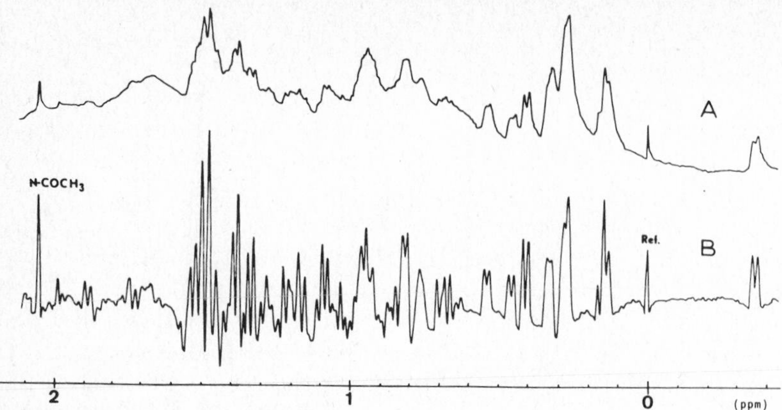

Fig. 9. Aliphatic region (−0.5 to +2.0 ppm) of the ^{1}H NMR spectrum at 360 MHz of an 8 mM solution of carp parvalbumin pI 4.25 in D_2O at pH 6.8 and 52° C. (A) Normal spectrum. (B) Spectrum after FID digital filtering with the "sine bell" technique [43]. Chemical shifts in ppm from Ref. = $TSPd_4$ or sodium 2,2,3,3-tetradeuterio-3(trimethylsily)propionate.

[8, 39]. Figure 8 shows a typical spectrum of carp parvalbumin $PaCa_2$ in D_20 at 270 MHz under Fourier transform conditions. Although the spectrum is well resolved the multiplicity due to spin–spin coupling is not observed. Coupling constants are usually less than 10 Hz and the natural broadening in proteins usually exceeds this value [40]. A detailed description of the spectrum of carp parvalbumin pI 4.25 is available [39]. If the FID signal* is treated mathematically the broadening of the resonances can be decreased substantially and spin–spin splitting can be observed on the ^{1}H NMR spectra of small proteins. The resolution enhancement shown in fig. 8B was obtained by convolution difference spectroscopy (CDS) [42]. The spin–spin multiplicity of many signals is thus apparent (the expanded spectrum of fig. 11 provides a better presentation).

An alternative method for resolution enhancement is the digital filtering of the FID with a sinusoidal window function or "sine bell" technique, which yields a similar resolution enhancement [43]. Figure 9 illustrates the resolution enhancement obtained with carp parvalbumin at 360 MHz. Spin–spin splitting is readily observed for many resonances. Resolution enhancement which is obtained either by CDS or by

*FID or free induction decay of the time-dependent magnetization after the radiofrequency magnetic field pulse. For further details the reader is referred to ref. [41].

the "sine bell" technique provides the possibility to analyze the ^{1}H NMR spectra of proteins by the spin decoupling techniques.

Figure 10 illustrates a series of decoupling experiments (double resonance) which yields the identification of the aromatic resonances of a given phenylalanine in carp parvalbumin. Irradiation of the triplet at 6.25 ppm (two proton intensity) affects the triplet at 5.95 ppm (one proton intensity), which is transformed into a singlet, as well as another resonance at 7.21 ppm (see fig. 10D signals P_1 and O_1 respectively). Since several resonances are present in the 7.2 ppm region it is difficult to recognize the multiplicity of the latter resonance. However, this is achieved by observing the difference between the non-irradiated spectrum and the irradiated one (difference spectroscopy): the signal at 7.21 ppm is a doublet which coalesces into a singlet on irradiation according to the difference pattern (fig. 10D).

Irradiation at 5.95 ppm as well as at 7.21 ppm affects the triplet at 6.25 ppm, which in both cases is transformed into a doublet (signal M_1 in figs. 10B and 10C, respectively). These results suggest that the triplet at 6.25 ppm correspond to two equivalent *meta* protons (M_1), the triplet at 5.95 ppm to the single *para* proton (P_1) and the doublet at 7.21 ppm to two equivalent *ortho* protons (O_1) of a phenylalanine residue arbitrarily labelled 1.

The aromatic region of the spectrum of carp parvalbumin was analyzed by the double resonance method. If the resonance frequencies of protons belonging to the same aromatic ring are sufficiently different the results of the decoupling experiments are usually unambiguous. This was the case for the phenylalanine residues labelled from 1 to 5 (see fig. 11). However, in the case of Phe 4 the para and meta proton resonances are distant only by 16 Hz and therefore do not give rise to a first-order spectrum (for a definition see refs. [23, 24]. Since no overlapping is occurring with other resonances the pattern corresponding to the *meta* and *para* protons of the Phe 4 could be identified by a theoretical simulation (see fig. 11).

Only partial assignments were possible between 7.0 and 7.5 ppm where most of the resonances of the phenylalanine residues labelled from 6 to 10 are present.

In all cases the equivalence of the two *meta* protons as well as that of the two *ortho* protons was observed for the phenylalanine aromatic protons of carp parvalbumin pI 4.25 (see fig. 11). Figure 12 illustrates the use of the triple resonance technique in order to identify the

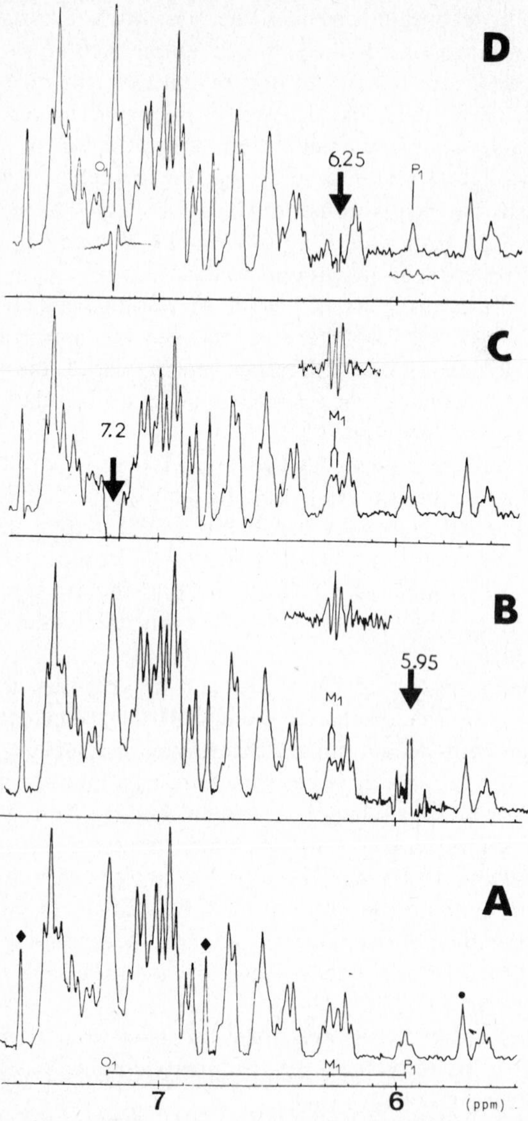

Fig. 10. Identification of resonances *meta* (M_1), *ortho* (O_1), and *para* (P_1) protons of Phe_1 (arbitrary numbering). Aromatic region of the CDS ^1H NMR spectrum at 270 MHz of carp parvalbumin pI 4.5 (8 mM) in D_2O at pH 6.8 and at 52° C. (A) Without irradiation. (B) *Para* irradiation at 5.95 ppm; inset: difference spectrum A–B for the *meta* resonance. (C) *Ortho* irradiation at 7.2 ppm; inset: difference spectrum A–C for the *meta* resonance. (D) *Meta* irradiation at 6.25 ppm; inset: difference spectrum A–D for the *ortho* and *para* resonances.

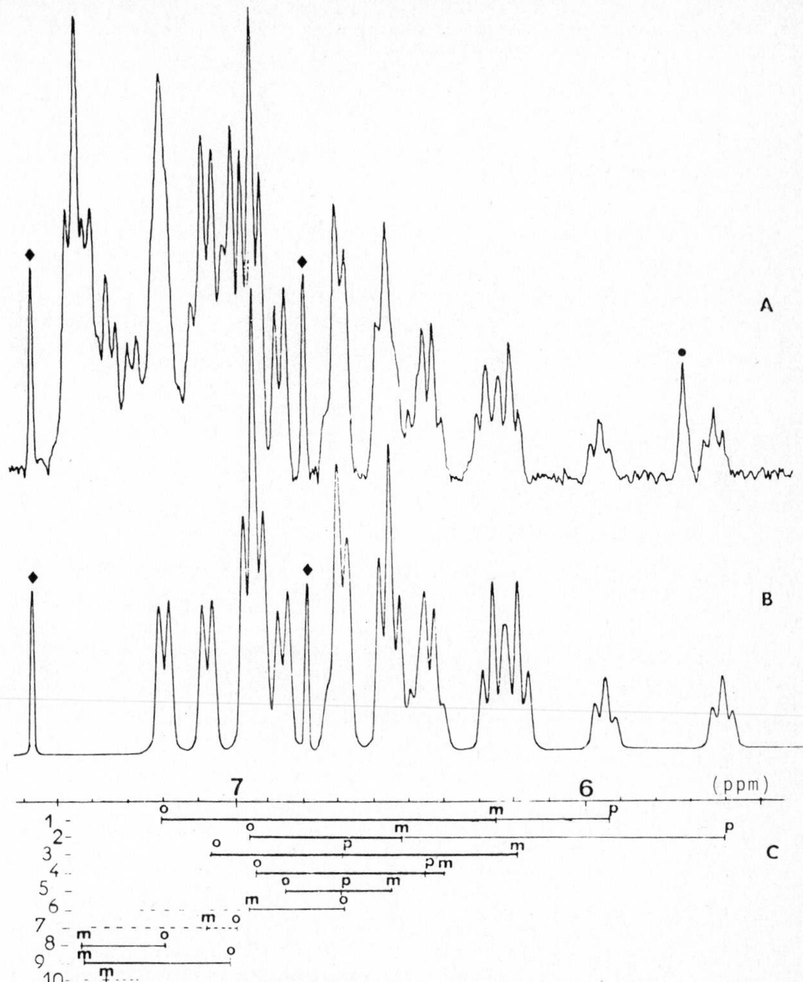

Fig. 11. Identification by double resonance of the *meta* (m), *ortho* (o), and *para* (p) proton resonances in the aromatic region (see A) of the CDS ^{1}H NMR spectrum at 270 MHz of carp parvalbumin pI 4.25 (8 mM) in D_2O at pH 6.8 and at 52° C. The final attributions are given in C (numbering of the 10 Phe residues is arbitrary). The spectrum in B was calculated for the first six Phe residues, whose aromatic resonances were fully identified, according to standard computering techniques (see fig. 4). (◆) imidazole proton resonances from His-26 (●) non-aromatic proton.

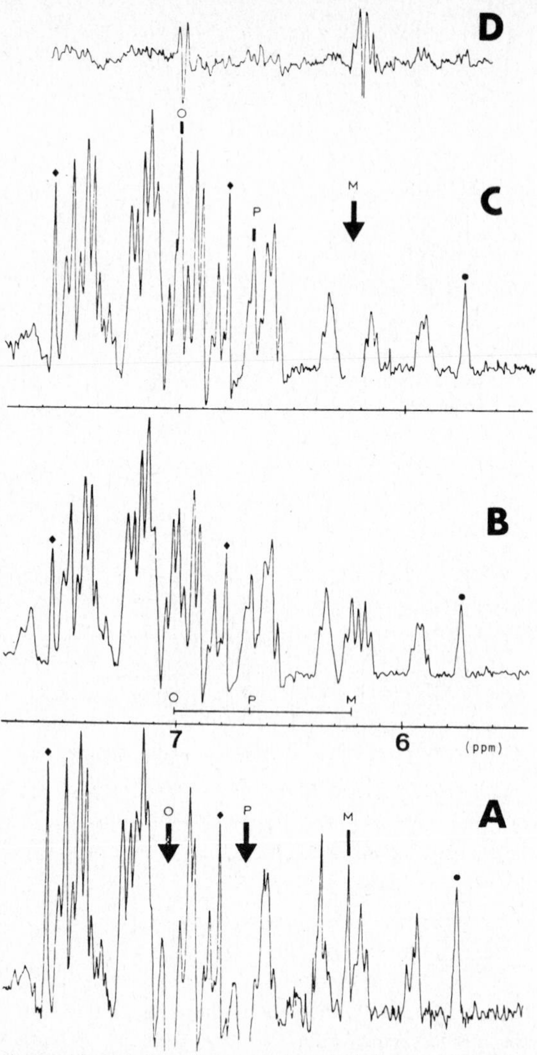

Fig. 12. Identification of the *meta* (*M*), *ortho* (*O*), and *para* (*P*) proton resonances of a given phenylalanine in the CDS ^{1}H NMR spectrum at 270 MHz of hake parvalbumin pI 4.36 (6.5 mM) in D_2O at pH 7.0 and at 52° C (1024 transients). (A) Simultaneous irradiation of *ortho* and *para* resonances affecting the *meta* resonance (singlet). (B) Without irradiation. (C) *Meta* irradiation. (D) Difference spectrum A–C showing the location of the *ortho* resonance.

aromatic resonances of a given phenylalanine residue in the case of hake parvalbumin pI 4.36. The simultaneous irradiation at 6.68 and 7.02 ppm (signals *P* and *O*, respectively in fig. 12) transforms the triplet at 6.2 ppm into a singlet (signal *M* in fig. 12A). A related double resonance experiment is also shown in fig. 12C.

3.3. *The fluid-like structure of the internal hydrophobic core of parvalbumins*

The decoupling experiments discussed above clearly establish that the two *ortho* protons as well as the two *meta* protons of the aromatic rings of almost all the phenylalanine residues of carp parvalbumin pI 4.25 are equivalent. Such an equivalence can be understood by considering rapid flipping movements about the C^{β}-C^{1} bonds of the phenylalanine residues of this protein. The same conclusion is valid for several other parvalbumins studied by ^{1}H NMR spectroscopy (see below). It can be argued that the observation of a chemical equivalence between the two *ortho* protons as well as the two *meta* protons of a phenylalanine ring (or tyrosine ring) in the proton NMR spectrum of a protein is not a proof per se that $\pm 180°$ rotations about the C^{β}-C^{1} bond do occur. However, the fact that 9 phenylalanine residues among the 10 of carp parvalbumin pI 4.25 are characterized by symmetrical patterns of the AA′BB′C type is difficult to reconcile with a full rigidity of the phenylalanine side-chains since the chemical environment around a given aromatic ring is to be rather asymmetric in the protein interior.

For the same reasons oscillations of relatively small amplitude about the C^{β}-C^{1} bonds ($\Delta\chi_2 = \pm 10$–$20°$) will not be able to produce a symmetrical pattern of the AA′BB′C type for the phenylalanine aromatic resonances. Such oscillations certainly occur in the interior of the protein and they are expected on theoretical basis to be very fast on the NMR time scale [1]. Therefore the observed chemical shifts are time-averaged values over a set of individual chemical shifts corresponding to a range of allowed χ_2 values.

Although almost all the phenylalanine side-chains of carp parvalbumin pI 4.25 are internally located according to X-ray crystallography, ^{1}H NMR spectroscopy clearly establishes that these side-chains are able to undergo a rapid conversion between two conformational states due to $\pm 180°$ rotations about the C^{β}-C^{1} bonds. The rates of interconversion are to be much more rapid than 10^3 s^{-1} (see fig. 15) even at temperatures near 0° C. This conclusion is certainly valid for parvalbumins in general since their tertiary structures are to be very similar according to NMR spectroscopy evidence, in particular the organization of their internal hydrophobic core [27, 44]. This internal core has therefore a fluid-like structure.

4. Relationship between the solid structure and the solution structure of parvalbumins

It is an open question whether the solid-state structure determined by X-ray crystallography is the same as that of the protein in solution. High-resolution NMR spectroscopy has often been used to give an answer to this question. The approach consists in predicting the proton NMR spectrum from the X-ray atomic coordinates. A detailed simulation is not really possible because of the great number of parameters which act on proton chemical shifts and whose effects are poorly understood at a theoretical level. However, the magnetic effects due to delocalized π-electrons of aromatic rings (as those of phenylalanine side-chains) are characterized by large amplitudes and, therefore, calculations can be restricted to these important effects. The magnetic perturbation (ring current effects) around the aromatic ring of a benzene molecule can be predicted satisfactorily by using the classical model of Johnson and Bovey [45]. A typical diagram is given in fig. 13 where the magnetic effects are presented under the form of some isoshielding curves which are relevant for chemical purposes. Two distinct zones are apparent in fig. 13. One above the zero isoshielding line is characterized by negative shielding values (i.e. resonances are displaced towards lower chemical shift values) and the other, below the zero shielding line, is characterized by positive shielding values (displacement towards higher chemical shift values). The effects are very important since the resonance of a proton in Van der Waals contact with the benzene ring along the Oz axis will be shifted upfield (negative shielding) by more than 2 ppm. This is a very large effect if one considers the resolution of the NMR method. Therefore, if contacts between chemical groups in the tertiary structure of a globular protein involve aromatic rings (from Phe, Tyr, or Trp) very important shifts of several proton resonances can be expected. A great number of aromatic contacts occur in the internal core of parvalbumins as indicated by the crystalline structure of carp parvalbumin pI 4.25. The position of each phenylalanine side-chain of this protein is given in fig. 14 according to refined X-ray atomic coordinates [31]. If the protein in solution retains

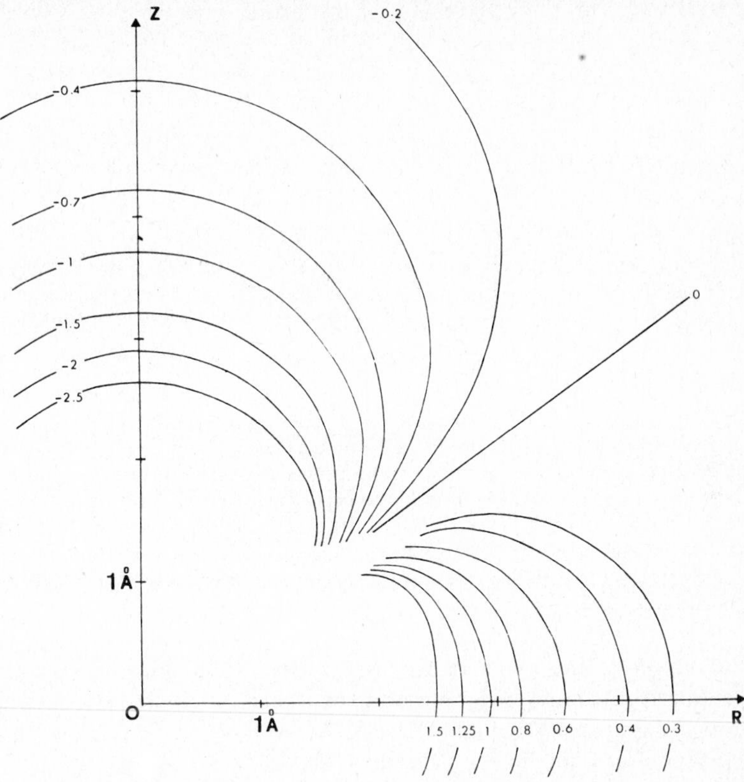

Fig. 13. Magnetic perturbation around a benzene ring according to the theoretical predictions of the model of Johnson and Bovey [45]. Some of the chemically relevant isoshielding curves are given. The negative sign corresponds to high field displacements (lower chemical shift values), while the positive sign corresponds to low field displacements (higher chemical shift values). The plane of the benzene ring contains the OR direction while the Oz axis of revolution is perpendicular to the benzene ring.

the same compact tridimensional structure as that observed in the crystalline state it can be anticipated that many proton resonances will be shifted from their "normal" positions as observed with the denatured protein. A detailed presentation of the proton NMR spectrum at 270 MHz of carp parvalbumin pI 4.25 at different temperatures is given in fig. 15. Actually the methyl proton resonances of Leu, Ile, and Val, which are all centered round +0.9 ppm in the denatured protein, are spread from −0.4 to +0.9 ppm in the native protein (fig. 15). Similarly

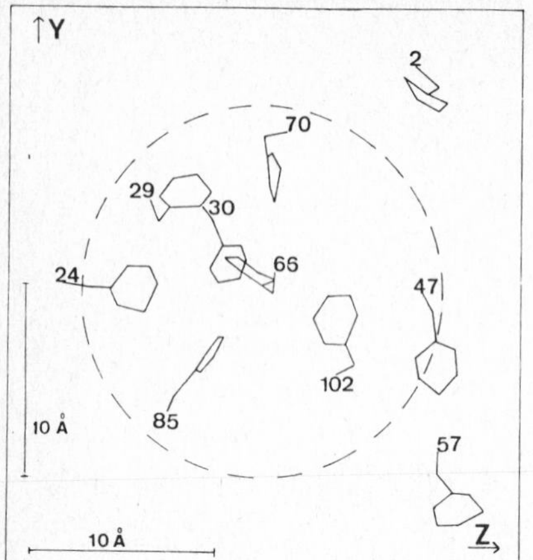

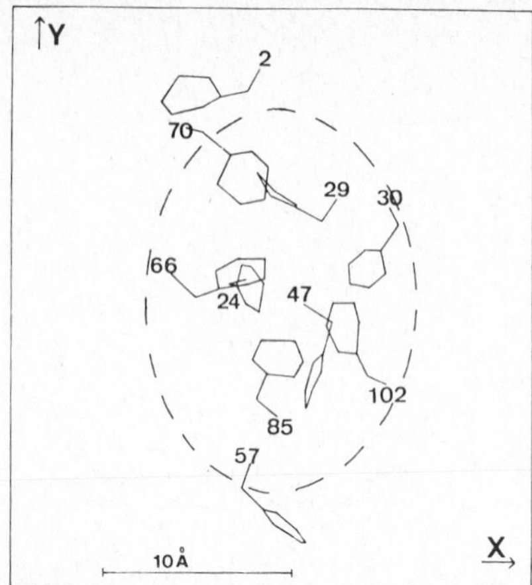

Fig. 14. Right-angle projections of the 10 phenylalanine side-chains of carp parvalbumin pI 4.25 according to refined X-ray atomic coordinates [Moews and Kretsinger, J. Mol. Biol. 91 (1975) 201.] It must be noticed that several aromatic rings are non-planar and have a slightly puckered shape (this certainly corresponds to spurious effects in the crystallographic analysis). All Phe residues expect Phe-2 and Phe-57 belong to the internal hydrophobic core.

the resonances of the 50 aromatic protons are shifted from their "normal" position at about +7.3 ppm and are spread over an extended area between +5.5 and +7.8 ppm. These shifts are likely to originate from ring current effects due to Phe–Phe as well as Phe–methyl contacts.

Above 80° C the shifts are no more observed as a consequence of the disorganization of the protein structure by thermal denaturation (see fig. 15). A similar effect is observed after removal of the calcium ions from $PaCa_2$ [39]. Ring current effects were calculated for the methyl resonances of aliphatic residues (Ala, Ile, Leu, Val) and the aromatic resonances of phenylalanine residues of carp parvalbumin pI 4.25 according to the Johnson and Bovey model*. The most important upfield shifts, which were calculated for methyl groups, mainly concern aliphatic residues whose side-chains are located within the hydrophobic core of the protein. Although the comparison between the calculated spectrum and the observed one does not provide a straightforward identification of the methyl resonances according to their location in the protein structure, it is remarkable to note that the predicted number of

*The validity of this model was tested with a series of polysubstituted benzenic compounds, resulting in good agreement between experiment and theory [46].

upfield shifted resonances is very close (12 methyl groups) to that observed experimentally (about 14 methyl groups) [39]. Similar calculations performed for the aromatic protons of the phenylalanine residues predicted important upfield shifts for 11 aromatic protons (chemical shifts below 6.6 ppm) in comparison to the 13 resonances observed experimentally. However, no strict identification of these shifted resonances can be done on the basis of such calculations. These results strongly suggest that the contacts between non-polar residues in the internal hydrophobic core of crystalline carp parvalbumin are also preserved in solution. Therefore the crystalline structure can be taken as a suitable reference for conformational studies of this protein in solution.

The main discrepancies between the calculated spectrum and the experimental one are likely to originate from the fact that the X-ray coordinates used in the calculations correspond to a unique protein conformation ("static" conformation) while the observed chemical shifts for the protein in solution are time-averaged values over a great number of allowed conformations due to fluctuations of the protein structure. Let us consider the dependence of the ring current effects on different rotational movements about the C^{β}-C^{1} bonds of phenylalanine residues. As an example let us take the case of the two neighboring phenylalanine residues, Phe-24 and Phe-29. According to the calculations based on the "static" model the most important shielding effect observed with the *meta* protons of the Phe-24 is due to the through-space influence of Phe-29 [39]. An important contribution from the Phe-29 also occurs for one of the methyl groups of Val-33. If the aromatic rings of Phe-24 and Phe-29 are allowed to oscillate about their C^{β}-C^{1} bonds ($\Delta\chi_2 = \pm 10°$), the *meta* proton of Phe-24 experiences important variations of its chemical shift (-0.4 to -0.8 ppm) from its unperturbed position according to the position of Phe-29 (see fig. 16). Similarly the variations of the chemical shift of the methyl group of Val-33 are comprised between -0.5 and -0.7 ppm. These are very important variations taking into account the relatively small amplitude of the aromatic ring oscillations. Since these oscillations are very rapid (see ref. [1]) on the NMR time scale averaged chemical shifts must be considered. Averaging of chemical shifts for the *meta* and the *ortho* protons of a phenylalanine residue during flipping about the C^{β}-C^{1} bond will be strongly dependent on the amplitude of the allowed oscillations. Furthermore, it is likely that these internal motions (oscillations, flipping) have a certain degree of correlation as indicated by theoretical studies

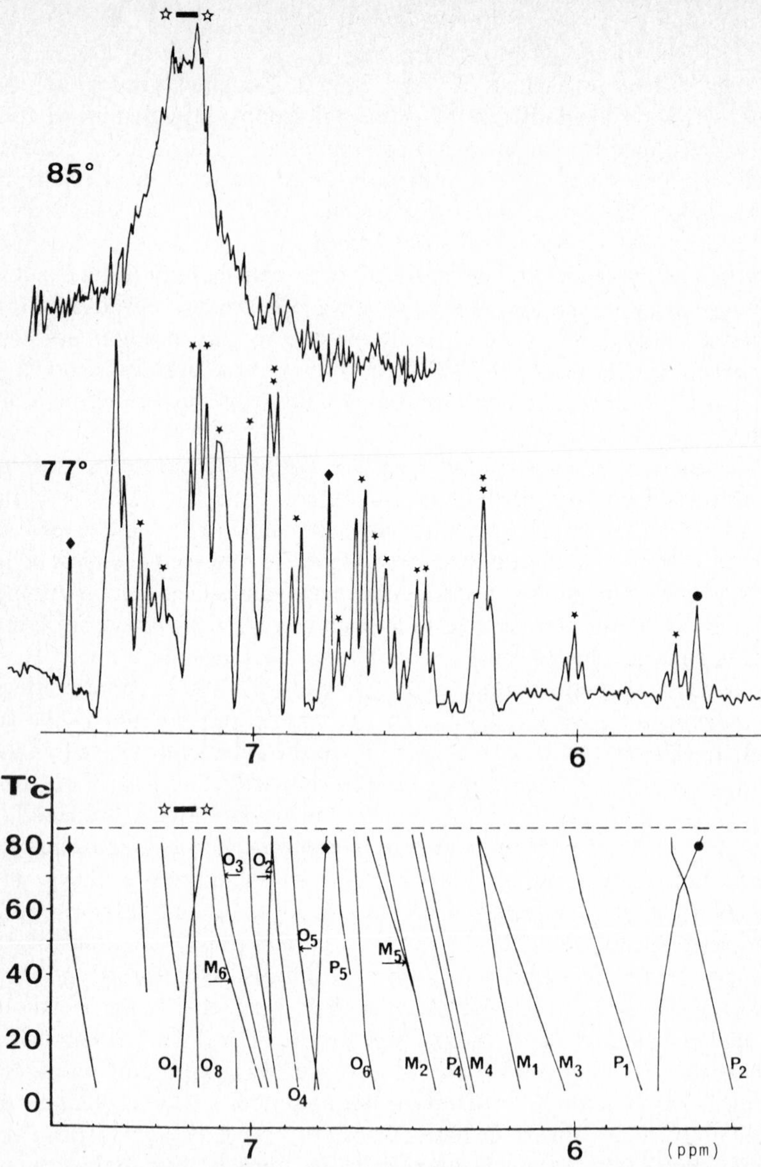

Fig. 15. Temperature dependence between 4° C and 85° C of the spectral regions from −1 to 3.5 ppm (left) and from 5.5 to 7.5 ppm (left) in the CDS ^1H NMR spectrum at 270 MHz of an 8 mM solution of parvalbumin pI 4.25 in D_2O at pH 6.8. (◆) Imidazole protons of His-26; (●) signal corresponding to a non-aromatic proton. The individual resonances or groups of resonances which are temperature dependent, are identified by stars. The spectra at 77° C and 85° C, respectively illustrate the conformational changes occurring on thermal denaturation. O_i, M_i, and P_1 ($i = 1, 2, \ldots$) indicate *ortho*, *meta*, and *para* protons belonging to the same phenylalanine i (i is an arbitrary number for a given Phe residue).

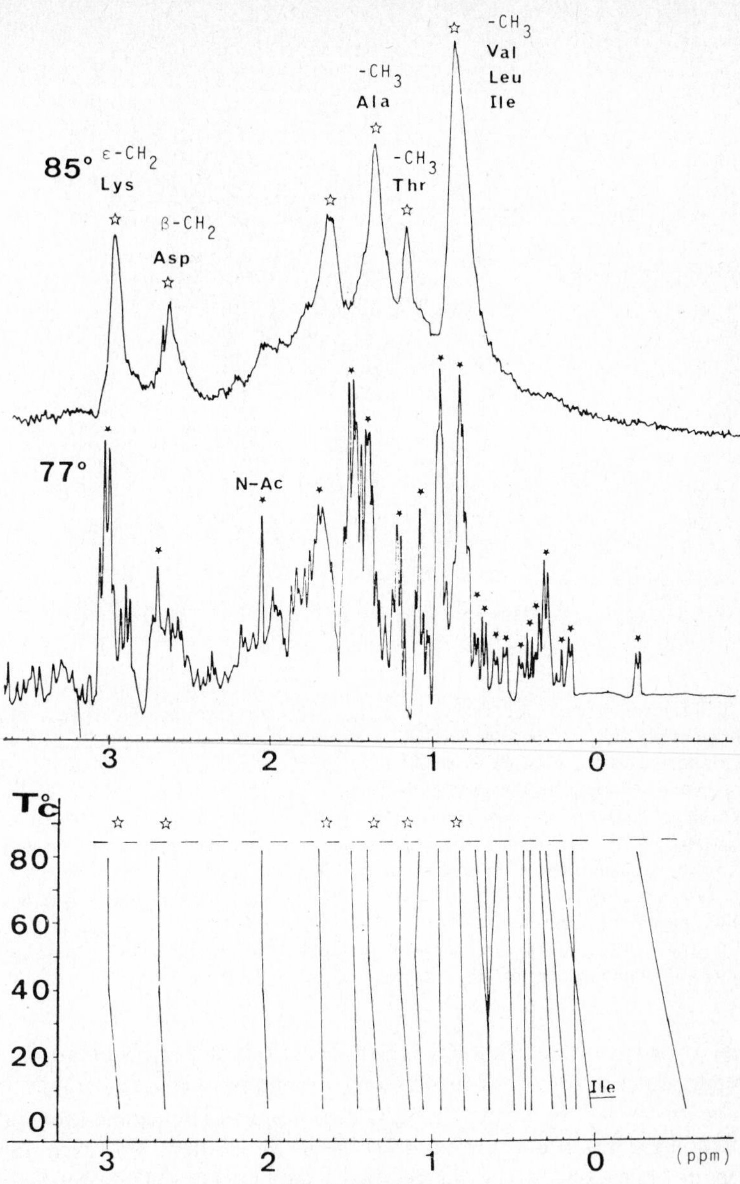

Fig. 15 Continued

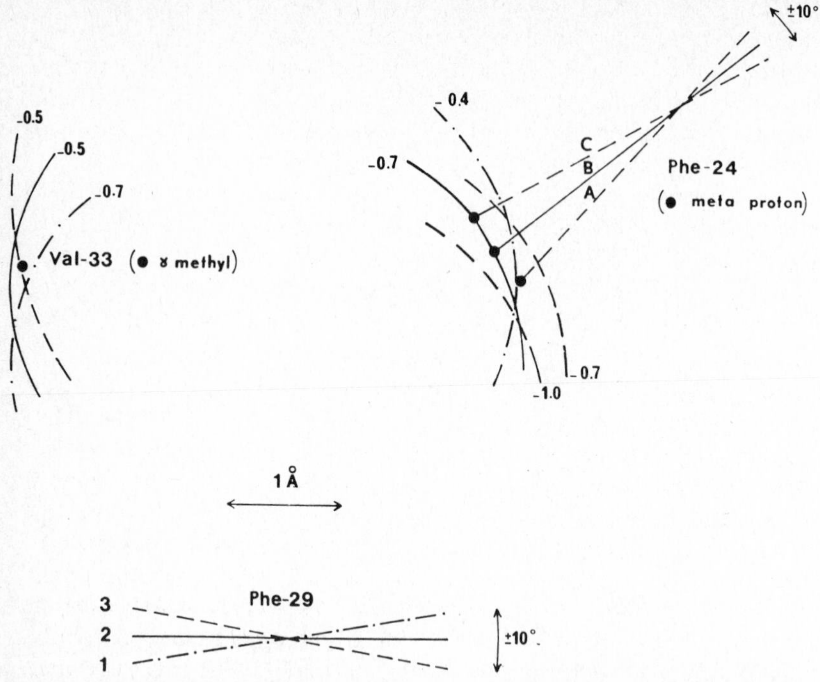

Fig. 16. Influence of small amplitude oscillations about phenylalanine C^{β}-C^{1} bonds on the NMR chemical shifts of protons located in the interior of carp parvalbumin pI 4.25. Phe-24 and Phe-29 are allowed to oscillate by $\pm 10°$ around their equilibrium position determined by X-ray crystallography. Magnetic isoshielding curves (see fig. 13 for a definition) are given at three different rotational positions of Phe-29 and are distinguished graphically by ----, ———, and –·–·–, respectively. Negative shielding values correspond to an upfield displacement of the perturbed proton, i.e. a lowering of the chemical shift value. The three dots for Phe-24 correspond to the positions during time of one of the *meta* protons according to the rotational state of Phe-24 about its C^{β}-C^{1} bond. The single dot for Val-33 corresponds to a geometrical point which is the center of the circle containing the three protons of the γ-methyl group of this residue.

[1]. Knowledge of the detailed mechanisms of internal fluctuations in globular proteins (amplitude, frequency, correlation between neighbours) will be necessary in order to carry out appropriate calculations for predicting the ^{1}H NMR spectra of proteins in solution. However, since the main features of the aromatic region of the ^{1}H NMR spectrum of carp parvalbumin pI 4.25 are well understood on the basis of the compact structure of the hydrophobic core of this protein (see fig. 14), the tertiary structure of parvalbumins in solution can be profitably

investigated by ^{1}H NMR spectroscopy. Comparative studies can be readily carried out using the decoupling techniques [44]. Figure 17 illustrates the results obtained with seven parvalbumins from different origins (carp, hake, nase, pike, ray), including five proteins of the phylogenetic β series and two proteins of the α series.

The observation of upfield shifted resonances in all the spectra indicates that the compactness of the hydrophobic core is kept for all these parvalbumins. The observation of a single resonance for the meta protons as well as for the *ortho* protons, which were identified on the spectra, establishes that the "fluidity" of the internal hydrophobic core is a general characteristic of parvalbumins.

Very similar characteristics are observed in the spectra of the β parvalbumins and are examined here. The signals of Phe 1 $(O \gg M > P)$ and Phe 3 $(O > M \gg P)$ are well recognized for all these proteins. It must be kept in mind that a distance variation of 0.1 Å can be accompanied by a chemical shift variation as high as 0.2 ppm (see fig. 13). The chemical shifts of Phe 1 and Phe 3 are practically unaffected except for the *para* proton of Phe 3 of hake parvalbumin which appears at 5.95 ppm instead of 5.6 ppm. Therefore the similarities observed in the aromatic patterns given in fig. 17 strongly indicate that the geometrical organization of the hydrophobic core is very well preserved during evolution. The spectral characteristics of pike parvalbumin pI 5.0, which belongs to the α series, differ markedly from those of parvalbumins of the β series. For instance one of the phenylalanine residues show the following order $(P \gg M > O)$ for its aromatic resonances and this is not observed with parvalbumins of the series. This is a very interesting observation since it suggests that parvalbumins of both series α and β differ by their tertiary structures. However, a more systematic study is necessary in order to establish a delineation between the two phylogenetic series on the basis of tertiary structure features.

5. Conformational internal mobility and biological function of proteins

Dynamic properties are likely to play a fundamental role in the biological function of proteins. Two examples will be considered: muscular parvalbumins and enzymes.

Parvalbumins are metalloproteins that interact with Ca^{2+} ions as well as with Mg^{2+} ions [34, 37, 38]. It is likely that the conformational mobility of their internal hydrophobic core is related to the ability of these proteins to adapt their tertiary structure according to the chemical

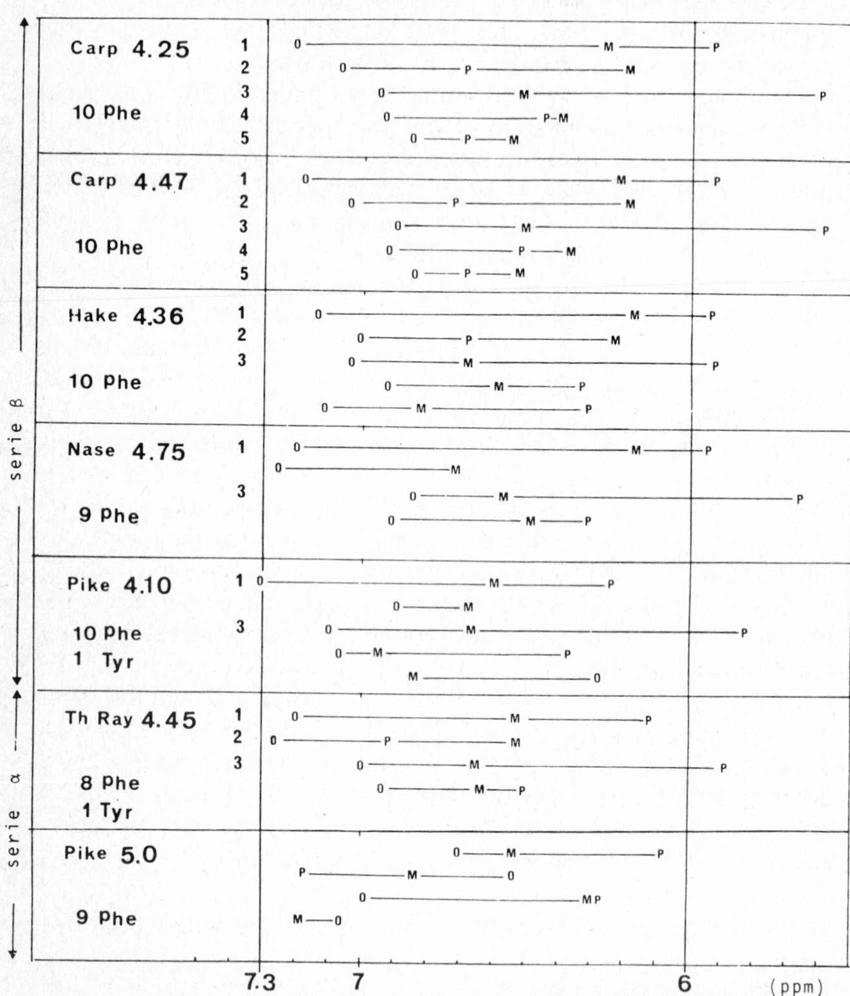

Fig. 17. Comparative patterns of the spreading of Phe aromatic resonaces in the ^{1}H NMR spectra of several parvalbumins, belonging to the α and β series. The numbering of Phe residues, which is independent of the sequence position, is done according to that adopted for carp parvalbumin pI 4.25 (see fig. 11) on the basis of chemical shift analogies.

nature of the bound cation. ^{1}H NMR spectroscopy indicates that Ca–Mg exchange is accompanied by structural modifications which although restricted in amplitude involve several chemical groups of the internal core of the parvalbumin molecule [47]. It is likely that the substitution of Ca^{2+} ($r = 0.99$ Å) by Mg^{2+} ($r = 0.65$ Å) is accompanied by a "contraction" of the coordination sphere around the protein-bound cation because of the difference between the ionic radii. Such a local contraction is to be followed by structural modifications of protein domains which are related to the cation-binding polypeptide loops CD and EF (see subsection 3.1).

Interactions between aromatic and polar groups of amino acids have been reported to have a functional aspect in enzymes. Chemical modifications of Trp 99, in the vicinity of His 46 and Ser 183, alter the catalytic activity of trypsin. Similarly in lysozyme Trp 108 and Glu 35 show a privileged interaction. These through-space interactions are able to affect the physicochemical properties of functional groups in the active site. Studies with model organic molecules clearly showed that the ionization properties of a carboxylic group are dependent on the immediate surrounding. The approach of a hydrophobic group at the vicinity of a carboxylic group is accompanied by a marked increase of the pK_a (about 0.5 unit) of this chemical group [48, 49]. If fluctuations were to occur in protein domain, where interactions between polar and non-polar groups occur, local pK_a fluctuations can be expected which would affect the reactivity of the enzyme during time. It is likely that the catalytic rates of enzymes are also sensitive to the dynamic properties of enzyme-substrate complexes [1]. Allosteric transitions are likely to involve the dynamic properties of proteins.

A careful experimental and theoretical approach to these structural questions is needed. NMR spectroscopy appears to be one of the most promising techniques used to investigate the dynamic properties of proteins in solution.

References

[1] M. Karplus and J. A. McCammon, C. R. C. Critical Reviews in Biochemistry (1980) in press.
[2] M. Saunders, A. Wishnia and J. G. Kirkwood, J. Am. Chem. Soc. 79 (1957) 3289.
[3] K. Wüthrich and G. Wagner, FEBS Lett. 50 (1975) 265.
[4] G. H. Snyder, R. Rowan, III, S. Karplus and B. D. Sykes, Biochemistry 14 (1975) 3765.
[5] G. Wagner and K. Wüthrich, J. Magnetic Res. 20 (1975) 435.

[6] C. M. Dobson, G. R. Moore and R. J. P. Williams, FEBS Lett. 51 (1975) 60.
[7] I. D. Campbell, C. M. Dobson and R. J. P. Williams, Proc. Roy. Soc. B 189 (1975) 503.
[8] A. Cavé, C. M. Dobson, J. Parello and R. J. P. Williams, FEBS Lett. 65 (1976) 190.
[9] F. R. N. Gurd and T. M. Rothgeb, Adv. Protein Chem., to be published.
[10] I. D. Campbell, C. M. Dobson and R. J. P. Williams, Adv. Chem. Phys. 39 (1978) 55.
[11] I. D. Campbell, in: NMR in Biology, eds. R. A. Dwek et al. (Academic Press, New York, 1977) p.33.
[12] K. Wüthrich, Nuclear Magnetic Resonance in Biological Research-Peptides and Proteins (North-Holland, Amsterdam, 1976).
[13] G. Wagner, A. DeMarco and K. Wüthrich, Biophys. Struct. Mech. 2 (1976) 139.
[14] I. D. Campbell, C. M. Dobson, G. R. Moore, S. J. Perkins and R. J. P. Williams, FEBS Lett. 70 (1976) 96.
[15] B. R. Gelin and M. Karplus, Proc. Natl. Acad. Sci. USA 72 (1975) 2002.
[16] R. Hetzel, K. Wüthrich, J. Deisenhofer and R. Huber, Biophys. Struct. Mech. 2 (1976) 159.
[17] J. Parello and J-F Pechère, Biochimie 53 (1971) 1079.
[18] S. J. Opella, D. J. Nelson and O. Jardetzky, J. Am. Chem. Soc. 96 (1974) 7157; D. J. Nelson, S. J. Opella and O. Jardetzlsy, Biochemistry 15 (1976) 5552.
[19] D. R. Bauer, S. J. Opella, D. J. Nelson and R. Pecora, J. Am. Chem. Soc 97 (1975) 2580.
[20] E. L. Eliel, Stereochemistry of Carbon Compounds (McGraw-Hill, New York, 1962).
[21] For a discussion of polypeptide conformation and the common nomenclature, see, e.g. (a) G. N. Ramachandran and V. Sasisekharan, Adv. Protein Chem. 23 (1968) 283; (b) IUPAC-IUB Commission on Biochemical Nomenclature, Biochemistry 9 (1970) 3471.
[22] R. H. Kretsinger and C. E. Nockolds, J. Biol. Chem. 248 (1973) 3313.
[23] R. J. Abraham, Analysis of High Resolution NMR Spectra, (Elsevier, Amsterdam, 1971).
[24] J. A. Pople, W. G. Schneider and H. J. Bernstein, High-Resolution Nuclear Magnetic Resonance (McGraw-Hill, New York, 1959).
[25] J. D. Baldeschwieler and E. W. Randall, Chem. Rev. 81 (1963).
[26] J. Parello, Bull. Soc. Chim. France (1964) 2033.
[27] A. Cavé, C. M. Dobson, J. Parello and R. J. P. Williams, to be published.
[28] J-F. Pechère, J-P. Capony and J. G. Demaille, Syst. Zoology 22 (1973) 533.
[29] J-F. Pechère, J. Demaille and J-P Capony, Biochim. Biophys. Acta 236 (1971) 391.
[30] M. Goodman and J-F. Pechère, J. Mol. Evol. 9 (1977) 131.
[31] P. C. Moews and R. H. Kretsinger, J. Mol. Biol. 91 (1975) 201.
[32] P. Lehky, M. Comte, E. H. Fischer and E. A. Stein, Analytical Biochem. 82 (1977) 158.
[33] A. Cavé, M-F. Daurès, J. Parello, A. Saint-Yves and R. Sempéré, Biochim. 61 (1979) 755.
[34] J. A. Cox, D. R. Winge and E. A. Stein, Biochim. 61 (1979) 601.
[35] F. J. Brinley, Jr., A. Scarpa and T. Tiffert, J. Physiol. 266 (1977) 545.
[36] G. Baron, J. Demaille and E. Dutruge, FEBS Lett. 56 (1975) 156.
[37] J. Haiech, J. Derancourt, J-F. Pechère and J. G. Demaille, Biochemistry 13 (1979) 2752.
[38] A. Cavé, J. Parello, T. Drakenberg, E. Thulin and B. Lindman, FEBS Lett. 100 (1979) 148.

[39] J. Parello A. Cavé, P. Puigdomenech, C. Maury, J.-P. Capony and J-F. Pechère, Biochimie 56 (1974) 61.
[40] C. C. McDonald and W. D. Phillips, J. Am. Chem. Soc. 91 (1969) 1513.
[41] D. Shaw, Fourier Transform NMR Spectroscopy (Elsevier, Amsterdam 1976).
[42] I. D. Campbell, C. M. Dobson, R. J. P. Williams and A. V. Xavier, J. Magn. Reson. 11 (1973) 172.
[43] A. De Marco and K. Wüthrich, J. Magn. Reson. 24 (1976) 201.
[44] A. Cavé and J. Parello, to be published.
[45] C. E. Johnson and F. A. Bovey, J. Chem. Phys. 29 (1958) 1012.
[46] P. Durand, J. Parello and N. P. Buu-Hoï, Bull. Soc. Chim. France (1962) 2438.
[47] A. Cavé, S. Kan and J. Parello, to be published.
[48] M. Beugelmans-Verrier, L. Nicolas, A. Gaudemer and J. Parello, Tetrahed. Lett. (1976) 361.
[49] J. Royer and M. Beugelmans-Verrier, Tetrahedron 35 (1979) 2369.

COURSE 3
(PART II)

MEMBRANE PROTEIN STRUCTURE

Richard HENDERSON

*Laboratory of Molecular Biology,
Hills Road, Cambridge, CB2 2QH
United Kingdom*

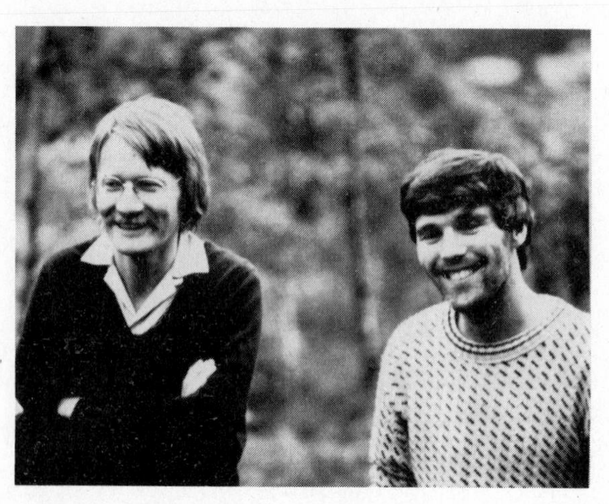

Contents

R. Balian et al., eds.
Les Houches, Session XXXIII, 1979 – Membranes et Communication Intercellulaire / Membranes and Intercellular Communication

1. Introduction

Proteins in membranes, just like soluble proteins, have many different structures and functions. Therefore, this chapter attempts to outline both structural features which may be general to membrane proteins because of their common membrane-bound state and those which are different because of the different function of each protein. By giving an account here of what is known about the structure of a few of the best studied membrane proteins, I hope that a coherent picture of current understanding of the structure of proteins in membranes will emerge.

2. Why are proteins in membranes?

The function of a protein which forms part of a membrane provides a strong constraint in any discussion of structure. A useful categorization of function is as follows: (a) information transfer (e.g. receptors); (b) physical transport of molecules and ions (e.g. pumps, channels); and (c) anchorage of a protein whose true function is in the aqueous phase (e.g. enzymes, antigens).

Only proteins in the second category which physically transport molecules from one side of the membrane to the other will need to provide a pathway or channel through the membrane along which the transported molecule can pass. In contrast, information can be transferred along covalent chemical bonds by a change of conformation, and anchorage can be performed by a fixed unchanging structure.

3. What do we want to know about membrane protein structure?

To answer the most interesting questions of function, we need to know the positions of most of the atoms in the protein and how they change. By analogy with the 150 soluble proteins and enzymes whose detailed structures have been determined by X-ray crystallographic analysis, we will only be able to formulate sensible molecular mechanisms once this level of analysis is reached. So far this has not been possible with membrane proteins though some progress is being made towards producing membrane protein crystals for analysis by X-ray diffraction.

Since we do not yet know the atomic structure from X-ray diffraction analysis, we can ask the following, more general questions about each membrane protein we consider:

(a) What is the relation to the bilayer? How far into the bilayer does it penetrate? How much polypeptide is exposed to the aqueous medium?

(b) What is the orientation or polarity in the cell? Normally the function of the protein will impose a requirement for orientation. Also, biosynthesis from the inside of the cell can provide a mechanism for the generation of polarity.

(c) Does the amino acid sequence of the membrane protein tell us more than the sequences of soluble proteins have? For example, large regions of hydrophobic amino acids may indicate a segment in contact with lipid hydrocarbon.

(d) Can secondary structure be determined? (e.g. β-sheet; α-helix; α-helix perpendicular to membrane; any other secondary structure, e.g. gramicidin A, see later).

(e) What is the nature of segments of the protein in the bilayer? Are hydrophilic residues allowed and if so are they charged or uncharged?

(f) What can be said about function (e.g. does a channel occur)?

4. Theoretical considerations

For the same reasons that the α-helix and β-sheet structures predicted by Pauling and Corey occur widely in soluble and fibrous protein structures, they are expected to be even more stable in the hydrophobic environment provided in a membrane by the central region of the lipid bilayer. This is because the solvation of peptide amido and carbonyl groups which occurs with an unfolded polypeptide in water could not occur at the level of the lipid hydrocarbon chains. The equilibrium towards the folded α-helix or β-sheet structure would, therefore, be greater when surrounded by hydrocarbon (by 5–6 kcal/mole of hydrogen bonds formed) than it would be in water. Structures such as those shown in fig. 1 would therefore be strongly favoured. Both the α-helical bundle structure and the β-sheet barrel structure are frequently found in soluble proteins. If the amino acid side chains exposed to the lipid hydrocarbons were hydrophobic, such structures would be expected to fit into a membrane perfectly. The function of the membrane protein could then be carried out by the amino acid residues at the two

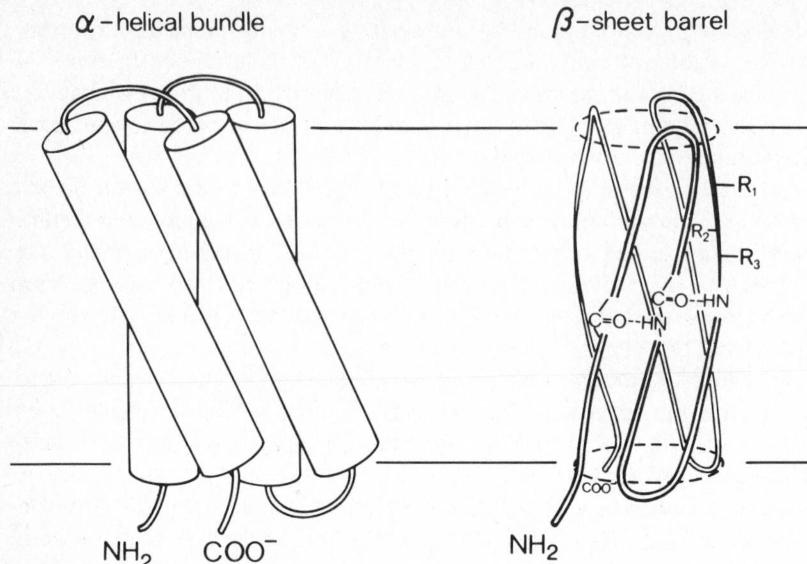

Fig. 1. α-helical bundle and β-sheet barrel structures.

surfaces and by those which form the centre of the α-helical bundle or the β-barrel. All backbone hydrogen bonds would be formed and the outside of the protein would be predominantly hydrophobic. (Some exceptions might be allowed, e.g. proline, serine, and threonine.)

One of the particular important features in the structures of fig. 1 is that the turns, which join together two segments of α- or β-structure, are at the aqueous interface. A characteristic of all turns in proteins, both simple turns (Venkatachalam 1968) and more complex ones, is that some backbone hydrogen bonding groups do not form intrapeptide hydrogen bonds. By having these in the aqueous phase, the loss of free energy which would otherwise occur is avoided. This is the main argument against the stable (as opposed to transient) existence of membrane proteins which are semi-integral or halfway through the membrane (Henderson 1979). Such proteins would necessarily require turns or bends to occur in the centre of the membrane where the contacts with the lipid hydrocarbon tails would be most hydrophobic. Moreover, the function of such semi-integral membrane proteins would be limited to anchorage or complexing with another protein which was semi-integral from the other side (to form an integral protein complex). Both of these functions could be carried out easily by proteins which were either truly transmembrane or superficially bound (e.g. ionically) to the lipid head groups. Thus, there is no functional necessity for the semi-integral membrane protein.

In soluble proteins with known structures, the predominant folding patterns are all based on fairly regular, internal secondary structures with the less regular turns and bends on the surface and are, therefore, in contact with water. Stretches of polypeptide that pass into the centre of the protein molecule, then turn and come out again, are never found. Since this type of feature is exactly equivalent to the structure which would be needed in a semi-integral membrane protein, the simplest conclusion must be that the formation of such proteins would be difficult.

Therefore, from the viewpoint of the energetics of protein folding, such structures as those shown in fig. 1, are to be expected, whereas semi-integral proteins of the halfway-through type are not. Of course more complicated arrangements, where only part of a protein is embedded and part is exposed to the water, are to be expected in abundance. The arguments given above apply only to the part of the protein which is positioned at the level of the hydrocarbon chains of the lipid bilayer.

5. Some examples of membrane proteins for which the amino acid sequence is known

Here we will consider a few membrane proteins which have sufficient chemical data from a wide variety of experiments including a knowledge of the amino acid sequence, that it is possible to propose a definite structure in the form of an arrangement of the polypeptide relative to the lipid bilayer. Only four are considered although considerable sequence information is available on a number of others. Two others that are worth further examination, but which are not discussed here are: (a) cytochrome b_5 which has a 50-residue hydrophobic tail which acts as an anchor (Ozols and Gerard 1977a,b, Fleming et al. 1978) and (b) the DCCD-binding subunit from mitochondrial H^+-ATPase which is probably in the membrane as a hexamer and may be a proton channel or part of it (Sebald and Wachter 1979).

5.1. Human erythrocyte glycophorin

This is the major glycoprotein of the red blood cell which has been shown (Bretscher 1971) to span the lipid bilayer. The structural work of

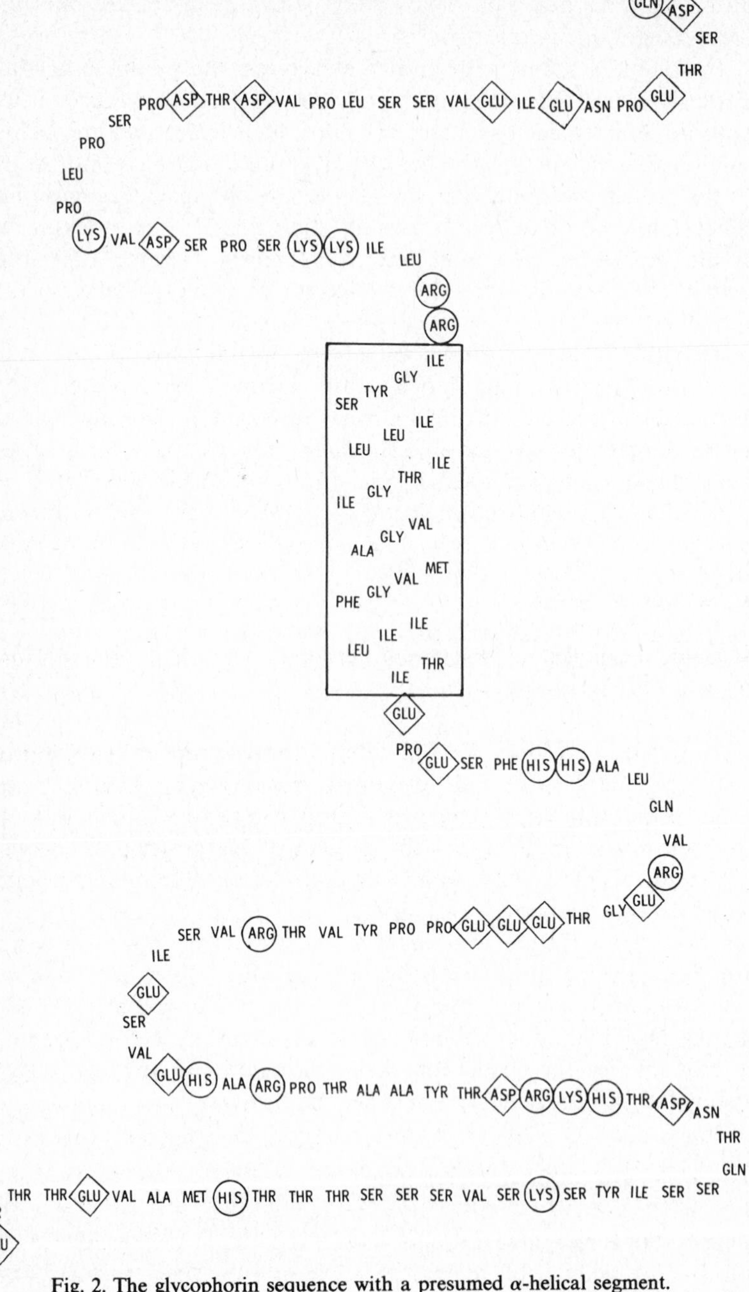

Fig. 2. The glycophorin sequence with a presumed α-helical segment.

Marchesi's group at Yale has resulted in the complete determination of the sequence of this 131 residue protein. The structural analysis has been reviewed recently by Furthmayr (1977). The function of the protein appears to be to act as an anchorage site for the enormous number of carbohydrate residues which are coupled at 16 positions to the polypeptide on the outside surface of the membrane. The function of the carbohydrate is a separate topic (see Sharon, this volume). Anchorage to the bilayer seems to occur by a very hydrophobic stretch of the polypeptide. The 23 residues from Ile-73 to Ile-95 are almost totally hydrophobic and contain only one serine and one threonine. The conformation of this section of the polypeptide is almost certain to be α-helical and its location at the level of the bilayer. Both ends of the protein, residues 1–72, on the outside of the cell and residues 96–131, on the inside contain a large number of charged and hydrophilic amino acid side chains.

In a recent paper, Schulte and Marchesi (1979) have examined the conformation of glycophorin and its constituent tryptic peptides by circular dichroism. They find that the hydrophobic peptide T6A, which includes the 23 residues mentioned above, is entirely α-helical, whereas the peptides corresponding to the amino and carboxyl termini are predominantly unordered. They also found that the sum of the circular dichroism spectra of all of the tryptic peptides was indistinguishable from the spectrum of the intact native molecule which contained only 27% α-helix. Thus, a structure along the lines of that shown in fig. 2 is indicated where the exact conformation of the parts of the molecule on the two sides of the membrane is uncertain, but likely to be substantially unordered. The α-helical stretch in the membrane fits well with its function as an anchor, and the parts of the peptide in the three different regions of the membrane (inside, within, outside) do not seem to interact with one another.

5.2. fd phage coat protein before association with DNA

The coat protein of fd is normally found surrounding the DNA of the filamentous fd phage and has a very high α-helical content. The structure of the whole virus has been the subject of detailed analysis by X-ray diffraction (Marvin and Wachtel 1975; Makowski and Caspar 1979). During assembly of the virus, however, the protein is first synthesized and is partitioned into the membrane of the infected bacterium (*E. coli*). Only later when the DNA (circular, single-stranded DNA) is replicated, does the coat protein combine with the DNA in a

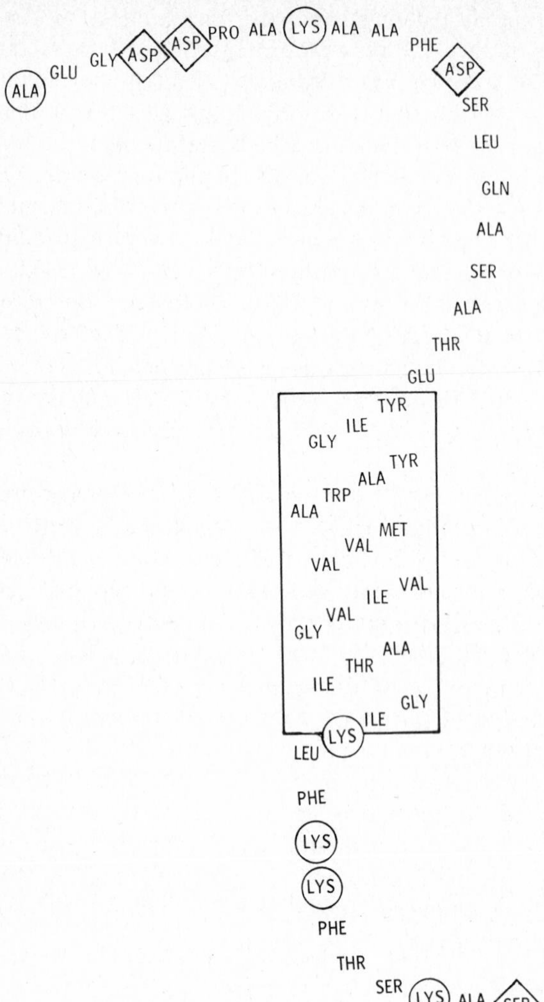

Fig. 3. The fd sequence with a presumed α-helical segment.

process believed to be one of combined virus extrusion and assembly (Marvin and Hohn 1969). Thus for a considerable time the fd coat protein is in the membrane of the bacterium. This is also true for the homologous phages pfl and Ml3.

The sequence of the 50 amino acid protein has been determined (Nakashima and Konigsberg 1974) and shows a hydrophobic stretch of 20 residues with hydrophilic segments at both amino and carboxyl termini. The arrangement suggests that in the membrane, as shown in fig. 3, the polypeptide would adopt a similar α-helical structure to that of glycophorin. The residues at the C-terminus are basic and are thought to combine with the acidic phosphate groups of the DNA in the centre of the virus after assembly whereas the more acidic residues at the *N*-terminus are thought to form the outside of the intact virus. Both these hydrophilic stretches would be expected to be in contact with water when the protein is in the membrane, the *N*-terminus being towards the outside of the cell (Wickner 1976).

Unfortunately, the experiments which have been carried out do not entirely support this simple view of the structure. Williams and Dunker (1977) find by circular dichroism that the spectrum and the extent of α-helicity depends on the history of the protein and the method of vesicle preparation. The work of Chamberlain et al. (1978), who have used proteolytic enzymes to digest away the soluble, hydrophilic parts of the molecule, seems to show that the remaining hydrophobic sequences have entirely β-structure. However, the experiments of Chamberlain et al. (1978) are not so complete as those of Schulte and Marchesi. They have not taken the spectra of the polypeptide segments which are released on proteolysis and, as they point out, the structure of the molecule may have been changed by proteolysis. The picture of the coat protein of fd as a simple α-helix when in the membrane is, therefore, not ruled out.

5.3. The gramicidin A channel

Gramicidin A is one of a related group of hydrophobic polypeptides which have antibiotic activity by means of forming membrane pores or channels which have some selectivity for cations like potassium. Its chemical structure, a sequence of 15 amino acids blocked at the amino end by a formyl group and at the carboxyl end by ethanolamine, is shown in fig. 4. Since the stereochemical configuration at the α-carbons of the amino acids alternates between L and D along the sequence, some rather unusual structures can be formed. These were proposed by Urry (1971) and are called π(L, D) helices. They can be described as sort of helical β-structures since the direction of the carbonyl (and amide) linkages alternates in direction from one amino acid to the next. Normally in β-structure, the side chains of the amino acids extend on both sides of the sheet, but with sequences like those of gramicidin with alternating L and D configurations, all side chains extend on the same

Gramicidin A

Formyl-L-Val-Gly-L-Ala-D-Leu-L-Ala-D-Val-L-Val-D-Val-L-Trp-D-Leu-L-Trp-D-Leu-L-Trp-D-Leu-L-Trp-$NHCH_2CH_2OH$

Fig. 4. The gramicidin sequence and blocking groups (Sarges and Witkop 1965).

side. This gives the sheet a tendency to curl, and the π(L, D) helices of Urry carry this to the logical conclusion in a helix. Urry et al. (1971) described a family of helices with 4.4, 6.3, 8.4, and 10.4 residues per turn. The structure of the gramicidin A channel as found in membranes is thought to have 6.3 residues per turn and to be made up of a head-to-head dimer in which there is hydrogen bonding between the *N*-terminus of each gramicidin monomer at the centre of the bilayer (Urry et al. 1971). The whole structure is about 25 Å long and can fit across bilayers of this and somewhat thicker dimensions if some local thinning of the lipid bilayer is allowed. Other structures based on this same type of stereochemistry have been proposed (e.g. Veatch and Blout 1974) but recent work using ^{13}C NMR has convincingly demonstrated that Urry's original model (Urry et al. 1971) is correct. Weinstein et al. (1979) have labelled both the *N*-formyl group and the C-terminus with carbon-13 labels for NMR observation, and used various paramagnetic probes (manganese ions, nitroxide free radicals) to relax the resonance from different levels of the bilayer. Their results show conclusively that the *N*-terminus is at the centre of the bilayer and the C-terminus on the surface when the gramicidin is in the form of a channel (at high concentration). Of course, at low concentration, most of the gramicidin in the membrane is monomeric, and only occasional conducting dimers are formed. The work of Veatch and Stryer (1975) showed the expected relationship between conductance and amount of gramicidin in the membrane under these conditions of low concentration (a slope of 2 in a log–log plot). The structure of the non-conducting, monomeric form of gramicidin is not known. It may form a helical structure at one surface of the membrane and parallel to it, where some hydration at each end can occur. The transient occurrence of a halfway through, correctly oriented gramicidin monomer must also occur on the pathway to dimer formation. The lifetime of this gramicidin conformation is not known. Further references and discussion on the gramicidin structure and evidence for dimer formation in the conducting state are given by Läuger (this volume). Figure 5 gives a schematic drawing of a gramicidin dimer.

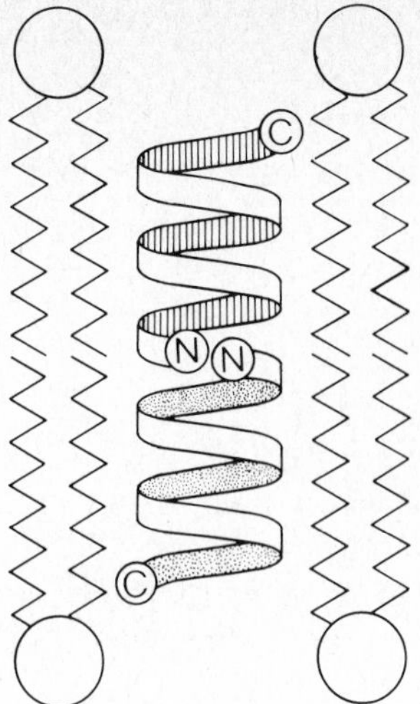

Fig. 5. Probable structure of gramicidin channel (*N*-to*N* dimer) (Urry et al. 1971, Weinstein et al. 1979).

5.4. Bacteriorhodopsin from the purple membrane of halobacterium halobium

The 247 residue protein, bacteriorhodopsin, is certainly the largest membrane protein to be sequenced to date (August, 1979). The sequence of Ovchinnikov et al. (1978) has been drawn in the form of a seven α-helix structure (Ovchinnikov et at. 1979) with respect to the bilayer using data from proteolytic enzyme accessibility experiments. The structure of Ovchinnikov et al. is reproduced in fig. 6.

Since the discovery of the simple composition (the single polypeptide) of the purple membrane by Oesterhelt and Stoeckenius (1971), much has been learned about its function and role in halobacterium. Recent reviews can bring the reader up to date on more detailed aspects (Stoeckenius et al. 1979, Henderson 1977). Briefly, bacteriorhodopsin with its purple-coloured retinal chromophore, is believed to function as a light-driven proton pump to provide energy for the cell in the form of an electrochemical gradient of hydrogen ions (Oesterhelt and Stoeckenius 1973). Light is absorbed by the retinal which is attached to the side chain of a lysine residue (lys-41) of the protein by a Schiff base linkage. Then, via a sequence of conformational changes in the protein–retinal complex, approximately one proton (per photon absorbed) is transferred across the membrane. The resulting ion gradient can then be used by other molecules in the membrane to carry out a multitude of different energy-requiring functions (e.g. Na^+ transport, ATP synthesis, amino acid transport).

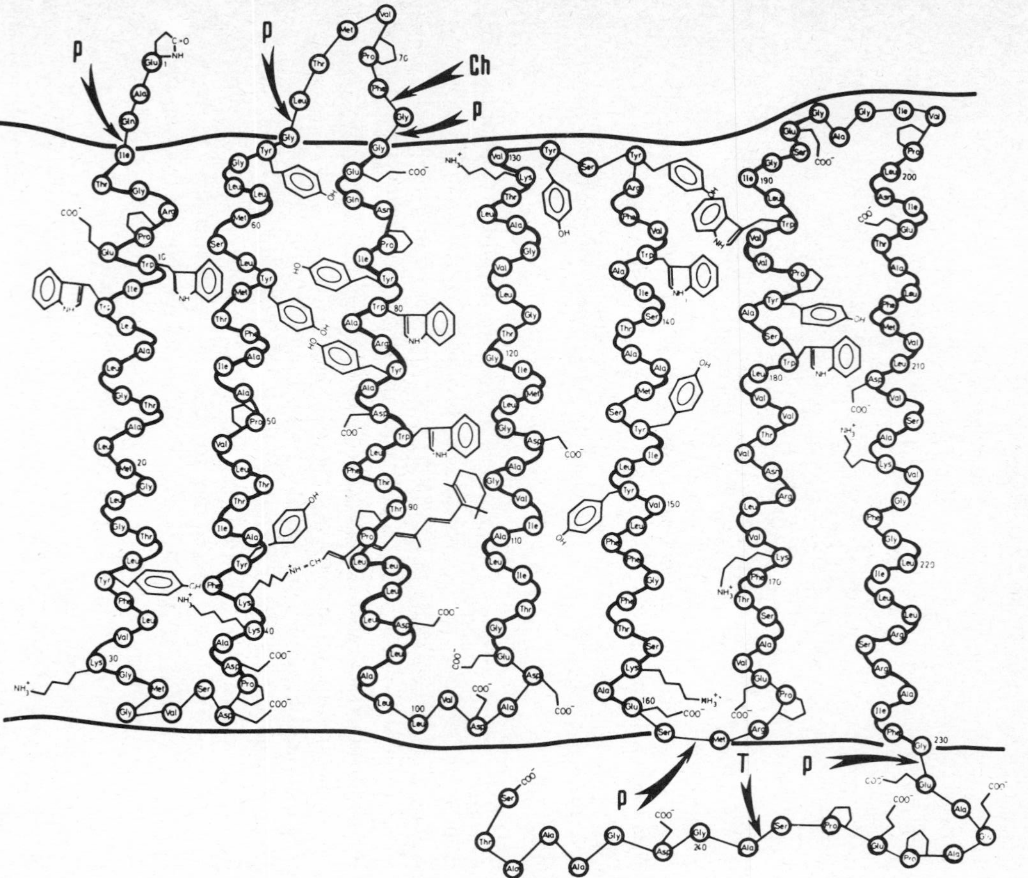

Fig. 6. Bacteriorhodopsin sequence and proposed polypeptide secondary structure (Ovchinnikov et al. 1978, 1979).

The structure of bacteriorhodopsin should therefore show features that help to explain how the pumping of hydrogen ions occurs. For example, there must be a pathway or channel along which protons can flow. The distribution of hydrophobic, hydrophilic, and charged residues shown in fig. 6 should provide some clues about the nature of this proton channel. Although the drawing of fig. 6 presents a hypothetical structure, some features occur which are almost certainly correct.

Most of the charged residues (lysine, arginine, aspartic acid, glutamic acid) occur at the membrane surface where they can come into contact with water. In particular, the majority occur on the cytoplasmic surface of the membrane (17–19 charged groups) and the minority (6 residues) on the extracellular surface. This would be consistent with the idea of the protein inserting itself by a self-assembly mechanism into the membrane from the inside of the cell where it is synthesized. In addition to these surface charges there seem to be 9 residues which are too far from the surface to be considered as being in the aqueous phase – they seem to be buried. Two pairs of charges occur on adjacent turns of two of the helices, so that they will be exactly juxtaposed in three-dimensions forming ion pairs. In this form, the energy which is required to bury them will be much reduced. Of the five remaining buried charges, perhaps two of the negative charges will be found to form salt bridges with the two positive charges in the completely folded structure. Another noteworthy feature is that where more than one charge occurs on a buried part of the same helix, all the charges seem to be on the same face of that helix when the polypeptide is folded into three-dimensional helices. Since this type of feature occurs on three of the seven helices, it may indicate that these helices form part of a channel through the membrane, and that the four helices with buried charges (these three plus the fourth, which has only a single charge) are all in the centre of the structure (however, see later).

6. Examples of membrane proteins forming two-dimensional crystals

Analysis of structure by X-ray diffraction and electron microscopy produces results which are entirely complementary to the sort of information gained by chemical studies such as those described above. The identification of the physical nature of a structure and the positions of features in three-dimensions produce a framework into which the chemically defined molecule can be fitted. This should eventually result in a model from which a chemically and physically explicit mechanism can be proposed. This stage of analysis has not been reached in most cases, but the examples given below indicate the present state of structural investigation for the two proteins bacteriorhodopsin and cytochrome oxidase.

These molecules are particularly suited to the methods of structural analysis because they form (naturally or by manipulation of the proteins in detergent solution) two-dimensional crystals to which the powerful methods of Fourier analysis can be applied. Something can be learned about the structure of membrane proteins even in the absence of crystallinity (see Chabre's analysis of rhodopsin in this volume), but the information is much less extensive. Two other membrane proteins for which some physical structural evidence is available from crystallography are the acetylcholine receptor from electroplax and the gap-junctional protein from mammalian cells. These are not discussed in detail here but the following papers can be referred to by those interested in recent developments. For the acetylcholine receptor, Klymkowsky and Stroud (1979) and Ross et al. (1977) provide a picture of the molecule as a multipeptide complex protruding largely from the outside of the cell membrane and having a shape like a horseshoe when viewed perpendicularly to the membrane. There appears to be a hole in the centre of the structure but it is not possible yet to correlate the physical and chemical aspects of the structure. For the gap junctional protein, the work of Caspar et al. (1977) shows the existence of a hexameric structure around each presumed channel. A more detailed analysis by Unwin and Zampighi (1980) will also be published shortly. Elsewhere in this volume (Benedetti) further references can be found. The 26 000 m.w. polypeptide of Benedetti is a good candidate and has approximately the right size to form one of the subunits of the hexamer that exists in each membrane.

6.1. Bacteriorhodopsin

In its naturally occurring purple membrane form, bacteriorhodopsin forms a p3 lattice in the plane of the membrane (Blaurock 1975, Henderson 1975). Using high angle X-ray diffraction (Henderson 1975) it can be shown that there are 4–7 α-helices in each bacteriorhodopsin molecule. Electron microscopy of unstained purple membrane (Henderson and Unwin 1975) further shows at 7 Å resolution the positions and orientations of seven rod-shaped features in the protein. From the evidence of the X-ray pattern and now from the seven hydrophobic segments of polypeptide found in the sequence (Ovchinnikov et al.

1979) it is fairly certain that these are seven α-helices which traverse the membrane from one side to the other in an orientation roughly perpendicularly to the plane of the membrane. The recent production and analysis of a second two-dimensional crystal form of bacteriorhodopsin (Michel et al. 1979) has allowed the definite identification of the polypeptide boundary in a single bacteriorhodopsin molecule, so that the model shown in fig. 7 (from Henderson and Unwin 1975) is now known to represent one molecule. The top of this molecule is the cytoplasmic side (Henderson et al. 1978, Hayward et al. 1978).

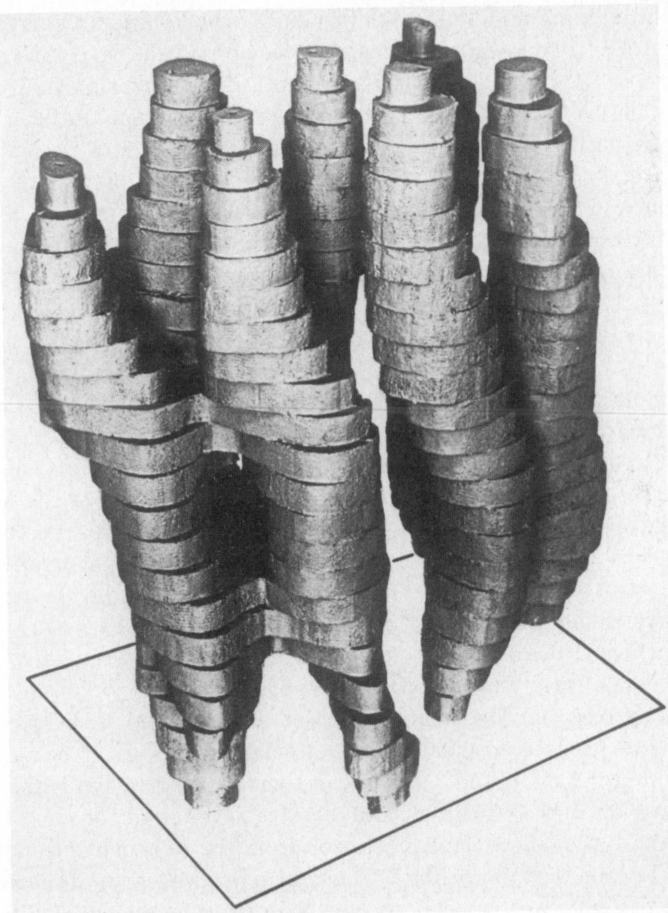

Fig. 7. Model of bacteriorhodopsin structure (Henderson and Unwin 1975).

Clearly, the seven hydrophobic segments found in the amino acid sequence must have a one-to-one correspondence with the seven rods of density in this low resolution model. Howerer, at the moment, there is not quite enough information to make the assignments and it is probably best to await the results of labelling experiments currently being performed. The remarks made in subsection 5.4, taken together with the model of fig. 7, would suggest that there is a channel containing a number of charged hydrophilic residues in the centre of the seven α-helices, and that the outside of the bacteriorhodopsin molecule is very hydrophobic. This would then provide a good pathway for the hydrogen ions (through the middle of each protein molecule) and an energetically satisfactory fit between the protein molecule and the lipid bilayer. The position of the retinal, despite the neutron diffraction analysis of King et al. (1979) seem likely to be near the cytoplasmic surface of the molecule but higher resolution structural analysis is now needed. Conformational changes in the protein together with pK changes of certain of the acidic or basic amino acid side chains are presumed to result in the proton pumping activity. Hopefully further work will result in a detailed understanding of the molecular mechanism.

6.2. Cytochrome oxidase from mitochondrial inner membrane

Two crystal forms of cytochrome oxidase can also be obtained. Both are two-dimensional crystals. One is produced with detergents of the Triton family and the other with deoxycholate. The analysis of these two crystal forms is described below to a resolution of about 25 Å using electron microscopy of negatively stained specimens. This resolution is insufficient to make any correlation with either the chemical polypeptide structure or with the function. To be complete, however, a brief summary of the function and chemical structure is given first.

Cytochrome oxidase is an enzyme in the mitochondrial inner membrane which catalyses the oxidation of (reduced) cytochrome c by molecular oxygen. The energy released in this oxidation reaction is thought to be used to create an electrochemical gradient of hydrogen ions across the membrane, which can then be used to synthesize ATP. The reaction of 4 cytochrome c molecules is required for each oxygen molecule so that the electrons released from the four cytochromes need first to be stored in the oxidase. The enzyme contains (as the monomer) two hemes and two copper ions which function as the sites of electron storage. The protein of the cytochrome oxidase monomer has been shown to contain at least seven distinct polypeptides with molecular weights between 5 000 and 36 000 (e.g. Chan and Tracy 1978). The molecular weight of the monomer based on one copy of each of the seven subunits is around 140 000. The enzyme *in vivo* may exist as a dimer since in Triton X-100 and other non-ionic detergents, the dimer is found to be the predominant species (Robinson and Capaldi 1977). This chemical description of the structure of cytochrome oxidase is quite independent of the physical description given below and at the moment the location of none of the components is known.

Of the two crystal forms, the one obtained by treatment of mitochondria with detergents of the Triton family shows the molecule to stick out a long way from one surface of the membrane (Henderson et al. 1977). This surface has been shown (Frey et al. 1978) to be the outside surface of the inner mitochondrial membrane using an antibody-binding method in which antibodies selective to one protein (known to be on one side) were used. The location of the membrane can also be seen in this crystal form.

A second crystal form obtained using the detergent deoxycholate in which the enzyme is monomeric, shows a clear boundary between monomeric units, and allows the relationship between monomers to be deduced (Fuller et al. 1979). Taking both crystal forms together, a model (fig. 8) of the cytochrome oxidase dimer can be constructed which shows the relationship between two monomers each shaped like a

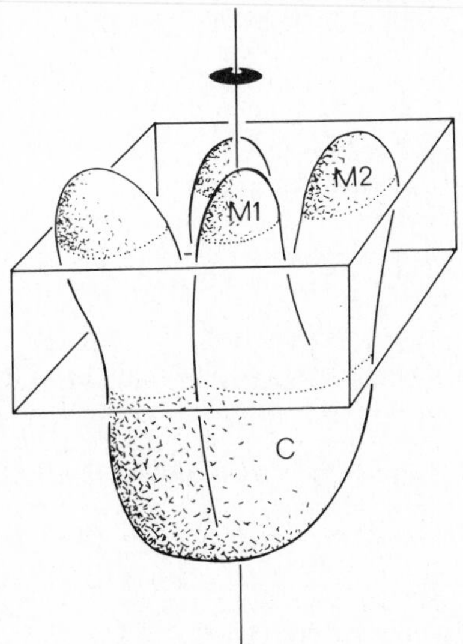

Fig. 8. Tentative model of cytochrome oxidase (Capaldi et al., unpublished work).

lopsided Y in which the arms of the Y stick into the bilayer as two separate domains, and the stem sticks out into solution (Capaldi et al. unpublished work). An unknown part of the stem interacts with the cytochrome c on the outside surface of the inner mitochondrial membrane. Perhaps each of the domains within the bilayer contains a number of α-helices with a structure much along the lines of bacteriorhodopsin.

7. Conclusions

I hope the above brief summary of what is known about the structures of five proteins in membranes is sufficient to convince you that there is nothing peculiar about membrane proteins. They come in different shapes and sizes just like soluble proteins. They may have one polypeptide or more. They may be dimeric. They certainly have extensive secondary structure particularly in the regions of the protein in contact with the lipid bilayer. Turns and bends in the course of the polypeptide are likely to occur at the water surfaces. So far only an α-helical conformation has been found in the part of the protein at the level of the bilayer. Perhaps this will be found for all sizeable membrane proteins – perhaps β-structure will also occur. What is certain, however, is that a more detailed knowledge of the structure of membrane proteins will provide a fascinating basis for explaining their mechanism of action.

References

Blaurock, A. E. (1975) J. Mol. Biol. 93, 139.

Bretscher, M. S. (1971) Nature New Biol. 231, 229.

Caspar, D. L. D., D. A. Goodenough, L. Makowski and W. C. Phillips (1977) J. Cell Biol. 74, 605.

Chamberlain, B. K., Y. Nozaki, C. Tanford and R. E. Webster (1978) Biochim. Biophys. Acta. 510, 18.

Chan, S. H. P. and R. P. Tracy (1978) Eur. J. Biochem. 89, 595.

Fleming, P. J., H. A. Dailey, D. Corcoran and P. Strittmatter (1978) J. Biol. Chem. 253, 5369.

Frey, T. G., S. H. P. Chan and G. Schatz (1978) J. Biol. Chem. 253, 4389.

Fuller, S. D., R. A. Capaldi and R. Henderson (1979) J. Mol. Biol. 134, 305.

Furthmayr, H. (1977) J. Supramol. Struct. 7, 121.

Hayward, S. B., D. A. Grano, R. M. Glaeser and K. A. Fisher (1978) Proc. Natl. Acad. Sci. U. S. A. 75, 4320.

Henderson, R. (1975) J. Mol. Biol. 93, 123.

Henderson, R. (1977) Ann. Rev. Biophys. Bioeng. 6, 87.

Henderson, R., R. A. Capaldi and J. S. Leigh (1977) J. Mol. Biol. 112, 631.

Henderson, R., J. S. Jubb, and S. Whyttock (1978) J. Mol. Biol. 123, 259.
Henderson, R. (1979) in: Membrane Transduction Mechanisms, eds. R. A. Cone and J. E. Dowling, Soc. Gen. Physical. Ser., vol. 33 (Raven Press, New York) pp. 3-15.
Henderson, R. and P. N. T. Unwin (1975) Nature 257, 28.
King, G. I., W. Stoeckenius, H. L. Crespi and B. P. Schoenborn (1979) J. Mol. Biol. 130, 395.
Klymkowsky, M. W. and R. M. Stroud (1979) J. Mol. Biol. 128, 319.
Makowski, L. and D. L. D. Caspar (1980) J. Mol. Biol., in press.
Makowski, L., D. L. D. Caspar, W. C. Phillips and D. A. Goodenough (1977) J. Cell Biol. 74, 629.
Marvin, D. A. and B. Hohn (1969) Bacterial Rev. 33, 172.
Marvin, D. A. and E. J. Wachtel (1975) Nature 253, 19.
Michel, H., D. Oesterhelt and R. Henderson (1980) Proc. Natl. Acad. Sci. U. S. A., 77, 338.
Nakashima, Y. and W. Konigsberg (1974) J. Mol. Biol. 88, 598.
Oesterhelt, D. and W. Stoeckenius (1971) Nature New Biol. 233, 149.
Oesterhelt, D. and W. Stoeckenius (1973) Proc. Natl. Acad. Sci. U. S. A. 70, 2853.
Ovchinnikov, Y. A., N. G., Abdulaev, M. Y. Feigina, A. V. Kiselev, N. A. Lobanov and I. V. Nasinov (1978) Bioorg. Khim. 4, 1573.
Ovchinnikov, Y. A., N. G., Abdulaev, M. Y. Feigina, A. V. Kiselev and N. A. Lobanov (1979) FEBS Lett. 100, 219.
Ozols, J. and C. Gerard (1977a) Proc. Natl. Acad. Sci. U. S. A. 74, 3725.
Ozols, J. and C. Gerard (1977b) J. Biol. Chem. 252, 8549.
Robinson, N. C. and R. A. Capaldi (1977) Biochemistry 16, 375.
Ross, M. J., M. W. Klymkowsky, D. A. Agard, and R. M. Stroud (1977) J. Mol. Biol. 116, 635.
Sarges, R. and B. Witkop (1965) J. Am. Chem. Soc. 87, 2011.
Schulte, T. H. and V. T. Marchesi (1979) Biochemistry 18, 275.
Sebald, W. and E. Wachter (1979) in: 29th Mosbacher Colloquium on Energy Conservation in Biological Membranes, eds. G. Schäfer and M. Klingenberg (Springer-Verlag, Berlin.) pp. 228–236.
Stoeckenius, W., R. H. Lozier and R. A. Bogomolni (1979) Biochem. Biophys. Acta. 505, 215.
Unwin, P. N. T. and G. Zampighi (1980) Nature 283, 545.
Urry, D. W. (1971) Proc. Natl. Acad. Sci. U. S. A. 68, 672.
Urry, D. W., M. C. Goodall, J. D. Glickson and D. F. Mayers (1971) Proc. Natl. Acad. Sci. U. S. A. 68, 1907.
Veatch, W. R. and E. R. Blout (1974) Biochemistry 13, 5257.
Veatch, W. R. and L. Stryer (1977) J. Mol. Biol. 113, 89.
Venkatachalam, C. M. (1968) Biopolymers 6, 1425.
Weinstein, S., B. A. Wallace, E. R. Blout, J. S. Morrow and W. Veatch (1979) Proc. Natl. Acad. Sci. U. S. A. 76, 4230.
Wickner, W. (1976) Proc. Natl. Acad. Sci. U. S. A. 73, 1159.
Williams, R. W. and A. K. Dunker (1977) J. Biol. Chem. 252, 6253.

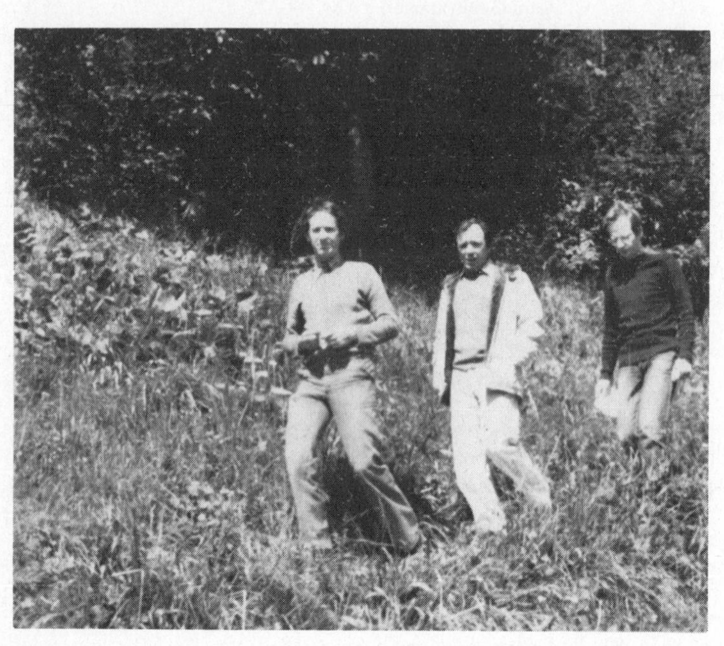

SEMINAR

STRUCTURAL STUDY OF AN INTRINSIC PROTEIN IN A FLUID MEMBRANE: RHODOPSIN

Marc CHABRE

Biophysique Moléculaire et Cellulaire
(Equipe de Recherche 199 C.N.R.S.), DRF, C.E.N.G., 85X
38041 Grenoble, France

1. Introduction

In the preceding chapter, R. Henderson has given beautiful examples of membrane protein structure determination, the outstanding one being that of bacteriorhodopsin. It must, however, be kept in mind that the precision of the structural information is directly related to the degree of two-dimensional crystalline ordering of the protein in the plane of the membrane. This crystalline ordering is by no means a general phenomenon and has, up until now, been obtained for few proteins only which were already packed with some ordering and little mobility in their native membrane. The extreme case is that of the purple membrane which is a natural rigid two-dimensional crystal and quite unique in this respect.

R. Balian et al., eds.
Les Houches, Session XXXIII, 1979 – Membranes et Communication Intercellulaire / Membranes and Intercellular Communication

Most membranes are highly fluid, and the membrane proteins enjoy a high degree of mobility. This mobility may be required for their function as it allows temporary assemblies of multicomponent systems in the membrane. The concentration of one protein species in the hydrophobic region of the bilayer may be very high in some specialized membranes, amounting, for example, to about 20% in volume in the case of rhodopsin in the retinal rod disc membrane. The natural formation of ordered arrays must then be hindered. Therefore, it seems unlikely that in such cases two-dimensional crystals will be easily, if ever, obtained. Then the alternatives are either to wait for a hypothetical crystal which as of yet no one knows how to obtain, or to try other structural approaches, certainly less powerful than crystallography. There is no general recipe; small pieces of information have to be gathered from as many biophysical and biochemical techniques as possible. I shall present a few approaches, attempted with partial success in a very favourable case – that of rhodopsin in the vertebrate retinal rod. One must be reminded that the homonimy with bacteriorhodopsin is due to the fact that both proteins bind retinal as a cofactor, but that does not imply any more structural or functional analogy: bacteriorhodopsin belongs to the most rigid membrane known, with a considerable amount of protein–protein interaction, and vertebrate rhodopsin to the most fluid membrane with the highest lateral diffusion coefficient [1, 2] and no protein–protein interaction (see, e.g., Devaux's contribution to this volume). Bacteriorhodopsin is a photoenergetic proton pump and vertebrate rhodopsin a phototransducer, whose only well demonstrated function up until now is to modulate cGMP level in the cell [3–7].

2. The retinal rod outer segment

The light sensitive rod cell of the vertebrate retina contains in its outer segment a fascinating membrane assembly which possesses many of the characteristics of a model system: (a) it contains only one species of membrane, and in this membrane, rhodopsin constitutes the near totality of the intrinsic proteins; (b) the membranes are stacked in a very regular array of flattened sacs – the discs; they are about 1500 discs in a frog rod, i.e. 3000 parallel membranes. The overall structure of a disc is centrosymmetric but the asymmetry of the individual membrane is preserved, which is not the case in artificial systems; and (c) the outer segment of the rod orients easily in magnetic fields of a few kilogauss

[8]. This property, related to the liquid crystalline ordering of the membranes, is experimentally very convenient; furthermore it is directly related to the structure of rhodopsin (see below).

3. Diffraction studies

The lamellar ordering of the disc membrane in native rods allows us to perform diffraction studies of the same type as those made on artificially stacked and oriented model systems (see the contribution by Seelig in this volume).

The main features of the diffraction pattern given by a retinal rod (or a collection of rods oriented parallel) are sketched on fig. 1.

The most intense signals are in the meridional direction, and arise from the quasi crystalline lamellar ordering of the disc membranes. The position of the peaks are related to the geometry of the membrane arrangement. The variation of the diffraction peak positions with the ionic strength of a perfusate is a measure of the osmotic response of the cell *in situ* and allows us to study, *in situ*, the permeability properties of the disc membrane [9].

From the relative intensities of the diffraction peaks, one obtains, through a Fourier analysis, the scattering density profile of the disc membrane. With X-rays, scattering is caused by electrons and the profile obtained is a projection of the electron density along the normal to the membrane plane. This analysis requires a phasing of the different reflections. The unit cell being centrosymmetric, phase angles are restricted to 0 and π. This phasing is based on some preliminary knowledge of the morphology of the cell (from electron microscopy) and on lattice swelling techniques [10, 11].

The information is limited by the fact that one does not get an absolute density scale, as one cannot vary the scattering density of the cytoplasm on a well controlled manner in the intact cellular structure. The scattering density profile obtained is dominated by the bilayer structure of the disc membrane: the only difference with that obtained with pure phospholipid bilayer models is that the whole pattern is shifted upward with respect to the cytoplasm scattering density and slightly asymmetric: those are indications that the protein mass is distributed through the whole thickness of the membrane and extends asymmetrically toward the cytoplasmic side. But this interpretation entirely relies upon the comparison with lipid model systems, and it would be hazardous to try to extract, from such data, quantitative information on the location of the proteins.

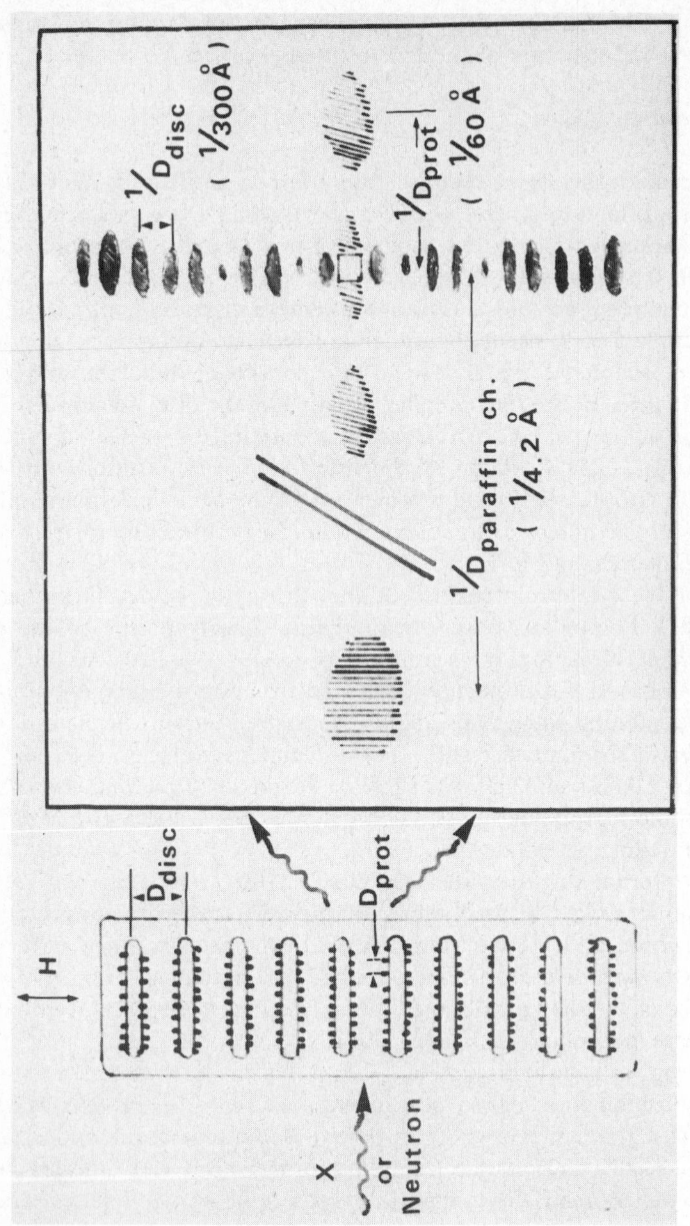

Fig. 1. Diffraction pattern of oriented retinal rods.

In the equatorial direction, various weak and diffuse bands are observed. The first one at smaller angles is the protein–protein correlation peak. The fact that it is broad is related to the non-crystallinity of the protein lateral distribution in the disc membrane plane. The position of the first maximum of this distribution is a good indication that rhodopsin molecules are dispersed in monomeric units. The intensity of this peak is related to the scattering density contrast between the proteins and their surrounding medium which, in this case, is far from being homogeneous: the proteins are in contact with the cytoplasmic solution, with the phospholipid's polar head region of high scattering density, and with the low density paraffin chain region inside the membrane. One cannot reliably evaluate the relative contributions of the three components to the total contrast, at least in X-ray diffraction. The situation is somewhat easier in neutron diffraction since one can vary, by very large amounts, the scattering density of the cytoplasm.

The experimental study of the equatorial signal is delicate as the signal is weak and can be partially contaminated by the strong lamellar diffraction if the orientation is not perfect. Furthermore, the large exposure times required in the early studies induced some degradation of the membranes. A very elaborate analysis [12, 13] could not correct for those experimental artifacts: the most sophisticated theoretical analysis will never compensate for a poor biological sample. The introduction of modern, position-sensitive, X-ray detectors reduced the data taking time from the range of hours to that of minutes. This, combined with the magnetic orientation, helped in clearing up quite a confused situation which now condenses into a very short story [14]: the protein equatorial signal is that of a two-dimensional disordered distribution in the disc membrane plane; it is characteristic of a monomeric dispersion of rhodopsin and is not measureably modified upon illumination.

At wider angles, corresponding to reciprocal distances around 10 Å, weak bands have been reported (not shown on our sketch). These bands are probably related to the quaternary structure of the protein (interchain distances). The next major band around 4.5 $Å^{-1}$ is given by the paraffin chain in the "liquid" disordered state. Upon cooling down, in rods from hot blooded animals (cattle), a partial transition to rigid crystalline state is observable, characterized by a sharp peak at 4.15 $Å^{-1}$, which corresponds to an hexagonal packing of the paraffin chains (see, e.g., Seelig's contribution to this volume). As it is always the case in natural membranes, there is no sharp transition, which might be harmful to the cell membrane, but only a very smooth and partial phase separation. This is related to the inhomogeneity of the membrane lipids in a natural membrane, and sets some limit to the biological interest of detailed studies of phase transitions in model systems constituted of synthetic and homogeneous lipids.

Correlated to the appearance of the sharp peak at 4.15 $Å^{-1}$, characteristic of ordered lipid patches, a shift of the protein equatorial signal is observable: this indicates a reduction of the average protein–protein distance in the membrane. It is due to a segregation of the proteins out of the ordered lipid patches. But there is no sharpening of the protein peak, which means that this closer packing of the proteins does not induce any ordering.

Neutron diffraction can often complement X-ray studies, and the two types of measurements should not be conducted independently, as information gained in one of the experiments may be helpful to interpret the other. Although the data taking time (at the Grenoble I.L.L. high flux reactor) are not much longer than with a standard X-ray generator, neutrons should not compete with X-rays for kinetic studies especially if the comparison is made with the new synchrotron radiation sources. Neutrons are scattered by nuclei and not by atomic electrons. The scattering density scale is therefore very different from that for X-rays. Hydrogen scattering is of the same order of magnitude as that of other nuclei. A nice feature of this nuclear scattering is that two isotopes of the same atom may have very different scattering powers. One of the largest differences observed is that found between the two isotopes of hydrogen: hydrogen and deuterium are as different in neutron scattering as carbon and lead are in X-ray scattering.

Therefore, the interest of neutrons arises from the fact that they allow us to obtain, for a given structure, an image with contrasts different from those obtained with X-rays; just as two different staining techniques give different pictures in electron microscopy. Furthermore, with neutron, the contrast can be varied at will by manipulating the isotopic ratio of hydrogen and deuterium in the solvant and/or in any of the components of the structure.

Contrast variation, the basic method of all neutron studies of biological material, is made most easily by manipulating the H_2O/D_2O ratio in the solvent. In fact, the most useful range of solvent scattering densities is that which spans the scattering densities of the main components of the biological material, i.e. for membranes this means between 0 and 40% D_2O, and therefore, one is always confronted with a high incoherent scattering from hydrogen. Nature was very kind in providing us

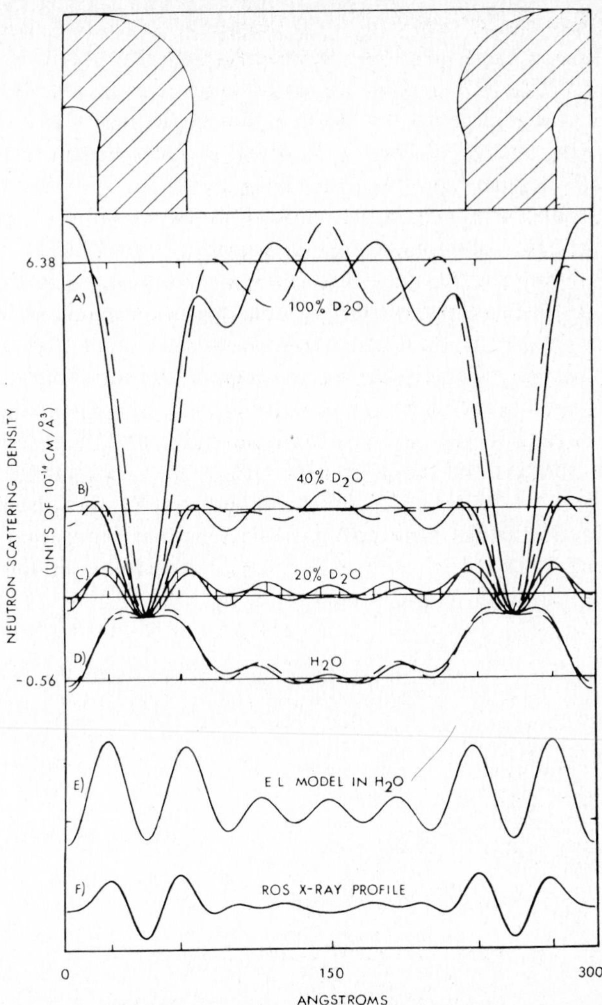

Fig. 2. Scattering density profiles of retinal rod disc membrane obtained from diffraction measurements. A, B, C, and D are the neutron scattering density profile obtained at various solvant contrasts in 100%, 40%, and 20% D_2O and in H_2O. These four profiles are obtained on a common and absolute scattering density scale. For comparison, but not normalised to the same scale, E shows the neutron scattering density profile of a pure lipid model system in H_2O; the comparison of D and E indicates that the proteins dominate the pattern in the disc membrane. F is the electron density profile obtained from X-ray diffraction. It should be compared to C. Reproduced from Nature 262 (1976) 266.

with two stable isotopes of hydrogen having very different scattering powers, but, on the other hand, it made us pay for this by giving the most common isotope a most undesirable nuclear spin dependence of the scattering which generates an enormous incoherent scattering. If not for that, neutrons would really be very tough competitors for X-ray studies on biological materials!

A comparison of scattering densities for neutrons and X-rays of the main components of biological membranes is shown in fig. 2. A very interesting feature is the fact that for a solvent containing about 20% D_2O, the relative neutron scattering densities of proteins, phospholipid headgroups, hydrocarbon chains, and solvents are close to their relative electron densities. Therefore, the relative diffraction amplitudes and phases of a membrane structure should be the same for neutron diffraction in 20% D_2O Ringer and for X-ray diffraction: in fact the neutron diffraction pattern of rods in 20% D_2O is very similar to the X-ray diffraction pattern [15]. One concluded that the phases of the main diffraction peaks were also similar. This matching point between neutron and X-ray work allows for the introduction, in the neutron

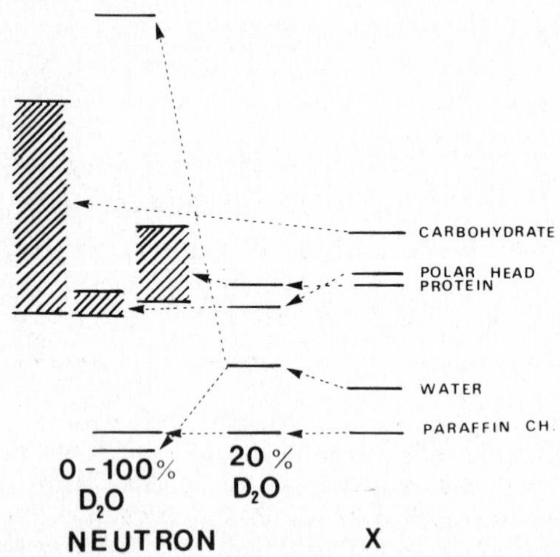

Fig. 3. Comparison of the relative scattering densities of the main components of a biological membrane for X-ray and for neutron. The scales have been adjusted by setting the paraffin chain scattering density at the same level. The dash region corresponds to the variation of scattering density observed in solvent of variable D_2O content. This is due to the exchange of labile hydrogen of the molecule with deuterium from the solvent. Only the paraffin chains are devoid of exchangeable hydrogen.

analysis, much of the phase information obtained more easily by swelling experiments in X-ray diffraction.

The results of the Fourier analysis of the lamellar diffraction data at various contrasts are shown on fig. 3. One sees that in H_2O the neutron scattering density pattern of the disc membrane is very different of that of a lipid bilayer, although both patterns are very similar in 20% D_2O. By obtaining an absolute density scale, it is now possible to locate the protein within the membrane thickness: about 50% of the protein is located in the bilayer, the longer hydrophilic part being on the cytoplasmic side.

4. Small angle scattering studies on rhodopsin in detergent micelles

Small angle scattering by macromolecules or macromolecular assemblies in dilute solution originates from the same elastic scattering phenomenon as diffraction. The technical approaches are very similar, since diffraction on membranes is limited to small angles, and both types of measurements can be performed using the same apparatus. X-rays and neutrons have the same complementarity for small angle scattering as for the diffraction. The structural information which is extractable from a small angle scattering measurement is limited, but significant if one cannot crystallize the macromolecule.

As intrinsic membrane proteins are not water soluble, a trick has to be used to disperse them: one replaces the continuous hydrophobic environment of the lipid bilayer by a local hydrophobic blob of detergent around each protein (see fig. 4). Careful biochemical preparations and controls by sedimentation equilibrium are necessary to ensure that such protein–detergent micelles are homogeneous in size, monomeric in protein, and devoid of lipids [16]. In X-ray small angle scattering [17], the solvent contrast could be varied by addition of large amounts of sucrose. There are no problems of compartments and of membrane impermeability as for the diffraction study. However the neutron approach [18] is more flexible, as the available range of contrast is larger, and one has the further possibility of varying, by deuteration, the scattering density of the synthetic detergent. This allows, in fact, to completely erace the contribution of the detergent to the scattering, and the hydrophobic protein scatters alone as if it would be water soluble. The analysis is done using the formalism developed by Stuhrmann [19]. The centers of mass of the protein and the detergent part of the micelle are found to be nearly coincident, as for the micelle (A) in fig. 4. The

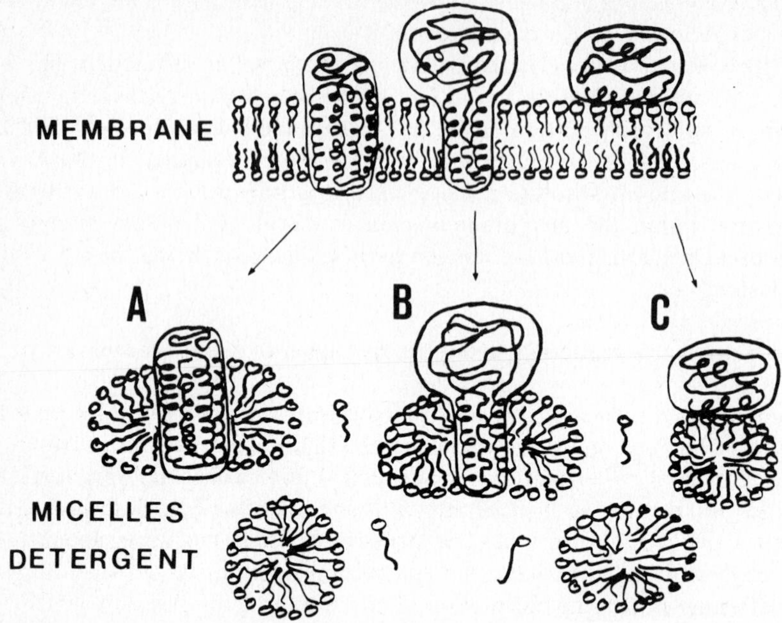

Fig. 4. Models of micelle formation with membrane proteins. The detergent is assumed to substitute for the lipids. An excess of free detergent micelles is always present in the preparation.

radius of gyration of the protein and its variation with contrast are characteristic of an elongated protein with an hydrophobic center and two hydrophilic ends.

5. Kinetics of peptide proton exchange

This technique, which has been extensively applied to soluble proteins, has been shown by Osborne [20, 21] to be of great interest in the study of membrane proteins: the kinetics of peptide proton exchange is an index of accessibility of water to a polypeptide chain. The determination by infrared, which specifically identifies the peptide N–H and N–D bands, is the most suitable. The technique can be applied to detergent solubilized proteins as well as to native membranes; this gives a control on the possible effects of the detergent on the protein conformation. Using this technique the existence of a highly hydrophobic core in rhodopsin was proven. This alone made it very unlikely that rhodopsin was a light controlled ionophore channel.

6. Magnetic anisotropy

The orientation of rod outer segments in magnetic field is related to a large diamagnetic anisotropy [22]. The anisotropy cannot be accounted for by the membrane lipids, and must therefore originate from the other main oriented component of the structure, rhodopsin. In a protein, the origin of diamagnetic anisotropy might be in a preferential orientation of the aromatic side chains, or in the case of rhodopsin in the orientation of the retinal cofactor. It was also pointed out, by Worcester [23], that α helical sections had a large diamagnetic anisotropy, i.e. the flat resonating structure of a peptide has a small diamagnetic anisotropy, but in an α helix, the anisotropy of all peptides sum up along the helix axis. In rhodopsin the contribution of aromatic side chains and of retinal could be excluded on the basis of linear dichroism measurements [24]. Circular dichroism measurements [25] indicate that rhodopsin is 50% α helix. Measurements of the diamagnetic anisotropy of the rods in a rotating field device suggested then that the major part of the α helical segments are oriented perpendicularly to the membrane plane [26].

7. Infrared linear dichroism

Infrared absorption bands related to stretching and bending vibrations of covalent bonds are highly anisotropic with respect to the bond direction (see fig. 5). In linear dichroism, one studies the ratio of

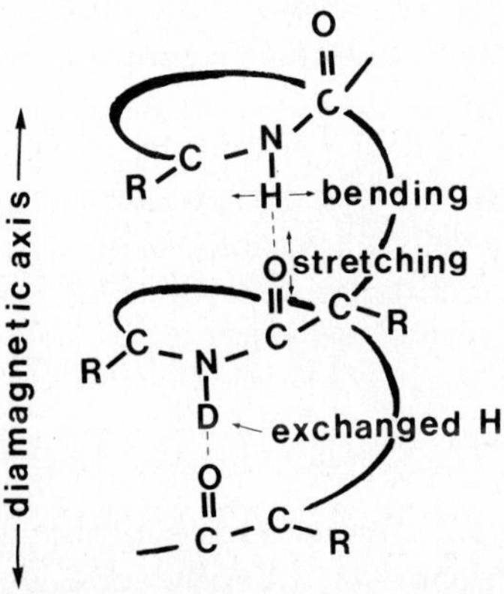

Fig. 5. Orientation of the main IR absorption dipoles in an α helix. Three major bands are observable: the C=0 stretch, N–H bend and, in D_2O, the exchanged N–D, which is also mainly a bending vibration. The helix axis is also the diamagnetic anisotropy axis.

absorbance of a given band for two orthogonal directions of linear polarisation of the incident beam. In proteins, peptide C=0 and N–H vibrations bands are strong and easily identified. As the sample must be in D_2O, to avoid excessive absorption by water, one also gets a N–D band resulting from the exchange of peptide protons with deuterium. Magnetically oriented samples of rod outer segments, suitable for IR studies are quite difficult to prepare. However, once they are obtained, the result is direct, i.e. both the C=0 (stretch) and N–H (bend) bands are dichroic, the latter to a greater extent, but the N–D is not dichroic. This confirms the preferential orientation of α helix segments in rhodopsin. It further indicates that these oriented α helix segments are concentrated in the hydrophobic core of the protein, unaccessible to exchange. The hydrophilic parts of the protein, accessible to exchange do not show any anisotropy [27].

8. Linear dichroism in the visible and uv

The technique of linear dichroism may also be used to study the orientations of various chromophores in the protein, essentially the aromatic residues and the retinal. The oriented samples are very easy to prepare for such studies and the orientation of the chromophores in the different photo-excited states of the protein, can be studied [24, 28].

9. Fluorescence transfer

When a molecule possesses a natural chromophore, fluorescence transfer is a powerful method. Fluorescence transfer between the retinal and specific probes bound externally to the protein indicated that the molecule had an elongated shape, and that retinal was far from most of the binding sites [29]. Fluorescent transfer between retinal and long-lived chromophore in solution recently showed that the chromophore is located close to the intradiscal (or extracellular) side of the membrane [30].

10. Electron microscopy

By the freeze etching technique (see contribution by Benedetti) it is demonstrated that the protein is deeply embedded in the hydrophobic layer of the membrane, as particles are observed in the fracture plane. The particles are observed only in the cytoplasmic half of the membrane, this indicates that the protein has stronger interaction with the cytoplasmic side and is probably related to the large extension of the protein in the cytoplasm.

By conventional method on thin sections the intradiscal location of glycoconjugates has been demonstrated, using concanavallin A – Ferritin conjugates [31].

11. Biochemical data, proteolysis, sequence

Although this protein can be easily isolated and purified in great quantities in the presence of detergent, precise biochemical data are scarce. It is only recently that a general agreement seems to be reached on the molecular weight (38 000) and amino acid composition. This stresses the specific difficulties encountered with intrinsic membrane protein.

But there is little information in the overall amino acid composition, as it makes an average between the hydrophilic and the hydrophobic parts of the protein. Controlled proteolysis, from one side only of the membrane or from both sides is a good approach to the topology of the polypeptide chain. It can be combined with chemical labelling. From this type of study it is concluded that the polypeptide chain crosses the membrane at least 3 times and that most of the markers, except that of the sugar moiety, are on the cytoplasmic side [32].

The sequence has been established for only small parts of the polypeptide chain; essentially the two hydrophilic ends, at the N terminal, where the sugars are linked, and at the C terminal on the cytoplasmic side [33]. A small hydrophobic segment including the retinal binding lysine is also sequenced; it bears no analogy with the retinal binding site of bacteriorhodopsin. The classical proteolytic method of sequencing encounters great difficulties in sequencing hydrophobic segments. But a breakthrough should soon occur, as the mRNA coding for rhodopsin has been recently isolated [34]. Sequencing a nucleotide chain is a much easier task.

12. Conclusions

Combining all the pieces of information, one may obtain the model shown in fig. 6, i.e. the hydrophobic transmembranous part of the protein would be constituted by an array of 5 or 7 α helical segments, oriented preferentially perpendicular to the membrane plane. As discussed by Henderson, this might be a general characteristic of all intrinsic membrane proteins. The retinal is probably in the hydrophobic

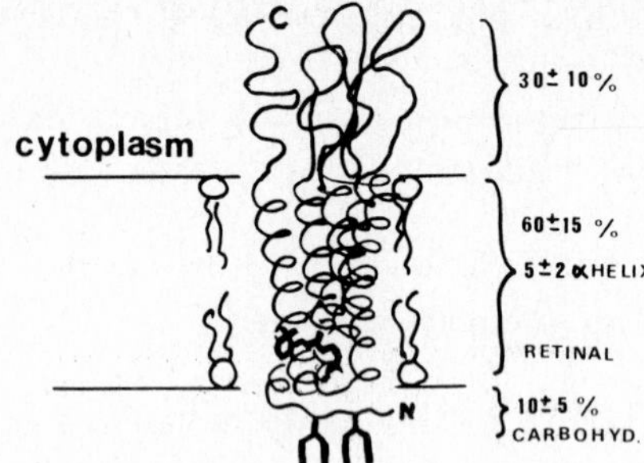

Fig. 6. Schematic model of rhodopsin in the disc membrane.

region, close to the extracellular side which bears the carbohydrate. The site which, after photoexcitation, recognises the cGMP controlling enzymatic chain is on the cytoplasmic side.

One is still far from a complete three-dimensional structural map of the protein, and there is little hope that it will be built soon. The next important step is certainly that of obtaining the full sequence, as it appears that for hydrophobic proteins, this brings much information, if the α helical hydrophobic segments can be identified.

Acknowledgements

It is a pleasure to acknowledge the collaboration of J. Breton, A. Cavaggioni, M. Michel-Villaz, H. B. Osborne, H. Saibil, C. Sardet and D. Worcester for the experiments in which the author was involved.

References

[1] R. A. Cone, Nature New Biol. 236 (1972) 39.
[2] M. Poo and R. Cone, Nature 247 (1974) 438.
[3] M. Woodruff and M. D. Bownd, J. Gen. Physiol. 73 (1979) 629.
[4] E. Bignetti, A. Cavaggioni and R. Sorbi, J. Physiol. 279 (1978) 55.
[5] G. L. Wheeler and M. W. Bitensky, Proc. Nat. Acad. Sci. USA 74 (1977) 4238.
[6] W. H. Miller and G. D. Nicol, Nature 280 (1979) 64.
[7] T. Shinozawa, I. Sen, G. Wheeler and M. Bitensky, J. Supramol. Struct. 50 (1979) 185.
[8] N. Chalazonitis, R. Chagneux and A. Arvanitaki, C. Rend. Acad. Soc. Paris D 271 (1970) 130.
[9] M. Chabre and A. Cavaggioni, Biochim. Biophys. Acta 382 (1975) 336.
[10] A. E. Blaurock and M. H. F. Wilkins, Nature 236 (1972) 313.
[11] J. M. Corless, Nature 237 (1972) 229.

[12] J. K. Blasie and C. R. Worthington, J. Mol. Biol. 39 (1969) 417.
[13] J. K. Blasie Biophys. J. 12 (1972) 191.
[14] M. Chabre, Biochim. Biophys. Acta 382 (1975) 322.
[15] H. Saibil, M. Chabre and D. Worcester, Nature 262 (1976) 266.
[16] H. B. Osborne, C. Sardet and A. Helenius, Eur. J. Biochem. 44 (1974) 383.
[17] C. Sardet, A. Tardieu and V. Luzzati, J. Mol. Biol. 105 (1976) 383.
[18] H. B. Osborne, C. Sardet, M. Michel-Villaz and M. Chabre, J. Mol. Biol. 123 (1978) 177.
[19] M. H. J. Koch and H. B. Stuhrmann, in: Methods in Enzymology, Vol. LIX, eds. K. Muldauer and L. Grossman (Academic Press, New York 1979) pp. 670–706.
[20] H. B. Osborne and E. Nabedryk-Viala, FEBS Lett. 84 (1977) 217.
[21] H. B. Osborne and E. Nabedryk-Viala, Eur. J. Biochem 89 (1978) 81.
[22] F. T. Hong, D. Mauzerall and A. Mauro, Proc. Nat. Acad. Sci. USA (1971) 1283.
[23] D. L. Worcester, Proc. Nat. Acad. Sci. USA 75 (1978) 5475.
[24] M. Chabre and J. Breton, Photochem. Photobiol. 30 (1979) 295.
[25] H. Schichi and E. Shelton, J. Supramol. Struct. 2 (1974) 7.
[26] M. Chabre, Proc. Nat. Acad. Sci. USA, 75 (1978) 5471.
[27] M. Michel-Villaz, H. Saibil and M. Chabre, Proc. Nat. Acad. Sci. USA 76 (1979) 4405.
[28] M. Chabre and J. Breton, Vision Res. 19 (1979) 1005.
[29] C. W. Wu and L. Stryer, Proc. Nat. Acad. Sci. USA 69 (1972) 1104.
[30] D. D. Thomas, W. F. Carlsen and L. Stryer, Proc. Nat. Acad. Sci. USA 75 (1978) 5746.
[31] P. Rohlich, Nature 263 (1976) 789.
[32] B. B. K. Fung and W. L. Hubbell, Biochemistry 17 (1978) 4403.
[33] P. Hargrave and S. L. J. Fong, J. Supramol. Struct. 6 (1977) 559.
[34] I. Schechter et al., Proc. Nat. Acad. Sci. USA 76 (1979) 2654.

COURSE 4

LATERAL MOLECULAR MOTION IN MEMBRANES: IMMUNE RECOGNITION AND RESPONSE

Harden M. McCONNELL

*The John Stauffer Laboratory for Physical Chemistry,
Stanford University, Stanford, CA 94305,
U.S.A.*

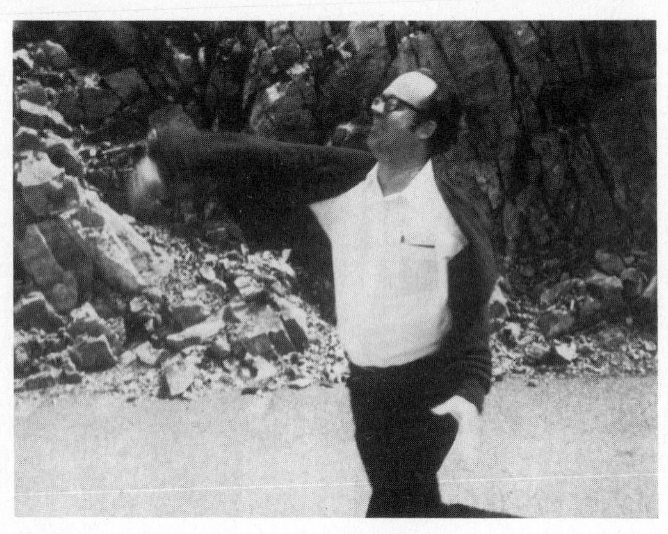

Contents

Abbreviations used:

DPPC, dipalmitoylphosphatidylcholine
DMPC, dimyristoylphosphatidylcholine
S-Con A, succinyl concanavalin A
NBD-PE, N-4-nitrobenzo-2-oxa-1,3-diazole phosphatidylethanolamine
FITC-IgG, fluorescein isothiocyanate rabbit antinitroxide antibodies

R. Balian et al., eds.
Les Houches, Session XXXIII, 1979 – Membranes et Communication Intercellulaire / Membranes and Intercellular Communication

1. Lateral molecular motion in membranes

1.1. Introduction

There can be little doubt that the lateral motions and distributions of molecules in membranes play significant roles in the biological functions of cells. One purpose of the present chapter is to describe a number of the experimental techniques that have been used to study and characterize some of these motions, especially lateral diffusion. A second purpose of this chapter is to suggest how reconstituted membranes ("model membranes") can be used to study immunological problems such as cell surface recognition, triggering, and target cell killing. Our choice of topics is selective rather than comprehensive, and particular emphasis is placed on techniques and results of special interest to the author.

At least three types of lateral molecular motions of membrane-associated molecules have been observed. These include protein and lipid diffusion (Frye and Edidin 1970, Poo and Cone 1974, Devaux and McConnell 1972, Sackmann and Träuble 1972), "patching," and "capping" (Raff 1976, Raff and de Petris 1973). Diffusion arises from thermal molecular motion (Brownian motion), and by definition, follows a diffusion equation. Membrane flow has also been proposed (Bretscher 1973) and, while the experimental evidence for it is not compelling, there remains a number of features of molecular motion on membrane surfaces that are not understood (Stern and Bretscher 1979). We begin with a discussion of lateral diffusion in model membranes (lipid bilayers) and biological cell membranes.

1.2. Lateral diffusion in a membrane that is isotropic and homogeneous in two dimensions

A given molecular species is said to undergo isotropic, homogeneous two-dimensional diffusion in a membrane if the concentration of that species follows the diffusion equation,

$$\frac{\partial c}{\partial t} = D\left(\frac{\partial^2 c}{\partial x^2} + \frac{\partial^2 c}{\partial y^2}\right), \tag{1}$$

where D is the diffusion coefficient and $c \equiv c(x, y, t) \equiv c(\boldsymbol{r}, t)$ is the two-dimensional concentration (e.g., molecules/cm^2). Here $\boldsymbol{r} = \boldsymbol{i}x + \boldsymbol{j}y$ where $\boldsymbol{i}$ and $\boldsymbol{j}$ are unit vectors in the x and y directions. Equation (1) may also be written

$$\frac{\partial c}{\partial t} = D\nabla^2 c, \tag{2}$$

where

$$\overline{\nabla} = \boldsymbol{i}\frac{\partial}{\partial x} + \boldsymbol{j}\frac{\partial}{\partial y}. \tag{3}$$

For present purposes an equivalent definition of the diffusion coefficient follows from the equation,

$$\overline{s^2} = 4Dt, \tag{4}$$

where $\overline{s^2}$ is the mean square displacement of a given molecule in a time t. Most current methods for measuring the diffusion constants for molecules on cell surfaces, and model membranes involve real-time kinetic measurements. That is, some technique is used to generate a non-uniform concentration distribution at time $t=0$ (i.e., $c(0, \boldsymbol{r}) \neq c(0, \boldsymbol{r}')$) and the time-dependent recovery of the system to a uniform concentration distribution is measured. This is then compared with the solution of the diffusion equation (1), with appropriate boundary conditions. The molecular species is then said to undergo isotropic, two-dimensional diffusion if the experimental recovery curve can be fit to the theoretical recovery curve using a single parameter, the diffusion coefficient, D.

The first experiment of this type for model bilayer membranes was carried out by Devaux in 1971 (Devaux and McConnell 1972). In this experiment the lateral diffusion coefficient of a head-group spin-labeled phospholipid (I) was measured in host lipid multilayers of egg phosphatidylcholine.

$$
\begin{array}{l}
\qquad\qquad\qquad\qquad \mathrm{O} \\
\qquad\qquad\qquad\qquad \| \\
\qquad\qquad \mathrm{H_2C{-}O{-}C{-}(CH_2)_{14}{-}CH_3} \\
\qquad\quad \mathrm{O} \qquad | \\
\qquad\quad \| \\
\mathrm{CH_3(CH_2)_{14}{-}C{-}O{-}CH} \qquad\qquad\qquad\qquad\qquad\qquad (\mathrm{I}) \\
\qquad\qquad\quad | \qquad \mathrm{O} \qquad\qquad\quad \mathrm{CH_3}{}_{+} \\
\qquad\qquad\qquad\quad \| \qquad\qquad\qquad | \\
\qquad\qquad \mathrm{H_2C{-}O{-}P{-}O{-}CH_2CH_2{-}N{-}}\langle\text{ring}\rangle\mathrm{N{-}O\cdot} \\
\qquad\qquad\qquad\quad | \qquad\qquad\qquad\quad | \\
\qquad\qquad\qquad\quad \mathrm{O^-} \qquad\qquad\quad \mathrm{CH_3}
\end{array}
$$

The non-uniform distribution was achieved by the careful introduction of a small spot ($\sim$1 mm diameter) of pure (I) into a coplanar multilamellar array of egg phosphatidylcholine bilayers. If we imagine an x, y, z Cartesian axis system, with the z-axis perpendicular to several hundred coplanar lipid bilayers, then the initial lateral concentration distribution of (I) at time $t=0$ was, at least approximately, $c(\boldsymbol{r}, 0)=c_0$ for $\boldsymbol{r} \leqslant R_0$ and $c(\boldsymbol{r}, 0)=0$ for $\boldsymbol{r}>R_0$. Here $|\boldsymbol{r}|=\sqrt{x^2+y^2}$ and R_0 is the radius of the spot. The solution of eq. (1) for these initial conditions is given in textbooks (Margenau and Murphy 1948, Carslaw and Jaeger 1959). It is sufficient to say that this solution describes how the concentration of spin-labeled lipids changes as the molecules diffuse away from the origin $x=y=0$. Because of dipolar and exchange interactions between the odd electrons of the spin labels, the paramagnetic resonance spectra of the sample also changes with time, and these changes can be compared quantitatively with those observed experimentally. This comparison leads to the determination of the lateral diffusion coefficient of (I) in egg phosphatidylcholine, $D=1.8 \pm 0.6 \times 10^{-8}$ cm^2/s.

A new technique for preparing non-uniform distributions of spin-labeled phospholipids has been developed by Sheats and McConnell (1978), and is particularly useful for measuring the lateral diffusion coefficients of spin-labeled phospholipids. In this method a photosensitive compound $\mathrm{Co(CN)_5^{\equiv}R}$ is introduced into the aqueous phase between the lipid bilayers containing head-group labels such as (I) at low concentrations (e.g., 0.1–1 mol %). On photolysis with 5180 Å radiation from an argon ion laser, this cobalt compound undergoes photolysis to yield a free radical,

$$\mathrm{Co(CN)_5^{\equiv}R} \xrightarrow{h\nu} \mathrm{Co(CN)_5^{\equiv}} + \mathrm{R}\cdot . \tag{5}$$

Radicals R$\cdot$ such as $\cdot\mathrm{CH_2COOH}$ produced in this way recombine very rapidly with $\mathrm{Co(CN)_5^{\equiv}}$ to produce the starting compound $\mathrm{Co(CN)_5^{\equiv}R}$, or react with the nitroxide radical to produce a diamagnetic species (Sheats and McConnell 1977, 1979)

$$N\text{–}O\text{–}CH_3COOH.$$

A "square wave" concentration distribution $c(\boldsymbol{r}, 0)$ of lipid spin labels such as (I) can be achieved by the optical irradiation of the multilayers through a grid, as illustrated in figs. 1 and 2. The concentration distribution at time $t = 0$ is depicted in fig. 3, and can be represented as a simple Fourier series,

$$c(x, 0) = A + \sum_k F_k \sin kx, \tag{6}$$

where $k = (n)(2\pi)/P$, $n = 1, 3, 5, \ldots$. Here P is the period of the pattern and F_k is the Fourier expansion coefficient. The solution of the diffusion equation, eq. (1), corresponding to one-dimensional motion, satisfying the boundary condition eq. (6), is

$$c(x, t) = A + \sum_k F_k \sin kx\ \mathrm{e}^{-k^2Dt}. \tag{7}$$

This equation then gives the spatial distribution following the initial burst of laser radiation. A second burst of laser radiation at a later time then produces further photochemical destruction of the lipid spin labels, the amount being destroyed being determined by the diffusion constant D. This method has been used to measure the lateral diffusion coefficient of (I) under a number of conditions (Sheats and McConnell 1978).

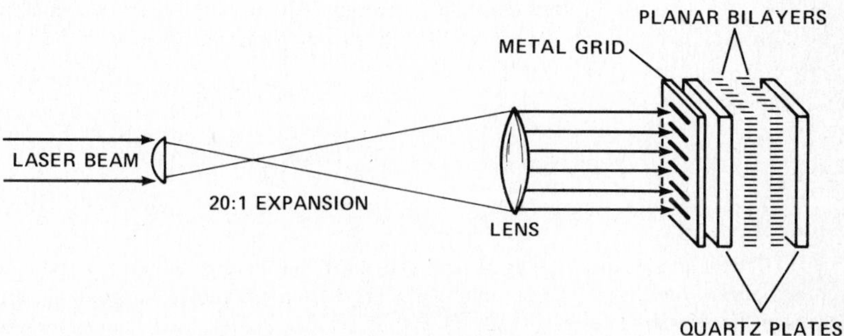

Fig. 1. Schematic representation of an apparatus used to create a non-uniform distribution of spin-labeled phospholipids in coplanar multibilayer samples.

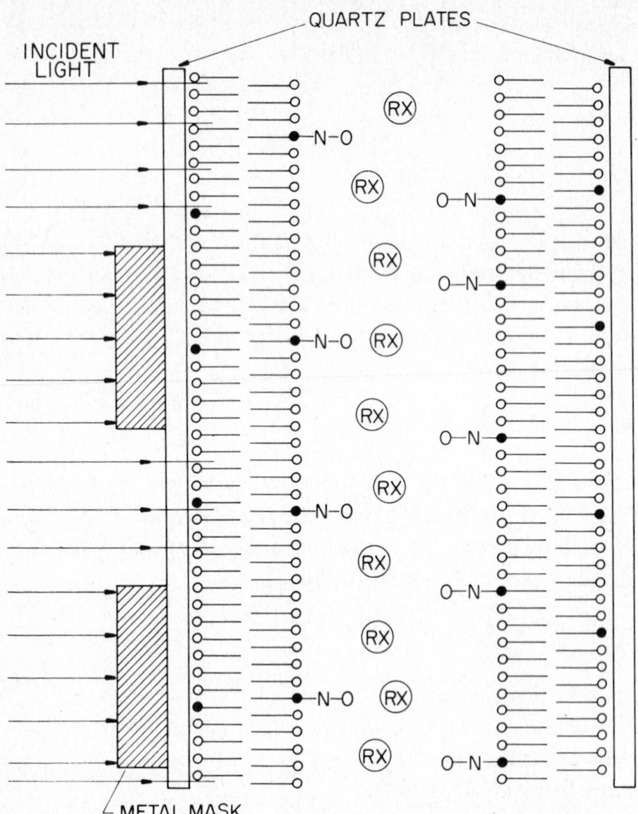

Fig. 2. Schematic representation of two coplanar bilayers, an enlargement (and simplification of fig. 1). Laser radiation which is not blocked by the metal mask dissociates the molecules RX into radicals that either rapidly recombine with one another, or destroy the nitroxide (NO) groups in the immediate vicinity. RX is the alkylcobalt complex $[Co(CN)_5CH_2CO_2^-]^{4-}$ and NO is the head-group spin-label phospholipid A.

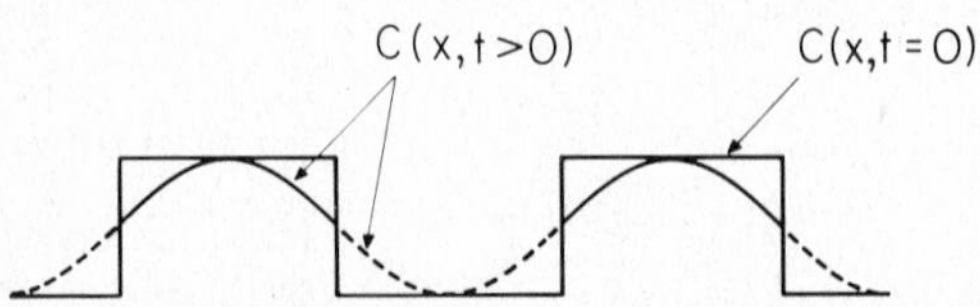

Fig. 3. Concentration distribution of the spin-label lipid A, as a result of periodic photochemical "bleaching." Before photolysis there is a uniform concentration, with paramagnetic resonance intensity proportional to $c(x, t<0)=c_0$. After brief photolysis, the concentration profile is square wave $c(x, t=0)$ and for times $t>0$ the label lipids diffuse into the zone where further photobleaching is possible, $c(x, t>0)$. From Sheats and McConnell (1978).

The photobleaching and diffusive recovery of fluorescent molecules can likewise be used to determine lateral diffusion coefficients. For example, the fluorescent probe NBD-PE (derived from egg phosphatidylethanolamine)

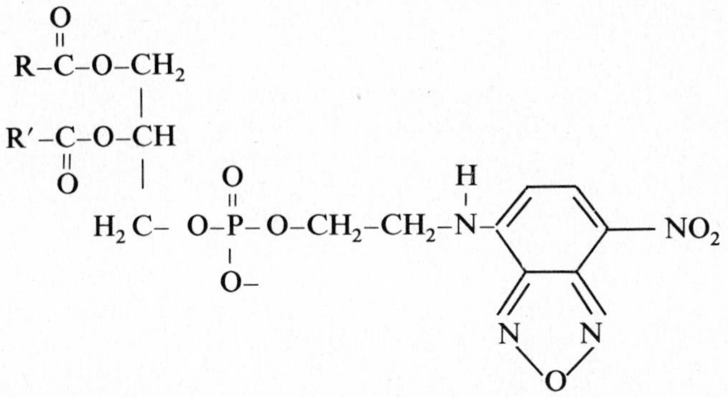

$$\begin{array}{l} R{-}\overset{O}{\overset{\|}{C}}{-}O{-}CH_2 \\ \qquad\quad\;\, | \\ R'{-}\underset{O}{\underset{\|}{C}}{-}O{-}CH \\ \qquad\quad\;\, | \\ \qquad\; H_2C{-}\,O{-}\overset{O}{\overset{\|}{P}}{-}O{-}CH_2{-}CH_2{-}\overset{H}{\overset{|}{N}}{-}(\text{benzoxadiazole ring: } N{-}O{-}N){-}NO_2 \\ \qquad\qquad\qquad\;\; \underset{O^-}{|} \end{array} \qquad \text{(II)}$$

can be incorporated into lipid bilayers and multibilayers. An intense focused laser beam can be used to "bleach" (photochemically destroy) a small region (e.g., ~5–10 μm) in lipid bilayers containing a fluorescent lipid probe, such as (II). The recovery of fluorescence in the bleached spot due to lateral diffusion can be monitored using an attenuated laser beam and photomultiplier detection of fluorescence. For a discussion of this method, see Axelrod et al. (1976) and Wu et al. (1977). From the point of view of the boundary conditions set up at the start of the experiment, this spot photobleaching-recovery technique is conceptually similar to the $t=0$ initial concentration distribution employed by Devaux and McConnell (1972).

B. Smith and McConnell (1978) have employed a periodic pattern photobleaching, fluorescence-recovery method that likewise bears a conceptual similarity to the periodic pattern spin–label method of Sheats and McConnell (1978) described above. The basic idea is illustrated in fig. 4. A Ronchi ruling is placed in a real image plane of a fluorescence microscope, and an intense laser beam is focused onto the plane of a lipid bilayer containing a fluorescent lipid such as (II). A short burst of laser radiation brings about the photochemical destruction of the fluorescent molecules in the irradiated region of the bilayer, yielding a concentration distribution (except for diffraction effects) similar to that shown in fig. 3. This concentration distribution can be recorded photographically, using a fluorescence microscope, as a function of time, as described by B. Smith and McConnell (1978).

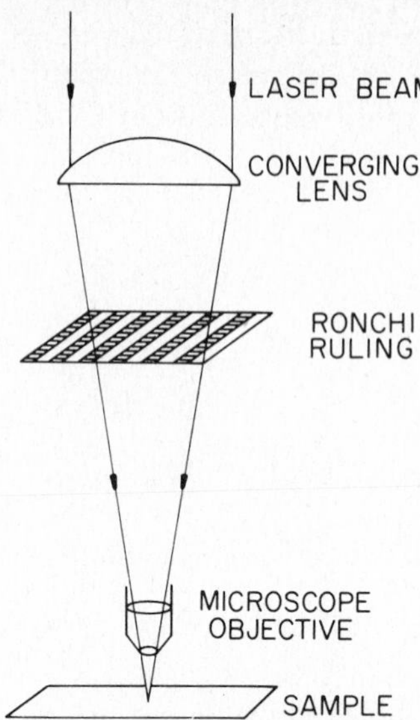

Fig. 4. Schematic diagram of optics for pattern photobleaching of fluorescent probe molecules. Light from an argon–ion laser is directed through a Ronchi ruling into the microscope objective which focuses an image of the ruling onto the sample. From Smith and McConnell (1978).

Densitometer tracings of these films provide a quantitative measure of $c(x, t)$, for which the general theoretical expression is again given in eq. (7). Since the higher order terms decay very rapidly compared to the first exponential term, plots of the log of the spatial amplitude of the concentration wave as a function of time yield straight lines, and thus the diffusion coefficients D. Examples of diffusion coefficients determined using this method will be given later. It is also possible to employ photomultiplier recording with periodic pattern photobleaching to determine lateral diffusion coefficients. [(See a study of the lateral diffusion of antibodies bound to lipid haptens by L. Smith et al. (1979b).]

1.3. Anisotropic lateral diffusion in plasma membranes of mouse embryo fibroblasts

In general, diffusion can be anisotropic. Perhaps the simplest example is thermal diffusion of heat in an anisotropic crystal (Carslaw and Jaeger 1959). It has now been found that the lateral diffusion of molecules on cell membranes can likewise be anisotropic, as shown by B. Smith et al. (1979) in the case of adherent mouse fibroblasts. In this study the cell surface was labeled with fluorescein isothiocyanate conjugated succinyl concanavalin A (S-Con A).

For anisotropic diffusion, the diffusion equation has the form,

$$\frac{\partial c}{\partial t} = \overline{\nabla} \cdot \boldsymbol{D} \cdot \overline{\nabla} c \tag{8}$$

where $\boldsymbol{D}$ is the diffusion tensor, which can be written for two dimensions in terms of a vector dyadic:

$$\boldsymbol{D} = \boldsymbol{ii}D_{xx} + \boldsymbol{jj}D_{yy} + \boldsymbol{ij}D_{xy} + \boldsymbol{ji}D_{yx}. \tag{9}$$

If we assume that $\boldsymbol{D}$ is homogeneous (i.e., does not depend on position x, y, but only on direction $\boldsymbol{i}, \boldsymbol{j}$), then the diffusion equation (8), takes the form

$$\frac{\partial c}{\partial t} = D_{xx}\frac{\partial^2 c}{\partial x^2} + D_{yy}\frac{\partial^2 c}{\partial y^2} + (D_{xy} + D_{yx})\frac{\partial^2 c}{\partial x\, \partial y}. \tag{10}$$

In general, the diffusion tensor is symmetric, $D_{xy} = D_{yx}$.

In the experiment of B. Smith et al. (1979) the fluoresceinated S-Con A fibroblasts were photobleached in a two-dimensional checkerboard periodic pattern. This periodic concentration pattern at time t can be represented in a Fourier series,

$$c(x, y, t) = \frac{1}{\sqrt{2\pi}} \int_{-\infty}^{+\infty} \int \exp\{i(k_x x + k_y y)\} F(k_x, k_y, t)\, \mathrm{d}k_x\, \mathrm{d}k_y. \tag{11}$$

The directions x and y are taken to be along the primative "unit cell" directions of the photobleached checkerboard pattern, which has the period $P = P_x = P_y$. Thus, $c(x + P, y, 0) = c(x, y, 0)$ and $c(x, y + P, 0) = c(x, y, 0)$. By "checkerboard pattern" we mean any pattern that has the translational and rotational symmetry elements of a two-dimensional square lattice. These periodic boundary conditions require that $\exp\{ik_x x\} = \exp\{ik_x(x + P)\}$. Thus, $\exp\{ik_x P\} = 1$ and $k_x = 2\pi n_x / P$ where $n_x = 0, \pm 1, \pm 2, \pm 3, \ldots$. Similarly $k_y = 2\pi n_y / P$ where $n_y = 0, \pm 1, \pm 2, \pm 3, \ldots$. By substitution of the above expression for $c(x, y, t)$ in the diffusion equation, eq. (10), we obtain

$$\frac{\partial F(k_x, k_y, t)}{\partial t} = -\left(k_x^2 D_{xx} + k_y^2 D_{yy} + 2k_x k_y D_{xy}\right). \tag{12}$$

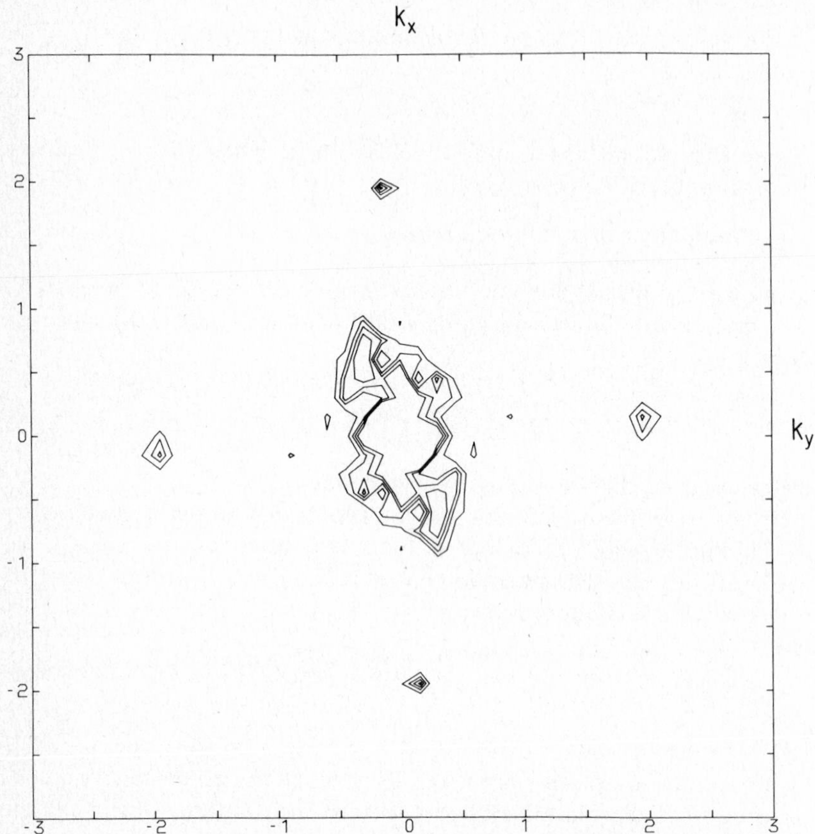

Fig. 5. Contour map of the Fourier amplitudes $F(k_x, k_y)$ of the Fourier transform of a pattern photobleached fibroblast. The contour lines connect points for which the amplitudes are equal. The units of k_x and k_y are spatial frequency (equal to 2π/distance) in μm^{-1}. Low frequencies, near the center of the figure, correspond to structures which cover long distances on the photograph. These low frequency amplitudes represent primarily the shape of the fibroblast itself and non-uniform laser illumination of the sample. The peaks in the Fourier amplitude which correspond to the photobleached pattern appear at $k_x = (1.95, 0.15)$ and $k_y = (-0.15, 1.95)$. Taken from B. Smith et al. (1979).

Thus,

$$F(k_x, k_y, t) = F(k_x, k_y, 0) \exp - \{k_x^2 D_{xx} + k_y^2 D_{yy} + 2k_x k_y D_{xy}\} t. \tag{13}$$

If there are many "lattice points" on the two-dimensional photobleach pattern of the cell, and sufficient contrast in this pattern, then the amplitudes of the Fourier components $F(k_x, k_y, t)$ will be large at the reciprocal lattice points k_x, k_y. The exponential decay of the amplitude corresponding to a reciprocal lattice point $k_x \neq 0$, $k_y = 0$ can be used to determine D_{xx} from eq. (13). Similarly, by measuring the decay of an amplitude $F(0, k_y, t)$ one can determine D_{yy}. Having determined D_{xx} and D_{yy}, the decay of a Fourier component $F(k_x, k_y, t)$ for $k_x = k_y \neq 0$ can be used to determine D_{xy}. If $D_{xy} \neq 0$, one can readily make a transformation to a principal axis system X, Y such that $\boldsymbol{D}$ is diagonal, i.e., $D_{XY} = 0$.

Figure 5 shows the Fourier amplitudes determined from the Fourier transform of densitometer tracings of photographs of fluorescent S-Con A labeled mouse fibroblasts bleached in a checkerboard pattern (B. Smith et al. 1979). In these experiments the principal axes for the diffusion coefficients were found to be parallel (X) and perpendicular (Y) to the stress filaments, with D_{XX} being typically larger than D_{YY} by a factor between two and ten, depending on the particular cell examined. The diffusion coefficients determined from the exponential decay of the Fourier amplitudes in fig. 5 were $D_{XX} = 1.4 \times 10^{-11}$ cm^2/s, and $D_{YY} = 3.8 \times 10^{-12}$ cm^2/s. For details, the reader is referred to the publication of B. Smith et al. (1979). The molecular basis of anisotropic diffusion is discussed in the next section.

1.4. Lateral diffusion in inhomogeneous membranes

The above study of lateral molecular diffusion in adherent mouse fibroblasts raises two interesting, general questions. Why is the diffusion anisotropic? The diffusion could be anisotropic if the host lipid bilayer were anisotropic. The diffusion could appear to be anisotropic, but is in fact isotropic, if the fibroblast membranes had a strongly scalloped profile. Neither of these possibilities appears likely. The most likely origin of this anisotropy is some interaction between the diffusing, labeled molecules and other membrane components that have an anisotropic distribution themselves. For example, if the diffusing, labeled molecules tended to avoid the fibroblast stress filaments, then a higher diffusion rate parallel to the stress filaments would be expected, as observed. In our study, we of course have no direct evidence for this interaction. However, the recent study by Ash et al. (1977) is certainly consistent with this interpretation.

The second question raised by the above study of fluorescent S-Con A labeled fibroblasts is: Why are the diffusion constants so low? Such low diffusion coefficients have been reported in many other photo-bleach-recovery experiments. For a leading reference, see Schlessinger et al. (1978). Our view that these diffusion constants are unexpectedly low is based on admittedly scanty data, and arguments that are far from compelling. First we note that the lateral diffusion coefficients of phospholipids are in the range 10^{-7}–10^{-8} cm/s for "fluid" host lipids in cell membranes. The lateral diffusion coefficient of rhodopsin in rod disc membranes is 0.4×10^{-8} cm^2/s (Poo and Cone 1974). The lateral diffusion coefficient of the M-13 phage coat protein in reconstituted lipid bilayers is $\sim 4 \times 10^{-8}$ cm^2/s (L. Smith et al. 1979a). The molecular weight of the M-13 phage coat protein is 5260. In an unpublished work, we have determined the lateral diffusion coefficient of a much higher mol wt intrinsic membrane protein, the vesicular stromatitus virus G-protein, and this has a comparably large ($\sim 10^{-8}$ cm^2/s) diffusion coefficient (Parce, Hale and McConnell unpublished work). On the basis of these results, it seems likely that other intrinsic membrane proteins (such as HLA and glycophorin) that span the lipid bilayer with one or two hydrophobic α-helices, should have comparably large diffusion coefficients in lipid bilayer membranes. Thus the low diffusion coefficients reported for many plasma membrane proteins indicate that these membrane components interact strongly with one another, and/or with extracellular and/or intracellular structures. This leads to the general problem of how to describe and interpret best the lateral diffusion of labeled molecular components of membranes that interact with other membrane components. [The reader should be cautioned, however, that some of the low diffusion coefficients reported in the literature for membrane proteins on cell surfaces may be in error due to photochemical damage. This effect has been demonstrated experimentally for antibodies bound to lipid haptens in model membranes. See L. Smith et al. (1979b).]

Unfortunately, the interpretation of experimental studies of lateral diffusion in inhomogeneous media is surprisingly complex, especially when an experiment is time-dependent, i.e. involves the creation of non-uniform distributions of spin labels, fluorescent probes, or nuclear spin polarizations, and the measurement of the relaxation of the system to equilibrium. The mathematical problems encountered in solutions of the diffusion equation are far more complex than those encountered for systems where diffusion takes place under steady-state conditions. (For examples, see Carslaw and Jaeger 1959, Crank 1957, Adam and Delbrück 1968). Below we briefly describe an example of a diffusion in an inhomogeneous model membrane.

There is experimental evidence that under certain conditions of temperature and composition, binary mixtures of cholesterol and phosphatidylcholines form regular alternating bands of "solid" phosphatidylcholine and "fluid", the fluid being a binary mixture containing approximately 20 mol % cholesterol (Copeland 1979, Copeland and McConnell unpublished). The widths of the solid bands remain constant, about 150 Å, and the widths of the fluid bands increase with increasing cholesterol concentration, and appear to approach infinity as the cholesterol concentration in the sample approaches 20 mol %, i.e. the system becomes entirely fluid. This conclusion is supported by the experiments of Rubenstein et al. (1979). These investigators observed an approximately tenfold sudden increase in the lateral diffusion coefficient of the fluorescent lipid probe (II) in binary mixtures of cholesterol and phosphatidylcholine as the cholesterol concentration is increased beyond 20 mol %, corresponding to the disappearance of the solid bands.

The problem of lateral diffusion as measured by pattern photobleaching in an inhomogeneous membrane of this type has been treated theoretically by Owicki and McConnell (1980). The theory assumes that on a microscopic scale, there are two isotropic lateral diffusion coefficients D_S and D_F, corresponding to the solid and fluid phases. If f_s represents the fraction of the membrane that is solid, and f_f represents the fraction of the membrane that is fluid, then Owicki and McConnell calculate that in a periodic pattern photobleach–recovery experiment (where the bleach repeat period P is much larger than the separation of the solid bands) the diffusion coefficient for a single membrane is anisotropic,

$$D_{\parallel} = f_f D_F + f_s D_S \qquad D_{\perp}^{-1} = f_f D_F^{-1} + f_s D_S^{-1} \tag{14}$$

where $D_{\parallel}$ and $D_{\perp}$ represent the diffusion coefficients parallel and perpendicular to the stripes. For multilayers having bands with all orientations in two dimensions, the diffusive recovery involves an average over all orientations (0–180°) of the angle between the bands and the direction of the bleach stripes. The calculated recovery curves are quite complex, and sometimes deviate strongly from a single exponential. These theoretical calculations are in semiquantitative agreement with the experimental data of Rubenstein et al. (1979).

2. Immunological aspects of lateral molecular motion

2.1. Introduction

As indicated in the introduction to section 1, lateral molecular motions in membranes are thought to play a number of roles in the biological functions of cells. In the present section we consider briefly the kinds of molecular motions that evidently do play significant roles in immune responses. Our approach is to use reconstituted membranes in which the lateral motions and distributions of specific molecules can, to a considerable extent, be controlled experimentally. Components of the immune system may "recognize", "attack", and even "kill" the reconstituted membrane. A reconstituted membrane vesicle is said to be "killed" if it is caused to be leaky by one or more components of the immune system, or if it is phagocytized. The reconstituted membrane may likewise stimulate the immune system to manufacture, or amplify, this recognition and killing equipment (afferent immune response). From the relation between the physical and chemical properties of the target membrane, and the immune response to it, we hope to infer something about the membrane-associated molecular events involved in immune response: recognition, triggering, and effector function (e.g., "killing"). For a number of years, progress using this approach seemed tortuously slow. Now, at the time of this writing this situation seems to have reversed itself completely, so that in this present chapter we can only briefly summarize some of the recent work.

2.2. Antibody recognition of haptens and antigens

The most studied example of recognition in the immune system is the binding of specific antibody to hapten or antigen. When this hapten and/or antigen is bound to the plasma membrane of a biological cell, or to the membrane of a lipid vesicle, this antibody binding may be followed by killing of the biological cell or lipid vesicle, provided additional molecular components (complement, see below) or cellular components (e.g., macrophages, *K*-cells) of the immune system are present. Since the paramagnetic resonance spectra of nitroxide spin labels are sensitive to their distribution (local concentration), rotational freedom, and lateral diffusion in membranes, we have chosen to use nitroxide lipid haptens in many of our studies. Three different nitroxide lipid haptens have been employed, having the chemical formulae,

$$\begin{array}{l} \quad\quad H_2C{-}O{-}CO{-}(CH_2)_{14}CH_3 \\ \quad\quad | \\ CH_3(CH_2)_{14}CO{-}O{-}CH \\ \quad\quad | \quad\quad O \quad\quad\quad\quad\quad H_3C \\ \quad\quad\quad\quad\;\; \| \quad\quad\quad\quad\quad\quad | \\ \quad\quad H_2C{-}O{-}P{-}O{-}CH_2CH_2{-}N^{+}{-}\text{(tetramethylpiperidine)}\;N{-}O \\ \quad\quad\quad\quad\;\; \| \quad\quad\quad\quad\quad\quad | \\ \quad\quad\quad\quad\;\; O^{-} \quad\quad\quad\quad\; H_3C \end{array} \tag{a}$$

$$\begin{array}{l} \quad\quad H_2C{-}O{-}CO{-}(CH_2)_{14}CH_3 \\ \quad\quad | \\ CH_3(CH_2)_{14}CO{-}O{-}CH \\ \quad\quad | \quad\; O \quad\quad\quad\quad\quad\quad H \quad\quad\quad O\;\; H \\ \quad\quad\quad\quad \| \quad\quad\quad\quad\quad\quad\;\; | \quad\quad\quad\;\; \| \;\;\; | \\ \quad\quad H_2C{-}O{-}P{-}O{-}CH_2CH_2{-}N{-}CH_2{-}C{-}N{-}\text{(tetramethylpiperidine)}\;N{-}O \\ \quad\quad\quad\quad | \\ \quad\quad\quad\quad O^{-} \end{array} \tag{b}$$

$$\begin{array}{l} \quad\quad H_2C{-}O{-}CO{-}(CH_2)_{14}CH_3 \\ \quad\quad | \\ CH_3(CH_2)_{14}CO{-}O{-}CH \\ \quad\quad | \quad\; O \quad\quad\quad\quad\quad\quad\quad\quad\quad\quad\quad\quad O\;\; H \\ \quad\quad\quad\quad \| \quad\quad\quad\quad\quad\quad\quad\quad\quad\quad\quad\quad\; \| \;\;\; | \\ \quad\quad H_2C{-}O{-}P{-}O{-}(CH_2)_2NH{-}CO{-}(CH_2)_3{-}C{-}N{-}\text{(tetramethylpiperidine)}\;N{-}O \\ \quad\quad\quad\quad | \\ \quad\quad\quad\quad O^{-} \end{array} \tag{c}$$

2.3. Antibodies to nitroxide lipid haptens

Although the production and isolation of antibodies to specific haptens is a highly developed art among immunologists, the antinitroxide antibodies used in our own work have some special properties that warrant comment. In fact, it was something of a surprise that antinitroxide antibodies could be prepared by conventional methods, e.g. immunization of rabbits. One might have anticipated rapid chemical degradation of the free radical. For example, chemical reduction of the nitroxide group to the corresponding hydroxylamine is particularly facile,

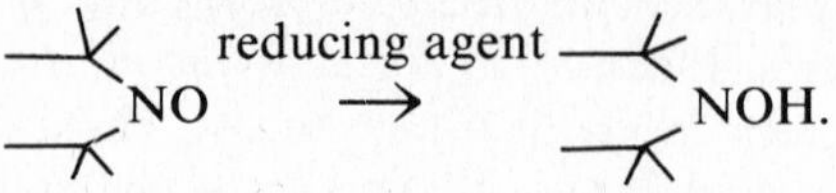

$$\mathrm{{>}NO} \xrightarrow{\text{reducing agent}} \mathrm{{>}NOH.}$$

Humphries and McConnell (1976) reported that it is possible to prepare specific rabbit IgG antibodies against the nitroxide group, using conventional techniques. The protein, keyhole limpet haemocyanine, was alkylated with the iodoacetamide label,

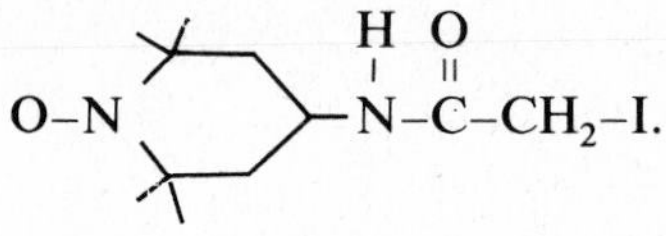

$$\mathrm{O{-}N\langle\ \rangle{-}N(H){-}C(=O){-}CH_2{-}I.}$$

The alkylated protein was used to immunize rabbits, using Freund's adjuvant. Affinity purified IgG antibodies, specifically directed against the above six-membered ring nitroxide group, have binding constants of the order of 10^5–10^6 l/mole. That is, if H designates a single haptenic molecule such as,

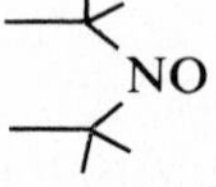

$$\mathrm{{>}NO}$$

then the two binding constants K_1 and K_2 are 10^5–10^6 l/mole

$$\mathrm{H + IgG \rightleftharpoons IgGH} \qquad K_1 = \frac{[\mathrm{IgGH}]}{[\mathrm{IgG}][\mathrm{H}]} \tag{15, 16}$$

$$\mathrm{IgGH + H \rightleftharpoons IgGH_2} \qquad K_2 = \frac{[\mathrm{IgGH_2}]}{[\mathrm{IgGH}][\mathrm{H}]}. \tag{17, 18}$$

It was then discovered that these antibodies bind to a given nitroxide

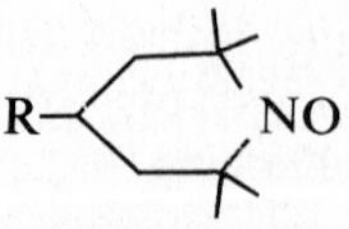

$$\mathrm{R{-}\langle\ \rangle NO}$$

nitroxide

and its corresponding hydroxylamine

R—(ring)—NOH

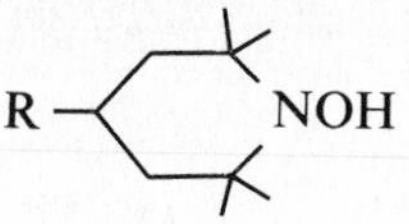

hydroxylamine

with very similar affinities (Rey and McConnell 1976). Irrespective of the explanation of this surprising result, it is extremely fortunate, since one can carry out paramagnetic resonance studies of antibody binding to nitroxide lipid haptens in model membranes under non-reducing conditions, and can then study specific antibody-dependent cellular interactions with bilayer membranes containing lipid haptens and not worry about cell-mediated chemical reduction of the nitroxide group to the corresponding hydroxylamine. The near equality of specific antibody binding to the nitroxide groups, and the corresponding hydroxylamines has also been found useful for the study of molecular motions of antibodies on cell surfaces.

2.4. Molecular motions of antibodies bound to lipid haptens in model membranes

Before discussing specific antibody-dependent immune attack against model membranes, it is of interest to first consider the kinetics and equilibria of the interaction of antibodies with model membranes containing lipid haptens. Various states of an antibody molecule at the membrane surface are depicted in fig. 6. Several points are noted below in connection with this figure.

2.4.1. Antibodies bound to lipid haptens in model membranes diffuse as rapidly as the lipids themselves

The data providing evidence for this statement are given in table 1, taken from L. Smith et al. (1979b). Note that this statement is valid for both the "fluid" and "solid" phases of dimyristoylphosphatidylcholine. Note also that the previously discussed sharp enhancement in lipid diffusion at 20 mol % cholesterol is also reflected in the diffusion of bound antibodies. The diffusion of the bound antibodies was determined using periodic pattern photobleaching and rabbit IgG anti-nitroxide antibodies labeled with fluorescein isothiocyanate. From these

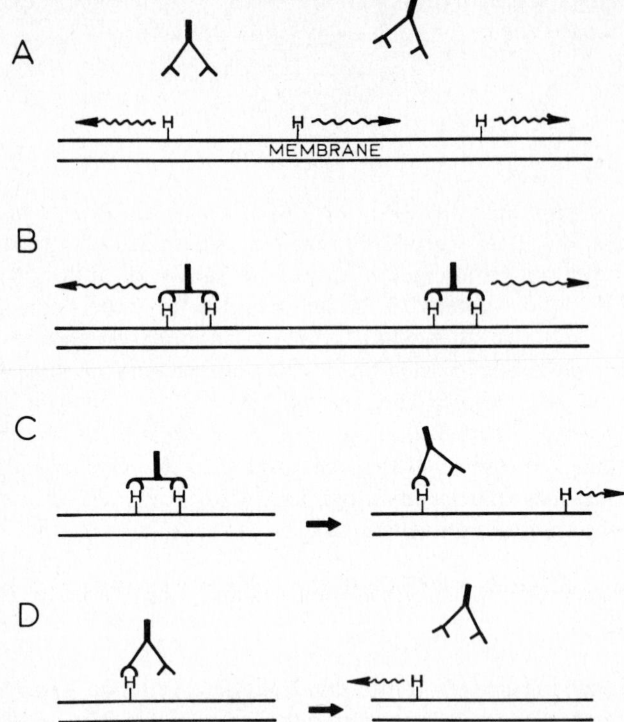

Fig. 6. Molecular motions of antibodies and haptens on model membranes. (A) Schematic illustration of lateral diffusion of lipids bearing the haptenic group H. IgG antibody molecules are depicted as dissolved in the surrounding aqueous solution. (B) Schematic illustration of specific IgG antibody molecules bound with both combining sites to a pair of lipid haptens. The bound antibody molecules are known not to cluster, and to diffuse laterally at nearly the same rate as the lipid haptens themselves (see text). (C) Schematic illustration of the dissociation of one antibody combining site from a lipid hapten, the antibody remaining bound with the second combining site. (D) Schematic illustration of the "complete" dissociation of antibody from the hapten-sensitized membrane surface. Taken from Parce et al. (1979).

data we conclude that the antibody molecules ($\sim$150 000 mol wt) interact with the membrane surface only at the hapten-combining site region. If the antibody molecules were to "lie down" or "submerge" on or in the lipid bilayer, then the lateral diffusion would have surely been found to be retarded in these experiments. Because of the chemical equivalence of the haptens in the bilayer, and the twofold symmetry of the IgG antibody molecules, the Fc tails of the antibodies are probably perpendicular to the membrane surface.

Table 1
Diffusion coefficients of membrane-bound antibodies and lipids

Sample	Temperature, (°C)	D^* (cm^2/s) $\times 10^9$
NBD-PE in DMPC liposomes	28	63 ± 12
NBD-PE in DMPC multibilayers	26	50
FITC-IgG on DMPC liposomes containing hapten I	28	57 ± 8
NBD-PE in DPPC liposomes	32	~0.01
FITC-IgG on DPPC liposomes containing hapten I	32	~0.01
NBD-PE in DPPC multibilayers containing 15 mol % cholesterol	21	0.012
FITC-IgG on DPPC liposomes containing hapten I and 15 mol % cholesterol	32	~0.01
NBD-PE in DPPC multibilayers containing 25 mol % cholesterol	21	1.2
FITC-IgG on DPPC liposomes containing hapten I and 25 mol % cholesterol	32	1.7 ± 0.6

*Error figures for the present work indicate standard deviations from the mean of these measurements.

2.4.2. Antibodies bound to lipid haptens in model membranes do not spontaneously aggregate

The diffusion data given in table 1 immediately rule out significant aggregation of the antibody molecules, which would also reduce their diffusion coefficients. Other evidence that antibody molecules bound to lipid haptens in model membranes do not spontaneously aggregate has been obtained from freeze-etch electron microscopy, where single, randomly distributed bound IgG molecules can be visualized on the membrane surface. For such studies it is important to remove auto-antibodies from the antibody preparation (Henry et al. 1978).

2.4.3. Antibodies bound to lipid haptens in model membranes bind with both combining sites. The rate of transfer of antibodies from one membrane to another

The evidence for the assertion above is based on kinetic data and kinetic arguments. Experiments have been carried out in which two populations of lipid membranes (liposomes) were mixed (Parce et al. 1979). One population contained fluorescent antibodies bound to lipid haptens, while the second population contained lipid haptens alone. The two populations were incubated for a given period of time, and then passed through a fluorescence activated cell sorter (FACS, Becton-Dickinson, Inc., New Jersey, USA). The strength of the resonance signals recorded as each lipid membrane (liposome) passed through the laser beam could then be used to measure the rate of antibody transfer from antibody-rich to antibody-poor liposomes. Under specified conditions the half-time for antibody transfer was of the order of one hour (Parce et al. 1979). Since the antibody exchange rate between liposomes is believed to be enhanced by membrane–membrane contact (liposome collisions), it can be concluded that the lifetime for these antibodies, bound to a given membrane, is at least of the order of one hour. This total dissociation is depicted in figs. 6A and 6D. An antibody molecule bound to a nitroxide hapten with only one combining site could hardly dissociate at this slow rate. The lifetime for the dissociation of a single nitroxide hapten from the antibody combining site in three-dimensional solution can be estimated to be of the order of 10^{-3}–1 s, assuming that the hapten "on" rate constant is 10^6–10^9 l/mole-s, and a single hapten binding constant $K_1 = 10^6$ l/mole. Thus, even when the probability of diffusive recombination of a dissociated antibody from its parent membrane is allowed for, we are left with the conclusion that the antinitroxide antibodies must be bound to the lipid membranes containing lipid hapten B with both combining sites. [For a treatment of the dissociation and diffusive recombination of molecules with a single membrane, see Berg and Purcell (1977).]

2.4.4. The rate of detachment of antibodies from single lipid haptens

Although we have concluded that the rabbit antinitroxide IgG antibodies bind to lipid hapten B with both combining sites, this of course does not preclude the kinetic events depicted in figs. 6C and 6D. Such processes are of interest in connection with the possibility that an antibody could diffuse laterally across a hapten-derivatized rigid membrane by "walking." The rate of the kinetic processes depicted in figs. 6C and 6D have been estimated using a chemical technique (Parce et al. 1979, Schwartz et al. 1979).

The following specially prepared nitroxide molecule has three properties,

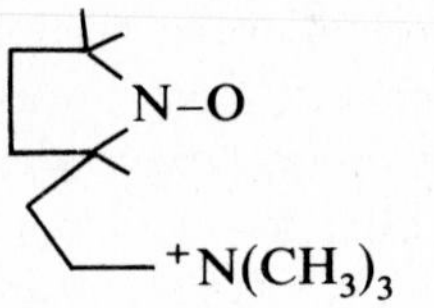

$$\text{N–O} \qquad {}^{+}\mathrm{N(CH_3)_3} \qquad \equiv \quad \mathrm{R_2{\frown}NO.}$$

(i) The hydroxylamine of $\mathrm{R_2{\frown}NO}$, namely $\mathrm{R_2{\frown}NOH}$, reacts chemically with the haptenic groups $\mathrm{R_1{\frown}NO}$ (see structures A, B, C):

$$\mathrm{R_2{\frown}NOH + R_1{\frown}NO \longrightarrow R_2{\frown}NO + R_1{\frown}NOH.}$$

The equilibrium constant for this reaction is greater than 10^4, favoring the reduction of the haptenic nitroxide group.

(ii) The nitroxide $\mathrm{R_2{\frown}NO}$ and its corresponding hydroxylamine $\mathrm{R_2{\frown}NOH}$ do not react significantly with the antinitroxide antibodies employed.

(iii) The paramagnetic resonance spectra of $\mathrm{R_1{\frown}NO}$ and $\mathrm{R_2{\frown}NO}$ are sufficiently displaced from one another, that one can measure the paramagnetic resonance intensity of one or the other.

Experiments were carried out by mixing solutions containing lipid membranes containing the lipid nitroxide hapten A, and the hydroxylamine $\mathrm{R_2{\frown}NOH}$ in the presence and absence of specific antinitroxide antibodies. It was found that the binding of the antibodies to the nitroxide lipid haptens significantly protected these haptenic groups against reduction by $\mathrm{R_2{\frown}NOH}$. The antibody-mediated depression of the oxidation rate of $\mathrm{R_2{\frown}NOH}$ (measured by paramagnetic resonance intensity) could then be used to estimate the net rate of exposure of haptens due to processes C and D in fig. 6. The half-time for the exposure of the haptenic groups obtained in this fashion is of the order of 30 min. Measured by this reaction, the rate of exposure of haptens is relatively slow, and of the same order as the antibody membrane-to-membrane transfer rate. Unfortunately this chemical hydrogen atom exchange rate is probably too low to detect every single site dissociation event (e.g., process C in fig. 6). Further experiments with more rapid reducing agents will be required to determine the single site dissociation rate with greater precision.

2.4.5. Antibody conformation changes on antibody binding to lipid haptens in model membranes

A problem of great interest is whether or not there is a functional antibody conformation change when antibody molecules bind to lipid haptens with both combining sites, as implied in the sketches in fig. 6. Preliminary evidence for such a conformation change has been obtained by Parce and McConnell (1979) for rabbit antidinitrophenyl antibodies, and the lipid hapten a dinitrophenyl-derivatized phosphatidylethanolamine. A spin label attached to the carbohydrate moiety indicated a surprising enhancement in the mobility of the nitroxide group on binding to the hapten-sensitized vesicles. Unfortunately, it has been difficult to reproduce this result which may be restricted to a particular rabbit allotype; allotypic diversity among rabbits is large.

2.5. Specific antibody dependent interactions of components of the immune system with lipid hapten-sensitized model membranes

Lipid hapten-sensitized vesicles of the type described above have been shown to elicit a variety of immune responses, including antibody-dependent afferent and efferent responses. The rather elaborate efforts described above to characterize the physical state of antibodies bound to lipid haptens has been made in the belief that these physical and chemical properties of the target vesicles are essential for understanding the various immune responses to them. There is now much evidence to support this view. However, the variety and complexity of these immune responses precludes a detailed discussion in this chapter. Instead we conclude with a listing of a few references that illustrate the use of reconstituted lipid membrane vesicles to study immune functions, where some special physical and/or chemical feature of the target membrane is delineated. For complement specific antibody-dependent depletion and Cl activation, see Esser et al. (1979) and leading references therein. For specific antibody-dependent activation of neutrophils and macrophages, see Hafeman et al. (1979), and Lewis, Hafeman and McConnell (to be published). For specific antibody-dependent *K*-cell "killing" of vesicles, see Geiger and Schreiber (1979). For antibody-independent T-cell mediated allogeneic killing of a reconstituted membrane vesicle, see Hollander et al. (1979). For H-2 restricted, virus-specific secondary stimulation of cytotoxic T cells, see Finberg et al. (1978). For *in vitro* B-cell stimulation by hapten-sensitized liposomes, see Yasuda et al. (1979) and Humphries (1979).

Acknowledgements

I am pleased to acknowledge the contribution of Dr. Philippe Devaux in his early determination of lipid lateral diffusion coefficients in my laboratory. I am likewise pleased to acknowledge Professor Roger Kornberg who, as a graduate student, synthesized the first nitroxide head-group phospholipid spin label and used this molecule in the first studies of transverse as well as lateral diffusion of phospholipids in bilayer model membranes.

The work described in this chapter has been supported by the National Science Foundation and the National Institutes of Health, most recently NSF Grant No. PCM 77-23586, and NIH Grant No. 5R01 AI13587.

References

Adam, G. and M. Delbrück (1968) Structural Chemistry and Molecular Biology, in: eds. A. Rich and N. Davidson (W. H. Freeman & Co., San Francisco) pp. 198–215.

Ash, J. F., D. Louvard and S. J. Singer (1977) Proc. Natl. Acad. Sci. USA 74, 5584.

Axelrod, D., D. E. Koppel, J. Schlessinger, E. Elson and W. W. Webb (1976) Biophys. J. 16, 1055.

Berg, H. C. and E. M. Purcell (1977) Biophys. J. 20, 193.

Bretscher, M. S. (1973) Science 181, 622.

Carslaw, H. S. and J. C. Jaeger (1959) Conduction of Heat in Solids, 2nd ed. (University Press, Oxford).

Copeland, B. R. (1979) Ph.D. Thesis (Stanford Univ., Stanford, Calif.).

Crank, J. (1975) The Mathematics of Diffusion, 2nd ed. (Oxford University Press, London).

Devaux, P. and H. M. McConnell (1972) J. Am. Chem. Soc. 94, 4475.

Esser, A. F., R. M. Bartholomew, J. W. Parce and H. M. McConnell (1979) J. Biol. Chem. 254, 1768.

Finberg, R., M. Mescher and S. Burakoff (1978) J. Exp. Med. 148, 1620.

Frye, L. D. and M. Edidin (1970) J. Cell Sci. 7, 319.

Geiger, B. and A. D. Schreiber (1979) Clin. Exptl. Immunol. 35, 149.

Hafeman, D. G., J. W. Parce and H. M. McConnell (1979) Biochem. Biophys. Res. Commun. 86, 522.

Henry, N., J. W. Parce and H. M. McConnell (1978) Proc. Natl. Acad. Sci. USA 75, 3933.

Hollander, N., S. Q. Mehdi, I. L. Weissman, H. M. McConnell and J. P. Kriss (1979) Proc. Natl. Acad. Sci. USA 76, 4042.

Humphries, G. M. K. H. (1979) J. Immunol., 123, 2126.

Humphries, G. M. K. and H. M. McConnell (1976) Biophys. J. 16, 275.

Margenau, H. and G. M. Murphy (1948) The Mathematics of Physics and Chemistry (D. van Nostrand Co., Inc., New York).

Owicki, J.C. and H.M. McConnell, Biophys. J., in press.

Parce, J. W. and H. M. McConnell (1979) Polym. Prepr. 20, 211.

Parce, J. W., M. A. Schwartz, J. C. Owicki and H. M. McConnell (1979) J. Phys. Chem., 83, 3414.

Poo, M.-M. and R. A. Cone (1974) Nature London 247, 438.

Raff, M. C. (1976) Sci. Am. 234, 30.

Raff, M. C. and S. de Petris (1973) Fed. Proc. 32, 48.

Rey, P. and H. M. McConnell (1976) Biochem. Biophys. Res. Commun. 73, 248.

Rubenstein, J. L. R., B. A. Smith and H. M. McConnell (1979) Proc. Natl. Acad. Sci. USA 76, 15.

Sackmann, E. and H. Träuble (1972) J. Am. Chem. Soc. 94, 4492.

Schlessinger, J., Y. Shechter, P. Cuatrecasas, M. C. Willingham and I. Pastan (1978) Proc. Natl. Acad. Sci. USA 75, 5353.

Schwartz, M. A., J. W. Parce and H. M. McConnell (1979) J. Am. Chem. Soc. 101, 3592.

Sheats, J. R. and H. M. McConnell (1977) J. Am. Chem. Soc. 99, 7091.

Sheats, J. R. and H. M. McConnell (1978) Proc. Natl. Acad. Sci. USA 75, 4661.

Sheats, J. R. and H. M. McConnell (1979) J. Am. Chem. Soc. 101, 3272.

Smith, B. A. and H. M. McConnell (1978) Proc. Natl. Acad. Sci. USA 75, 2759.

Smith, B. A., W. R. Clark and H. M. McConnell (1979) Proc. Natl. Acad. Sci. USA, in press.

Smith, L. M., B. A. Smith and H. M. McConnell (1979a) Biochemistry 18, 2256.

Smith, L. M., J. W. Parce, B. A. Smith and H. M. McConnell (1979b) Proc. Natl. Acad. Sci. USA 76, 4177.

Stern, P. L. and M. S. Bretscher (1979) J. Cell Biol. 82, 829.

Wu, E.-S., K. Jacobson and D. Papahadjopoulos (1977) Biochemistry 16, 3936.

Yasuda, T., T. Tadakuma, C. W. Pierce and S. C. Kinsky (1979) J. Immunol. 123, 1535.

COURSE 5
(Part I)

BASIC ELEMENTS OF IMMUNOLOGY

Michel FOUGEREAU,

Centre d'Immunologie I.N.S.E.R.M.–C.N.R.S.
de Marseille-Luminy, Case 906,
13288 Marseille Cedex 2,
France

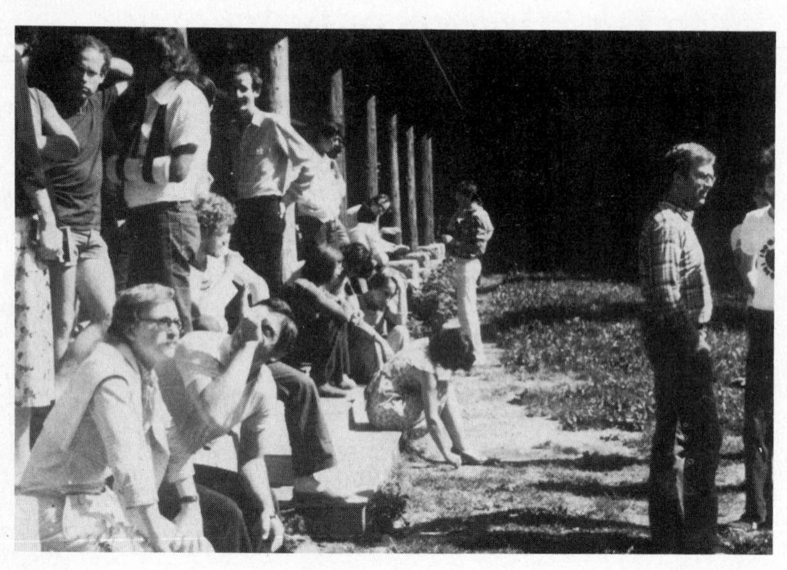

Contents

R. Balian et al., eds.
Les Houches, Session XXXIII, 1979 – Membranes et Communication Intercellulaire / Membranes and Intercellular Communication

1. Main recognition systems in immunology

1.1 Historical background

Immunology emerged from microbiology at the end of the 19th century, after the pioneering observations of Louis Pasteur, who described immunization against various microbial and viral diseases. The last 20 years of the 19th century were devoted to the description of many basic immunological reactions. The common belief, based on the exquisite specificity of immune reactions, was that the vertebrates had a powerful tool to fight against microorganisms. It was only much later that the real significance of this physiological system started to emerge, as centered on the self–non-self distinction. Even nowadays, the deep reason of the immune system significance is not entirely understood.

1.2. Some examples of humoral responses

1.2.1. Protective antibodies: specific effects and non-specific aspects of the immune response

The specificity of the protective effect observed *in vivo* was clearly established in 1890 by von Behring and Kitasato, for the diphtheria and tetanus toxins. The passive transfer of specific immunity could be obtained with serum, which indicates that "humoral" substances are responsible for this protection. Specific reactions were then extended to various observations made *in vitro*, i.e. precipitation, lysis, agglutination, etc.

Bacteriolysis and then hemolysis were shown, by Bordet (1895), to result in one specific reaction mediated by the antibodies and one non-specific factor, the complement, which has since been described as a complex series of substances.

It was next realized that non-microbial agents could induce the production of antibodies, and a large variety of antigens was systematically injected to many animal species. Non-pathogenic substances could induce an excellent production of antibodies, which led to the essential notion that the central condition for a substance to be "antigenic" was that it had to be foreign to the organism to which it was injected.

In fact, this requisite, which announced the latter clear distinction between "self" and "non-self," deserves some comments that can be summarized in the nomenclature of antigenic specificities defined by Oudin:

(a) isotypic specificities, which apply to the antigenic determinants that all individuals have in common, within a given animal species;

(b) allotypic specificities, which are shared by individuals within a group of a given animal species; and

(c) idiotypic specificities, which are characteristic of a given antibody synthesized by a given animal (or a group of animals) specific for a precise antigen.

Finally, it should be stressed that in certain circumstances, most often of pathological significance, a given organism can raise antibodies against some of its own antigens (autoimmunity). Therefore, this notion of "foreign" to the organism must be well tempered.

1.2.2. Phagocytosis and opsonisation

Aside from the protective effect of antibodies, which was claimed by the "humoral" immunologists, another means of protection against the foreign invaders consisted in phagocytosis, put forward by Metchnikoff. The great fight between the two schools cooled considerably when it was realized that antibodies could help the activity of the phagocytosing cells, by attaching both to the antigen and to the macrophage. As in the case of the complement fixation, it was shown that only the attachment onto the antigen was specific, whereas the fixation on the phagocytic cell was not. Thus, one would say that the antibody molecule exerts a dual function: recognition (specific) and effector (non-specific). This functional duality will be of prime importance to the molecular organization of the antibody molecule.

1.2.3. Anaphylaxis and immediate hypersensitivity

By the turn of the 20th century, every immunologist probably thought that antibodies were the absolute weapon against microbial disease; and that the immune response was inscribed in a wonderful finalism. Until, in 1902, Richet and Portier showed that immunization of dogs with actinocongestin (a toxin extracted from sea anemones) resulted in a severe reaction of the "patients" that just died upon a second injection, instead of being protected. This "reverse" protection, or anaphylaxis, is the first example of immediate hypersensitivity, and has been since described through a variety of clinical conditions, such as asthma, hay fever, etc. Here again, passive transfer was obtained, thus gaining evidence for the presence of a humoral substance, which was specific for the antigen, later called in that case, "allergen". The antibodies have a special property to bind to cells specialized in the liberation of toxic substances (histamine, tryptamine, . . .) responsible for the observed symptoms.

1.3. Some examples of cell-mediated immunity

A large spectrum of immune reactions cannot be passively transferred by the immune sera. It is possible, however, to transfer these immune statuses by lymphoid cells which are of primary importance in immunology: the lymphocytes.

1.3.1. Delayed hypersensitivity

This immune reaction can be induced by a variety of antigens, and is well illustrated by the hypersensitivity that appears upon tuberculosis, or that is induced upon immunization with the BCG. The delayed type hypersensitivity (DTH) is thus called because it takes several hours (i.e. 24–48 h) before reaching its maximum, as opposed to the immediate hypersensitivity (which is due to antibodies), the symptoms of which occur within minutes after the challenge with antigen. The DTH is detected after intradermal injection of the sensitizing antigen (the tuberculin, or P.P.D., in the case of tuberculosis).

1.3.2. Graft rejection

This reaction is typically represented by skin graft in the mice. When a skin fragment is grafted to an animal that has an identical genetical background, the graft is successful, whereas there is a rapid rejection (12 days upon the first graft, 2–3 days upon subsequent grafts) whenever donor and recipient differ in their genetic characteristics. It was shown by Gorer and Snell, in the 30s, that the genetical basis for graft rejection relied on specialized loci that encoded for "histocompatibility antigens" which are present on most cells of the organisms. Over 18 such loci have been identified in the mouse, among which, the major one is the H2 system. This complex locus has been located on the 17th chromosome, and has been divided in several subregions that play a central role in the immune system. This section is about 15 centimorgans long, and represents an extremely complex multigenic and multiallelic series of genes,

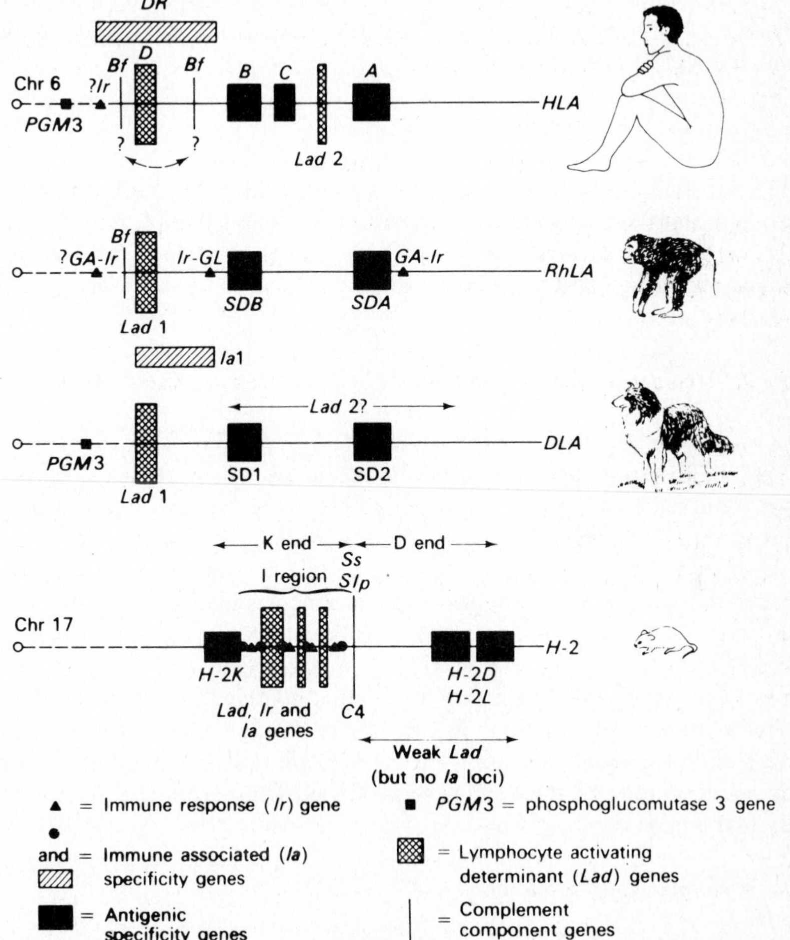

Fig. 1. The major histocompatibility complex genes in various animal species. [From H. Festenstein and P. Démant, HLA and H-2. Basic Immunogenetics Biology and Clinical Relevance (E. Arnold).]

limited between the H2K and the H2D regions, expressed on most cells, whereas the inner I region contains genes (IA, IB, IJ, IE, IC) the products of which are mostly expressed on lymphocytes (at least on some subpopulations) and play a major role in the self–non-self recognition and in the genetical control of the immune response. In addition, in this complex region genes are also found which encode for some serum substance and for constituents of the complement system.

In the human system, the counterpart is represented by the HLA system, which also plays a central role in self–non-self recognition, including graft rejection (fig. 1).

1.3.3. Graft vs host reaction (GVH)

This reaction is a particular situation in which the grafted tissue belongs to the immune system itself (bone marrow, thymus, lymph nodes, etc.). In that case the grafted lymphocytes will attack the tissues of the host, which results in a severe reaction which may lead to the host death (runt disease).

1.3.4. Mixed lymphocyte reaction (MLR) and cell mediated lympholysis (CML)

The MLR represents a reaction *in vitro*, in which there is mutual stimulation of two populations of lymphocytes that are derived from two animals of different genetical background. This stimulation, that can be rendered "one-way" by irradiating one population, which behaves as the stimulator. The other responding population will proliferate as a result of this stimulation. The proliferation may be quantified by the DNA synthesis, as appreciated from labeled-thymidine incorporation. The genes which are implicated in this reaction belong to the I region already defined. Among cells which have been thus stimulated, a fraction will acquire the ability to specifically kill the stimulator cells, upon recognition of their H2 gene products. This reaction of cytotoxicity is the CML.

1.3.5. Immunological tolerance

In 1953, it was shown by Brent, Billingham and Medawar, that if a newborn mouse was injected with tissues of an adult mouse from a different strain, once mature, it would accept skin graft from an animal of the same strain as the donor. It has become tolerant. This status, which plays a very important role in immunology (both for the physiology of the immune system and for the development of concepts) may result in the immature state of the newborn. In that case, the contact with the antigen would lead either to the elimination of the potentially responding lymphocytes ("forbidden clones"), or to the raising of lymphocytes having special "suppressor" functions.

1.4. Humoral and cellular immunity: unicity or duality of the recognition system?

1.4.1. B and T lymphocytes

The existence of antibodies was established long ago, however, the importance of the lymphocyte in the immune response has come up only much more recently, i.e. about 25 y ago, when it was shown (Miller) that the thymus played a central role in both the humoral and the cellular responses, and when Glick and Chang showed that the removal of the Bursa of Fabricius (lymphoid organ of the cloacal region in birds) led to the specific abolition of humoral responses. These observations provided the basis for the existence of 2 distinct cell lines of primary importance in immunology: the B (for bursa) and the T (for thymus) lymphocytes.

1.4.2. The B-cell lineage and the antibody molecules

A variety of experiments (discussed in the next sections) clearly indicated that, upon antigenic stimulation, the B lymphocytes differentiate into plasma cells (through successive steps), which secrete the antibody molecules. In some cases ("T-independent antigens"), the triggering of B cells directly induces this differentiation, thus immediately leading to the synthesis and excretion of antibodies. Thymectomy will not affect this humoral response, which thus occurs as a pure B cell stimulation.

1.4.3. The T-cell lineage and the cellular responses

Similarly, bursectomy will not affect typical cellular responses, which are selectively abolished upon thymectomy. This indicates that T-cell triggering directly leads to cellular responses, the variety of which (DTH, MLR, CML, . . .) is the consequence of the existence of subpopulations of T cells that may exert discrete effector functions (vide infra).

1.4.4. *Cellular cooperation: interrelationship of B- and T-cell lineages*

As already mentioned, thymectomy also affects, in most cases, the humoral response. This is because, most antigens require intervention of T cells to allow the B cells to be triggered ("T-dependent antigens"). This B–T cellular cooperation (Claman, Miller, Mitchison, . . .) is of crucial importance in contemporary immunology. It implies that the antigen must somehow be recognized by the two cell lineages, and, evidently, this raises the important question of the "repertoire" (Jerne) of both the B and T cells. Are there two discrete sets of recognition systems, one B and one T, or is there a unique one, distributed onto both types of cell membranes? This has direct, genetic implications, which may be summarized in the following simple scheme: (a) How many sets of discrete gene systems? (b) How many genes for each set? (c) If several sets – does any kind of relationship exist between them?

1.4.5. *Classical theories of antibody formation*

Long before the duality of the cell lineages was described, i.e. at the turn of the 20th century, Ehrlich proposed, in his "side chain theory", that the cell receptors and the antibody molecule were the same entity. The antigen just selected the right receptors and, following this first interaction, the proliferation of the complementary receptor was favored within the stimulated cell, according to a mechanism which was not (and which is still not) understood. This is a typical Darwinian selective theory. Later on, after the extensive work of distinguished chemists (Landsteiner) who showed that it was possible to raise antibodies against a huge variety of odd "invented" molecules, it was largely considered by the scientific community that the existence of preprogrammed receptors against such fancy inventions of organic chemists was not tenable, and most distinguished scientists (Pauling et al.) then proposed that the antigen had to give a direct information at the folding level of chain synthesis. This view, in turn, became obsolete with the current view imposed by the central dogma in molecular biology, and by crucial observations in immunology (tolerance, secondary response, . . .). The proposals that receptors (antibodies) preexisted in large numbers on a huge collection of cells, each having a unique one expressed, was first put forward by Jerne, in his "natural selection theory". The antigen comes in merely to induce those cells which have the appropriate receptors to proliferate. Then, Burnet modified this view into the clonal selection theory, which also takes into account the elimination of immature clones and provides an explanation for immune tolerance with this notion of forbidden clones. Most immunologists would still think along with the clonal theory, although minor adjustments may be required. The problem of the duality of the recognition B and T systems would, however, bring some complications into the picture. This expresses the need for a clarification of the repertoire, i.e. for the elucidation of the structure of the molecules involved in the immune response. This is well engaged for the antibody molecules, although the origin of this diversity is still not completely established, but it remains to be done almost entirely for the T-cell receptors, which may be of some distinct nature. This central problem will be presented and discussed in the following lectures, together with the genetical implications which seem of central importance in this field of contemporary biology.

2. Antigens and antibodies. The diversity problem

2.1. Antigens, antigenicity, immunogenicity

2.1.1. Definitions

An antigen is a substance that can induce the synthesis of a specific antibody, with which it can combine through a variety of reactions *in vivo* and *in vitro*. Isotypic, allotypic, and idiotypic specificities allow us to define the limits of the “foreign” character of an antigen. Antigenicity refers to those structures of the antigen that can combine with the antibody molecule, whereas immunogenicity stresses the property of a substance to induce the production of antibodies (or to elicit a cell-mediated reaction).

2.1.2. Typical primary and secondary responses

Conditions that allow us to define immunogenicity and antigenicity (antigenicity is very often used in the sense of immunogenicity) depend upon a variety of factors including the nature of the antigen, its molecular characteristics, its pertaining to the self or non-self system, etc., but, operationally, it is of crucial importance to precisely define the dose conditions, according to which a positive response or a negative response (tolerance and paralysis) will be observed. Whenever correct doses of antigen are used, it is possible to define a primary response, and a secondary response, which implies the notion of immunological memory, and the existence of a "memory cell". This applies to both the humoral and the cellular response.

2.1.3. *What is an antigen?*

Natural antigens. Proteins are considered as the "best" natural antigens. Polysaccharides also provide good antigens. Nucleic acids can elicit antibody formation, although some manipulations may be required. Lipids are very poor immunogens. What is antigenic in an antigen molecule, such as a protein or a polysaccharide? Inhibition of the antigen–antibody reaction has clearly shown, in many systems, that each antigen was composed of a "mosaic" of "antigenic determinants". The average shape and size of one single determinant has been found for both the polysaccharides and the proteins, thanks to inhibition techniques using oligosaccharides or polyaminoacids, respectively. More precise definition of what an antigenic determinant might look like came from the utilization of models, which have been studied extensively.

Models for the study of antigenicity. An important breakthrough has been gained by the use of small, well-defined molecules – the haptens (Landsteiner). A hapten refers to a small molecule which can be recognized by an antibody, but which does not induce the synthesis of antibodies itself. It thus requires to be attached to a larger molecule, commonly a protein, which is then referred to as the "carrier". Another possibility is to use a well-defined and monotonous structure as a carrier such as a polyaminoacid or branched synthetic polypeptides, that have been of major importance in defining genetical control of the immune responses.

2.2. *Antibodies and immunoglobulins*

It has been established long ago (in the beginning of the 1930s) that antibody molecules were proteins, rapidly characterized as very heterogeneous in nature (electrophoretic migration, mol wt, . . .). This heterogeneity is certainly expected if one considers that antigenic determinants, which are potentially recognized by the immune system, are extremely numerous, however, it appears much more complex in that, even for a simple antigenic structure, there is ample evidence that stimulation leads to the production of many discrete antibody structures which may be simply explained on the grounds that many clones are stimulated by a given antigenic structure. Therefore, the central underlying idea is that the antigen recognition (or the antibody function) is largely degenerate, and that the primitive and precise formulation, anchored on the one key–one lock image, is no longer acceptable. Evidently this situation is more compatible with the idea that the antibody repertoire must be of finite size. In fact, for a given human being, at a given time, the overall number of lymphocytes averages 10^{12} and the total number of immunoglobulin molecules would be around 10^{20}, among which all molecules that have been produced by the same clone are alike.

2.2.1. Models for studying the antibody structure

Aside from the theoretical considerations concerning the heterogeneity of a "purified" preparation of antibody molecules, one obvious difficulty in analyzing the repertoire from a chemical point of view, is linked to this very heterogeneity. Models have been defined, which are a consequence of the clonal theory. Most popular models, aside conventional preparations of heterogeneous antibodies, are:

Myeloma proteins which represent the monoclonal product synthesized by a cancerized plasma cell. This may result in a spontaneous event (in the human for instance), or may be induced and the tumor transplanted (in the mouse).

"*Homogeneous*" *antibodies* that may be fortuitously produced in a number of cases such as some antipolysaccharide antibodies in the rabbit, antiphosphoryl choline in the mouse.

Hybridomas, a most powerful and recent technique which allows to "clone" an antibody-producing cell, by somatic hybridization of a stimulated lymphocyte with a myeloma cell line. This allows for the production of, *in vivo* or *in vitro*, large amounts of monoclonal antibodies of well-defined specificity.

2.2.2. Multichain structure of immunoglobulins

Classical results in this field have been gained at the end of the 1950s, due to the leading efforts of Porter in England and Edelman in the U.S.A. (Fig. 2). The well-known model of Porter remains a valid representation of the basic four-chains structure of the IgG molecule,

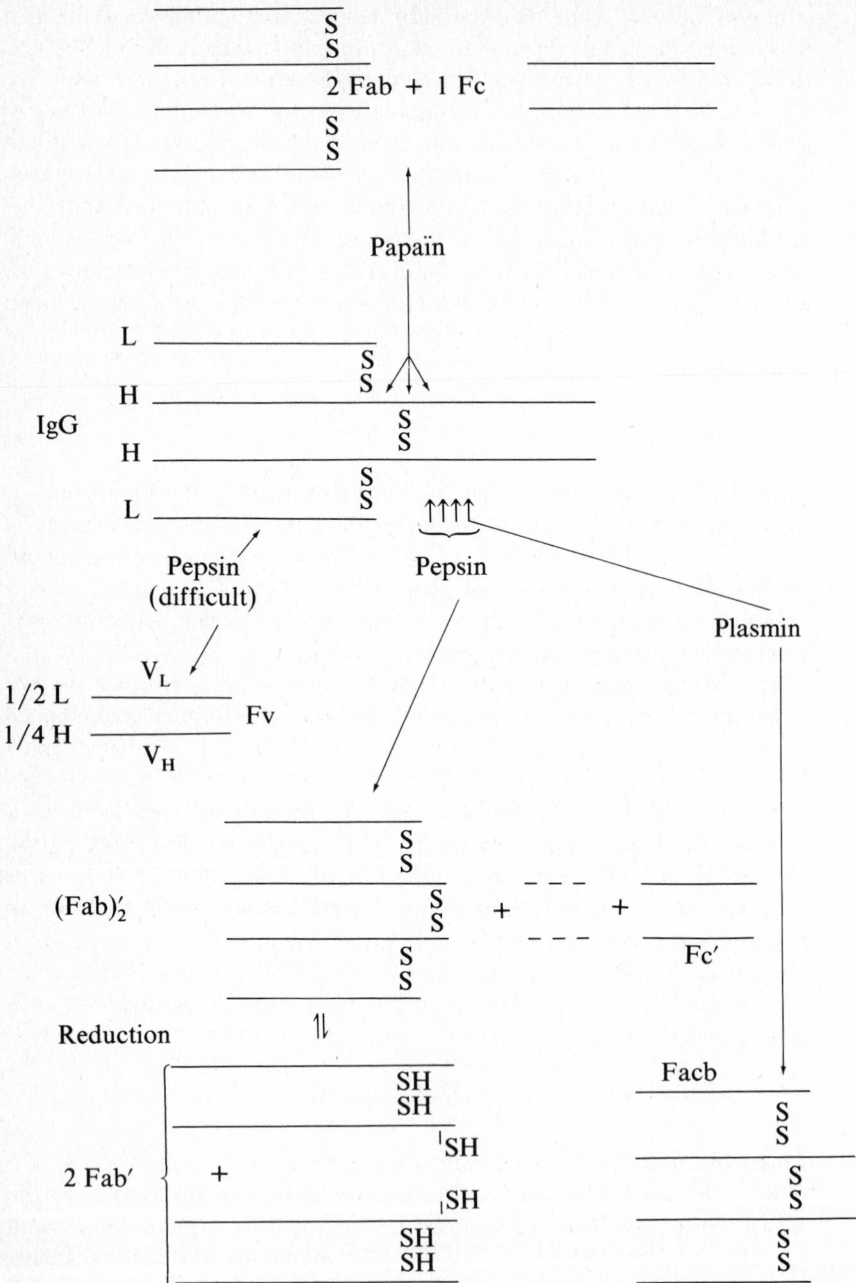

Fig. 2. Enzymatic cleavage of the IgG molecule.

which is the "classical" antibody molecule, and which represents over 70% of the circulating antibodies. This molecule contains two identical heavy (γ) chains and 2 identical light chains (χ or λ). Cleavage with papain allows the separation of 2 Fab (antigen binding) fragments and one Fc (crystallizable) fragment. The mol wt of the IgG molecule is 50 000 Daltons (53 000 for the H and 22 000 for the L chains). Each papain fragment averages 50 000 Daltons, the Fc being formed by a dimer of the COOH-terminal halves of the H chains. The molecule has a symmetrical structure, a feature which is compatible with the existence of 2 identical combining sites for the antigen, each being located on the Fab fragments. In addition the molecule contains a carbohydrate which is attached on the H chain, and that accounts for about 2% of the mol wt.

2.2.3. Classes of immunoglobulins

Aside the IgG molecule, other classes of immunoglobulins have been described (table 1). They are all organized on the basic H2L2 structure, but differ from one another by the structure of their heavy chain, and the carbohydrate content, that may reach over 10%. In the human species, and apparently in most higher vertebrates, 5 classes have been defined: the IgG (with the γ chain), the IgM (μ chain), the IgA (α chain), the IgD (δ chain), and the IgE (ε chain). The IgM is a pentamer of the basic H2L2 structure, it first occurs in the immune response, but also in ontogeny. The IgA is most often a dimer or a trimer, and is found in secretions (intestinal, collostrum, tears, . . .) and is of primary importance in ensuring a protection of the newborn, whenever the placenta does not allow an active transfer from maternal antibodies. The IgD, which seems to exist as a monomer is a typical membranous immunoglobulin, which is found on the B-cell membrane. The IgE is specialized in supporting immediate hypersensitivity.

In addition, subclasses have also been described that differ by minor modifications of the basic structure of the H chains, that bring an additional functional specialization on the side of the effector functions, and that necessitate distinct subsets of germ-line genes to operate for the Ig synthesis.

2.2.4. The diversity problem

The existence of classes and subclasses provides a structural basis for the effector functions mediated by immunoglobulins. But they do not

Table 1
Main characteristics of human immunoglobulins classes

	Light chains		Heavy chains				
Chains	κ	λ	γ	α	μ	δ	ε
mol wt	22 000	22 000	53 000	55 000	60 000	55 000	61 000
Ig classes	All classes		IgG	IgA	IgM	IgD	IgE
Mol formula			$L2_{\gamma}2$	$L2_{\alpha}2$ or $(L2_{\alpha}2)n$, SC, J[a] with $n=2$ or 3	$(L2_{\mu}2)5$, J	$L2_{\delta}2$	$L2_{\varepsilon}2$
Ig mol wt			150 000	152 000 385 000 . . .	870 000	160 000	185 000
Number of domains	1V + 1C	1V + 1C	1V + 3C	1V + 3C	1V + 4C	1V + 3C(?)	1V + 4C
% CHO	–	–	2.5	5–10	5–10	5–10	12
Average serum conc (mg/ml)			12	1.8	1.0	0/03	0.0003
Effector functions			Complement fixation Active placental transfer	External secretions (milk, mucus, tears . . .)	Complement fixation agglutinating "natural" antibodies	B-lymphocytes receptors	Immediate hypersensitivity Attachment to mast-cells
Subclasses	–	λ1–λ3	IgG1 to IgG4 (γ1 to γ4)	IgA1 and IgA2 (α1 and α2)	IgM1 and IgM2 (μ1 and μ2)	?	?

[a]J: J chain (found in IgA and IgM polymers), SC: Secretory Component (found in IgA polymers).

bring any basis to the antigen recognition. This results in the existence, for both the H and the L chains of variable regions, the description of which has been given in 1965 by Hilschmann, while working on the structure of Bence–Jones proteins, Ig light chains that are found in the urine of patients with myeloma disease. Light chains isolated from the urines of two patients were found to have an identical COOH-half, whereas extensive differences were present when the amino acid sequences of the NH_2-terminal halves were compared. A few years later, a similar situation was described for the heavy chains, the V-region of which had a similar length as that of the light chains (i.e. about 115 amino acid residues), the constant region being 3 times longer (for the γ chain) or 4 times (for the μ chain). In addition, sequence studies allowed us to propose (Hill et al.) that immunoglobulins had evolved from a common ancestor gene that would have encoded for a segment about 110 amino acid residues long, on the basis of internal homologies found within the H and L chains. This structure (internal repetition of a pseudosubunit) led Edelman to propose that the Ig molecule was organized in discrete domains, each centered on the 3-D structure of a basic segment of 110 residues, that would have been selected in evolution for a given effector function.

The chemical basis for antigen recognition and antibody diversity was then at hand. Since a variety of techniques (affinity labeling, chain reconstitution experiments, X-ray diffraction) clearly indicated that the antigen-combining site resulted in the interaction of both the V_H and the V_L domains, the sequence analysis pointed out that whatever the origin of the fine diversity, the overall number of genes encoding for the V-regions of Ig would probably not exceed about 20 000 (i.e. 10 000 for the H and 10 000 for the L chains, assuming the possibility of a random association of H–L pairs and taking 10^8 as a possible number of antibody of discrete Ag-binding properties). The problems that remain unresolved bear, therefore, on: (a) The exact number of germ-line genes that encode for Ig chains. (b) The mechanism by which the V and C regions are joined in order to provide a functional Ig chain.

As for the first problem, two theories have been proposed to account for the fine antibody diversity, which primarily concerns the complementarity-determining regions (CDR), three (or four) of each being found on each V-region chain, and which are contributing to the antibody combining site. The so-called germ-line gene theories propose that all different chains are encoded by germ-line genes, which implies that, aside from allotypic differences, the complete repertoire is transmitted to the progeny. On the other hand, somatic theories propose that a limited number of genes are present in the germ line, and that somatic mechanisms (either mutations or recombinations) operate to amplify the repertoire up to the required size. It is hardly possible to decide whichever theory is right merely on amino acid sequence data. The recent breakthrough in the field comes from the isolation of Ig genes, both from differentiated lymphoid cells and from embryonic DNA (Tonegawa, Leder). The observations may be summarized as follows:

(a) The information for Ig synthesis is localized on three "translocons", which are presumably on discrete chromosomes (this has been shown to be the case in the mouse κ and H system), in agreement with an already old observation that H, κ, and λ chain genes were not genetically linked.

(b) Within each translocon, three sets of genes are physically separated in the embryonic DNA: the V genes, that cover residues 1 to 96 for the L chains, the J genes (J for "junction") that extends from residue 97 to residue 112, and the C genes, that might be unique for the κ and the λ of mouse Ig. In the functional plasma cell, the joining of V and J has occurred, so that only two genes are still separated on the DNA: the VJ and the C. When heavy chain genes are being considered, the same type of organization has been found, except that for each discrete C region (i.e. γ, μ, α, . . .) each domain is separated from the next one by an intron that has been detected, both by sequence studies and by R-loop electron microscopy. The discontinuous structure of DNA is, therefore, a basic fact in Ig genes organization.

(c) Although the exact number of V germ-line genes has not been determined so far, it seems likely that fine diversity results from a limited number of somatic recombinations, involving both the V and the J sets (there appears to be several J genes as well).

(d) Translocation, allowing to join V–J takes place in ontogeny. As to the final attachment of the V–J ensemble onto the C gene, although a rearrangement has already taken place at the DNA level during ontogeny, the final events that lead to a functional mRNA molecule take place after the precursor RNA has been synthesized.

3. B and T lymphocytes

3.1. Two distinct populations of lymphocytes are implicated in immune responses

As already and briefly described in the first section, thymectomy and bursectomy have allowed a clear distinction between two cell lineages:

the T and the B cells, which may be involved separately ("pure B" or "pure T" cell responses) upon various antigen stimulations. The repertoire problem of the B cell may be attacked through the analysis of the antibody molecules, whereas that of the T cells, being expressed solely through membranous receptors still remains largely unknown. Cellular immunology, and more precisely T-cell immunology, although of primary importance, is still largely dominated by a complex phenomenology, since clearcut models are lacking, mostly because of the inability to clone and expand *in vitro* T-cell populations of individual specificity and function. Most efforts tend to characterize T-cell populations and functions, using antigenic markers, T-cell hybridomas, and by identification of the specific receptors for the antigen.

3.2. *General notions on the origin and differentiation of T and B lymphocytes*

3.2.1. *Stem cells*

Upon X-irradiation, an animal loses the ability to make new blood cells, including lymphocytes. But it can be restored if bone marrow cells are injected. The bone marrow contains the "stem-cell" which can differentiate, according to its environment, to various cell lineages, including the T and the B lymphocytes.

3.2.2. *Primary lymphoid organs*

The environmental factors that will allow differentiation of stem cells into B and T cells are provided by the primary lymphoid organs. The T-cell characters are acquired in the thymus, thanks to epithelial cells, whereas B cells differentiate in the bursa in birds, or in its equivalent, which have not been anatomically individualized in mammals. Bone marrow, or gut-associated lymphoid tissue might provide, in a more diffuse manner, the suitable environment required for this differentiation. It must be stressed that primary organs are never the site for encountering the antigen, nor a place where antibodies are synthesized.

3.2.3. *Secondary lymphoid organs*

Lymphocytes leave the thymus and the bursa-equivalent tissues, and circulate through blood and lymph vessels to populate the secondary lymphoid organs, i.e. the spleen and the lymph nodes. Contact with antigen takes place in the secondary lymphoid organs, which possess some degree of histological organization, and some other auxilliary cells, such as macrophages. Lymphocytes may be short- or long-lived and recirculate.

3.3. Cellular interaction in antibody synthesis (B–T cooperation)

3.3.1. Experimental models

In vivo, the classical model is provided by the X-irradiated mice that behave as "living test tubes", in which the appropriate reagents are introduced: i.e. bone marrow cells, thymus cells, spleen or lymph node cells which have been treated according to the experimental design. Neonatally thymectomy and nude mice are also used.

In vitro, complementation by various cell populations can be used, among them mixture of adherent (macrophages) and non-adherent (lymphocytes) are largely used.

3.3.2. Basic reconstitution experiments

When irradiated mice receive thymus cells with antigen (sheep red blood cells or SRBC), or bone marrow cells with SRBC, the ability of forming antibodies against SRBC is not restored. When both the thymus cells and the bone marrow cells are injected with the antigen, antibody is produced (Claman).

3.3.3. Identification of effector and helper cells

A CBA mouse ($H2^k$) is neonatally thymectomized, and reconstituted 8 weeks later with thymus cells of a C57 B1/6 mouse ($H2^b$). After immunization with SRBC, spleen cells are removed and tested for antibody production as such, or after treatment with anti-$H2^k$ or anti-$H2^b$ serum with complement. Only in the second case (when the $H2^k$ cells of the CBA, which must be the B cells, were destroyed) was the antibody production abolished. Therefore the thymus cells help, but do not synthesize the antibody. Identification of the antibody forming cells was done, using a chromosomal marker (T6T6). This latter experiment showed clearly that the antibody producing cell originated in the bone marrow (Miller). In addition, it can be shown that adherent cells (macrophages) are necessary for the antibody synthesis to take place.

3.4. Cellular interaction in cell-mediated immune responses (T–T cooperation)

3.4.1. Cellular cooperation in GVH reactions

In 1970, Cantor and Asofsky showed that a 100 times potentiation in GVH was obtained, when a mixture of parental thymus and peripheral blood cells were injected in a newborn Fl, as compared with the index obtained with the isolated cells' populations. The use of specific anti-T cell serum abolished the effect when isolated populations were treated (anti-theta serum, see next section).

3.4.2. Cellular cooperation in CML

This experiment requires the ability to separate two subpopulations of T cells. This was achieved by using anti-Ly 1, or anti-Ly 2 + Ly 3 serum,

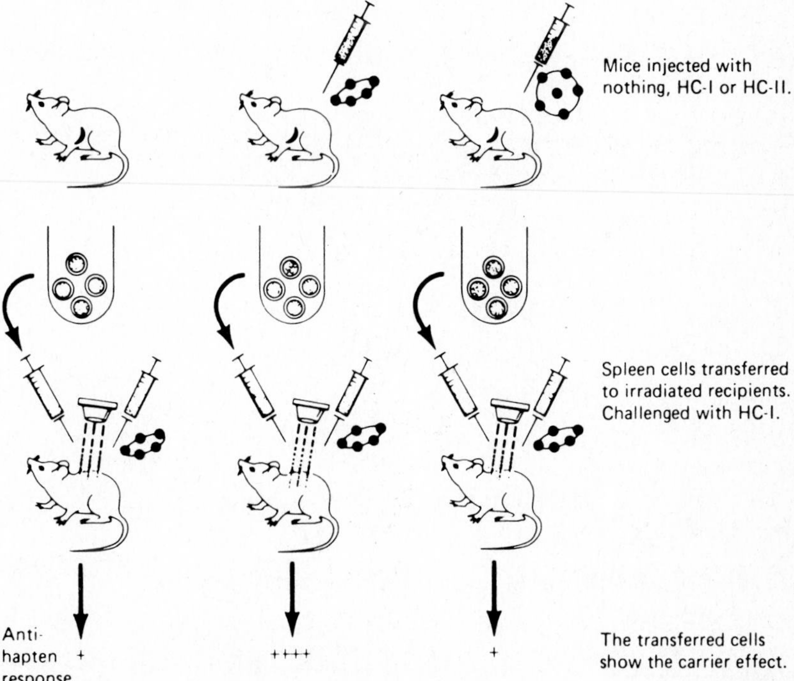
Mice injected with nothing, HC-I or HC-II.
Spleen cells transferred to irradiated recipients. Challenged with HC-I.
Anti-hapten response
+
++++
+
The transferred cells show the carrier effect.

Fig. 3. [From E. S. Golub, The Cellular Basis of the Immune Response (Sinauer Associates, Inc., Sunderland, Mass.).]

which can kill, in the presence of complement either the Ly-1 or the Ly-2 + Ly-3 subpopulations of T cells. Whenever one population is killed, generation of cytotoxic cells *in vitro* was abolished or greatly impaired. When both cell types were used, full restoration of the cytotoxic cell generation was obtained. Finally, when cytotoxic cells were treated with anti-Ly 2 + anti-Ly 3 serum, the lysis was selectively abolished, which provides a clear indication that the Ly-1 cells are the helper cells, whereas the Ly 2–Ly 3 cells behave as the effectors. This experiment therefore, shows both the T–T cooperation in CML, and the existence of functionally different T-cell subpopulations.

3.5. *The carrier effect in the B–T cooperation*

3.5.1. *The basic carrier effect*

It has been said (see section 2) that a hapten alone was not able to induce antibody formation (fig. 3). For this reason coupling to a

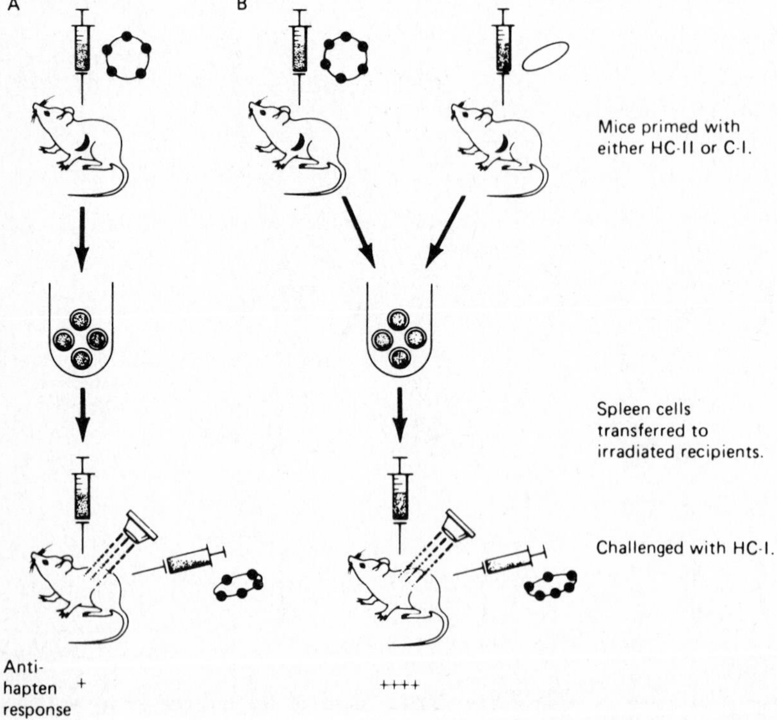
A
B
Mice primed with either HC-II or C-I.
Spleen cells transferred to irradiated recipients.
Challenged with HC-I.
Anti-hapten response
+
++++

Fig. 4. [From E. S. Golub, The Cellular Basis of the Immune Response (Sinauer Associates, Inc., Sunderland, Mass.).]

carrier-protein must be achieved. When an animal has been primed with a hapten coupled to a given carrier, the secondary response is clearly obtained only whenever the second injection is made with the hapten coupled to the same carrier (fig. 4).

3.5.2. T cells are responsible for the carrier effect

The carrier effect can be transferred to irradiated mice, with spleen cells of donors that had been primed with the relevant hapten-carrier (fig. 5).

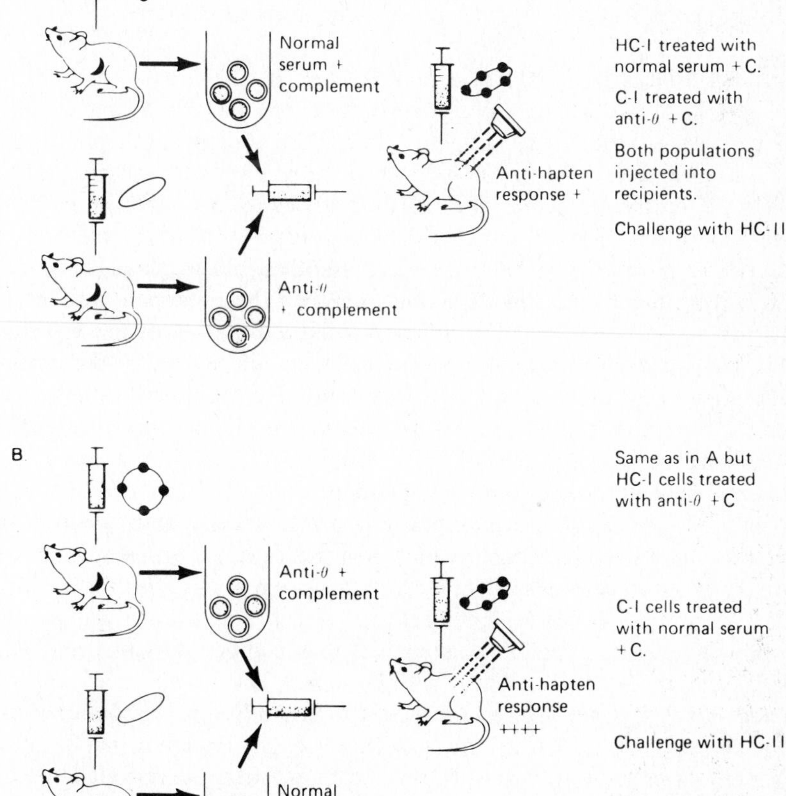

Fig. 5. [From E. S. Golub, The Cellular Basis of the Immune Response (Sinauer Associates, Inc., Sunderland, Mass.).]

It is also possible to prime one set of mice with hapten–Carrier I, and another set with Carrier II alone. Reconstitution of irradiated (or simply syngeneic) mice with this mixture of primed spleen cells, and challenge with hapten–Carrier II will result in antibody production. Whenever cells primed to Carrier II were treated with anti-theta + complement prior transfer, antibody production was abolished, thus indicating that T cells were responsible for the carrier recognition, whereas B cells would recognize the haptenic part of the molecule. This situation may be generalized to classical T-dependant antigens. When natural protein antigens are used, some determinants will be recognized as "carrier determinants" by the T cells and "hapten-like determinants" will stimulate the B cells. Furthermore, it should be recalled that macrophages are also required in some critical steps of cellular cooperation.

3.6. T-cell markers and T-cell subpopulations

Since T cells, aside from antigenic determinant recognition, may exert various functions such as B help or T help, cytolytic activity in the CML, T suppression, etc., the question arises to establish the cellular basis for these different aspects of T-cell activity. Markers have been identified, mostly by raising specific antibodies in allogeneic (or sometimes in xenogeneic) animals (table 2). When the precursor cell enters the thymus, it bears by definition no specialized marker of the T-series. Upon maturation in the thymus (which takes place first in the cortex where epithelial cells synthesize various "thymic hormones") all T cells will acquire the Thy-1 antigen (or theta), the TL antigen ("Thymus Leukemia") and 3-Ly antigens: Ly 1, Ly 2, and Ly 3, the two latter being genetically linked, and independant of Ly 1. Later on, once the thymic cells have fully differentiated into true T cells, all of them have retained the Thy-1 antigen, but have lost the TLA. Ly antigens allow us to distinguish three subsets of T cells: those expressing, as thymic cells, all 3 Ly antigens, those expressing only Ly 1, and a third group that expresses only Ly 2, 3. The existence of these subpopulations corrolates with special T-cell functions. For instance, Ly-1 cells are helpers, whereas Ly 2, 3 are effectors in the CML. Additional subpopulations can be described, taking the presence of Fc Receptor (FcR) into account or not, or the contribution of Ia markers to various subsets. Again, each subpopulation thus characterized seems to exert a discrete function, either helper, suppressor, or effector in nature. Markers have also been described for the B cell. The hallmark of B cells remains to be,

Table 2[a,b]

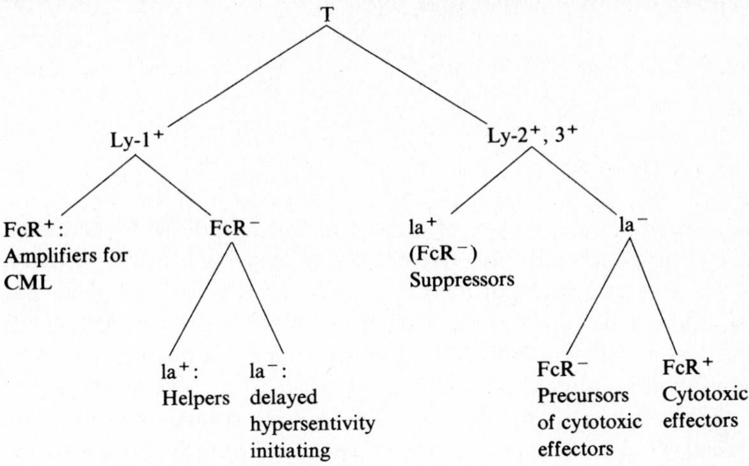

T cells of different subsets cooperate as:

1. helpers for antibody formation
2. amplifiers of cell-mediated immunity
3. suppressors for cell-mediated immunity and antibody production.

The T cell subsets which perform the various functions carry different Ly (lymphocyte) differentiation antigens. They are divided into three kinds:

1. Ly-1 + ve, ($Ly\text{-}1^+$) : 30%
2. Ly-2 + ve, Ly-3 + ve ($Ly\text{-}2^+$, 3^+) : 7%
3. Ly-1 + ve, Ly-2 + ve, Ly-3 + ve ($Ly\text{-}1^+$, 2^+, 3^+) : 50%.

N.B. All three kinds of $Ly\text{-}1^+$ cells in the above Table have helper activity – i.e. $Ly\text{-}1^+$, FcR^+; $Ly\text{-}1^+$, FcR^- (Ia^+, $Qa\text{-}1^+$) and $Ly\text{-}1^+$, FcR^- (Ia^-, $Qa\text{-}1^-$). Ly-2, 3^+, $FcR^- Ia^-$ cells are precursors of alloreactive cytotoxic effectors (Cantor, personal communication).

a) After Feldman, Beverley and Dunkley (1975) and Shiku et al. (1976).
b) From H. Festenstein and P. Démant, HLA and H-2. Basic Immunogenetics Biology and Clinical Relevance. (E. Arnold).

however, the presence of membrane Ig at their surface (mIg), which will be discussed with the receptor problem.

3.7. Identification of receptors specific for the antigen on both the B and the T cells

3.7.1. Suggested evidence

If a cell which possesses a specific receptor for an antigen is incubated with the corresponding radioactive antigen of very high specific activity, it will be killed as a result of its interaction with the "hot" antigen, due to irradiation. This type of inactivation can be obtained for both the B and the T cell, which suggests that both cell types do possess a specific receptor for the antigen. It is also possible to retain selectively on an immunoadsorbant column that contains a given antigen adsorbed on glass beads T and B cells that are able to specifically attach to the antigen (Wigzell).

3.7.2. Characterization of membrane receptors

B-cell receptors. B cells bear genuine Ig molecules, which are to some extent anchored by their Fc moiety into the bilayer membrane. However, details for a structural relationship between mIg and the membrane are not known. mIg is removed from the cell surface only when non-ionic detergents or chao-tropic agents are used, but the known structure of seric Ig (sIg) does not allow us to find, on the COOH-terminal portion of the H chain, an amino acid sequence with sufficient length (i.e. higher than 20) of hydrophobic residues, that would be necessary for the Ig to be truly transmembrane in nature. Only two main classes are found associated with the B-cell membrane: the IgM, which is a monomer (H2L2), called mIgM, and the IgD, which is solely found on B lymphocytes, and which is present in only minute amounts in the blood. IgG and IgA may occasionally be found on B cells, but their contribution does not seem to account for more than 2 or 3%. IgM and IgD molecules appear on separate B cells, but a fair number of cells are found with both isotypes expressed at the same time. In that case they would express the same V-regions, an observation which is therefore compatible with the clonal selection theory. Finally, it cannot be excluded that mIg may be slightly different of sIg.

T-cell receptors. The search for mIg molecules on T cells has been the subject of a long controversy amoung those who found Ig and those who did not. Although the issue is still not entirely clear, more and more immunologists tend to conclude the absence of complete Ig on T cells. The presence of V regions, however, seems to meet with the approval of most groups working in the field.

Presence of idiotypic determinants. Rajewsky and Eichmann have shown that T cells and antibodies produced against cross-reactive haptenic structures presented the same pattern of cross-reactivity. They could specifically stimulate T helper cells by injecting small amounts of antiidiotypic antibodies (a larger amount would stimulate T suppressors). Finally, a molecule of about 100 000 mol wt. was isolated from the T cells, that would bind the hapten, and that bear idiotypic determinants of the heavy chain, but not of the light. Binz and Wigzell have raised an antiidiotypic antibody against idiotypic determinants of an antibody specific for a MHC component. These receptors, specific for the MHC were isolated and partially characterized. Here again, isotypic determinants of the Ig system were not found, although idiotypic determinants were present, and, indeed initiated the antiidiotypic response in the animal.

Helper factors. Helper factors have been isolated by several groups of authors, and have been shown to replace the T-cell helper activity either *in vivo* or *in vitro* (Taussig, Feldmann, Tada) (fig. 6). These factors are specific for the stimulating antigen. They may act either directly on the B cell, or via the macrophage, or via another T cell, that would, upon factor activation, bring help to the B cell eventually through the macrophage. It must be stressed that characterization of these factors has been obtained essentially by antiserum, the specificity of which is rather difficult to be sure of, mainly because of the uncertainty as to the nature of the immunizing material itself (fig. 7).

3.8. A few notions about the lymphocyte membrane

Nothing specific is known concerning the lymphocyte membrane. Signals by which cells might be turned on upon contact with the antigen, are completely ignored. A partial list of markers and receptors has been described, and given previously. Among phenomena that have been described, receptors redistribution has been amply investigated without bringing any decisive issue. Ig molecules can be induced to

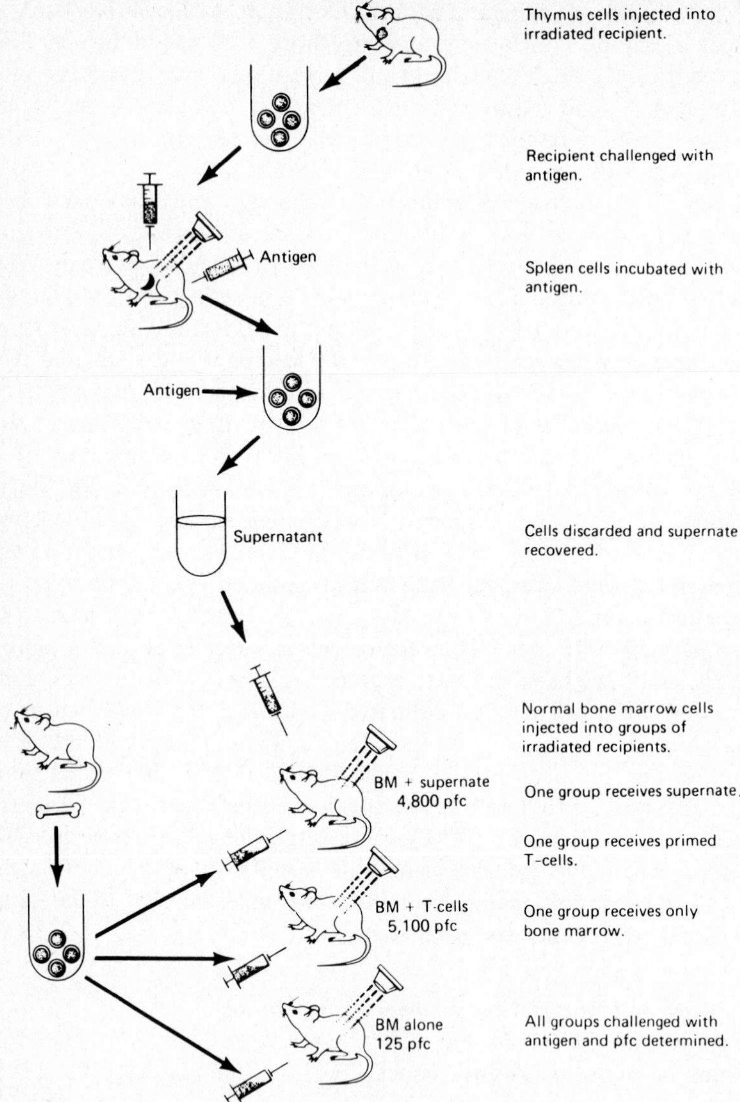

Fig. 6. [From E. S. Golub, The Cellular Basis of the Immune Response (Sinauer Associates, Inc., Sunderland, Mass.).]

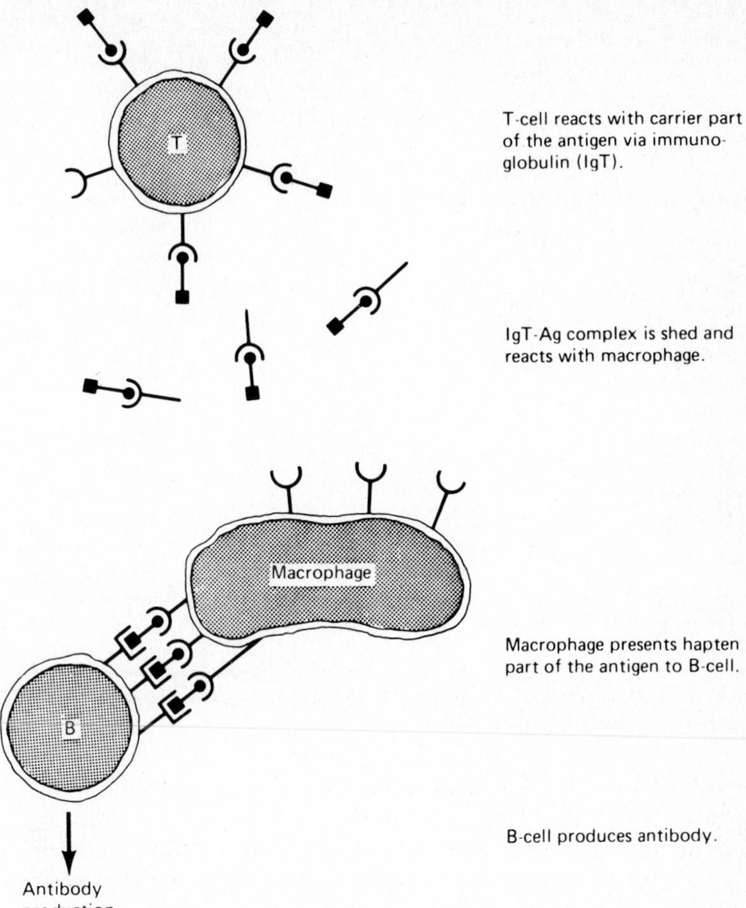
T
T-cell reacts with carrier part of the antigen via immunoglobulin (IgT).
IgT-Ag complex is shed and reacts with macrophage.
Macrophage
Macrophage presents hapten part of the antigen to B-cell.
B
B-cell produces antibody.
Antibody production

Fig. 7. [From E. S. Golub, The Cellular Basis of the Immune Response (Sinauer Associates, Inc., Sunderland, Mass.).]

patch and to cap after contact with anti-Ig antibodies. As usual, patching is not energy-dependent, whereas capping appears to be a metabolic process. Capping is generally followed either by endocytosis, or by shedding. New mIg receptors reappear within about 3 h. The complete set seems to be replaced after 8 h.

Other markers or receptors may be redistributed upon interaction with specific antibodies: H2K and H2D antigens (that would cap

Table 3
Some membrane structures on lymphoid and other cells[a)]

	T cells	B cells	Other
Antigen-binding receptors	?	Immunoglobulins (IgD; IgG) M	
Fc receptor	+ (activated)	+ + +	Macrophage K cell
Ly-1, Ly-2, Ly-3 specificities	+ + (suppressors; helpers; killers)	–	–
Ly-(b)-4 specificities	(activated)	+	–
Thy-1 antigen	+ +	–	Brain
C3d (complement) receptor	+	+ + +	Macrophage
H-2 specificities	+ +	+ + +	Platelets Red cell
Mls determinants	–	+ + +	Macrophage
Ia specificities	+ + in some subclasses	+ + +	Macrophage Sperm
Lads	±	+ +	Macrophage Sperm
Specific antigen receptor	+	+	

a)From H. Festenstein and P. Démant, HLA and H-2. Basic Immunogenetics Biology and Clinical Relevance. (E. Arnold).

independently, but which require a second anti-Ig antibody to be used, presumably because of the low affinity of the anti-H2 antibodies), $\beta 2$ microglobulin, a 12 000 mol wt chain, which contributes to the H2 molecule, and presents some homologies with the 3rd constant domain of the γ chain, TLA, theta antigens, FcR, C3R, will cap.

Various lectins will induce capping in lymphocytes and a correlation between capping and mitogenicity was looked for, but, unfortunately not found. For instance, conA will induce capping both in B and T cells, but is mitogenic for the T cell only. Conversely succinyl conA (which is divalent), or, even monomeric derivatives of conA will be mitogenic for T cells although they cannot induce capping.

Capping has been obtained with various antigens, such as polymerized flagellin (an antigen extracted of Salmonella adelaide) or KLH (keyhole limpet hemocyanin). No relationship has been, however, established so far, between such events and the exact nature of signals that condition lymphocytes specific triggering.

General references

Books

Roitt, Essential Immunology (Blackwell, London, 1974).
E.S. Golub, The Cellular Basis of the Immune Response (Sinauer Ass., Sunderland, MA, 1977).
Fougereau, Eléments d'Immunologie Fondamentale, 2nd ed. (Masson, Paris, 1977).
H. Festenstein and P. Demant, HLA and H2, Current Topics in Immunology, (No. 9) (Arnold, London, 1978).

Periodical reviews

Advances in Immunology (Academic Press).
Immunological Reviews (Munksgaard, Copenhagen).

COURSE 5
(PART II)

T LYMPHOCYTES IN IMMUNITY

Jacques F. A. P. MILLER

Walter and Eliza Hall, Institute of Medical Research,
Melbourne 3050, Australia

Contents

R. Balian et al., eds.
Les Houches, Session XXXIII, 1979 – Membranes et Communication Intercellulaire / Membranes and Intercellular Communication

1. Evolution of the T cell system

The two board categories of lymphocytes, T and B cells, are now well defined. Each is derived from the same ancestral stem cell which can differentiate to more mature forms in one or another of the specialized microenvironments of the primary lymphoid organs, the thymus and bursa or bursa equivalent. These two distinct families of lymphocytes constitute a physiological basis for the differences between cellular and humoral immunity. Classically, the distinction between these two categories of immune response arose from a practical and clinical concern with the treatment of infectious disease. These could be classified into two major groups according to the nature of the infectious agent or parasite and whether or not it was susceptible to immune serum. In general, extracellular microbes, such as the Pneumococcus, are sensitive to serum antibodies whereas intracellular agents, such as Listeria are not, but can be inactivated as a result of cooperation between immune T cells and phagocytic cells. It is worthwhile speculating on how this dichotomy arose as this will lead to considerations such as the distinction between self and non-self, the phenomena of tolerance and suppression, the question of antigen recognition by T cells and the influence of the major histocompatibility complex on T cell recognition and T cell repertoire selection. The main theme to be developed is that resistance to infectious agents must have been the driving force for the evolution of the T cell system. More detailed reference to the influence of the major histocompatibility complex on T cell function will be covered later. This will entail a discussion of the phenomenon known as H-2 restriction and the possible ways by means of which the T cell repertoire is selected. The final topic will deal primarily with immunoregulation by T lymphocytes.

Unicellular organisms such as the amoeba can distinguish between self and non-self. They engulf foreign particles and digest them. If one cell is analogous to such a primitive unicellular organism in multicellular species, it is the macrophage. Its major function is phagocytosis and it, too, can distinguish between self and non-self. In its most basic form, the mechanism of such discrimination may require the recognition of a self marker (H) by a receptor which is complementary to H (anti-H).

Binding of H to anti-H activates an off signal to prevent phagocytosis. Thus macrophages will engulf foreign material including parasites since these do not possess the self marker. To avoid phagocytosis, the parasite must therefore invade the cell, replicate intracellularly, not alter the self marker so as to be protected by it. Evolution thus demands that the host acquire the capacity to earmark, as it were, the infected cell [via some parasite product or metabolite displayed on the membrane (X)] and to recognize such infected cells, presumably by a receptor complementary to X (anti-X). The simplest way in which anti-X might arise would be by duplicating the gene coding for anti-H. Some alteration would have to take place, however, not only in the specificity of recognition (from anti-H to anti-X) but also in biological function: anti-X must become coupled to the signal for phagocytosis, not to the off signal, as in the case of anti-H. Thus binding of anti-X to X leads to an ON signal for phagocytosis and this must override the OFF signal resulting from the binding of anti-H to H. Since the parasites will develop some heterogeneity and various form of X (X_1, X_2, X_3 . . . X_n) will be produced, there must occur a rapid expansion of the host anti-X repertoire. This in turn, allows the parasite to develop further stratagems to evade host responses: those parasites that produce a form of X which tends to mimic the self marker H will activate a host response that not only destroys infected cells but also healthy cells bearing the self marker. It is therefore essential that the host learns to purge any antiself specificity from its anti-X repertoire: this will ensure tolerance to self and guard against self destruction (autoimmunity). The mechanism of such self tolerance will be discussed in detail and is briefly summarized below.

Once antiself reactivities have been purged from the anti-X repertoire, parasites cannot tempt the defence system to self destruction. They can, however, divert the attention of anti-X bearing cells away from infected cells by simply releasing extracellular forms that could predominate over the intracellular forms. To cope with this, hosts must have evolved two separate cellular systems – one to deal primarily with infected cells, the other with extracellular forms. At this stage the function of phagocytosis and specific recognition of the various forms of X could have become separated; T cells, which only recognize cell-bound forms of antigen (by taking over both anti-H and anti-X functions, but not phagocytosis), could be specialized to kill (directly or indirectly) infected cells. Intracellular forms would then be released to be dealt with by other cell defence systems, including phagocytosis. B cells, which secrete anti-X (antibodies), on the other hand, would be specialized to deal with the extracellular forms.

The simplest mechanism to explain tolerance is to delete antiself reactivities from the repertoire by making each cell express only one receptor specificity (clonal expression of anti-X) and killing off those cells that express antiself reactivities. Since, for any cellular activity, the flow of information is from the gene (DNA) to the protein, it is not possible to purge from the membrane of a cell expressing a multiplicity of receptors differing only in specificity, one particular receptor whilst retaining all others. It is simpler to have one receptor specificity per cell so that the whole cell can be signaled to responsiveness or unresponsiveness via interaction of its receptor. Interaction with self-antigens leads to unresponsiveness, interaction with other antigens to responsiveness. How then do self antigens differ from other antigens and how is unresponsiveness achieved? Self antigens cannot differ from non-self antigens in physicochemical terms since they have the same basic composition and since what is self for one individual is non-self for another. Self antigens can be distinguished from non-self antigens only in their temporal relationship to the immune system. Self exists prior to the development of the system and persists throughout the life of the individual. Non-self enters the individual generally after the development of the system and does not usually persist. Since T cells acquire immunocompetence within the thymus, it is likely that the thymus is the site where self-reactive clones are eliminated. T cells with self-reactivities would be stimulated to divide within the epithelial framework of the thymus by contact with self components and then acquire their competence to become killer cells. Since after cell division in a confined space, both daughter cells would also bear the same self components, it is quite possible that they would eliminate one another. Self tolerance would thus be primarily a property of the T cell system. In fact, there is good evidence that B cells with self reactivities exist.

2. Influence of the major histocompatibility complex on the activities of T lymphocytes

The major stimulus for the activation of certain subsets of T lymphocytes is not antigen alone but antigen in association with one or the other of the gene products of the major histocompatibility complex (MHC). These products are expressed on the surface of the body's own cells and some of these, e.g. macrophages or macrophage-like cells, are particularly well equiped to present antigen in the appropriate form to T lymphocytes and to deliver the activating signal. This section will deal with the association of antigenic determinant and MHC gene product as an essential element in T cell activation and the role of the MHC in the selection of the T cell repertoire.

The MHC exerts a profound influence on T cell function. This is clear from the following:

(a) The frequency of alloreactive T cells, i.e. of T cells with specificities directed against other MHC gene products, is of the order of 100 to 1000 times higher than the frequency of T cells with specificities directed to non-MHC antigens (e.g. antigen X).

(b) A T cell response to a foreign antigen (X) is stimulated not by X alone, but by an antigenic pattern dependent on both X and an appropriate MHC gene product. This leads to the phenomenon of MHC (or H-2) restriction as discussed later.

(c) Genes linked to the MHC (MHC-linked Ir genes) determine the level of T cell responsiveness and hence the high or low responder status of a particular strain for a particular antigen.

(d) T cell-derived products involved in helper or suppressor functions are said to bear I region determinants.

Most phenomena associated with T cells are subject to H-2 restriction. To illustrate this, consider a CBA mouse (H-2^k) infected with LCM virus. As a result, cytotoxic T cells (T_C cells) are generated which kill LCM-infected H-2^k targets but not LCM infected targets of any other H-2 type nor uninfected H-2^k targets. The T cells are thus specific for both virus and H-2^k. The restriction of T_C cell activity was mapped to the H-2K and H-2D loci. It applied to T_C cells directed against virus-infected cells, cells bearing minor histocompatibility antigens foreign to their host, or cells modified chemically in some way. For both helper T cells and cells involved in delayed type hypersensitivity (DTH) the restriction was mapped to the I-A region (and I-E/I-C in some cases). For suppressor T cells no restriction was apparent in some cases, but in others it was imposed by the I-J region. Experiments performed with T cells involved in various activities gave results inconsistent with a hypothesis which would explain MHC restriction on the basis of a requirement for matching between like MHC-coded cell interaction molecules on activated T cells and their targets. On the contrary, the results were consistent with a model which states that the T cell may have one receptor directed towards both antigen and the MHC component involved in restriction or two distinct receptors, one for antigen and the other for the MHC component.

The fact that MHC genes govern T cell recognition has been apparent for some time since the discovery of the MHC-linked Ir genes. Thus, for example, the immune response of helper T cells and of T cells involved in DTH to a large number of antigenic substances was found to be governed by genes which mapped in the I region of the MHC. On the other hand, genes controlling T_C cell responses mapped in the H-2K or H-2D loci. For example, association of various virus molecules, or virus products of infected cells, with defined H-2K or H-2D allelic products provoked better cytotoxic responses than association with other alleles. The exact manner by which the MHC produces such effects is not known, but one possible mechanism is that MHC gene products are intimately involved in delivering an activating signal to T cells. Only antigenic determinants able to associate effectively with such products would thus be immunogenic. The existence of several MHC gene loci and of multiple allelism at each locus would ensure effective association of antigenic determinants with MHC gene products in most members of a given species. Polymorphism thus allows most individuals to respond adequately to one or other determinants of a complex antigen.

It seems likely that both MHC restriction and MHC-linked immune responsiveness are basically the same phenomenon. They depend essentially on whether an associative interaction has occurred between antigenic determinant and certain MHC gene products on the membrane of cells capable of stimulating T cells and on whether these T cells can recognize the "associative" antigen. Recent experiments using chimeric mice and thymus grafts suggest that differentiation of pre-T cells to T cells within the thymus could be one level at which the MHC immune responsiveness genes exert their action. Low responsiveness could occur because there is a defect in the T cell receptor repertoire that is linked to the recognition of an MHC gene product. Thus, expression of a receptor for such a gene product would preclude the expression of a second receptor for a particular antigenic determinant. This implies that reactivities for such determinants arise from somatic diversification of genes coding for anti-MHC receptors. Models, according to which the T cell repertoire is generated and selected, can thus be constructed and may be tested experimentally. This in turn may shed light on the actual mechanism of T cell recognition.

3. Immunoregulation by T lymphocytes

A major goal in basic immunological research is to sufficiently understand the forces that regulate the immune system to allow one to predict the outcome of a particular response and thus learn how to control this.

For example, in many clinical situations it would seem highly desirable to enhance the immune response or some of its manifestations, in particular in resistance to infectious agents and to antigenically distinct tumours. In other situations, it would be valuable to suppress the immune system, e.g. in allergic disorders, autoimmune disease and transplantation of alien skin or organs. Unfortunately there are numerous complexities that must be overcome before we can ever hope to achieve these goals. Thus, an immune response is not a simple reaction but results after the activation of an elaborate network of interacting cells. In addition, each response is a highly amplified reaction and, as is the case with other amplification systems, each step must be subjected to a multitude of control mechanisms. A modest beginning was made in unravelling the complexities of immune induction some ten years ago when the existence of cell-to-cell interactions was demonstrated. It was originally shown that T cells were essential to assist B cells produce antibody to many antigens. Later, other investigations showed the reverse: a suppressive influence of T cells on B cell responsiveness. Evidence then accumulated for a functional heterogeneity in the T cell pool: distinct subsets of T lymphocytes performed distinct immunological tasks. The existence of a complex network of interacting cells soon became apparent. It is now evident that various T cells can exert control at several levels. Hence, the potential for immunoregulation is enormously increased.

This section will concentrate on T cell-dependent suppression, since helper T cells involved in cooperation with B cells have been covered elsewhere. It is well documented that specific or non-specific stimulation of the immune system generates a population of T lymphocytes with suppressive activities. Such T_S cells have been demonstrated following priming, tolerance induction, mitogen stimulation, in MHC-linked low responsiveness, and idiotype suppression. Those activated by mitogens non-specifically suppress both cell-mediated and humoral immune responses. In most other cases, T_S cells are specific and inhibit immune reactions only against the antigen which activated them. T_S cells play a crucial role in regulating a variety of immune responses, in antigenic competition, in the induction and maintenance of immunological tolerance and in the prevention of allergic and autoimmune phenomena.

T_S cells may be distinguished from other T cell subsets by their distinct surface phenotypes. They are also highly radiosensitive and easily inactivated by low doses of antilymphocyte serum and cyclophosphamide. In contrast to other T cell subsets, T_S cell activities do not generally appear to be H-2 restricted. Thus, they can function in allogeneic hosts and they are able to bind to native antigen, being selectively enriched by adsorption to antigen-coated dishes. It would appear, therefore, that antigen which bypasses the macrophage system (e.g. excess antigen, highly deaggregated forms of antigen, antigen which fails to associate with I-region gene products on macrophages in low-responder strains) activates T_S cells selectively. Such antigen was generally held to induce tolerance and, in fact, the induction and maintenance of tolerance could well be due to the activation of T_S cells.

An antigen-specific suppressive factor has been extracted from T_S cells obtained from a variety of sources. The factor has specificity and affinity for antigen, is a protein of molecular weight ranging from 35 000 to 55 000 Daltons, does not have Ig determinants but possesses a determinant coded by the I–J region of the MHC. It can replace T_S cells both *in vivo* and *in vitro*.

The exact mechanism of action of T_S cells or of suppressive factors extractable from these is not clear. In view of the complexities of the cell interactions which operate in immune responses and of the amplification loops involved, it is difficult at this stage to present a comprehensive scheme of the manner in which T_S cells influence other lymphocytes. The target cells of suppression may vary in different systems. Macrophages or T cells, themselves, may be suppressible targets in cell-mediated immunity. In antibody responses, the B cells may be targets in some cases and the T_H cells in others. An understanding of the mechanism of T cell dependent suppression is urgently required as this phenomenon must certainly play a crucial role in immune homeostasis and in self-surveillance against autoantigens.

These considerations lead us to a reappraisal of the phenomena of self-tolerance and autoimmunity. Is tolerance the result of clonal abortion or deletion or of the activation of some control mechanism, such as the T_S cell system? Does autoimmunity result from somatic mutation which leads to the generation of aberrant clones or from the failure of the T_S cell control mechanism? It is, of course, not possible to offer categorical answers to these questions.

Tolerance to self-MHC components is primarily "learned" when T cells differentiate in the thymus, as discussed before. Tolerance of T cells to other components and antigens, and tolerance in B cells, may not result from clonal deletion but rather from an active suppression imposed by T_S cells. Pure deletion allows no flexibility and this is incompatible with the proper functioning of a system which must encounter new self-antigens, self-antigens previously sequestered, antigens cross-reactive with self-antigens, etc. "Pure" B cell tolerance may well be a laboratory artifice. Indeed B cells with receptors for autoantigens have been demonstrated. It is thus more likely that "apparent" B cell tolerance results from B cell antigen-blockade or from active suppression by T_S cells. Hence, a loss in T_S cell function (which may occur with age, or due to genetic, viral and hormonal factors) would be associated with the production of an increased antibody response, allergic reactions and autoimmune manifestations. On the other hand, an enhanced T_S cell function could be the cause of some forms of hypogammaglobulinaemia. It may also be associated with a decrease in other T cell activities. In leprosy, for example, it may tip the balance towards the lepromatous form. In other cases, it may increase cancer risks, particularly when T_C cell activity may normally be required to limit tumour growth (as has been demonstrated experimentally with manoeuvres that diminish T_S cell function).

Unravelling the numerous and complex regulatory events that occur in immune responses is clearly an urgent task if we are ever to learn to manipulate the immune system for our benefit.

General references

Acquisition of the T cell repertoire, Immunol. Rev. 42 (1978).

Idiotypes on T and B cells, Immunol. Rev. 34 (1977).

R. E. Langman, The role of the major histocompatibility complex in immunity: a new concept in the functioning of a cell-mediated immune system, Rev. Physiol. Biochem. Pharmacol. 81 (1978) 1.

J. F. A. P. Miller, Influence of the major histocompatibility complex on T cell activation, Adv. Cancer Res. 26 (1979) 1.

R. M. Zinkernagel and P. C. Doherty, MHC-restricted cytotoxic T cells, Adv. Immunol. (1979) in press.

COURSE 6
(PART I)

TRANSDUCTION OF HORMONAL SIGNALS THROUGH THE MEMBRANE: KINETIC ANALYSIS OF HORMONE BINDING TO MEMBRANE RECEPTORS

Serge JARD

Laboratoire de Physiologie Cellulaire, Collège de France, 75231 Paris Cedex 05, France

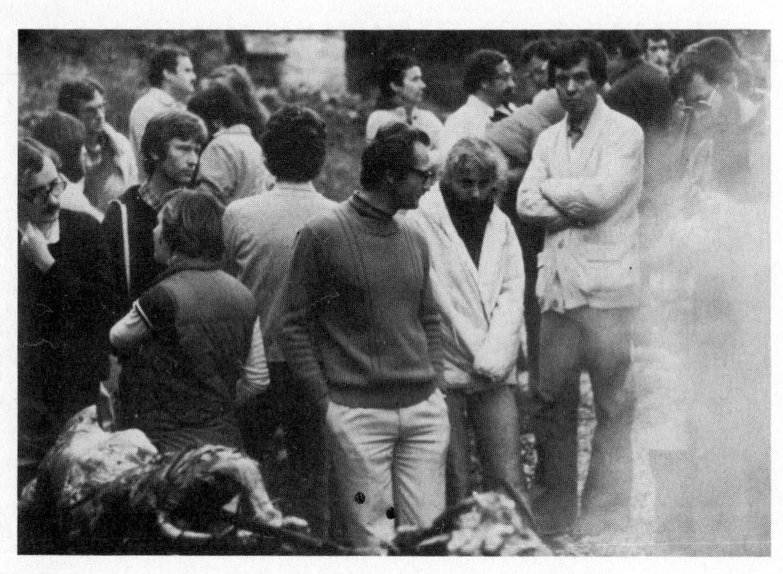

Contents

R. Balian et al., eds.
Les Houches, Session XXXIII, 1979 – Membranes et Communication Intercellulaire / Membranes and Intercellular Communication

0. Introduction

Hormones are regulatory signals that are present in the blood at very low concentrations, usually less than 1 nM. For a given hormone, the actual blood concentration is determined by the balance between the rate of hormone secretion by a group of specialized endocrine cells and the rate of hormone elimination by excretion or metabolic conversion into inactive products; it varies depending on the physiological status of the organism. Changes in blood hormone concentration are usually triggered by changes in the hormone secretion rate in response to specific stimuli.

Most hormonal actions exhibit a high degree of cellular specificity, i.e. a given hormone is active on a limited number of cell types. To account for this cellular specificity it has been suggested, from the early beginning, that target cells contain structures or components called "receptors" which are responsible for specific recognition of the hormonal signal and transduction of the signal into a physiological response.

Depending on the localization of receptors in the cell, two types of hormonal actions can be distinguished. A group of hormones derived from cholesterol called steroid hormones are able to cross the cellular plasma membranes and interact with intracellular receptors. The site of action of these hormones is the nucleus where they contribute to the regulation of gene expression. Thyroid hormones which are iodinated derivatives of tyrosine apparently act in a similar fashion. A second group of hormones including most of the polypeptide hormones and catecholamines interact with membrane receptors accessible from the external surface of the membrane. A major achievement in our understanding of the mechanism of hormonal action was the introduction by Sutherland and colleagues of the "second messenger" concept [1]. These authors initiated a series of studies leading to the conclusion that many hormones exert their specific actions through a common mechanism. Membrane receptors for a large number of hormones as well as membrane receptors for several neurotransmitters are functionally coupled to adenylate cyclase, a membranous enzyme which catalyzes the conversion of ATP into cyclic adenosine 3′–5′-monophosphate (cyclic AMP). Hormone binding to receptors triggers either activation or inhibition of adenylate cyclase leading to the corresponding changes in intracellular cyclic AMP. Hormonal regulation of adenylate cyclase activity can be demonstrated *in vitro* using purified membranes prepared from hormone-responsive target cells. By a cascade of biochemical events including, activation or inhibition of cyclic AMP-dependent protein kinases [2], with subsequent modifications in the phosphorylation of key regulatory proteins, these changes in intracellular cyclic AMP, acting as a "second messenger", are responsible for the production of the cellular response to the initial hormonal stimulation. Sutherland's discovery that the role of cyclic AMP in hormonal action had a great impact in the field of endocrinology. The possibility of measuring a hormonal action *in vitro* using purified membrane preparations and rather simple biochemical techniques greatly facilitated biochemical and functional characterization of hormonal receptors. In the present status of knowledge, it seems reasonable to extend the "second messenger" concept to all hormones acting through the intermediacy of membrane receptors. However, it must be emphasized that cyclic AMP is not the only intracellular messenger of hormonal action. Cyclic 3′–5′-guanosine monophosphate (cyclic GMP) was found in all cell types so far studied. In several hormone-responsive cells, variations in intracellular cyclic GMP content subsequent to hormonal stimulation have been demonstrated [3]. However, very little is known yet about the functional coupling between hormonal receptors and guanylate cyclase, the enzyme responsible for the formation of cyclic GMP from GTP. Up to now, it was not possible to demonstrate guanylate cyclase activation or inhibition by hormones in acellular preparations. Among other possible transduction mechanisms of hormone receptor interactions are: changes in membrane permeability to calcium or other ions with subsequent modifications in the ionic composition of the intracellular compartment [4] and activation or inhibition of other membrane enzymatic activities involved in the metabolism of phospholipids and prostaglandins [5–7].

Present knowledge of hormone receptors was mainly derived from a kinetic analysis of hormonal binding to intact target cells or to purified membranes prepared from these cells. As will be shown in the following sections, this approach was extensively used for: characterizing receptors in terms of binding capacity, apparent affinity for the hormonal molecule, and structurally related molecules; analyzing the relation of hormonal binding to a physiological response; studying the effects of several modulators like nucleotides and ions on hormone-responsive systems; and establishing the existence of regulatory mechanisms that control receptor number and function in the intact target cells.

1. Basic principles underlying kinetic analysis of hormone binding to receptors

1.1. Theory of hormone–receptor interactions

In this section, an attempt has been made to present simple derivations of the mathematical formulations that were found to be a useful framework for practical analysis of hormone binding data. Most of the concepts presented here are derived from the mass action law and from the classic Michaelis–Menten analysis of enzyme substrate kinetics. Five of the more frequently discussed models will be described in equations (1)–(5):

Model I corresponds to the simplest mechanistic assumption that can be made, i.e. reversible binding of a single ligand molecule [L] to a single receptor molecule [R]. It is assumed that each molecular interaction is independent of other interactions and that the populations of hormonal and receptor molecules are homogeneous:

$$\mathrm{L} + \mathrm{R} \longleftrightarrow \mathrm{RL}.$$

A direct application of the mass action law is

$$\frac{[\mathrm{R}]\,[\mathrm{L}]}{[\mathrm{RL}]} = Kd \tag{1}$$

in which [R], [L], and [RL] are the concentrations of free receptor, free ligand, and ligand–receptor complex, respectively. *Kd* is the equilibrium dissociation constant of the complex. Rearrangement of eq. (1) gives:

$$[\mathrm{RL}] = [\mathrm{Rt}]\frac{[\mathrm{L}]}{[\mathrm{L}] + Kd} \tag{2}$$

in which [RT] is the total concentration of receptor molecules ([R]+[RL]). The saturation function of the receptor is:

$$\bar{Y} = \frac{[\mathrm{RL}]}{[\mathrm{Rt}]} = \frac{[\mathrm{L}]}{[\mathrm{L}] + [\mathrm{Kd}]}\,. \tag{3}$$

Models II and III, cooperative models, correspond to situations in which the assumption that each molecular interaction is independent of other interactions is not fulfilled. Quite generally for a series of n interacting sites on a receptor molecule, the saturation function can be adequately described by:

$$\bar{Y} = \frac{[\mathrm{L}]^n}{[\mathrm{L}]^n + K}. \tag{4}$$

From a purely phenomenological point of view two types of cooperative behaviour can be distinguished depending on the value of n: positive cooperativity ($n > 1$) and, negative cooperativity ($n < 1$). Note that for $n = 1$ relations 3 and 4 are identical.

Models IV and V, these correspond to situations in which the assumption about homogeneity of the population of receptor molecules is not fulfilled. Two situations will be considered: (1) existence (Model IV) of n independent populations of receptors molecules. The saturation function is:

$$\bar{Y} = \sum_1^n \frac{N_i}{NT} \frac{[\mathrm{L}]}{[\mathrm{L}] + Kd_i} \tag{5}$$

in which N_1, N_2, N_i, N_n are the total numbers of receptors in the different subpopulations and Kd_1, Kd_2, Kd_i, Kd_n the corresponding equilibrium dissociation constants. (2) Situations (Model V) in which the receptor is viewed as existing in two interconvertible states:

$$\begin{array}{ccc} \mathrm{L} + \mathrm{R} & \overset{\alpha}{\rightleftharpoons} & \mathrm{R}' + \mathrm{L} \\ K \updownarrow & & \updownarrow K' \\ \mathrm{RL} & \rightleftharpoons & \mathrm{R'L} \end{array}.$$

In the case, one can easily derive the saturation function as:

$$\bar{Y} = \frac{[\mathrm{L}]}{[\mathrm{L}] + [\mathrm{K}'(\alpha + 1)/(\alpha c + 1)]}, \tag{6}$$

in which α is the equilibrium constant between the R' and R states ([R]/[R′]) and c, the ratio of the microscopic dissociation constants (K'/K). Note that relation (6) is equivalent to relation (1) with an apparent dissociation constant:

$$Kapp = \frac{K'(\alpha + 1)}{(\alpha c + 1)}.$$

Figures 1 to 3 illustrate the three classical plots which are the more frequently used to describe hormone–receptor binding isotherms. (Models I and V which predict identical saturation functions (1) and (6) have not been distinguished). Plotting $\bar{Y}$ vs [L] (fig. 1) leads to a simple hyperbola for Models I and V. Half maximal saturation $\bar{Y}=0.5$ is obtained for a free ligand concentration equal to *Kd*. Positive cooperativity is characterized by a sigmoidal curve; complete saturation occurs in a rather narrow range of free ligand concentrations (usually less than two orders of magnitude). Negative cooperativity is characterized by a flattened curve; complete saturation occurs in a large range of free ligand concentrations (more than two orders of magnitude). Receptor heterogeneity (or ligand heterogeneity) and negative cooperativity lead to qualitatively similar curves. The classic Scatchard plot, $\bar{Y}/[\mathrm{L}]$, versus $\bar{Y}$ (fig. 2) leads to a linear relationship in the simplest cases (Models I and V). The slope equals $-1/Kd$ and the X intercept equals maximal binding capacity. For the other models discussed the Scatchard plots are non-linear. Existence of an upward directed convexity is generally considered as an index of positive cooperativity. A downward directed convexity being considered as an index of negative cooperativity or receptor heterogeneity. Hill plots (log $[(\bar{Y}/(1-\bar{Y})]$ vs log [L]) lead, in most instances, to linear relationships. Relation (4) which applies to Models I to IV can be transformed to

$$\bar{Y}/(1-\bar{Y}) = [\mathrm{L}]^n/K. \tag{7}$$

From fig. 3, one can note that Models III (negative cooperativity) and IV (receptor heterogeneity) are hardly distinguishable.

In principle, experimental determination of the time-courses for ligand–receptor complex formation and dissociation allows the calculation of individual rate constants. In fact, the appropriate relations can be easily derived only for very simple models in situations where the ligand concentration [L] is high as compared to the concentration of total receptor. Hence [L] can be considered as a constant throughout the duration of the binding reaction. In the case of an homogeneous population of non-interacting binding sites:

$$\mathrm{L} + \mathrm{R} \underset{k_2}{\overset{k_1}{\rightleftharpoons}} \mathrm{RL},$$

integration of the differential equation

$$\mathrm{d}[\mathrm{RL}]/\mathrm{d}t = k_1[\mathrm{L}][\mathrm{R}_t - \mathrm{RL}] - k_2[\mathrm{RL}] \tag{8}$$

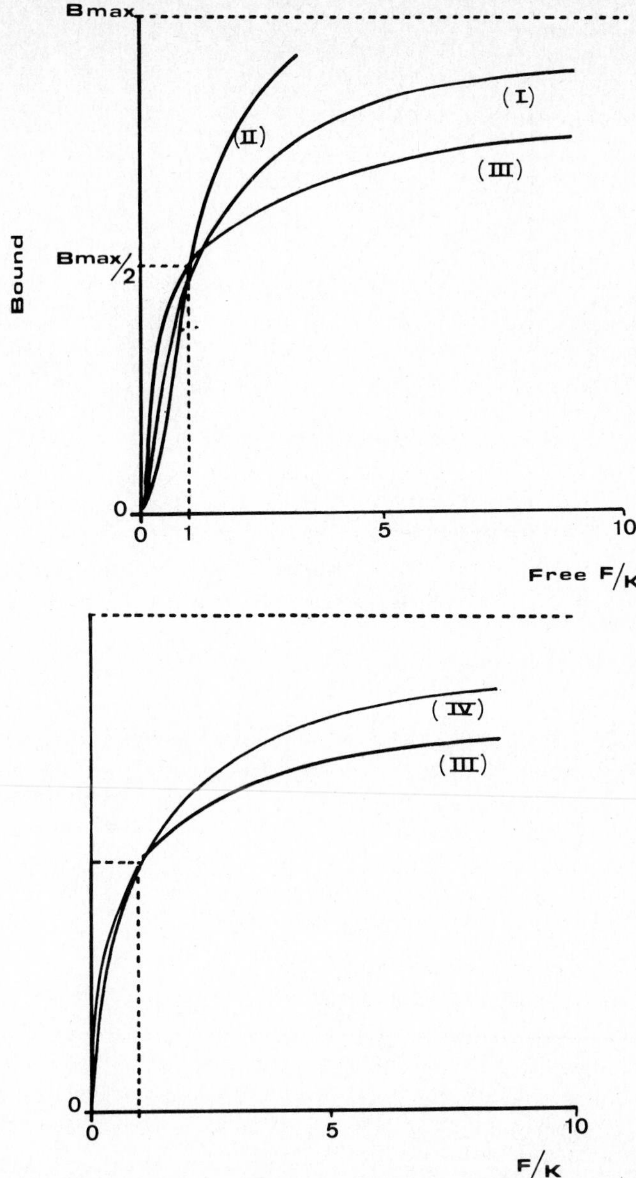

Fig. 1. Dose-dependency for ligand binding to receptors. The curves on the graph were calculated from eqs. (3), (4), (5), and (6). Concentrations of free ligand $[F]$ are normalized concentrations $[F/K]$. The amount of bound ligand is expressed in arbitrary units. Bmax = maximal binding capacity. Indications on the curves refer to the different models considered (see text). For Models II and III the values of n (see eq. 4) chosen to construct the curves were 1.25 and 0.75, respectively. The curve IV corresponds to a situation where two categories of binding sites are present.

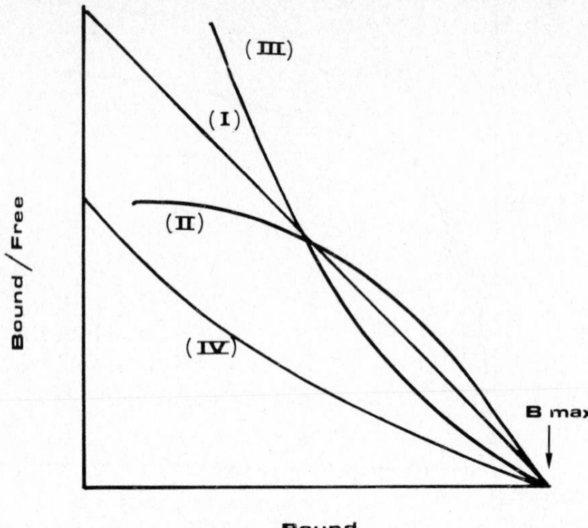

Fig. 2. Scatchard plots of binding isotherms. For symbols, see caption to fig. 1.

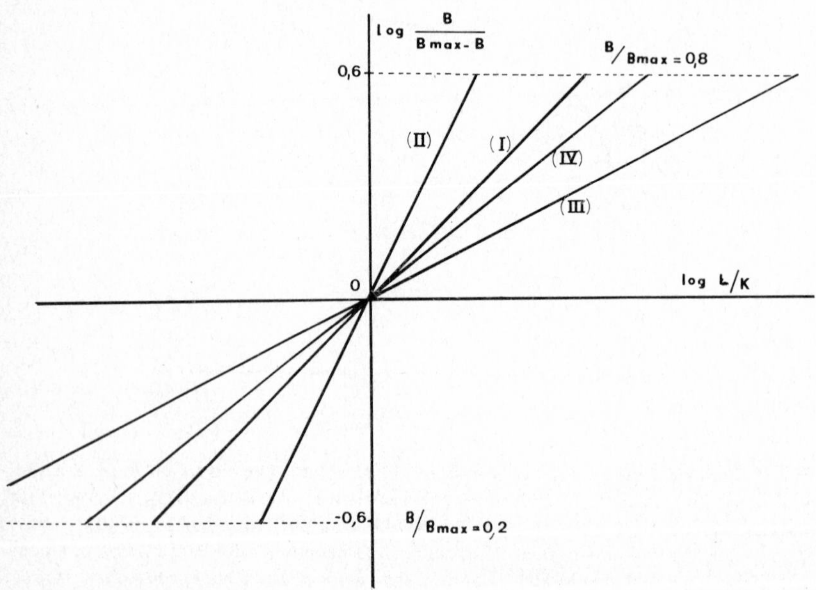

Fig. 3. Hill plots of binding isotherms. For symbols, see caption to fig. 1.

gives when the reaction is started by addition of L to R:

$$(\mathrm{RL}) = (\mathrm{RLeq})\ (1 - e^{-(k_1[\mathrm{L}]+k_2)t}) \tag{9}$$

in which [RLeq] is given by eq. (2). Equation (9) can be rearranged in the form of:

$$\ln\left([\mathrm{RLeq}]/[\mathrm{RLeq}-\mathrm{RL}]\right) = (k_1[\mathrm{L}]+k_2)t. \tag{10}$$

Plots of eqs. (9) and (10) are illustrated by fig. 4. The figure also shows how the values of the rate constants k_1 and k_2 can be deduced from the determination of binding-time courses for two different values of [L].

When the formation of RL is blocked either by eliminating L or introducing a large amount of a competitor eq. (9) reduces to:

$$\mathrm{d}[\mathrm{RL}]/\mathrm{d}t = k_2[\mathrm{RL}] \tag{11}$$

integration of which gives:

$$[\mathrm{RL}] = [\mathrm{RL}_0]e^{-k_2 t} \tag{12}$$

in which $[\mathrm{RL}_0]$ is the ligand–receptor complex concentration at $t=0$.

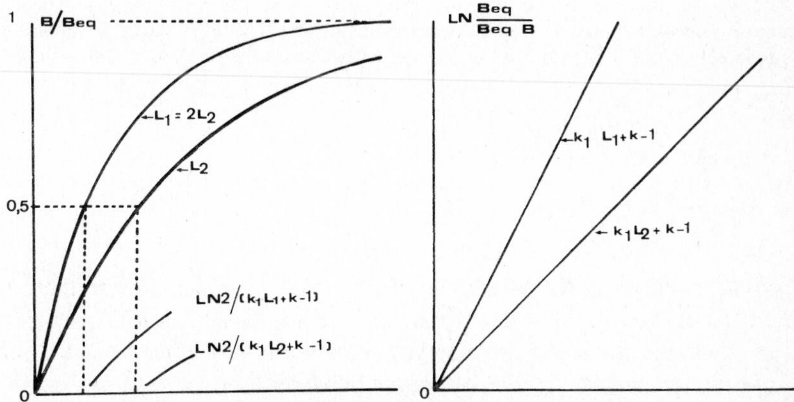

Fig. 4. Time-course of ligand binding to receptors. The curves on the graph were calculated from eqs. (9) and (10) which apply to the reversible binding of a ligand to an homogeneous population of non-interacting binding sites in a situation where the total amount of binding sites is negligible as compared to the total amount of ligand molecules present in the system. As indicated in the right panel, the rate constants for the reactions of formation and dissociation of the complex (k_1 and k_{-1}) can be deduced from the slopes of the two curves. Note that the difference in slope and as a consequence the precision of an experimental determination of k_1 and k_{-1} will depend on the ligand concentrations used.

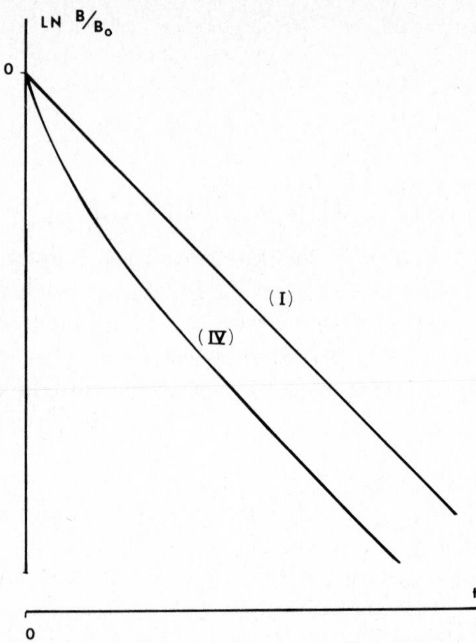

Fig. 5. Dissociation time-course of ligand–receptor complex. The curves were constructed from eq. 13, which applies to Model I described in the text. The figure shows that receptor heterogeneity (Model IV) will lead to a deviation from the expected linear relationship.

Rearrangement of eq. (11) gives:

$$\ln([\mathrm{RL}]/[\mathrm{RL}_0]) = -k_2 t. \qquad (13)$$

Plot of eq. (13) (see fig. 5) allows a very simple graphical determination of k_2. As shown by the figure a deviation of the dissociation time-course from a simple monoexponential law is an index of either receptor (or ligand) heterogeneity or of cooperative behavior.

1.2. Measurement of hormonal binding to receptors

The total number of hormonal receptors present on a target cell is in most cases very small (in the range of 10^4 receptors per cell). Plasma membranes prepared from hormone-responsive cells or tissues do not contain usually more than 1 pM receptor/mg protein. For practical reasons, it is difficult to use more than 0.1 mg membrane protein per assay. Hence, to be able to measure an hormone–receptor complex concentration corresponding to 1% of the total binding capacity it is necessary to detect as low as 10^{-15} mole of bound hormone. Radioactive ligands of high specific radioactivity allow us to reach this high detection sensitivity. In most cases, it is very difficult to work with radioligands having a specific radioactivity of less than 5–10 Ci/mmole. This prerequisite strongly limits the choice of the radioactive isotopes which can be used for ligand labeling. Both tritiated and iodinated ligands are currently used. Tritiated ligands offer the advantages of a rather long half-life and no significant alteration of the chemical structure because of the presence of the isotope. The principle advantage of iodinated ligands over tritiated ligands is the high radioactivity attainable. Incorporation of one ^{125}I atom per molecule would give a maximal specific activity of 2175 Ci/mM, whereas incorporation of one ^{3}H atom would produce a compound with a specific radioactivity of 29 Ci/mM. The main disadvantage of using iodinated ligands for binding studies is the potential alteration of biological activity caused by iodination.

Besides a high specific radioactivity there are a number of characteristics that a good radioligand for a given receptor should have: (1) Demonstrable biological activity as an agonist or antagonist; (2) High homogeneity and radiochemical purity. When using iodinated peptides it is frequently necessary to carefully purify one particular subpopulation of iodinated molecules (usually a monoiodinated species); and (3) High affinity for the receptor sites, thus permitting the use of the radioligand at low concentrations and facilitating the physical separation of bound ligand from free ligand (see below).

The biological material used for hormone–receptor binding studies is either intact isolated cells or plasma membrane fractions prepared from the hormone-responsive tissue. Whatever the type of biological preparation used, it is imperative to carefully check the chemical stability of the radioligand in its presence. A variety of methods have been used to quantify specific radioligand binding. In general, these methods take advantage of the relatively high stability of hormone–receptor complexes. Half-lives (time required for dissociation of half the complexes present immediately before elimination of free ligand from the incubation medium) are currently of several minutes and can be increased to much larger values by rapid lowering of the temperature. Hence, it is possible to accurately determine the concentration of ligand–receptor complexes in a given situation by physically separating bound from free ligand. Association of receptors with a particulate material (membranes) greatly facilitates this separation. The two most widely used techniques are rapid centrifugation and filtration on an appropriate matrix.

Radioligands used for receptor characterization, like many other compounds, non-specifically adsorb to glass, paper, cellular membranes, and other substances. Thus, the amount of radioactivity bound to a receptor preparation is the sum of radioactivity bound to the receptor molecules (specific binding) and radioactivity bound to other constituents (non-specific binding). Schematically:

$$\text{total radioactivity bound} = R_t \frac{[\mathrm{L}]}{[\mathrm{L}]+Kd} + N_t \frac{[\mathrm{L}]}{[\mathrm{L}]+Kns}, \qquad (14)$$

in which the first term represents radioactivity bound to the receptor [see eq. (1)], and the second term, radioactivity non-specifically bound with (N_t = total number of non-specific binding sites and Kns = mean dissociation constant for these non-specific sites). If the radioligand has a high affinity for the specific receptor sites, it can be used at low concentrations. ([L] and Kd of the same order of magnitude). If, in addition, it has a much lower affinity for the non-specific sites ($Kns \gg Kd$), [L] will be negligible as compared to Kns. Hence, eq. (14) can be reduced to:

$$\text{total radioactivity bound} = R_t \frac{[\mathrm{L}]}{[\mathrm{L}]+Kd} + N_t \frac{[\mathrm{L}]}{Kns}. \qquad (15)$$

From eq. (15), it is easy to show that reduction of the specific activity of the ligand by addition of an excess of unlabeled ligand will reduce to a very low value the specific component of binding and leave the non-specific component unchanged. The specific binding is usually determined by the difference between radioactivity bound in the presence of the labeled ligand only and radioactivity bound in the presence of labeled ligand plus an excess (usually equivalent to 100 Kd) of unlabeled ligand. For a given system, an individualized set of experimental conditions should be established that optimizes the accuracy of specific binding measurement.

As it will be discussed later, one important aspect of the characterization of an hormonal receptor is a precise analysis of its specificity towards a series of structurally related ligand molecules (agonists, partial agonists, and antagonists). In most instances, all those molecules are not available in a labeled form. Methods have been devised which allow determination of the equilibrium dissociation constants for unlabeled ligands. They are based on a kinetic analysis of the inhibition of radioactive ligands by unlabeled ligands. In the case one radioactive ligand [L] and one unlabeled ligand [I] competing for binding to a single population of independent binding sites, the saturation function of the receptor by L is rendered by:

$$\bar{Y} = \frac{[\mathrm{L}]}{[\mathrm{L}] + Kd[1 + ([I]/Ki)]}, \tag{16}$$

in which [I] is the concentration of the unlabeled ligand and Ki its equilibrium dissociation constant. For a given value of [L], the fractional inhibition: $\bar{Y}/\bar{Y}_0$ ($\bar{Y}_0$ is the value measured in the absence of unlabeled ligand) varies according to:

$$\bar{Y}/\bar{Y}_0 = \frac{[\mathrm{L}] + Kd}{[\mathrm{L}] + Kd[1 + ([I]/Ki)]} \tag{17}$$

which can be rearranged to give:

$$(\bar{Y}_0/\bar{Y} - 1) = [I](1/Ki)(Kd/(Kd + [\mathrm{L}]). \tag{18}$$

Relation (18) allows a simple graphical determination of Ki if the value of Kd is known. Note that when [L] is very small as compared to Kd, eq. (18) can be reduced to: $[\bar{Y}_0/(\bar{Y} - 1)] = [I]/Ki$.

1.3. Functional characterization of hormonal receptors

At present, there is no other possible definition of a hormonal receptor than a functional definition. A receptor is characterized by two fundamental properties: its capability to specifically interact with a regulatory ligand and its capability when liganded to trigger a physiological response.

Hence complete characterization of a given receptor always implies the demonstration that the putative target structure contains specific binding sites and the demonstration that the binding process and physiological response are closely correlated.

The criteria currently used for the functional characterization of hormonal receptors are the following:

(1) The radioligand used for binding studies must be physiologically active either as an agonist or as an inhibitor of the response induced by an agonist.

(2) Dose-dependencies for hormonal binding and response must be compatible. However, in most systems, the magnitude of the response is not linearly related to receptor occupancy. Therefore, one cannot expect the dose-response and dose-binding curves to be superimposable.
(3) The order of potency of a series of agonists in eliciting the biological response should be reflected in their order of potency in competing for the binding sites. Any competitive inhibitor of the labeled ligand must either be able to elicit a biological response or behave as a specific blocker of the response to an agonist.

2. Hormonal receptors coupled to adenylate cyclase

As already mentioned, a large variety of biological effects elicited by peptidic hormones, catecholamines, and other regulatory agents as prostaglandins are triggered by an activation of membrane adenylate cyclase. It is now clearly established that hormone-responsive adenylate cyclases contain at least three components [8–12]: a catalytic unit which is the site of cyclic AMP production from ATP; a receptor unit responsible for specific recognition of the hormonal signal; and a coupling unit which is necessary for the formation of an activated state of the catalytic unit when the receptor is occupied by an active ligand. The coupling unit is the site of action of GTP which plays an obligatory role in the process of adenylate cyclase activation by hormones (see below). The three components of hormone-responsive adenylate cyclases are integral membrane proteins. They can be extracted from the membrane under the influence of non-ionic detergents and physically separated using conventional biochemical techniques. Variants of hormone responsive cells lacking one or several components of the adenylate cyclase system could be selected thus indicating that these components are the products of different genes [13]. The adenylate cyclase components are minor constituents of the membrane and yet have not been purified to homogeneity. Most of the available data on the properties of membrane receptors and adenylate cyclase were derived from studies using intact membranes.

2.1. Kinetics of hormonal binding: effects of GTP and other nucleotides on hormone binding to receptors

The role of GTP in hormonal action was discovered by Rodbell and colleagues during the course of their studies on the glucagon-sensitive adenylate cyclase from rat liver membranes [14, 15]. On this system, GTP has two different, but very likely related effects. The nucleotide is necessary for the transduction of hormone–receptor binding into a biological response (activation of adenylate cyclase). GTP or GMP–PCP (5′-guanylyl diphosphonate) does not markedly influence adenylate cyclase activity measured in the absence of glucagon while the glucagon-sensitive activity is markedly increased by the two nucleotides in a dose-dependent manner. GTP also influences (^{125}I) glucagon binding to rat liver membranes. In the absence of nucleotide hormone binding is very slowly reversible upon dilution of the incubation medium or addition of unlabeled glucagon. In the presence of GTP, the hormone–receptor complex is rapidly dissociated. The overall effect of GTP on hormone–receptor interaction is to increase the equilibrium dissociation constant. The effect of GTP on the rate of dissociation is dose-dependent. The maximal effect of GTP is obtained for a nucleotide concentration which is at the lower limit of the nucleotide concentration found in the intact tissue. Therefore, it seems unlikely that under physiological conditions the magnitude of adenylate cyclase activation could be modulated through variations of intracellular GTP concentration. The GTP effect on hormonal binding and adenylate cyclase activation does not require nucleotide hydrolysis; it can be elicited by non-hydrolyzable derivatives of GTP such as 5′-guanylyl-imidodiphosphate (Gpp(NH)p).

Recent extensive studies of the guanyl nucleotide effect on specific ligand binding to beta-adrenergic receptors revealed an important and possibly general characteristic of the action of guanyl nucleotides. Using radioactively-labeled antagonists to study the receptors, Maguire et al. [16] and Lefkowitz et al. [17] have demonstrated that guanyl nucleotides reduce the affinity of agonists for beta receptor sites from frog erythrocyte membranes. This conclusion was reached by measuring the abilities of agonists and antagonists to compete for binding sites labeled by the radioactive antagonists (^{125}I) hydroxybenzylpindolol and (^{3}H) dihydroalprenolol. The results obtained with a large series of drugs acting on the beta receptor as full agonists, partial agonists, or pure antagonists are summarized in table 1. For the full agonists large (20-fold) shift in affinity is observed. The values obtained for partial agonists were substantially less and varied as a function of their respective intrinsic activities. The nucleotide effect on agonist binding could be directly studied by the use of the radioactive agonist (^{3}H) hydroxybenzylisoproterenol. The effect was found identical to that initially described for

Table 1

Effect of guanyl nucleotide on the binding of agonists and antagonists to beta-adrenergic receptors [a)]

Agent	Intrinsic activity	Shift in (−)-(^{3}H) dihydro-alprenolol displacement curve (fold)
(−)-Isoproterenol	1.0±0	19.1±4
(±)-Cc-34	1.0±0.1	18.0±6
(−)-Epinephrine	1.0±0.1	21.0±1
(±)-Isoetharine	0.72±0	15.7±0
(±)-Cyclopentylbutanephrine	0.64±0.05	9.6±1
(±)-Salbutamol	0.26±0.02	5.4±2
(±)-MJ9184-1	0.23±0.02	2.0±0
(−)-Soterenol	0.21±0.03	2.9±0.8
(−)-Propranolol	0±0	1.0±0
(−)-Alprenolol	0±0	1.0±0
(−)-Oxprenolol	0	1.0
(±)-Nylidrin	0	1.0
(±)-Dicholrisoproterenol	0±0	1.0±0

[a)]The dissociation constants of the listed compounds for the beta-adrenergic receptors from frog erythrocytes were determined from competition experiments using (^{3}H) dihydroalprenolol as the labeled ligand. Determinations were performed both in the absence and presence of Gpp(NH)p (50 μM). The nucleotide-induced change in receptor affinity was estimated by the ratio *Kd* in the presence of Gpp(NH)p/*Kd* in its absence. The experimental values obtained are indicated in the right column. Intrinsic activities were measured by the magnitude of maximal adenylate cyclase activation. Values indicated in the table are relative activities using intrinsic activity of isoproterenol as a reference. Modified from Lefkowitz et al. [17].

glucagon binding to rat liver plasma membranes, i.e. guanyl nucleotides markedly increase the rate of dissociation of the ligand–receptor complex.

Nucleotide effects similar to those described above have been found for many but not all membrane receptors coupled to an adenylate cyclase. It is likely that for some "unresponsive systems" the observed lack of nucleotide effect is only apparent. It might be a consequence of a contamination of the biological preparation by endogeneous nucleotides.

2.2. Receptor occupancy – adenylate cyclase activation relationship

Hormone-sensitive adenylate cyclases represent rather unique systems for which hormonal binding to the receptor and one early consequence of this interaction, i.e. activation of adenylate cyclase, can be measured on membrane fractions incubated *in vitro* under reasonably well controlled and identical experimental conditions. This provides the possibility of a rather precise analysis of the quantitative relationships existing between binding and response, i.e. what is currently referred to as the coupling function.

One obvious question which can be raised concerns the choice of the parameters which could be used for the quantification of the hormone–receptor interaction on the one hand and of the response on the other hand. As far as the response is concerned, the situation is rather simple. There is no real reason to suspect the validity of measuring the magnitude of the response by the hormone-induced changes in the rate of cyclic-AMP production by adenylate cyclase. The response is currently measured either as the absolute increase in enzyme activity over basal activity measured in the absence of hormone or, as the ratio of the activities measured in the presence and absence of hormone (activation ratio). Usually the parameter used to quantify the hormone–receptor interaction is the actual number or concentration of hormone–receptor complexes present in the system at a given time. The validity of this choice has sometimes been questioned in view of a theory referred to as the rate theory, which has been developed by pharmacologists. In this theory the possibility is considered that the response to a pharmacological agent acting through specific receptors might be triggered by the rate of ligand receptor interaction. The magnitude of the response is supposed to be a function of the number of ligand molecules which bind to the receptors during a given period of time. One prediction of this theory is that the magnitude of the response reaches maximal value immediately after addition of the active ligand. Indeed the rate of ligand–receptor interaction is maximal at the early beginning of the reaction when the concentration of unoccupied receptors is maximal. It then decreases towards an equilibrium value as the degree of receptor occupancy increases. In fact, time-course studies of adenylate cyclase activation by hormones failed to reveal any clear initial burst of activation. Therefore, it appears that the response is better related to receptor occupancy than to the rate of hormone–receptor interaction.

The coupling function can be studied under two main types of experimental conditions: steady-state conditions or transient-state conditions. In one case, the evolution patterns of the steady-state level of receptor occupancy and enzyme activation as a function of the concentration of free hormone concentration are compared. In the second case, the time-courses of hormone binding and enzyme activation are compared.

The coupling function under steady-state conditions has now been determined for a great number of hormone-responsive adenylate cyclases. Marked differences have been observed from one system to the other. In some systems, the dose-dependent binding curve and dose-dependent activation curves are more or less superimposable suggesting the existence of a simple linear relationship between binding and response (linear coupling). More frequently, the dose-binding curve and dose-response curve are not superimposable but parallel, maximal response being achieved for a fractional receptor occupancy less than one. The coupling function is non-linear. Such a situation was found for instance in the case of the glucagon-sensitive adenylate cyclase from rat liver membranes [18]. A rather simple explanation can be found within the general framework of the so-called "floating receptor hypothesis". According to this hypothesis, the activated form of adenylate cyclase is viewed as a complex between the hormone–receptor complex and the enzyme at least one of the two partners being able to diffuse within the plane of the membrane. The simplest reactional scheme of that type is the following:

$$L + R \overset{K_B}{\rightleftharpoons} RL + E \overset{K_A}{\rightleftharpoons} RLE \tag{19}$$

in which L, R, and E are the hormone, the hormonal receptor, and the enzyme, respectively. RL and RLE are the binary (receptor–hormone) and ternary (hormone–receptor–enzyme) complexes respectively; and K_B and K_A are the equilibrium constants for reactions I and II, respectively. In a condition in which there is an excess of receptor molecules as compared to adenylate cyclase molecules and the constant K_A is small (high affinity of RL for E), it is easy to account for a non-linear coupling.

In most systems, there is no obvious relation between the nature of the hormone–receptor occupancy relationship and the dissociation constant characteristic of the agonist used to induce the activation. Thus Lucas and Bockaert [19] found in C_6 glioma cells that the coupling of beta-adrenergic receptors to adenylate cyclase was non-linear. However the ratio *Kd* for binding/*Ka* for enzyme activation (a good index for evaluating the degree of non-linearity in coupling) was the same for a series of beta-adrenergic agonists with different *Kd* values.

As indicated above, specific effects of guanyl nucleotides on hormone–receptor interaction could be demonstrated in several systems. The overall nucleotide effect results in an increase in the rate of dissociation of the hormone–receptor complex. The domain of hormonal concentrations for which a dose-dependent increase in binding is

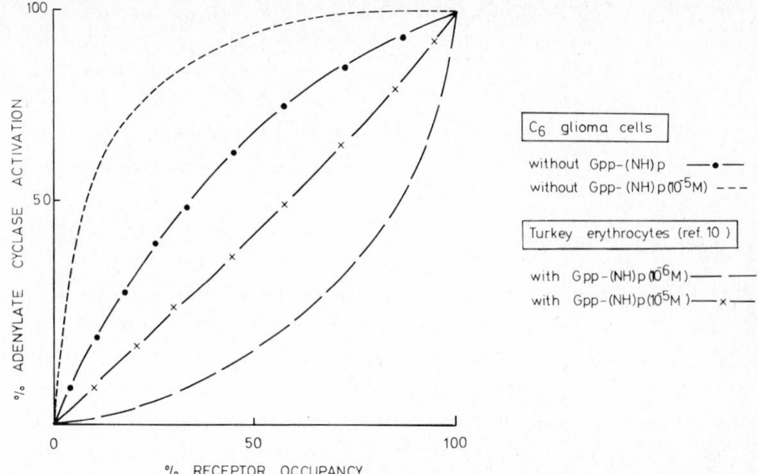

Fig. 6. Effect of Gpp(NH)p on the relationship between receptor occupancy and adenylate cyclase activation. Fractional activation of adenylate cyclase by isoproterenol is plotted as a function of fractional receptor occupancy. The figure shows the effect of Gpp(NH)p on two systems: C_6 gliomal cells and turkey erythrocytes. The figure is reproduced from Lucas and Bockaert [19]. It includes data from Brown et al. [37].

observable is shifted towards a higher value (increase in steady-state dissociation constant). In most systems, guanyl nucleotides were also found to affect the dose-response relationship. The apparent *Ka* for activation is decreased. These two opposite effects of guanyl nucleotides on binding and response leading to a marked accentuation of the usual non-linear character of the coupling function. These conclusions are illustrated by fig. 6 in the case of beta-adrenergic, agonist-sensitive adenylate cyclase from C_6 glioma cells.

2.3. *Relation of hormonal binding to final biological response*

As indicated before, it seems very likely that in several systems binding of the active ligand to only a small fraction of the total number of receptors present is sufficient to induce maximal adenylate cyclase activation. The apparent affinity (or sensitivity) is higher when tested at the level of effector (adenylate cyclase) than when tested at the receptor level. Such an apparent increase in sensitivity can occur at intermediary steps following the adenylate cyclase activation state (production of more cyclic AMP than needed to maximally activate intracellular protein kinases for instance). Summation of such effects can lead to rather paradoxical situations like that depicted in fig. 7. In rat testes, binding

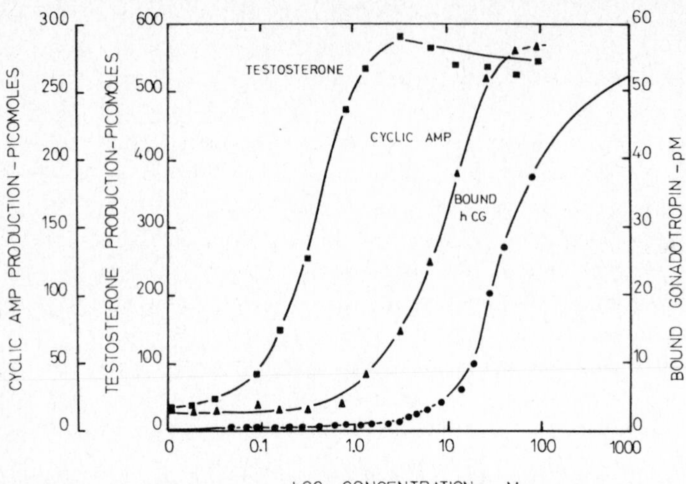

Fig. 7. Relation of gonatropin binding to response in interstitial cells from the rat testis. Correlation of human chorionic gonotropin (picomoles/liter, ●–●), cyclic AMP production (picomoles, ▲–▲) and testosterone production (picomoles, ■–■) during incubation of collagenase-dispersed interstitial cells with increasing concentrations of hormone (hCG). Reproduced from Dufau and Catt [20].

of gonadotropin to half the total number of receptors present is sufficient to maximally stimulate intracellular cyclic AMP accumulation. Apparently a small fraction of cyclic AMP which can be generated by maximally stimulated adenylate cyclase is sufficient to induce a maximal increase in testosterone production which is the final response [20]. Finally, it appears that occupation of a very small fraction of the total number of receptors present can induce a full biological response. It must be noted that it has been convincingly demonstrated: (1) that the binding sites detected are effectively those receptors involved in adenylate cyclase activation and (2) that stimulation of cyclic AMP production is an obligatory step in hormonal stimulation of steroidogenesis.

Usually hormonal concentrations in circulating blood are lower than the value which would be needed to saturate their specific receptors. One consequence of the existence of the so-called "receptor reserve" phenomenon is that distinct biological effects of an hormone acting on a target cell through the intermediacy of the same set of receptors can exhibit rather different dose-dependencies.

3. Other membrane receptors

The nature of the primary effects of several hormones acting through the intermediacy of membrane receptors is at least partially unknown. Among these hormones are insulin, alpha-adrenergic agonists, angiotensin, vasopressin, and prostaglandins.* Even in situations where the sole measurable consequence of hormone–receptor interaction is the magnitude of the final response a satisfactory correlation between binding and response could be demonstrated (see, e.g., [21]).

It has been recently shown that the nucleotide effect on ligand–receptor interaction is not restricted to those receptors which are functionally coupled to an adenylate cyclase or more exactly for systems in which an agonist-induced stimulation of adenylate cyclase can be demonstrated using acellular preparation. Thus U'Prichard and Snyder [22] have provided clear evidence for an effect of guanyl nucleotides on ligand binding to alpha-noradrenergic receptors from calf brain membranes. GTP induces a dose-dependent reduction in receptor affinity with no change in maximal binding capacity. GTP significantly reduces the apparent affinity of agonists but not that of antagonists for the (^{3}H) epinephrine binding sites. These results resemble those described above for the adenylate cyclase-coupled beta receptor from frog erythrocytes. Guanyl nucleotides were also found to affect ligand binding to brain opiate receptors [22], angiotensin receptors from the adrenals [24], and vasopressin receptors from liver [25].

4. Regulation of membrane receptors

An important consequence of the widely used radioligand binding techniques for the characterization and quantification of membrane receptors for hormones and neurotransmitters was the discovery that receptors are dynamic components of the plasma membrane that can be functionally altered by a variety of endocrine and genetic factors. In this section, some of these dynamic aspects of membrane receptor functions will be described and some of the current hypothesis on the molecular basis of these control mechanisms of receptor function will be rapidly discussed.

*Depending on the type of target cell considered, prostaglandins or peptidic hormones like vasopressin, act either through an activation of adenylate cyclase or through other mechanisms.

4.1. The down regulation concept

The idea that concentration of membrane hormone receptors in target cells might be regulated by homologous hormones originating from studies with genetically obese mice. In those mice it was found that obesity is associated with hyperinsulinemia and insulin resistance [26]. Insulin resistance could be correlated to a decrease in insulin receptor concentration per insulin target cell of per unit of cell surface. Correction of the hyperinsulinemia is associated with amelioration of the metabolic abnormalities and a restoration of insulin binding to normal. Further studies *in vivo* in both rodents and man [27–28] have demonstrated under many circumstances a remarkable inverse correlation between the chronic (but not acute) concentration of circulating insulin and the concentration of insulin receptors on target cells. Regulation of receptor concentration by homologous hormone currently designated as "down regulation" of receptors was found to occur for a large variety of hormone responsive tissues and cultured cells. The main characteristics of this down regulation phenomenon are the following:

(1) Down regulation is hormone specific. This could be convincingly demonstrated using cells which respond to several hormones through specific and independent sets of membrane receptors. For example it has been shown that human lymphocytes contain membrane receptors for insulin and growth hormone. These receptors are highly specific; insulin does not interfere with the binding of labeled growth hormone and conversely growth hormone does not interfere with the binding of labeled insulin. As reported by Lesniak and Roth [29], exposure of human lymphocytes to growth hormone but not exposure to insulin resulted in a loss of growth hormone receptors. Exposure to growth hormone alone and exposure to a combination of growth hormone and insulin gave similar results.

(2) Down regulation is dose- and time-dependent. The magnitude of the reduction in receptor number is dependent on the hormonal concentration to which the cells are exposed. The dose-dependent receptor loss is usually observed over a concentration range comparable to that needed to obtain dose-dependent receptor occupancy under steady-state conditions. Down regulation of receptors is a rather slow process as compared to the process of hormone binding to receptors. In most systems, continous exposure of the target cells for hours is needed to produce receptor loss.

(3) Down regulation is agonist specific. In situations where large series of compounds with agonistic and antagonistic properties are available, it could be shown that down regulation could be induced by agonists but not by antagonists. The relative potencies of agonists for the induction of receptor loss is fairly well reflected by their relative potencies for eliciting a biological response [30].

Data obtained with mutant lines of the S49 lymphoma cells sensitive to beta-adrenergic agonists suggest that down regulation can only be induced by agonist binding to a "functional" receptor [31]. One of these mutant lines referred to as $(AC)^-$ appears to lack adenylate cyclase activity but does contain beta-adrenergic receptors. When these cells are exposed to agonist, no fall in beta-adrenergic receptor number occurs despite the fact that such an agonist-induced fall in receptor number can be readily demonstrated in wild type cells.

(4) It has been currently observed that the fall in receptor number induced by chronic exposure of target cells to homologous hormone is spontaneously reversible upon removal of the hormone from the incubation medium [29].

4.2. Possible mechanisms involved in down regulation of hormonal receptors

It was suggested from the early beginning that the loss of receptors induced by agonists might reflect internalization of activated receptors through an endocytotic mechanism. If such a mechanism is operating, it seems necessary, in order to account for the specificity of the down regulation process, to also assume that receptors are primarily or secondarily concentrated onto membrane portions which become or are preferential loci for the formation of endocytotic vesicles. Using insuline derivatives formed by covalent association of one insuline molecule and one lactalbumin molecule bearing a large number of fluorophores, Schlessinger et al. [32] studied the fluorescence distribution on the plasma membranes of isolated fibroblasts incubated with these insulin derivatives. When the binding of the fluorescent insulin derivative was performed at temperatures lower than 23° C, the fluorescence was found to be diffusely distributed over the cell membrane surface. When the cells were incubated at higher temperatures (between 23° C and 37° C) a redistribution of bound fluorescence was observed; fluorescence became concentrated into patches. The patching was followed by internalization, increasing portions of bound fluorescence becoming associated with intracellular endocytotic vesicles. Similar results were obtained with fluorescent derivatives of epidermal growth factor.

The physiological significance of down regulation of receptor as a regulatory mechanism of target cell sensitivity to hormonal stimulation has frequently been questioned especially in those systems where the so-called receptor reserve phenomenon is highly operative, i.e. in systems where a low fractional receptor occupancy is sufficient to induce a full biological response. In fact, one must realize that for any given hormonal concentration the number of hormone–receptor complexes formed under steady-state conditions is directly proportional to the total number of receptors present in the target cell. Therefore, even if a large receptor reserve exists, a reduction in receptor number will lead to an increase in the hormonal concentration for which the number of hormone–receptors complexes reaches the value needed for the expression of a full biological response. Reduction in total receptor number effectively reduces the sensitivity of the target cell to hormonal stimulation.

Down regulation of hormone receptors appears to be a widespread phenomenon. However, it does represent the sole type of receptor regulation by homologous hormone. In several systems like the vasopressin-sensitive renal adenylate cyclase [33], prolactin-sensitive liver cells from hypophysectomized rats [34], it appeared that minimal levels of circulating hormone are necessary for the expression of maximal sensitivity of specific target cells. Thus an inherited defect in the production of vasopressin observed in mutant rats from the Brattleboro strain is associated with a decreased sensitivity of renal adenylate cyclase to vasopressin stimulation [33]. Chronic treatment of those rats with low doses of vasopressin restored a normal sensitivity of renal adenylate cyclase. In normal rats experimental reduction of the basal rate of vasopressin secretion reduces the sensitivity of renal adenylate cyclase to vasopressin stimulation. A slight increase in basal vasopressin secretion rate had an opposite effect.

4.3. Other factors that influence receptor function

A rapidly increasing set of experimental data clearly indicate that membrane-receptor number and function are influenced by a variety of factors and regulatory mechanisms. In this subsection, a small number of selected examples of such regulations will be rapidly described and discussed.

4.3.1. Heterologous hormonal control of receptor function

Thyroid hormones and steroid hormones were found to influence the sensitivity of several hormone-sensitive tissues of cells to their specific regulatory hormones. Thus experimental hyperthyroidism in the rat provoked by treatment with thyroid hormones results in a highly significant increase in number of beta-adrenergic receptors present on cardiac plasma membranes with no significant alteration in receptor affinity for agonists and antagonists. Similarily, oestrogen treatment in the rabbit (oestrogen dominance) markedly increases the number of alpha-adrenergic receptors in uterine membranes [35]. Hormonal regulation of hormonal responsiveness is not always reflected by changes in the total number of receptors. Thus we observed that, adrenalectomy reduces and glucocorticoid therapy increases the magnitude of maximal renal adenylate cyclase activation by vasopressin [36]. These changes were not accompanied by marked modifications in the number and properties of vasopressin receptors in the kidney. The overall effect of glucocorticoids is to increase the efficiency of receptor adenylate cyclase coupling.

4.3.2. Developmental factors

The developmental pattern of several hormonal receptors has been studied with some detail. In general, a good synchrony was observed between the appearance of the receptors and that of intracellular mechanisms involved in the transduction of hormone–receptor interaction into a final biological response. For hormone-sensitive adenylate cyclases, it was found in several systems that the binding properties and functional properties (i.e. capability of inducing adenylate cyclase activation) are expressed simultaneously.

4.3.3. Genetic influences and other factors

As already mentioned, it has been clearly demonstrated in the case of hormone-sensitive adenylate cyclases that the three main components of the system, i.e. receptor, the adenylate cyclase itself and the component(s) involved in the functional coupling between these two, are under independent genetic control. Mutants lacking one of these components could be selected.

It has also been shown that neoplasia or viral transformation of hormone-sensitive cells are in general associated with alterations in receptor number and function. Analysis of receptor function alterations in those variant or transformed cell lines is obviously of primary importance for further studies. It has already been proved [13] that such cell lines provide unique materials for dissecting the molecular components of membrane receptor–effector systems.

References

[1] E. W. Sutherland and T. W. Rall, Pharmacol Rev. 3 (1960) 265.

[2] P. Greengard and J. F. Kuo, On the Mechanism of Action of Cyclic AMP, in: Advances in Biochemical Psychopharmacology, vol. 3, eds. P. Greengard and E. Costa (Raven Press, New York, 1970) pp. 287–306.

[3] N. D. Goldberg, R. F. O'Dea and M. K. Haddox, Cyclic GMP, in: Advances in Cyclic Nucleotide Research, vol. 3, eds. P. Greengard and G. A. Robison (Raven Press, New York, 1973) pp. 155–223.

[4] H. Rasmussen and A. Tenenhouse, Proc. Natl. Acad. Sci. USA 59 (1968) 1364.

[5] L. M. Jones, S. Cockcroft and R. H. Michell, Biochem. J. 182 (1979) 669.

[6] F. Hirata, W. J. Strittmater and J. Axelrod, Proc. Natl. Acad. Sci. USA 76 (1979) 368.

[7] P. W. Ramwell and J. E. Shaw, Rec. Prog. Hormone Res. 26 (1970) 139.

[8] J. Orly and M. Schramm, Proc. Natl. Acad. Sci. USA 73 (1976) 4410.

[9] L. E. Limbird and R. J. Lefkowitz, J. Biol. Chem. 252 (1977) 799.

[10] G. Vauquelin, P. Geynet, J. Hanoune and A. D. Strosberg, Proc. Natl. Acad. Sci. USA 74 (1977) 3710.

[11] T. Pfeuffer, J. Biol. Chem. 252 (1977) 7224.

[12] A. G. Welton, P. M. Lad, A. C. Newby, H. Yamamura, S. Nicosia and M. Rodbell, J. Biol. Chem. 252 (1977) 5947.

[13] T. Haga, E. M. Ross, H. J. Anderson and A. G. Gilman, Proc. Natl. Acad. Sci. USA 74 (1977) 2016.

[14] M. Rodbell, H. J. Krans, S. L. Pohl and L. Birnbaumer, J. Biol. Chem. 246 (1971) 1872.

[15] M. Rodbell, L. Birnbaumer, S. L. Pohl and H. M. J. Krans, J. Biol. Chem. 246 (1971) 1877.

[16] M. E. Maguire, P. M. Van Arsdale and A. G. Gilman, Mol. Pharmacol. 12 (1976) 335.

[17] R. J. Lefkowitz, D. Mullikin and M. G. Caron, J. Biol. Chem. 251 (1976) 4686.

[18] M. Rodbell, M. C. Lin and Y. Salomon, J. Biol. Chem. 249 (1974) 59.

[19] M. Lucas and J. Bockaert, Mol. Pharmacol. 13 (1977) 314.

[20] M. L. Dufau and K. J. Catt, Gonadal Receptors for Luteinizing Hormone and Chorionic Gonatotropin, in: Cell Membrane Receptors for Viruses, Antigens and Antibodies, Polypeptide Hormone and Small Molecules, eds. R. F. Beers and E. G. Basset (Raven Press, New York, 1976).

[21] M. F. El-Refai, P. F. Blackmore and J. H. Exton, J. Biol. Chem. 254 (1979) 4375.

[22] D. C. U'Prichard and S. H. Snyder, J. Biol. Chem. 253 (1978) 3444.

[23] A. J. Blume, Proc. Natl. Acad. Sci. USA 75 (1978) 1713.

[24] H. Glossmann, A. Bavkal and K. J. Catt, J. Biol. Chem. 249 (1974) 664.

[25] B. Cantau, S. Keppens, H. de Wulf and S. Jard, in preparation.

[26] C. R. Kahn, D. M. Neville and J. Roth, J. Biol. Chem. 248 (1973) 244.

[27] A. J. Soll, C. R. Kahn, D. M. Neville and J. Roth, J. Clin. Invest. 56 (1975) 769.
[28] J. A. Archer, P. Gorden and J. Roth, J. Clin. Invest. 55 (1975) 166.
[29] M. A. Lesniak and J. Roth, J. Biol. Chem. 251 (1976) 3720.
[30] C. Mukherjee and R. J. Lefkowitz, Mol. Pharmacol. 13 (1977) 291.
[31] M. Shear, P. A. Insel, K. L. Melnon and P. Coffino, J. Biol. Chem. 251 (1976) 7572.
[32] J. Schlessinger, Y. Shechter, M. C. Willingham and I. Pastan, Proc. Natl. Acad. Sci. USA 75 (1978) 2659.
[33] R. M. Rajerison, D. Butlen and S. Jard, Endocrinology 101 (1977) 1.
[34] M. J. Waters, H. G. Friesen and H. G. Bohnet, Regulation of Prolactin Receptors by Steroid Hormones and Use of Radioligand Assays in Endocrine Research, in: Receptors and Hormone Action III, eds. L. Birnbaumer and B. W. O'Malley (Academic Press, New York, 1978)
[35] L. T. Williams, D. Mullikin and R. J. Lefkowitz, J. Biol. Chem. 252 (1976) 6915.
[36] R. M. Rajerison, J. Marchetti, C. Roy, J. Bockaert and S. Jard, J. Biol. Chem. 249 (1974) 6390.
[37] E. M. Brown, S. A. Fedak, C. J. Woodward, G. D. Aurbach and D. Rodbard, J. Biol. Chem. 251 (1976) 1239.

COURSE 6
(PART II)

THE ROLE OF HORMONE RECEPTORS AND GTP – REGULATORY PROTEINS IN MEMBRANE TRANSDUCTION

Martin RODBELL

Laboratory of Nutrition and Endocrinology
National Institute of Arthritis,
Metabolic and Digestive Diseases,
National Institutes of Health,
Bethesda, MD 20205,
U.S.A.

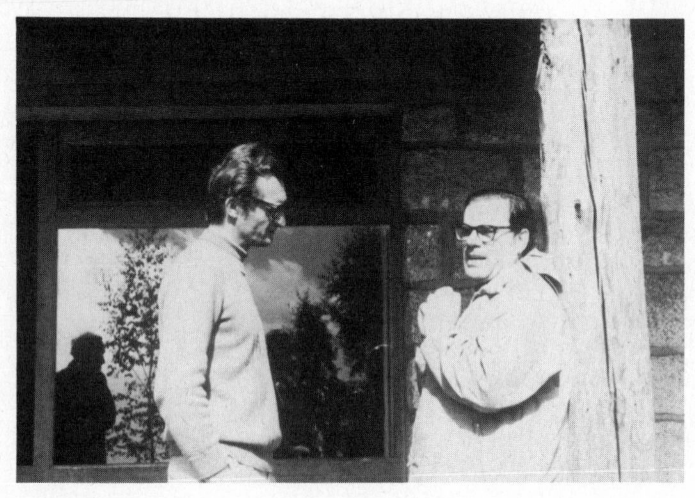

Contents

R. Balian et al., eds.
Les Houches, Session XXXIII, 1979 – Membranes et Communication Intercellulaire / Membranes and Intercellular Communication

0. Introduction

Adenylate cyclase, the enzyme that produces cyclic AMP, is part of a complex regulatory system that mediates the actions of hormones and neurotransmitters on their target cells. Structured within the lipid framework of the cell membrane, the enzyme system is composed of at least three classes of components. Located at the outer surface are the variable receptor (R) components each containing specific sites for binding of hormones and neurotransmitters. At the inner face of the membrane are the catalytic units (C), and what are termed nucleotide regulatory components (N). The latter contain sites for the binding of GTP and are responsible for mediating the effects of GTP and the various hormones on the activity of C [1]. Two types of N units have been distinguished functionally. One mediates stimulation (termed N_s), the other inhibition (N_i) of the enzyme's activity by GTP. As discussed below, each type seems to be linked to separate classes of receptors for hormones and neurotransmitters.

Here I present a theoretical framework for the role of hormone receptors and N units in regulating adenylate cyclase activity and which may be useful as a general model for membrane transduction. Illustrated in fig. 1, the theory suggests that R and N exist separately from C in the membrane as a multimeric complex. In this complex, R inhibits interaction of N with GTP. Hormone binding to R (step 1) triggers release of the structural constraints imposed on N with resultant enhanced reaction with GTP, breakdown of the multimers to monomers (step 2), and formation of RNC (step 3), the holoenzyme. Depending on the type of R and N unit attached to C, the holoenzyme exhibits either increased or decreased production of cyclic AMP. In developing this theory, I review evidence for the existence of N_s and N_i and their complexes with R and C, describe the properties of the various components, give recent evidence that RN complexes exist as multimers, and discuss the possibility that the theory may be generalized to include R and N units that regulate membrane transduction processes other than adenylate cyclase.

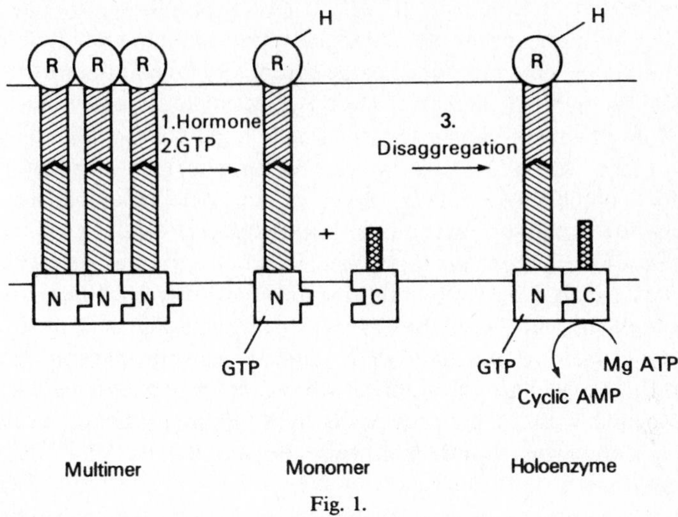

Fig. 1.

1. The role of N_s in activation of adenylate cyclase

Before the discovery that GTP is the essential activator of adenylate cyclase [2] and that hormones enhance the nucleotide's action [3], it was thought that hormone receptors interacted directly with the catalytic unit and that fluoride ion, an ubiquitous activator, affected the catalytic unit directly [4]. It is now clear that GTP acts through a separate protein from receptors and enzyme; this protein is responsible for mediating the actions of hormones and fluoride ion. First identified [5, 6] with GTP photoaffinity analogues as a heat-stable 42 000 Dalton protein in detergent extracts of avian erythrocytes, the protein (N_s) has been shown to exist in a variety of cell membranes. Cholera toxin, long known to stimulate the production of cyclic AMP in animal cells [7, 8], has played an important role in identifying N_s. Toxin treatment of membranes potentiates the activating effects of GTP even in the absence of hormones and affects other characteristics of the enzyme that suggest that it acts directly on N_s [10–14]. The toxin contains in its A_1 subunit an ADP-ribosylating enzyme that labels preferentially the 42 000 Dalton protein in the presence of labeled NAD [16–18]. Cells genetically deficient in N_s by functional criteria or from toxin-labeling studies, but which contain hormone receptors and the catalytic unit have been especially useful for reconstitution studies [18, 19]. Addition of extracts of membranes containing N_s from a variety of cell types restores the ability of hormones, guanine nucleotides, fluoride ion, and cholera toxin to stimulate the enzyme. Thus, judged from several standpoints, N_s is an essential component in the activation of adenylate cyclase. Though its structure remains unknown, N_s must have highly conserved recognition units or sites that allow it to activate C derived from a variety of cells and to "couple" with several types of hormone receptors known to mediate the stimulatory actions of hormones.

A few of the properties of N_s and C, when separate and combined, are listed in table 1 (combinations with R are discussed below). When not complexed with N_s, C uses MnATP preferentially as a substrate [20, 21]. Only when combined with N_s does C use the natural substrate, MgATP [21]. N_s has a low affinity for guanine nucleotides when it is unassociated with C but acquires a tight-binding, guanine nucleotide-binding state when complexed with the enzyme [6, 22]. N_sC is not

Table 1
Properties of adenylate cyclase components

Components	Properties	Selected references
C	Preferential reaction with MnATP as substrate	[20, 21]
NC	MgATP or MnATP as substrate activated by Gpp(NH)p, cholera toxin and NAD in presence of GTP; and by fluoride ion	[16, 23]
R	Low affinity for hormone agonists; no heterotropic effects of GTP	[19]
RN or	GTP reduces affinity of R for hormone agonists	
$(RN)^n$	Hormones form tight-binding complex	[24, 31, 35]
RNC	Same as NC but responds to hormones and GTP; binds GDP tightly in absence of hormones; hormones stimulate exchange of GDP and GTP at N site	[64]

affected by hormones since it is not linked to R units. The complex seems to preexist in some membranes (see below) but it is not clear whether it is present as an artifact of isolation of membranes and/or that it plays any role in cellular regulation. From the standpoint of hormone action, the RN complexes formed from R and N units appear to be essential for the regulation of C by GTP and hormones.

2. The role of the RN complex

In classical theories of hormone action, the binding event leads to a shift in receptor structure to one favorable for action. The relationship between hormone binding (K_D) and action (K_{act}) on adenylate cyclase systems is more complicated owing to the fact that two ligands, hormone, and GTP, are required for action [2]. This complexity is exemplified by studies of the glucagon-sensitive cyclase system in liver membranes [23–25]. During activation of the enzyme the two ligands exerted positive heterotropic effects on each other's K_{act}. However, direct binding studies with labeled glucagon revealed that GTP, at concentrations required for activation in the presence of hormone, converted 90% of the receptors to a state with a higher K_D than K_{act}; the remaining 10% displayed both the kinetic and thermodynamic properties commensurate with hormonal activation of the enzyme. A similar distribution of glucagon receptor states is seen in intact hepatocytes [26] which presumably contain sufficient GTP to interact with N_s at the internal face of the cell membrane. A plausible explanation for the opposing effects of GTP on K_{act} and K_D is the following set of reactions (modified from ref. [27]):

(i) $H + R \cdot N \rightleftharpoons H \cdot R \cdot N^*$
(ii) $H \cdot R \cdot N^* + GTP \rightleftharpoons H \cdot R \cdot N \cdot GTP \rightleftharpoons H + R \cdot N \cdot GTP$
(iii) $H \cdot R \cdot N \cdot GTP + C \rightleftharpoons H \cdot R \cdot \underset{\substack{\cdot \\ GTP}}{N} \cdot C$ (active holoenzyme),

in which hormone [H] binding to RN promotes interaction of N with GTP (ii); at this step the negative heterotropic effects of GTP on hormone binding occurs. Preferential interaction of the transient quaternary complex [RN occupied by both GTP and hormone] with C results in formation of the holoenzyme complex (iii); this structure is presumed to display the positive heterotropic effects of GTP on K_{act} of glucagon and vice versa. In this "uncoupled" equilibrium model, the final concentration of the activated holoenzyme is a function of the relative concentrations both of the macromolecular components [R, N, C] and the small ligands (hormones and GTP). In the overall equilibrium, all RN complexes are involved in activation of C but the amount of RNC formed is limited by the concentration of C. In the case of the liver system, the latter may be 10% or less of R and N.

Studies of the beta-adrenergic receptor have contributed supportive evidence for the above reaction scheme. For example, agonists but not antagonists promote the negative heterotropic effects of GTP on catecholamine binding [28–32]. This is consistent with an ordered reaction in which hormones promote interaction of N in the RN complex with GTP. Evidence that the negative heterotropic effects derive from the RN complex rather than the holoenzyme stems from findings that cells lacking C but containing N_s and R display negative heterotropic effects of GTP on hormone binding [20]. Furthermore, RN complexes have been isolated following detergent extraction of membranes and separation from C (or NC); such complexes show the same negative heterotropic effects of GTP seen in the intact membrane [33, 34]. As an indication of the importance of the RN complex in hormone and GTP action, it has been noted [35] that cyclase systems showing high ratios of hormone activation to hormone binding (so-called "tightly-coupled" systems) are those which display marked negative heterotropic effects of GTP on agonist binding. Finally, as evidence that the same N_s is associated with R and C, extracts containing the same factors that restore guanine nucleotide, hormone, and fluoride stimulation of C restore the ability of GTP to affect agonist binding to R in cell membranes of mutants lacking N_s [32]. Identity is also suggested from studies showing that cholera toxin affects GTP action both on hormone binding and cyclase activity [13].

It is evident from the above that R units not associated with N units are non-functional with respect to adenylate cyclase activation by hormones. Free R units in membranes have a lower affinity for agonists than RN units (when unreacted with GTP) [28]. Perhaps R when unassociated with N is destined for endocytotic removal, as seems to be the case for a number of external membrane receptors [36, 37].

Table 2 lists receptors reported to show negative heterotropic effects of GTP on hormone binding and which are presumed, therefore, to represent RN complexes. Note that they distribute into three categories: those which are involved in stimulation of adenylate cyclase (RN_s), those known to mediate inhibition of cyclase (RN_i) in the membranes

Table 2
Hormone receptors regulated by GTP (the RN complex)[a)]

Receptor type	Source	Type of N unit[b)]	Comments	Selected refs.[c)]
Glucagon	Rat liver	N_s	GTP=GDP; Gpp(NH)p; and Gpp$(CH)_2$p less potent	1)
Catecholamines (beta receptors)	Several cell types	N_s	Divalent cations promote binding of agonists; only agonist binding affected	2)
Prostaglandin E	Thyroid, frog erythrocyte	N_s	Binding promoted by calcium ions	3)
Dopamine	Corpus striatum	N_s, N_x	GTP=GDP>Gpp(NH)p; agonist specific	4)
Muscarinic	Canine and rat myocardium	N_i	Methacholine inhibits GTP effects on beta receptor; Na^+ probably affects binding	5)
	Neuroblastoma *x* glioma cells	N_i	Mg^{2+} enhances agonist binding	6)
Catecholamines (alpha-receptors)	Brain	N_x	GTP=Gpp(NH)p>GDP; Na^+ affects agonist binding	7)
	Rat liver	N_x	Agonist specific	8)
Angiotensin	Adrenal cortex	N_x	Agonist binding affected by Na^+ in same manner as by GTP	9)
Opiates	Brain	N_x	Na^+ affects binding of agonists and antagonists. Two distinct opiate receptors	10)

a) In all cases addition of guanine nucleotides decreases binding of hormone or neurotransmitter to specific receptors in isolated membrane preparations.
b) N_s is N unit linked to stimulation of adenylate cyclase; N_i affects inhibition of the enzyme; N_x is an N unit that is either not related to cyclase activity or has an undetermined relationship to a specific signal-processing system in the cell membrane.
c) 1) = ref. [24], 2) = [28–32], 3) = [92, 93], 4) = [94–95], 5) = [96, 97], 6) = [99], 7) = [100, 101], 8) = [102], 9) = [78], 10) = [50, 98, 103].

investigated, and those (RN_x) to which a specific function either has not been assigned and/or the receptor is known not to be involved with cyclase.

3. Role of RN_i in inhibition of adenylate cyclase by neurotransmitters and GTP

In addition to its activating role, GTP inhibits adenylate cyclase systems. First observed [38] and characterized [39–42] in rat adipocyte membranes, inhibitory effects have been noted in other cell types [43, 44]. The GTP-inhibitory process (N_i) resembles N_s in that it requires a nucleotide triphosphate and is seen with Gpp(N)p, indicating that neither production of GDP nor phosphorylation is mechanistically involved. Recent studies [45–47] indicate that the resemblance to N_s ends there. For example, adenosine promotes inhibition whereas a different set of hormones or neurotransmitters promote activation by GTP. Moreover, the GTP-inhibitory process is selectively affected by sulfhydryl agents and by proteolytic enzymes. The close functional linkage between the adenosine receptor (R-site [48]) and N_i in the adipocyte suggests that, as with RN_s, there is an RN_i complex for adenosine in fat cells. It appears that RN_i and RN_s complexes in the fat cell interact with a common C unit [47] indicating that cyclase activity is governed by independent GTP-regulatory components linked to different sets of receptors for hormones and adenosine. Receptors for such neurotransmitters as opiates, dopamine, catecholamines (alpha), and cholinergic agents (muscarinic) also mediate inhibition of adenylate cyclase by a GTP-dependent process [49–52], suggesting that the linkage of neurotransmitter receptors to N_i may be widespread. In the few cases examined, the GTP-dependency of cyclase inhibition correlates with negative heterotropic effects of GTP on agonist binding (table 2), suggesting that RN_i complexes are involved in the inhibitory process by analogy with the role of RN_s complexes in the stimulation of adenylate cyclase. Note that in table 2 sodium ion exerts marked effects on the binding of neurotransmitters to receptors involved in inhibition of adenylate cyclase; RN_s complexes are not similarly affected by sodium ions.

4. The structure of RN

The information gathered above suggests that the various RN units are the regulatory complexes responsible for hormone or neurotransmitter and GTP-regulation of adenylate cyclase. What are the structures of these complexes before and after association with the enzyme and the small ligands (hormones and guanine nucleotide)? This problem has been addressed recently with the use of the technique of target size analysis (for its application and theory see reference [53]). Results obtained from target analysis of adenylate cyclase systems in liver [54], adipocytes [55], and turkey erythrocyte membranes (unpublished) are shown in table 3. In the liver system, the minimal size unit expressing activity is that obtained with MnATP as substrate and no activating ligands; it is presumed to represent C. The functional size increases

Table 3
Functional sizes of adenylate cyclase components[a)]

Enzyme source	Components				
	RN_s	C	N_sC	RN_sC	RN_i
	$\times 10^5$ Daltons				
Rat liver: R = glucagon	6–13[b)]	1.5	2.3	3.5	–
Fat cell (rat) R = catecholamine, ACTH	13	[d)]	2.3	[d)]	> 13
Turkey erythrocyte R = cathecholamine	N.D.[c)]	[d)]	[d)]	3.5	–

[a)]Sizes were determined by Target Size Analysis using high energy irradiation. See reference [54] for methods for determining size and rationale for assigning components to size. Data for fat cell in reference [55]; turkey erythrocyte data are unpublished.
[b)]Estimated both from GTP-sensitive glucagon binding and from adenylate cyclase activity of "ground-state" enzyme.
[c)]N.D. = not detected.
[d)]Not determined.

significantly with preactivation by Gpp(NH)p or fluoride ion (N_sC). Activation by glucagon and GTP, which should reflect the holoenzyme (RNC), is accompanied by a further increment in size commensurate with this premise. The sizes of the regulatory complexes (RN_s) were estimated from studies of the binding of labeled glucagon in the presence of GTP and from the "ground-state" cyclase activity; i.e. the size of components present before coupling. Both studies indicate that the RN_s in the liver ranges in size from $6–13 \times 10^5$ Daltons or from 3 to 6 times the estimated size of the RN unit associated with the holoenzyme. The conclusion from these findings is that RN_s exists in multimers prior to linkage to the C unit. The unit (presumably RN_i) through which adenosine and GTP inhibit the adipocyte cyclase enzyme (determined under conditions in which GTP is inhibitory) is significantly larger in size than the RN_s unit that mediates the effects of stimulatory hormones and GTP in the adipocyte. Although target analysis cannot give the structure and composition of the target, it can be inferred from the size differences that the stimulatory and inhibitory processes reflect different structures which are multimers of the units comprising the holoenzyme.

Preliminary findings with the turkey erythrocyte cyclase system indicate the surprising result that the multimer unit is not detected; i.e. the functional size remains identical before and after activation with catecholamines and guanine nucleotides; it approximates that of the hormone-GTP activated holoenzyme observed in liver membranes. Existence of a precoupled RNC unit in the turkey erythrocyte membrane is consistent with the report [56] that there is a stoichiometric (rather than hyperbolic) relationship between hormone activation and receptor occupation in this system.

5. A model for hormone and GTP action on adenylate cyclase

The existence of multimer complexes of RN provides a structural basis for the uncoupled equilibrium reactions described above. Assuming that the multimer complex of RN cannot react with C unless dispersed to monomers, the reaction scheme translates in simplified form to the following sequence:

$$
\begin{array}{ccccccc}
(\mathrm{R}\cdot\mathrm{N})^{p} & \xrightarrow{\mathrm{H}} & (\mathrm{H}\cdot\mathrm{R}\cdot\mathrm{N})^{p} & \xrightarrow{\mathrm{GTP}} & p(\mathrm{H}\cdot\mathrm{R}\cdot\mathrm{N}\cdot\mathrm{GTP}) & \xrightarrow{\mathrm{C}} & \mathrm{H}\cdot\mathrm{R}\cdot\overset{\mathrm{GTP}}{\dot{\mathrm{N}}}\cdot\mathrm{C}_{\mathrm{active}} \\
\uparrow & & & & & & \downarrow \\
\llcorner & \xleftarrow{\quad ? \quad} & & \longleftarrow & & \longleftarrow & \mathrm{H}\cdot\mathrm{R}\cdot\overset{\mathrm{GDP}}{\dot{\mathrm{N}}}\cdot\mathrm{C}_{\mathrm{inh.}} + \mathrm{P}_{\mathrm{i}}
\end{array}
$$

in which the hormone promotes changes in N (designated by N*) that facilitate the ability of GTP to react with and disperse the multimeric structure; the resultant monomer complex interacts with C to yield the activated holoenzyme. In broad terms, this "disaggregation" model for hormone and GTP action can be likened to the manner by which cyclic AMP controls, through its receptor, the activity of protein kinase; the latter involves a change in the association of dimeric regulatory and catalytic subunits [57]. In the case of hormone receptors associated with adenylate cyclase systems, their interaction with N units constrains the ability of the latter to react with GTP, thus preventing the formation of the "active" form of the regulatory unit (N_s^* or N_i^*). It follows that cyclase systems devoid of receptors linked to N should display high reactivity with GTP. This has been reported recently [58] with a strain of Hela cells deficient in beta-adrenergic receptors; when the same cells become enriched with these receptors, GTP-stimulation decreases and the addition of catecholamines is required to restore the level of activity seen with GTP alone in receptor-deficient cells.

The model predicts a non-linear relationship between receptor occupation and activation of adenylate cyclase since N is an intermediate in the overall process. The degree of non-linearity ("tight" versus "loose" coupling) is a function of p (the number of N units in the multimer) and, if there are homologous subunit interactions, in the extent of cooperativity of hormone binding to the multimer. Thus, amplification of the hormone–receptor interaction is an important and natural consequence of the aggregate form of the RN complex.

Incorporated in the model is a GTPase associated with formation of the active holoenzyme [14, 59] and which accounts for the so-called "turn-off" reaction that occurs with GTP but not with non-hydrolyzable analogues of the nucleotide [60, 61]. The latter form stable complexes that sustain the activated state [62, 63]. Hydrolysis of GTP to GDP at the activation site leads to a stable inhibited state of the holoenzyme [64]. At saturating concentrations of the activating ligands (hormone and GTP), relief of this inhibited "rigor" state of the holoenzyme is likely to be a rate-limiting step in the overall reaction scheme; i.e. restoration of the RN complex – presumably released from the inhibited GDP occupied holoenzyme – to the multimer is a key step in maintaining the enzyme in its activated form at steady state. Possibly, separate factors control the latter step(s). There is suggestive evidence of a second site that binds guanine nucleotides (GTP, GDP, or GMP) and which affects both the binding of hormones to receptors [27, 65] and the release of bound nucleotides at the nucleotide activation site on N_s [64–66]. Additionally, there are several reports [67–71] of cytosolic factors (other than GTP) that affect the activity and response of adenylate cyclase to hormones.

The assembly of RN complexes as multimers suggests that R and N components may be concentrated in domains on the outer and inner aspects, respectively, of the cell membrane. Such structures may have logistic advantages over randomly-dispersed (or "floating") receptors, particularly if the RN multimer and C are in common domains (as depicted in fig. 1) within the lipid matrix of the membrane. Support for this possibility comes from studies [72–73] with phospholipases that destroy the lipid matrix. Hormone action on cyclase remains intact even after 85% of the lipid matrix is destroyed; steep losses in hormone response occurs when a fraction of the remaining phospholipids is hydrolyzed. These findings can be accommodated by having RN multimers and C contained in a selective domain of interacting phospholipids and possibly other proteins [74] that effectively shield against phospholipase-destruction of the structurally-bound lipids.

Finally, the possibility can be considered that, in addition to the quaternary structure of the multimer complex, higher orders of structural complexity may stabilize the multimer structure in its domain and control its dispersion and interaction with C. Among the higher orders of structure for consideration are cytoskeletal elements that indirectly or directly associate with the cell membrane [75]. It is of interest that agents that disrupt cytoskeletal structures have been reported to enhance cellular production of cyclic AMP in response to hormones [76, 77].

6. Generalization and problems

To the extent that the multireceptor adenylate cyclase system in adipocytes displays evidence of multimers of RN_s and RN_i, the theory may have general applications to the actions of hormones. Critical assessment of the multimeric structures determined by target analysis must await independent biochemical analysis. If the postulated dispersion of multimers to monomers is the basis of the negative heterotropic effects of GTP (or GDP) on hormone binding, such effects of the nucleotide may be a useful means of probing the existence of multimeric structures. However, in view of the findings that more than one type of N unit (in the functional sense) mediates the actions of hormones, there are other interesting problems to be considered.

Note that in table 2 GTP affects the binding of agonists to receptors for angiotensin [78] and catecholamines (alpha-receptors in liver) [80] that do not affect cyclic AMP production in the particular target cells examined. These findings suggest that GTP affects (through N_x) receptors coupled to membrane transduction processes other than adenylate cyclase. Thus, the generalization that GTP acts on adenylate cyclase through N_s and N_i may be extended to a broader role of GTP and of the N units responsible for whatever primary effects catecholamines and angiotensin may have on their target cells. Assuming that N_s, N_i, and N_x are separate proteins, what determines whether a particular type of receptor is linked to these regulatory proteins?

There are hints that a given receptor can interact with each type of N unit. For example, it has been reported that catecholamines, acting through alpha-adrenergic receptors, both stimulate [80] and inhibit [49, 52] cyclic AMP production, and induce effects unrelated to adenylate cyclase activity [79]. Similar examples of the same hormone exerting multiple effects on membrane processes include adenosine [46, 48], dopamine [51, 81–83], opiates [84, 86], vasopressin [87, 88], and serotonin [89]. What are the variable elements–receptors, N units, or both? It is doubtful that pharmacological studies (specificity, potency, antagonist, or hormone binding to receptors) can uniquely resolve this question. Heterotropic effects of GTP on agonist binding have the merit of indicating that the receptor is linked to an N unit but does not distinguish the type of N unit. I have noted in table 2 that certain RN complexes are affected by sodium ions, others by divalent cations, and that guanine nucleotides have different potencies on agonist binding. Perhaps such differences can be used to classify the N unit associated with the receptor. Even the testing of biological effects is not necessarily the means of determining the type of RN unit. A bizarre example of problems encountered is the action of cholecystokinin on pancreatic acinar cells [90]. In the cell, the hormone stimulates zymogen secretion, calcium release, and cyclic GMP production, but not the production of cyclic AMP; after breakage of the cell, the hormone stimulates adenylate cyclase in a GTP-dependent fashion. Although other explanations are possible, these findings raise the possibility that "redistribution" of receptors and N units occurs upon cell breakage owing to the breakdown of stationary domains that normally segregate these units in the cell. "Lateral domain redistribution" might be a physiologically regulated process due either to changes in the structural relationship of the cytoskeleton to the ordered domains or to propagated disturbances in the membrane structure. A possible example of the latter is the report [91] that catecholamines, acting through a beta-adrenergic receptor, stimulate a phospholipid methylating enzyme by a process affected by GTP but which does not involve the production of cyclic AMP; associated with methylation is an apparent "flip" of the internally methylated lipids to the outer face of the membrane and a change in lipid microviscosity. Pleitropic effects of the hormone could thus be generated by localized changes in lipid structure being propagated laterally and modifying the postulated domain structures of the membrane. In any event, these findings overthrow the commonly held view that beta-adrenergic receptors are uniquely linked to stimulation of adenylate cyclase. Moreover, the dependency of the hormone effect on GTP suggests again the versatility of the N units in mediating the actions of hormones.

In conclusion, by introducing a new theory of hormone action I have raised a number of questions relating to fundamental problems in the receptor field. The constraining role of hormone receptors postulated here differs from the role of the receptor postulated in other theories of hormone action. More importantly, the theory places in perspective the role of another set of regulatory proteins (the N units) hitherto given relatively scant attention, particularly with regard to their apparent multiple and fundamental roles in the regulation of membrane-associated processes. Hopefully, this rather brief article will stimulate investigation of the new problems to be faced in ascertaining the structures and functions of the GTP-regulatory proteins, and how these units are involved in the transduction of hormone binding at cell membrane receptors into physiological action.

References

[1] M. Rodbell, in: Molecular Biology and Pharmacology of Cyclic Nucleotides, eds. G. Folco and R. Paoletti (Elsevier, Amsterdam, 1978) pp. 1–12.
[2] M. Rodbell, L. Birnbaumer, S. L. Pohl and H. M. J. Krans, J. Biol. Chem. 246 (1971) 1877.
[3] M. Rodbell, M. C. Lin, Y. Salomon, C. Londos, J. P. Harwood, B. R. Martin, M. Rendell and M. Berman, Adv. Cyclic Nucleotide Res. 5 (1975) 3.
[4] J. P. Perkins, Adv. Cyclic Nucleotide Res. 3 (1973) 1.
[5] T. Pfeuffer, J. Biol. Chem. 252 (1977) 7224.
[6] T. Pfeuffer, FEBS Lett. 101 (1979) 85.
[7] R. A. Finkelstein, Crit. Rev. Microbiol. 2 (1973) 553.
[8] D. M. Gill, Adv. Cyclic Nucleotide Res. 8 (1977) 85.
[9] G. L. Johnson and H. R. Bourne, Biochem. Biophys. Res. Comm. 78 (1977) 792.
[10] J. Fischer and G. W. G. Sharp, Biochem. J. 176 (1978) 505.
[11] D. Cassel and Z. Selinger, Proc Natn. Acad. Sci. USA 74 (1977) 3307.
[12] S. L. Levinson and A. J. Blume, J. Biol. Chem. 252 (1977) 3766.
[13] M. C. Lin, A. F. Welton and M. F. Berman, J. Cyclic Nucleotide Res. 4 (1978) 159.
[14] D. Cassel and Z. Selinger, Biochim. Biophys. Acta 452 (1978) 538.
[15] D. M. Gill and R. Meren, Proc. Natn. Acad. Sci. USA 75 (1978) 3050.
[16] D. Cassel and T. Pfeuffer, Proc. Natn. Acad. Sci. USA 75 (1978) 2669.
[17] G. L. Johnson, H. R. Kaslow and H. R. Bourne, Proc. Natn. Acad. Sci. USA 75 (1978) 3113.
[18] G. L. Johnson, H. R. Kaslow and H. R. Bourne, J. Biol. Chem. 253 (1978) 7120.
[19] E. M. Ross, A. C. Howlett, K. M. Ferguson and A. G. Gilman, J. Biol. Chem. 253 (1978) 6401.
[20] A. C. Howlett, P. C. Sternweiss, B. A. Macik, P. M. Van Arsdale and A. G. Gilman, J. Biol. Chem. 254 (1979) 2287.
[21] C. Londos, P. M. Lad, T. B. Nielsen and M. Rodbell, J. Supermol. Struct. 10 (1979) 1031.
[22] T. Nielsen, P. M. Lad and M. Rodbell, J. Biol. Chem. (1979) in press.
[23] M. Rodbell, H. M. J. Krans, S. L. Pohl. and L. Birnbaumer, J. Biol. Chem. 246 (1971) 1872.
[24] M. Rodbell, M. C. Lin and Y. Salomon, J. Biol. Chem. 249 (1974) 59.
[25] M. C. Lin, S. Nicosia and M. Rodbell, Biochemistry 15 (1976) 4537.
[26] O. Sonne, T. Berg and T. Christoffersen, J. Biol. Chem. 253 (1978) 3203.
[27] P. M. Lad, A. F. Welton and M. Rodbell, J. Biol. Chem. 252 (1977) 5942.
[28] M. E. Maguire, P. M. Van Arsdale and A. G. Gilman, Mol. Pharmacol. 12 (1976) 335.

[29] E. M. Ross, M. E. Maguire, T. W. Sturgill, R. L. Biltonen and A. G. Gilman, J. Biol. Chem. 252 (1977) 5761.
[30] L. T. Williams and R. J. Lefkowitz, J. Biol. Chem. 252 (1977) 7207.
[31] R. J. Lefkowitz and L. T. Williams, Adv. Cyclic Nucleotide Res. 9 (1978) 1.
[32] P. C. Sternweiss and A. G. Gilman, J. Biol. Chem. 254 (1979) 3333.
[33] A. F. Welton, P. M. Lad, A. C. Newby, H. Yamamura, S. Nicosia and M. Rodbell, J. Biol. Chem. 252 (1977) 5947.
[34] L. E. Limbird and R. J. Lefkowitz, Proc. Nat. Acad. Sci. USA 75 (1978) 228.
[35] M. E. Maguire, E. M. Ross and A. G. Gilman, Adv. Cyclic Nucleotide Res. 8 (1977) 1.
[36] K. J. Catt, J. P. Harwood, G. Aquilera and M. L. Dufau, Nature 280 (1979) 109.
[37] J. L. Goldstein, R. G. W. Anderson and M. S. Brown, Nature 279 (1979) 679.
[38] P. E. Cryer, L. Jarett and D. Kipnis, Biochim. Biophys. Acta 177 (1969) 586.
[39] J. P. Harwood, H. Löw and M. Rodbell, J. Biol. Chem. 248 (1973) 6239.
[40] M. Rodbell, J. Biol. Chem. 250 (1975) 5826.
[41] J. Pairault, Eur. J. Biochem. 62 (1976) 323.
[42] R. Ebert and U. Schwabe, Naunyn-Schmiedberg's Arch. Pharmacol. 286 (1974) 297.
[43] L. Birnbaumer, T. Nakahara and P. Yang, J. Biol. Chem. 249 (1974) 7857.
[44] N. Narayanan and P. V. Sulakhe, Arch. Biochem. Biophys. 185 (1978) 72.
[45] H. Yamamura, P. M. Lad and M. Rodbell, J. Biol. Chem. 252 (1977) 7964.
[46] C. Londos, D. M. F. Cooper, W. Schlegel and M. Rodbell, Proc. Natn. Acad. Sci. USA 75 (1978) 5362.
[47] D. M. F. Cooper, W. Schlegel and M. Rodbell, J. Biol. Chem. (1979) in press.
[48] C. Londos and J. Wolff, Proc. Natn. Acad. Sci. USA 74 (1977) 5482.
[49] S. L. Sabol and M. Nirenberg, J. Biol. Chem. 254 (1979) 1913.
[50] A. J. Blume, D. Lichtshtein and G. Boone, Proc. Natn. Acad. Sci. USA (1979) in press.
[51] P. DeCamilli, D. Macconi and A. Spada, Nature 278 (1979) 252.
[52] K. H. Jacobs, in: Molecular Biology and Pharmacology of Cyclic Nucleotides, eds. G. Folci and R. Paoletti (Elsevier, Amsterdam, 1978) pp. 265–278.
[53] E. S. Kempner and W. Schlegel, Anal. Biochem. 92 (1979) 2.
[54] W. Schlegel, E. S. Kempner and M. Rodbell, J. Biol. Chem. 254 (1979) 5168.
[55] W. Schlegel, D. M. Cooper and M. Rodbell, J. Biol. Chem. (1979) in press.
[56] E. M. Brown, S. A. Fedak, C. J. Woodward, G. D. Aurbach and D. Rodbard, J. Biol. Chem. 251 (1976) 1239.
[57] H. G. Nimino and P. Cohen, Adv. Cyclic Nucleotide Res. 8 (1977) 145.
[58] M. C. Lin, C.-S. Lin and J. P. Whitlock, Jr., J. Biol. Chem. 254 (1979) 4684.
[59] M. Rendell, M. Rodbell and M. Berman, J. Biol. Chem. 252 (1977) 7909.
[60] D. Cassel, H. Levkovitz and Z. Selinger, J. Cyclic Nucleotide Res. 3 (1977) 393.
[61] D. Cassel and Z. Selinger, Biochem. Biophys. Res. Comm. 77 (1977) 868.
[62] M. Schramm and M. Rodbell, J. Biol. Chem. 250 (1975) 2232.
[63] C. Londos, Y. Salomon, M. C. Lin, J. P. Harwood, M. Schramm, J. Wolff and M. Rodbell, Proc. Natn. Acad. Sci. USA 71 (1974) 3087.
[64] D. Cassel and Z. Selinger, Proc. Natn. Acad. Sci. USA 75 (1978) 4155.
[65] A. F. Welton, P. M. Lad, A. C. Newby, H. Yamamura, S. Nicosia and M. Rodbell, J. Biol. Chem. 252 (1977) 5947.
[66] T. Pfeuffer and E. J. M. Helmreich, J. Biol. Chem. 250 (1975) 867.

[67] C. O. Brostrom, Y. Huang, B. McL. Breckenridge and D. J. Wolff, Proc. Natn. Acad. Sci. USA 72 (1975) 64.
[68] J. Moss and M. Vaughan, Proc. Natn. Acad. Sci. USA 74 (1977) 4396.
[69] F. Pecker and J. Hanoune, J. Biol. Chem. 252 (1977) 2784.
[70] J. J. Egan, R. J. Majeska and G. A. Rodan, Biochem. Biophys. Res. Comm. 80 (1978) 176.
[71] M. S. Katz, T. M. Kelly, M. A. Pineyro and R. I. Gregerman, J. Cyclic Nucleotide Res. 5 (1978) 389.
[72] B. Rubalcava and M. Rodbell, J. Biol. Chem. 248 (1973) 3831.
[73] P. M. Lad, S. Preston, A. F. Welton, T. B. Nielsen and M. Rodbell, Biochim. Biophys. Acta 551 (1979) 368.
[74] A. F. Welton, P. M. Lad, A. C. Newby, H. Yamamura, S. Nicosia and M. Rodbell, Biochim. Biophys. Acta 522 (1978) 625.
[75] G. M. Edelman, Science 197 (1976) 218.
[76] P. A. Insel and M. J. Kennedy, Nature 273 (1978) 471.
[77] S. A. Rudolf, P. Greengard and S. E. Malawista, Proc. Natn. Acad. Sci. USA 74 (1977) 3404.
[78] H. Glossman, A. Baukal and K. J. Catt, J. Biol. Chem. 249 (1974) 664.
[79] P. F. Blackmore, F. T. Brumby, J. L. Marks and J. H. Exton, J. Biol. Chem. 253 (1978) 4851.
[80] T. M. Chan and J. H. Exton, J. Biol. Chem. 252 (1977) 8645.
[81] J. W. Kebabian and D. B. Calne, Nature 277 (1979) 93.
[82] J. W. Kebabian, G. L. Petzold and P. Greengard, Proc. Natn. Acad. Sci. USA 69 (1972) 2145.
[83] P. F. Spano, S. Govoni and M. Trabucchi, Adv. Biochem. Psychopharmac. 19 (1977) 155.
[84] R. G. Van Inwegen, S. J. Strada and G. A. Robison, Life Sci. 16 (1975) 1875.
[85] S. K. Puri, J. Cochin and L. Volicer, Life Sci. 16 (1975) 759.
[86] D. H. Clouet and H. Iwatsubo, Life Sci. 17 (1975) 35.
[87] S. Jard and J. Bockaert, Physiol. Rev. 55 (1975) 489.
[88] C. S. Kirk and D. A. Hems, FEBS Lett. 47 (1974) 128.
[89] J. Macdermot, H. Higashida, S. P. Wilson, H. Matsuzawa, J. Minna and M. Nirenberg, Proc. Natn. Acad. Sci. USA 76 (1979) 1135.
[90] J. D. Gardner, Ann. Rev. Physiol. 41 (1979) 55.
[91] F. Hirata, W. J. Strittmatter and J. Axelrod, Proc. Natn. Acad. Sci. USA 76 (1979) 368.
[92] W. V. Moore and J. Wolff, J. Biol. Chem. 248 (1973) 5705.
[93] R. J. Lefkowitz, D. Mullikin, C. L. Wood, T. B. Gorde and C. Mukherjee, J. Biol. Chem. 252 (1977) 5295.
[94] N. R. Zahniser and P. B. Molinoff, Nature 275 (1978) 453.
[95] I. Creese, T. Usdin and S. H. Snyder, Nature 278 (1978) 577.
[96] A. M. Watanabe, M. M. McConnaughey, R. A. Strawbridge, J. W. Fleming, L. R. Jones and H. R. Besche, Jr., J. Biol. Chem. 253 (1978) 4833.
[97] C. P. Berrie, N. J. M. Birdsall, A. S. V. Burgen and S. C. Hulme, Biochem. Biophys. Res. Comm. 87 (1979) 1000.
[98] C. B. Pert and D. Taylor, in: Endogenous & Exogenous Opiate Agonists and Antagonists, ed. E. L. Way (Pergamon Press, 1979) in press.

[99] A. J. Blume, G. Boone and D. Lichtshetein, in: Modulators, Mediators, and Specifiers in Brain Function, eds. Y. H. Erlich, J. Volavka, L. F. Davis and E. Brunngreben (Plenum Press, New York, 1979) pp. 163–173.

[100] D. C. U'Prichard and S. H. Snyder, J. Biol. Chem. 253 (1978) 3444.

[101] H. Glossman and P. Presek, Naunyn-Schmiedeberg's Arch. Pharmacol. 306 (1979) 67.

[102] M. F. El-Rafai, P. F. Blackman and J. H. Exton, J. Biol. Chem. 254 (1979) 4375.

[103] S. R. Childers and S. H. Snyder, Life Sci. 23 (1978) 759.

SEMINAR

ROLES OF CYCLIC NUCLEOTIDES IN SYNAPTIC TRANSMISSION

Joël BOCKAERT

Laboratoire de Physiologie Cellulaire,
Collège de France, 11 pl. Marcelin Berthelot,
75231 Paris, France

0. Introduction

Cyclic nucleotides (cyclic AMP and cyclic GMP) appear to be implicated in several physiological processes in neurons such as: neurotransmitter synthesis, microtubular function, and synaptic transmission (for a review see reference [1]). In this conference we will draw our attention to the role of cyclic AMP (cAMP) and cyclic GMP (cGMP) in synaptic transmission. Two major pathways of intercellular communication exist in multicellular organisms: the endocrine system and the nervous system.

In the endocrine system, specialized cells secrete hormones (1st messenger) which are carried in the bloodstream and influence the activity of other cells generally localized far from the secreting cells. In

R. Balian et al., eds.
Les Houches, Session XXXIII, 1979 – Membranes et Communication Intercellulaire / Membranes and Intercellular Communication

previous conferences, you have learned that two types of hormones do exist:

(1) The steroid hormones (sexual hormones, cortisone, . . .) which go into the cells and influence their activity.

(2) The peptide and amino acid-derived hormones which have their receptors outside the cell membranes. A great number of the latter influence their target cell activity by producing an intracellular compound "second messenger" which has been identified by Sutherland as being the cyclic AMP.

In the nervous system, cells (neurons) communicate by a mechanism called synaptic transmission. A neurotransmitter is released from one cell, goes through the tiny gap of the synaptic cleft (15×10^{-7} cm) and, by interacting with a receptor of the receiving cell, changes its electrical activity. Both in the endocrine and nervous systems, the communication between cells involves (1) release of molecules (messengers) and (2) modification of the target cell activity. In view of these similarities and assuming that nature has selected a minimal number of chemical processes to perform a similar pattern of activities, one can postulate that cyclic AMP plays an important role in synaptic transmission as it does in hormonal action. We will now summarize the different evidence for such a role.

1. Adenylate and guanylate cyclases in the nervous system

1.1. General characteristics

Original papers by Sutherland [2] on adenylate cyclase, the enzyme which catalyzes the formation of cyclic AMP from ATP, pointed out on the interest of this enzyme in brain biochemistry. With the activity (per mg protein) of liver homogenate set equal to unity (1 μmole cyclic AMP in 15 min at 30° C, table 1), it can be observed that the activity of cerebral cortex is much higher (activity 22) than that of any tissues studied (for example 4 for skeletal muscle; 2 for the kidney). The guanylate cyclase activity is also very high in the brain and especially in the cerebellum. Except for these high specific activities and the nature of receptors which are able to modulate their activity, the general characteristics of adenylate and guanylate cyclases are similar in the brain and other organs.

I shall recall that adenylate cyclase is mostly localized in the plasma membrane and we will see that in many instances it is possible to

Table 1
Distribution of adenyl cyclase in dog tissues

Tissue	Units per 100 g (wet wt)[a)]	Relative activity
Liver	11	1
Kidney	13	2
Intestinal muscle	11	2
Adipose tissue	0.53	2
Lung	23	3
Cardiac muscle	28	4
Skeletal muscle	32	4
Brain	91	22

[a)] 1 unit = 1 μmole cAMP/15 min mg protein from ref. [2].

demonstrate, in brain homogenates, a neurotransmitter stimulation of the enzyme in isolated membranes. On the contrary, guanylate cyclase is mostly found in soluble extracts. Attempts to demonstrate a neurotransmitter or hormonal effect on guanylate cyclase in cell-free preparations have been unsuccessful. This failure, together with the demonstration that extracellular calcium is required in order to raise cGMP in target tissues with neurotransmitter hormones, had led to the suggestion that these compounds increase cGMP by causing an influx of Ca^{++} into the cell.

1.2. Synaptic localization

In 1967, De Robertis et al. [3] found that when brain tissue was disrupted by homogenization and the resulting subcellular components were separated according to their density, those fractions containing the largest amount of nerve endings also showed the highest level of adenylate cyclase activity. This observation is interesting since these nerve endings contained fragments of membranes from both sides of the synaptic junction and hence represent the precise areas of the brain where nerve cells communicate.

2. Neurotransmitter receptors involved in adenylate or guanylate cyclase activation

If some neurotransmitters act on their target cell as some peptidic hormones do, they must be able to increase cAMP or cGMP in those cells. Dopamine, which is well known to be implicated in Parkinson's disease and possibly in schizophrenia, has been one of the most studied. This neurotransmitter increase cAMP in the sympathetic ganglia [4] as well as in brain slices or homogenates of several brain areas especially the striatum [5] (fig. 1). Other dopaminergic agonists such as apomorphine or LSD also activate a dopamine-sensitive adenylate cyclase whereas neuroleptics are competitive antagonists (fig. 1). Table 1 summarizes the effects of several neurotransmitters on adenylate or guanylate cyclases. Norepinephrine, serotonin, histamine, and adenosine all increase cAMP formation. Norepinephrine (NE) and histamine which both act on two receptors (α and β for NE and H_1 and H_2 for histamine), only stimulate cAMP formation by acting on one of these receptors β for NE and H_2 for histamine (table 2). For each of these receptors, classical antagonists block the formation of cAMP induced by agonists (table 2). As basal adenylate cyclase, neurotransmitter-sensi-

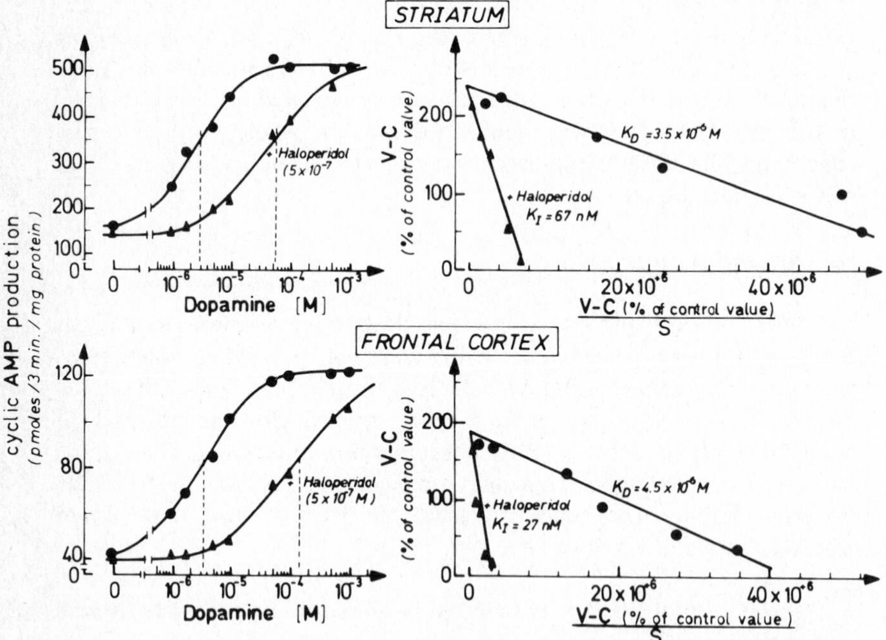

Fig. 1. Stimulation of adenylate cyclase from rat striatum and frontal cortex by dopamine and its competitive inhibition by the neuroleptic haloperidol. Left part: dose activation curve in the absence or the presence of a constant dose of haloperidol (5×10^{-7} M). Right part: Hofstee's plots of the dose-activation curves. In this plot the slope gives the apparent activation constant (taken from ref. [5]).

Table 2
Neurotransmitters and their relation to cyclic nucleotides

Neurotransmitters	Type of receptor	Evidence for mediation by a cyclic nucleotide		Drugs acting at the neurotransmitter receptor	
		Cyclic AMP	Cyclic GMP	Agonists	Antagonists
Dopamine (DA)	Dopamine	Yes	No	Dopamine Apomorphine LSD, . . .	Neuroleptics
Norepinephrine (NE)	α-adrenergic	No	No	NE, phenylephrine	Phentolamine
	β-adrenergic	Yes	No	NE, adrenaline, . . .	Propranolol
Serotonin	Serotonin	Yes	No	Serotonin, . . .	LSD, . . .
Histamine	H_1	No	Yes	Histamine, . . .	Diphenhydramine
	H_2	Yes	No	Histamine, . . .	Metiamide Imipramine (Antidepressant)
Acetylcholine	Muscarinic	No	Yes	Acetylcholine, . . .	Atropine
	Nicotinic	No	No	Acetylcholine	Hexamethonium
Adenosine	Adenosine	Yes	No	Adenosine	Theophylline

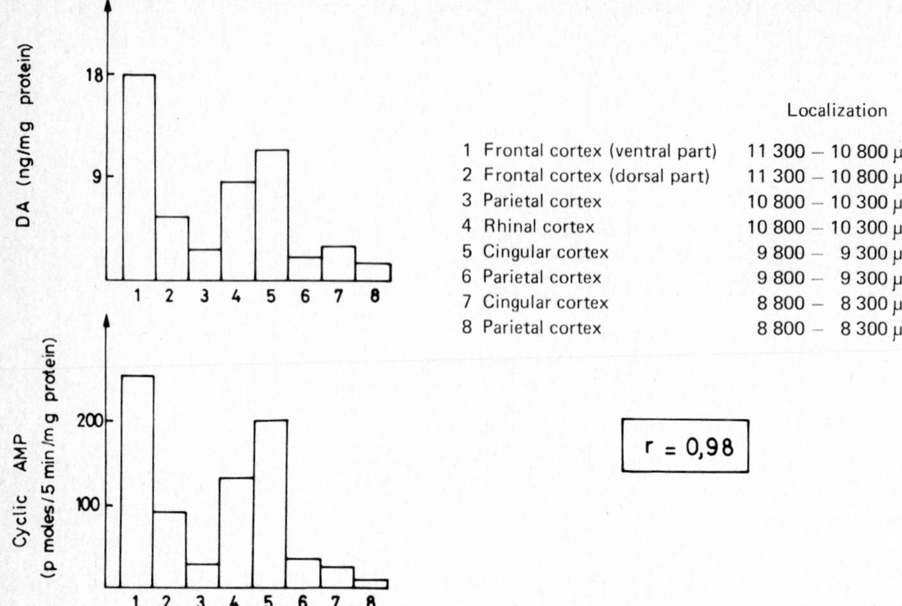

Fig. 2. Correlation between dopamine-sensitive adenylate cyclase and endogenous dopamine in the anterior cortex. The different areas of anterior cortex were dissected on frozen slices and both dopamine-sensitive adenylate cyclase and endogenous dopamine were measured on homogenates.

tive adenylate cyclases are localized at the synaptic level. Subcellular fractionation of striatum homogenates clearly indicates that dopamine [6] and adenosine-sensitive adenylate cyclases [7] are associated with synaptic membranes. For the dopamine-sensitive adenylate cyclase, it has been demonstrated that in the striatum, the enzyme is localized on postsynaptic cells whereas in the substantia nigra the same enzyme is localized presynaptically [8]. For both serotonin- and dopamine-sensitive adenylate cyclases, it has been demonstrated that their topographical distribution in several brain areas are in close correlation with topographical distributions of serotonin and dopamine terminals, respectively [9]. One example of such a correlation is shown in fig. 2. In taking together these findings the idea was strongly supported that neurotransmitter-sensitive adenylate cyclase are indeed part of the synaptic element and that cyclic AMP might mediate intracellular action of some neurotransmitter at certain synapses.

3. Biochemical characteristics and localization of enzymes implicated in the cAMP machinery

In addition to adenylate cyclase, three other enzymes are necessary to complete cAMP machinery, phosphodiesterase, protein–kinase, and phosphoprotein–phosphatase.

Phosphodiesterase localization in the brain has been studied both by subcellular fractionation and cytochemical procedure. Both methods indicate a synaptic localization. Futhermore, the cytochemical method localizes clearly phosphodiesterase on the postsynaptic membrane. Protein–kinase is also a key enzyme in cAMP machinery since it is the only enzyme which interacts directly with cAMP. Cyclic AMP is thought to interact with protein–kinase by binding to an inhibitory subunit of the kinase in such a way as to cause its dissociation from the catalytic component of the enzyme. The loss of the inhibitory subunit enhances the kinase activity which then phosphorylates its substrate. The phosphorylated substrate has different properties than the non-phosphorylated one (e.g., activated phosphorylase or lipase). In order to be reversible, the system needs to be dephosphorylated by a phosphoprotein–phosphatase. As adenylate cyclase and phosphodiesterase, cyclic AMP dependent protein–kinase and phosphoprotein–phosphatase are highly concentrated in synaptic membranes.

4. An hypothesis for the mechanism of action of cAMP in neurotransmission

It is known that a nerve cell responds to a neurotransmitter with a brief change in its membrane permeability to one or several ions. Depending on the nature of the ion which moves and the direction of the movement, the change in electrical potential induced by the neurotransmitter will make it more or less likely that the cell will reach the threshold of excitation necessary to induce an impulse. At a given time, one neuron can receive several messages and has to integrate them before knowing whether to fire or not.

The hypothesis put forward a few years ago by Greegard et al. [11] is that cAMP or cGMP, by interacting with a protein–kinase, will cause the phosphorylation of a membrane-bound protein implicated in ion-movement (fig. 3). The transfer of a phosphate group to such a protein could conceivably change the permeability of the membrane to ions, either directly by changing its configuration or indirectly by affecting

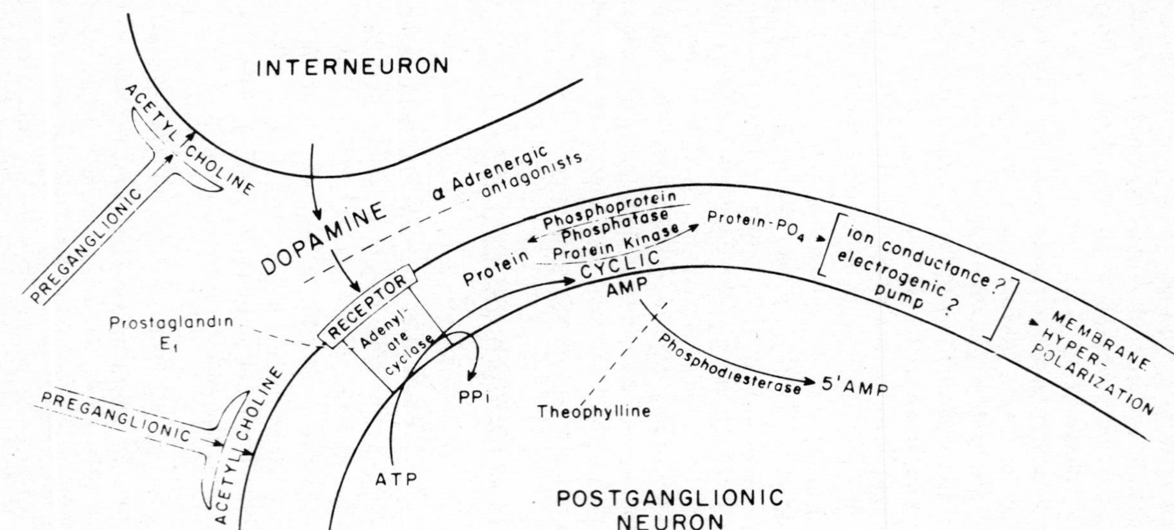

Fig. 3. Model proposed by Greengard et al. for the mechanism of action of cAMP at synaptic level (taken from ref. [11]).

the activity of a "pump" which can transfer ions across the membrane (fig. 3). This simple hypothesis is rather difficult to verify. However, a few years ago, the Greengard group started work on protein phosphorylation in relation to synaptic transmission. In brain homogenate, the subcellular fraction which has the greatest amount of substrate proteins for protein–kinase is the synaptic membrane. When synaptic membranes were incubated in a solution containing ATP $\gamma^{32}P$ in the presence or absence of cyclic AMP, they found that phosphorylation of only two of the numerous proteins in the membrane was greatly increased by cyclic AMP (protein I and II), see fig. 4 [12]. The mol wt of proteins I and II are 86 000 and 48 000, respectively. Subsequently, the same group found that protein I is composed of two subunits.

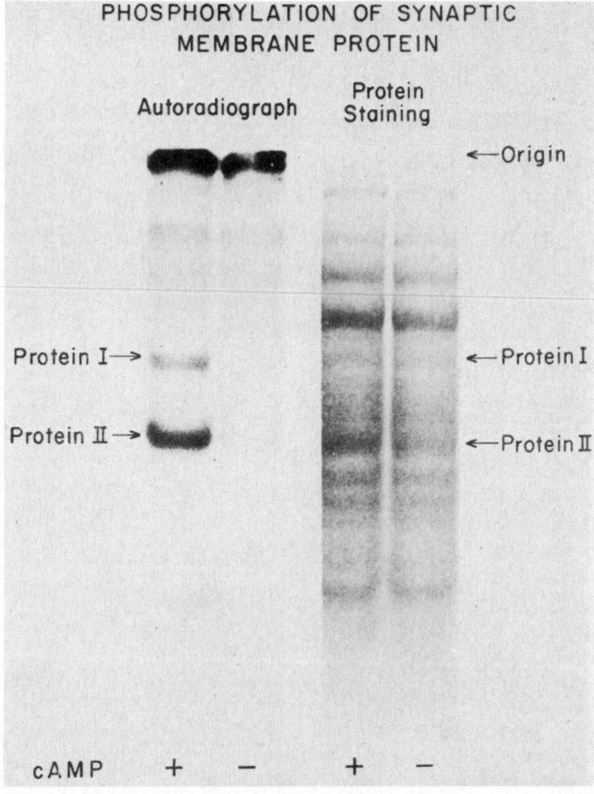

Fig. 4. Effect of cAMP on the endogenous phosphorylation of synaptic membranes preparation from rat cerebrum. Mol wt of protein I and protein II were 86 000 and 48 000, respectively (taken from ref. [12]).

In contrast with protein II, protein I was only found in tissues containing synapses whereas neuronal or non-neuronal tissues devoided of synapses did not contain protein I. Protein I is absent from the brain of foetal animals before the formation of connections between nerve cells. This protein has been purified to homogeneity and antibodies have been raised. Cytoimmunochemistry reveals that this protein is localized both pre- and postsynaptically. The physiological meaning of this finding is unknown. The phosphorylation of protein I is very rapid (less than 5 s). However, it is very difficult to know if the speed of this reaction is high enough to account for the change in ion permeability giving a rise in some slow postsynaptic potentials (few hundred milliseconds).

5. Electrophysiological evidence for a role of cyclic nucleotides in synaptic transmission

5.1. Effect of NE and cAMP on spontaneous firing of cerebellar Purkinje cells

A Purkinje cell is a classical cell of cerebellar cortex which has a great number of dendrites making 100 000 synapses with different afferent neurons. In particular it receives NE fibers from the locus coeruleus

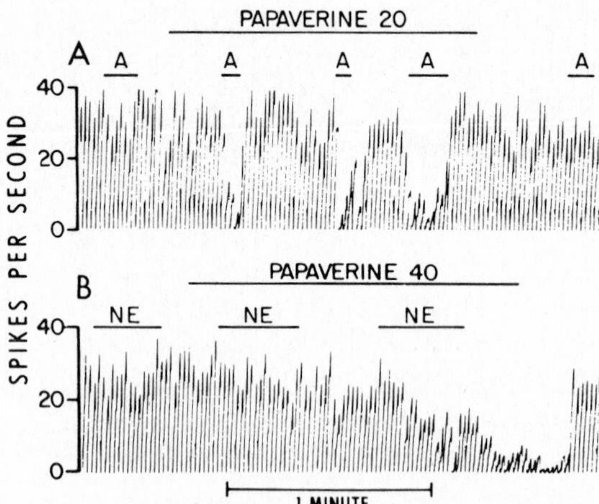

Fig. 5. Potentiation of microelectrophoretically administered cAMP (A) and NE by microelectrophoratic administration of papaverine. Numbers indicate duration of ejection (taken from ref. [13]).

(LC). The role of cAMP on the Purkinje cell has been studied by Hoffer et al. [13]. Microiontophoresis of NE reduces the spontaneous discharge of these cells. NE produces long pauses between single spikes. As expected stimulation of locus coeruleus produces a similar effect. The effects of NE and locus coeruleus stimulation are all blocked by a β-adrenergic antagonist propranolol. Microiontophoretic application of cAMP in the presence of papaverine, a known phosphodiesterase inhibitor, gives similar results than either NE iontophoresis or locus coeruleus stimulation (fig. 5). Furthermore, papaverine potentiate the NE effects (fig. 5). As expected if cAMP is the intracellular messenger of NE action on Purkinje cells, propranolol does not block cAMP action.

5.2. *Effect of cAMP and cGMP on the superior cervical ganglia*

5.2.1. *The work of Greengard et al. in the superior cervical ganglion of the rabbit*

The ganglion contains preganglionic cholinergic fibers whose perikarya lie in the spinal cord and make synapses with two kinds of neurons:

The postganglionic neurons sending axons in the peripheral organs.

Small interneurons, SIF cell (small intensely fluorescent) which contain catecholamines which could be either norepinephrine or DA- depending of the species considered.

Terminations on the postganglionic neurons: acetylcholine (ACh) released from preganglionic fibers interacts with either a nicotinic receptor (blocked by hexamethonium) generating fast excitatory postsynaptic potential (fEPSP) or a muscarinic receptor blocked by atropine and generating a slow excitatory postsynaptic potential (sEPSP).

Terminations on SIF cells: ACh can also interact with another muscarinic receptor localized on SIF cells. Following this interaction, DA which is released from SIF cells will cause the generation of a slow hyperpolarization on the postsynaptic neuron (sIPSP) fEPSP is very rapid (few ms), on the contrary, SIPSP and SEPSP can last for several seconds and thus cAMP and cGMP machinery can be involved.

Greengard et al. [10] have presented evidence that cAMP is involved in sIPSP:

(1) Stimulation of preganglionic fibers but not stimulation of postganglionic fibers increases cAMP in the ganglion.

(2) DA but not ACh increases cAMP in ganglion.

(3) The increase in cAMP following preganglionic stimulation, as sIPSP are blocked by either antimuscarinic or α-adrenergic blocking agents. Antimuscarinic agent blocks muscarinic receptor on SIF cells whereas α-adrenergic blocking agent blocks DA receptors on postganglionic cells.

(4) McAfee and Greengard [14] have shown that theophylline, a known inhibitor of phosphodiesterase, potentiates sIPSP triggered either by electrical stimulation or DA.

(5) Monobutyryl cAMP produces hyperpolarization.

Similar evidence has been provided by the same group for a role of cGMP in mediating sEPSP [14].

5.2.2. Discussion of the role of cAMP in mediating sIPSP

The possibility to produce sIPSP with monobutyl cAMP or theophylline has been questioned by several groups in particular by Libet et al. [15]. This group was not able to reproduce monobutyryl-cAMP experiments.

The theophylline effect was reproducible in their hand but possibly due to a non-specific effect of this agent. Indeed RO 201724, a new and potent phosphodiesterase inhibitor, did not enhance sIPSP [15].

On the contrary, Libet et al. found that sEPSP is enhanced both by RO 201724 and theophylline. They proposed that cAMP is not mediating sIPSP but is modulating sEPSP.

5.2.3. Modulation of sEPSP by cAMP

Kobayashi et al. [16] have shown that intracellular injection of cAMP enhances the sEPSP obtained by preganglionic stimulation for a time period of 2 h. This "facilitation" of the sEPSP is also obtained after conditioning stimulation of preganglionic nerve which is known to increase cAMP (fig. 6).

5.2.4. Discussion of the role of cGMP in mediating sEPSP

Hashigushi et al. [17] have recently reproduced the primary observation by McAfee and Greengard [14] that cGMP induces sEPSP in the superior cervical ganglia. This has been done by using intracellular recording.

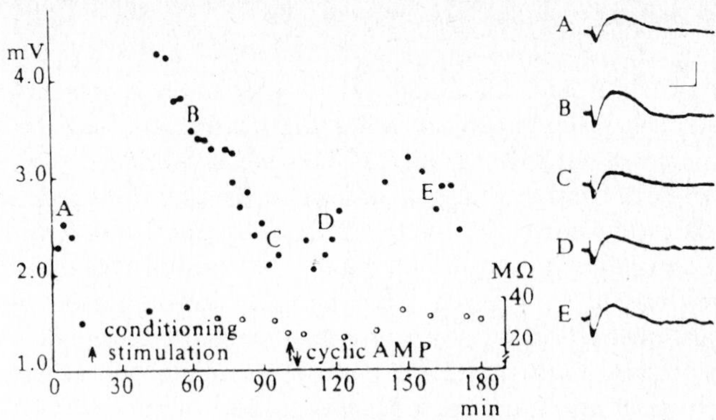

Fig. 6. Potentiation of sEPSP after conditioning stimulation of preganglionic nerve [(20/s) supramaximal for 1 min at the arrow] and after intracellular injection of cAMP (between arrow.) The resting potential was −52 mV. The resting membrane potential and resistance did not change. (Schematic representation of the data presented in ref. [16].)

In conclusion, there is an agreement to propose that cGMP induced sEPSP in the sympathic ganglia. On the contrary, the effect of cAMP on sIPSP is a subject of controversy. For Greengard's group cAMP mediates sIPSP for Libet's group cAMP potentiates sEPSP.

5.3. *Peptidic effect on neurons F_1 in Helix. Role of cyclic nucleotides*

F_1 neurons in parietal ganglia of Helix pomatia exhibit a characteristic "bursting" pattern of electrical activity in which an oscillating membrane potential gives rise to alternating periods of action potential bursts and interbursts hyperpolarization. Peptidic extracts as well as oxytocin and vasopressin produce an increase in the frequency of bursts and amplitude and duration of interburst hyperpolarization. Peptidic extracts, enhance cAMP and cGMP production in the ganglion. Their electrophysiological effects are reproduced by 8-benzyl-thio-cAMP which has been shown to increase both cAMP and cGMP (by inhibiting phosphodiesterases). Futhermore, after intraneural injection of Gpp(NH)p, which is known to stimulate irreversibly adenylate cyclase, there is a continue hyperpolarization of the neurons that last for hours. In this system it is proposed by Levitan [18] that an elevation in both cAMP and cGMP modifies the frequency of bursts whereas an elevation of cAMP alone induces an increase in hyperpolarization.

5.4. Role of cAMP in presynaptic facilitation

In aphysia californica, stimulation of the siphon leads to a withdrawal of the gill. This reflex is subject to habituation that is to say that stimuli are less and less efficious until a stable level is obtained (fig. 7). The reflex can be abruptly enhanced for several minutes if a single stimulus is applied to the head (fig. 7). It has been demonstrated by Kandel's group [19] that this is due to a presynaptic facilitation. Neurons coming from the head make synapses with nerve terminals coming from the siphon and increase the release of neurotransmitter from these terminals. This results in an increase in the postsynaptic potential recorded in L7. Both serotonin and cAMP can produce this facilitation. The

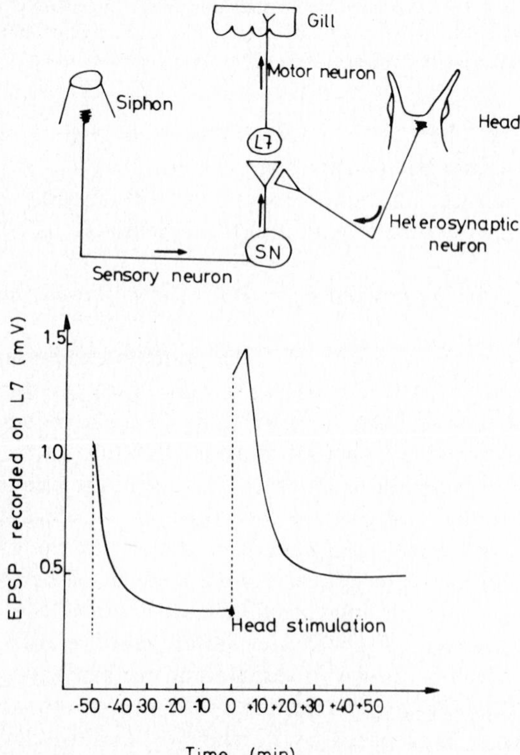

Fig. 7. Neuronal network of the gill reflex underlying habituation and facilitation (upper panel). Time-course of habituation (– 50 to 0 min) and facilitation (starting at time 0) by stimulation of the head (modified from ref. [19]).

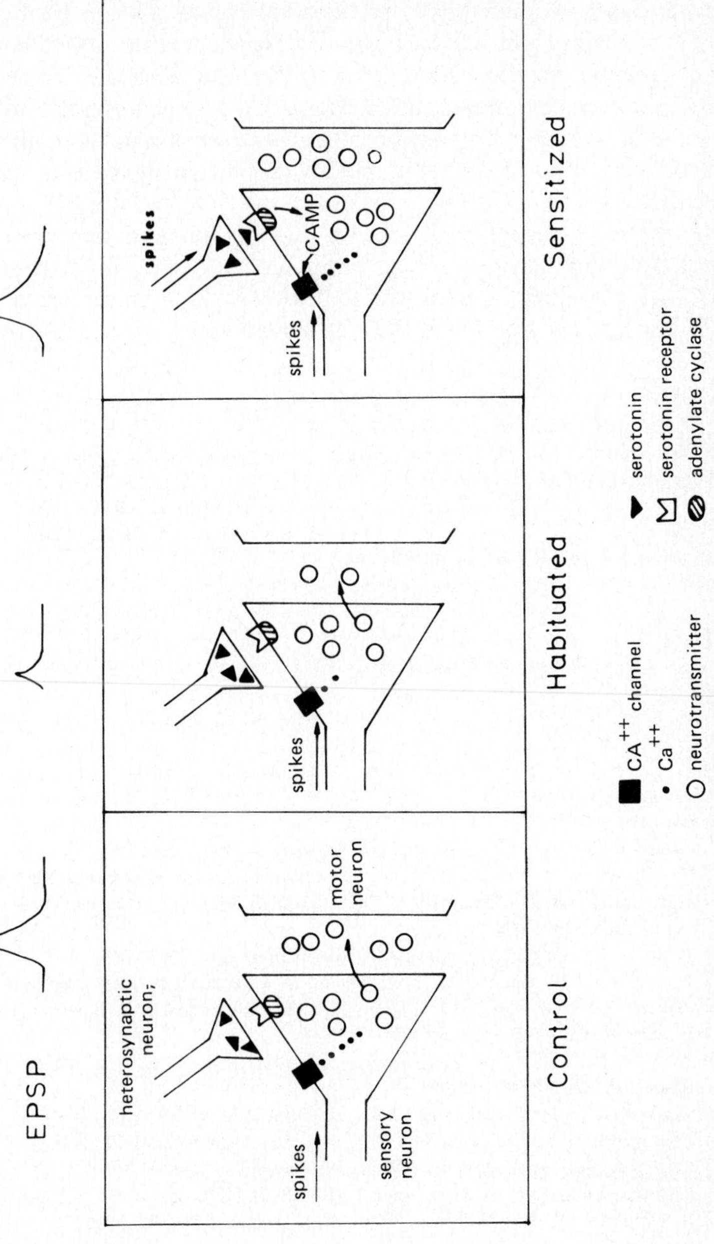

Fig. 8. Speculative model for habituation and facilitation (modified from ref. [20]).

mechanism by which serotonin and cAMP increase the release of neurotransmitter is probably a modification of the calcium current of the action potential in the terminals. Indeed, Klein and Kandel [20] have shown that electrical stimulation of the head, serotonin, cAMP or phosphodiesterase inhibitors, all increase the peak amplitude and the plateau of sensory neuron's action potential in experimental conditions in which this action potential is mainly due to an increase in Ca^{++} permeability.

The attractive model proposed for habituation and facilitation is presented in fig. 8.

In conclusion, there is no doubt that cAMP plays an important role in synaptic transmission but also in its modulation.

References

[1] J. W. Kebabian, in: Advances in Cyclic Nucleotides Research, vol. 8, eds. P. Greengard and G. A. Robison (Raven Press, New York, 1977) pp. 421–508

[2] E. W. Sutherland, T. W. Rall and T. Menon, J. Biol. Chem. 237 (1962) 1220.

[3] E. de Robertis, G. R. De Lores Arnaiz, M. Alberici, R. W. Butcher and E. W. Sutherland. J. Biol. Chem. 242 (1967) 3487.

[4] J. W. Kebabian and P. Greengard, Science 174 (1971) 1346.

[5] J. Bockaert, J. P. Tassin, A. M. Thierry, J. Glowinski and J. Premont, Brain Res. 122 (1977) 71.

[6] Y. C. Clement-Cormier, R. G. Parrish, G. L. Petzold, J. W. Kebabian and P. Greengard. J. Neur. Chem. 25 (1975) 143.

[7] J. Premont, M. Perez, G. Blanc, J. P. Tassin, A. M. Thierry, D. Herve and J. Bockaert, Mol. Pharmacol. 16 (1979) 790.

[8] J. Premont, A. M. Thierry, J. P. Tassin, J. Glowinski, G. Blanc and J. Bockaert, FEBS Lett. 68 (1976) 99.

[9] J. Bockaert. J. Physiol. Paris 74 (1978) 527.

[10] P. Greengard and J. W. Kebabian, Fed. Proceed. 33 (1974) 1059.

[11] P. Greengard, D. A. McAfee and J. W. Kebabian, in: Advances in Cyclic Nucleotide Research vol. 1, eds P. Greengard, R. Paoletti and G. A. Robison (Raven Press, New York, 1972) pp. 337–355.

[12] T. Veda, H. Maeno and P. Greengard, J. Biol. Chem. 148 (1973) 8295.

[13] B. J. Hoffer, G. R. Siggins, A. P. Oliver and F. E. Bloom, in: Advances in Cyclic Nucleotide Research, vol. 1, eds P. Greengard, R. Paoletti and G. A. Robison (Raven Press, New York, 1972) pp. 411–423.

[14] D. A. McAfee and P. Greengard, Science 178 (1972) 310.

[15] B. Libet. Life Sci. 24 (1979) 1043.

[16] H. Kobayashi, T. Hashigushi and N. S. Ushiyama. Nature 271 (1978) 263.

[17] T. Hashigushi, N. S. Ushiyama and H. Kobayashi, Nature 271 (1978) 267.

[18] I. B. Levitan. J. Physiol. Paris 74 (1978) 521.

[19] V. Castellucci and E. R. Kandel, Science 194 (1976) 1176.

[20] M. Klein and E. R. Kandel, Proc. Natl. Acad. Sci. USA 74 (1978) 35.

SEMINAR

CONFORMATION BIOLOGICAL ACTIVITY RELATIONSHIP IN THE SERIES OF ANGIOTENSIN II

Serge FERMANDJIAN

Service de Biochimie, Département de Biologie, CEA, Saclay, B.P. n° 2, 91190 Gif-sur-Yvette, France

Recognition of a biologically active molecule by its receptor site must be considered as the first event of the interaction process, while binding and signal release are subsequent phenomena. In physiological conditions, it is likely that during the approach of a peptide hormone to the cell membrane the change of surroundings modifies the conformation (s) such as a "recognizable" conformation is selected. It is assumed that in a given set of experimental conditions, e.g. solvent, ionic strength, and pH, etc., the peptides showing similar physical properties to that the parent hormone, may survive the conformational selection procedure during their approach to the cell membrane. The study of the hormone angiotensin II having pressor activity (Asp-Arg-Val-Tyr-$^{\mathrm{Val}}_{\mathrm{Ile}}$-His-Pro-Phe) and several of its structural analogues provides evidence for this

R. Balian et al., eds.
Les Houches, Session XXXIII, 1979 – Membranes et Communication Intercellulaire / Membranes and Intercellular Communication

hypothesis. Conformational analysis was performed by using circular dichroism and proton nuclear magnetic resonance spectroscopy for peptides dissolved in aqueous solution at several pH.

Two types of analogues were examined more specifically: (a) The antagonist (1-sarcosine, 8-isoleucine) angiotensin II and its derivatives obtained by replacing the residues in positions 4 (tyrosine) and 5 (isoleucine) with the corresponding *N*-methylated amino acids – the later analogues showed drastically reduced antagonistic properties; and (b) Those deriving directly from the hormone by substituting positions 3 (valine), 5, and 7 (proline) with residues of different types. The results indicate:

(1) For maximum agonistic and antagonistic activity the conformation of the analogue should resemble, at each pH, that of the parent hormone so as it could mimic angiotensin II in recognizing and binding with the receptor site on the cell.

(2) Drastic decrease in antagonistic activity obtained with *N*-methylated amino acids in position 4 or 5 in (1-sarcosine, 8-isoleucine) angiotensin II seems due to rotational restriction of the tyrosine-4 and histidine-5 side chains.

(3) The residue in position 5 must be β-branched. It plays a controlling influence in orienting the tyrosine and histidine side chains and in maintaining the backbone of the central segment 4-5-6 either in extended or β-sheet form. Whereas proline in position 7 has a strong directing influence on the immediately preceding residue (histidine) in the sequence, valine in position 3 seems only weakly involved in the organization of the succeeding tyrosine.

(4) Nuclear magnetic resonance and circular dichroism spectroscopy are appropriate in studying conformation biological activity relationship in peptides. The ellipticities (circular dichroism signals) and the fractions of rotamer populations (nuclear magnetic resonance) as well as their magnitude of change against pH characterizing the surroundings and side-chain arrangement of histidine and tyrosine in angiotensin II and its antagonist, must be a standard property of analogues possessing the same biological activity.

References

M. C. Khosla, R. R. Smeby and F. M. Bumpus, in: Handbook of Experimental Pharmacology, vol. 37, eds. I. M. Page and F. M. Bumpus (Springer Verlag, Berlin/Heidelberg/New York, 1973) pp. 126–161.

D. Regoli, W. K. Park and F. Rioux, Pharmacol. Rev. 26 (1974) 69.
M. C. Khosla, H. Munoz-Ramirez, M. M. Hall, R. R. Smeby, P. A. Khairallah, F. M. Bumpus and M. J. Peach, J. Med. Chem. 19 (1976) 244.
M. C. Khosla, M. M. Hall, R. R. Smeby and F. M. Bumpus, J. Med. Chem. 17 (1974) 431.
R. R. Smeby and S. Fermandjian, in: Chemistry and Biochemistry of Amino Acids, Peptides and Proteins, ed. B. Weinstein (M. Dekker, Inc., New York, 1978) ch. 4, pp. 117–162.
S. Fermandjian, K. Lintner, W. Haar, P. Fromageot, M. C. Khosla, R. R. Smeby and F. M. Bumpus, in: Peptides 1976, ed. A. Loffet (Editions de l'Université de Bruxelles, Bruxelles, 1976) pp. 339–352.
K. Lintner, S. Fermandjian, P. Fromageot, M. C. Khosla, R. R. Smeby and F. M. Bumpus, Biochemistry 16 (1977) 806.
K. Lintner, S. Fermandjian, P. Fromageot, M. C. Khosla, R. R. Smeby and F. M. Bumpus, FEBS Lett. 56 (1975) 366.
S. Fermandjian, K. Lintner, F. Piriou, F. Toma, H. Lam-Thanh and P. Fromageot, in: Peptides 1978, eds. I. Z. Siemon and G. Kupryszewski (Wydawnikwa Uniwersytetu Wroclawskiego, Wroclaw, Poland, 1979).
S. Fermandjian, F. Piriou, K. Lintner, F. Toma, H. Lam-Thanh, P. Fromageot, M. C. Khosla, R. R. Smeby and F. M. Bumpus, in: Proc. 6th American Peptide Symposium, Washington (1979).
F. Piriou, K. Lintner, S. Fermandjian, P. Fromageot, M. C. Khosla, R. R. Smeby and F. M. Bumpus PNAS (Jan. 1980).

SEMINAR

CELL SURFACE DOMAIN FORMATION AND CELL COMMUNICATION*

E. Lucio BENEDETTI
and
I. DUNIA

Laboratoire de Microscopie Electronique
Institut de Recherche en Biologie Moléculaire
de l'Université Paris VII et du C.N.R.S.
2, Place Jussieu, 75221 Paris Cedex 05, France

*Lectures delivered at Les Houches by E. L. Benedetti.

1. Introduction

Molecular genetics supports the concept that the genome contains all coded instructions required to govern the developmental program of a living organism and to regulate cell growth and differentiation by the production of chemical constituents and by their assembly in time and space [1]. The latter epigenetic aspect of the control mechanism – the assembly – might also imply that the properties of a system would not be determined by the totality of the chemical constituents but rather by a sorting out of a number of compounds that have the opportunity, at least temporarily, to merge and interact in an appropriate pattern whereby they become operative [2, 3]. The behaviour of any chemical constituent in the random dispersed state would contrast dramatically

R. Balian et al., eds.
Les Houches, Session XXXIII, 1979 – Membranes et Communication Intercellulaire / Membranes and Intercellular Communication

with the performance of the same compound in a topologically, well-defined domain. This notion has been reinforced by several lines of evidence derived from experiments on the modulation of membrane receptors, antigenic and enzymatic activities by regulatory ligands [4–6]. The plasma membrane is indeed a viscous, heterogeneous, fluid lipid bilayer, but specific membrane functions are only expressed by the emergence of integral protein lipid supramolecular domains. Essentially, the membrane proteins constitute gateways and carrier systems across the lipid core and generate stereospecific recognition, ion selectivity, active transport, electrical excitability, and photoelectric effects. In this line the plasma membrane acts as sensor, channel and transducer [7].

A key step of cell surface domain formation arises when the plasma membranes of individual cells become mutually in contact and various types of cell-to-cell interactions take place. These surface domains generally ensure stable physical association, ionic coupling and metabolic cooperation between cells. Another type of tight interaction controls the traffic of water-soluble constituents of the extracellular medium along paracellular routes of permeation [8].

Some clues have recently emerged, indicating that from the early stage of embryonic differentiation, positional information is dependent on the acquisition of cell surface adhesion properties, the budding of microprojections and, in particular, upon the assembly of intercellular junctions. At the eight cell stage of mouse embryo, the initial step of segregation of inner and outer blastomers, presumptive for inner cell mass and trophoblast respectively, is coupled with the recruitment of junctions. The formation of these cell surface specialized domains educes the compaction of blastomers by generating distinctive "inside" and "outside" embryonal microenvironments [9–17].

Intercellular junctions are characterized by a variety of morphological forms. They include a type that can be purported as a candidate for the structural specialization responsible for the transfer of ions and active metabolites directly from one cell to another. This private cell-to-cell pathway, widely present in most metazoan animals, has been the object, in the recent past, of a number of diverse investigations. It is called "gap" or "nexus" and belongs to the category of cell interaction in which the plasma membranes of neighbouring cells come into close contact.

Several reviews have extensively summarized and critically evaluated the fundamental structural and functional aspects of the "gap" junction [18–25]. Many of the physiological and morphological characters have been positively assessed. Yet the gap junction chemical nature, and the assembly program and its control remain wide open questions. The purpose of this contribution is to report on some of the selected biochemical and structural grounds which may be relevant to our knowledge of the gap junction design principles.

2. The morphology of the gap junction

The gap junctions described in a variety of animal tissues have the shape of plaques of various extension. In the thin section of fixed and embedded material, two opposite outer layers of each trilaminar junctional plasma membrane appear in close proximity. A minute "gap" (2 nm) is visible between the membranes. In routine-stained thin sections, the fence appears to be occupied by an amorphous plug. Only by introduction, through intercellular space, of colloidal electron opaque tracers (lanthanum hydroxide, potassium pyroantimoniate) as it was originally applied by Karnowsky and Revel in 1966 [26], is the subunit pattern of the interlocking device between the junctional membranes discovered (fig. 1). Following the isolation of intact plasma membranes and fractions containing mainly "gap" junction fragments [27], negative staining reveals a similar bidimensional lattice of repeating subunits in the plane of the junctional membranes with a center-to-center distance of 8 to 9 nm [28]. The application of the freeze-fracture technique has brought forth new information showing that the lattice subunit penetrates the lipid hydrophobic core of both junctional membranes. In the gap junctions, the freeze-fracture simultaneously splits the two junctional membranes in a stepwise fashion. The cleavage passes along one of the bilayers and exposes the inner aspect of the leaflet adjacent to the cytoplasm (PF), then the adjacent membrane is cleaved and the exposed fracture surface corresponds to the inwardly directed face of the outer membrane leaflet (EF). The junctional *P* fracture face is characterized by a polygonal lattice of 9 nm particulate entities (IMPs) (fig. 2). The corresponding fracture face *E* displays a complementary arrangement of pits or depressions (see fig. 2). The interpretation of the freeze-fracture features of the gap junction in terms of molecular model, however, is not easily apparent.

A distinct asymmetric distribution of particulate entities is constantly found in freeze-fractured gap junctions* [18, 20]. This might suggest, at

*The gap junctions are "inverted" only in arthropods since the inner membrane half (PF) comprises the pitted aspect, whereas the particulate entities remain associated with the outer membrane leaflet (EF) and are larger (11 nm) than in other animal [19, 20] phyla.

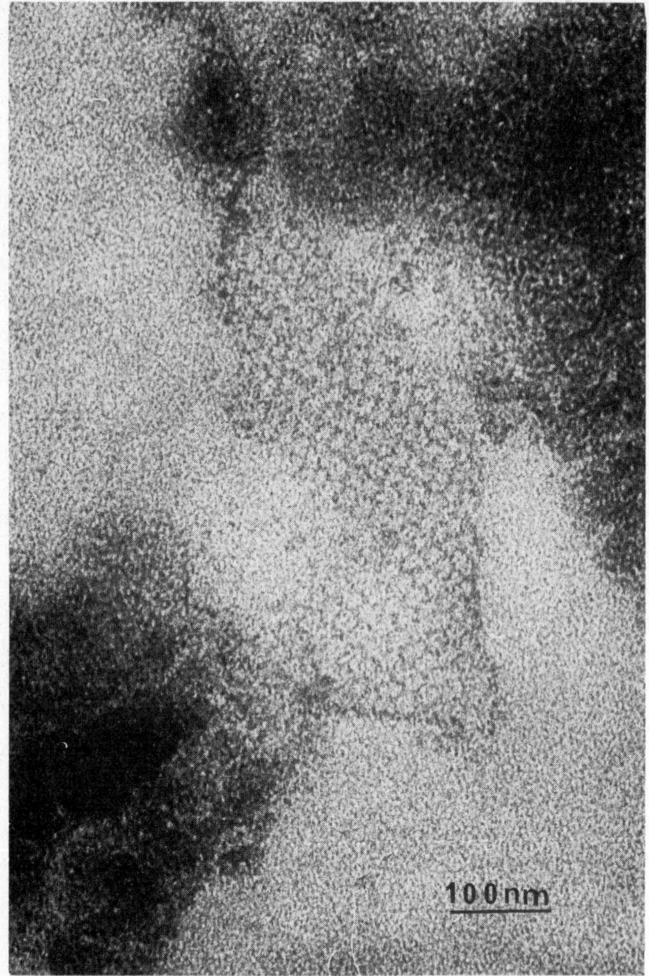

Fig. 1. Eye lens fibers impregnated with lanthanum nitrate. In the thin section, the electron dense marker filling the intercellular spaces has outlined the gap junctional region. Note the two-dimensional geometric pattern of repeating subunits with a center-to-center space of 9 nm.

least, that the transmembrane units or connections interact more strongly with the cytoplasmic halves of the bilayer and/or with extrinsic constituents associated with the protoplasmic surface (PF) of the junctional membranes. Although this assumption is corroborated by a variety of data provided by other membrane systems showing that the

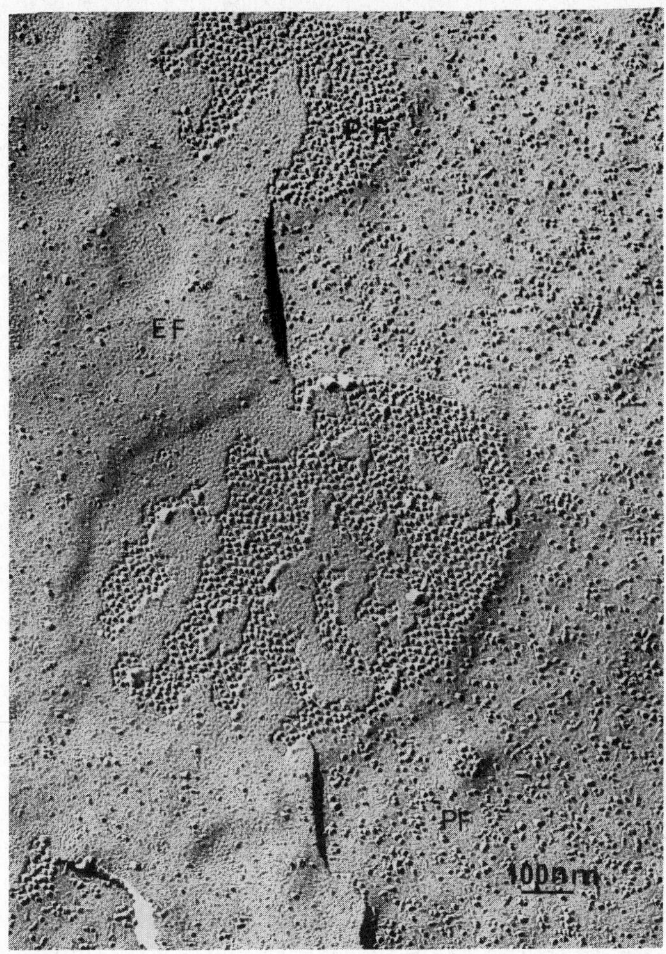

Fig. 2. Replica of freeze-fractured lens fiber plasma membrane. Junctional domains are characterized by polygonal clusters of IMPs on PF and pits on EF.

"stabilization" of transmembrane entities and their asymmetric freeze-fracture distribution rely upon a multimeric association of plasma membrane constituents localized at various levels of the cell border [29] the explanation of gap-junction, asymmetric distribution of particulate entities in freeze-fracture replicas remains merely speculative. In fact the biochemical nature of the junctional domain and its interaction with cytoplasmic constituents are far from being explained. On the other hand, some controversy exists as to whether the particulate entities forming the polygonal lattice which spans the junctional membrane hydrophobic core comprise only proteins which, during the cleavage, have been unplugged from the outer half of the bilayer leaving the hollow pits on the fracture face (EF). According to Verkleij and Ververgaert [30], the complementarity – the particulate entities on PF and pits on EF – is a strong indication that the particles comprise lipid and not only protein. It is surprising that protein–lipid interactions have almost been neglected in the interpretation of the chemical nature of the intramembranous particles generated by the freeze-fracture of biological and artificial membranes. The lipid micelles may form, themselves, particulate entities visualized on fracture faces of artificial lipid membranes in water [31]. Hence, it is conceivable that a consistent amount of lipid fragments might remain associated with the transmembrane proteins and contribute to the particulate aspect of the fracture faces. This asumption, however, does not necessarily refute the junctional unit concept based on the protein nature of the permeable transmembrane device [23, 32].

3. The permeable path

One viewpoint is that the communicating units are pairs of protein oligomers aligned on the two adjoined membranes spanning the lipid bilayer and comprising a central hydrophilic channel of about 2 nm in diameter with cytoplasmic resistivity [32, 35]. Each individual, junctional membrane possesses a set of repeating units packed in a polygonal lattice. A pair of opposite units matching one another forms the connecting transmembrane device in the middle of the extracellular gap and in perfect register [22]. A crucial question concerns the nature of the chemical and/or physical bonds that make the two merging units strongly associated with one another and leak-proof to the outside once the assembly process is completed. The splitting of the gap junction into two halves down the middle of the extracellular gap occurs upon perfusion of tissues with hypertonic solutions (0.5 M sucrose or 0.9% sodium propionate [19]. The gap junctional domain splits symmetrically, according to freeze-fracture evidence, in the middle of the gap and each of the separated membranes comprises one lattice of repeating units. It is remarkable that, according to Gilula [19], the splitting of the junction can be easily reversed by replacing the hypertonic sucrose with a normal salt solution. Conversely, the withdrawal of divalent cations and the action of several other inhibitors of the junctional communication [19], are not followed by the splitting of the junctional membranes. If one of these actions is associated with cell separation, the gap junction domain usually stays with one cell while the disrupted plasma membrane of the other cell is rapidly sealed off [19, 24]. Similar events also occur when the cells are dissociated by proteases. The gap junction which is resistant to this treatment is held either by one or the other cell [19, 24].

Owing to the strong evidence for a gap junction as the site of intercellular traffic, one may ask whether a minimum size of the junctional areas exists which is compatible with the transfer of ions and active metabolites, and what kind of structural organization of the membrane correlates with junctional competence. Once the junction has been initiated, the establishment of a low-resistance pathway, monitored by the increasing junctional conductance, seems to be a progressive event; this reflects the gradual apposition of junctional units in parallel with the increase of the junctional competence [23]. The experiment of Loewenstein et al. provides evidence that each quantal up-step of conductance correlates with the complete opening of a junctional channel [36].

There is probably more than one unique kind of gap junction and the architectural pleomorphism [20] may well fit with a physiological diversity which is not easily assessed by electrical measurements alone. The size of individual gap junctions as well as the total areas per cell-to-cell interface may vary considerably. For instance, in mammalian heart, the cell surface area occupied by gap junction is approximately 3.7%, in liver 1.5%, in brown fat 1%, in fibroblasts 0.05% and in smooth muscle 0.2% [35, 37]. In reassociated Novikoff hepatoma cells, the mean area of gap junction was 0.187 μm^2 to 0.269 μm^2 with a junctional conductance of 1.13×10^2 mho/cm^2 and 0.78×10^2 mho/cm^2 [25, 35]. A direct approach would be to correlate the changes of the ultrastructural features of gap junctions after treatment with uncouplers which increases the junctional resistance. It has been claimed that the increase in junctional resistance following the treatment with uncouplers is associated with a more regular geometrical packing of the repeating units in the plane of the junctional membrane, with considerable reduction of the lattice constant [22, 38, 39]. In other tissues, complex structural features, i.e. formation of particle-free "aisles" interspaced with particulate rows [22] and internalization and shedding of the gap junctions have been implicated in the physiological uncoupling [40].

4. The molecular model of the permeable path

A molecular model of gap junctions which may indicate how the pore size of the junctional channels is regulated, has been recently provided by Unwin and Zampighi [33, 34]. These authors, by tilting negatively-stained specimens at various angles to the incident beam and by analyzing the electron microscopic pictures by Fourier and image reconstruction techniques, have obtained an 18-Å resolution, three-dimensional map of the isolated liver gap junctions. Several interesting implications can be derived from this investigation. The junctional unit can be depicted as an annular oligomer comprising 6 protein rod-shaped subunits (2.5 nm in diameter and 7.5 nm long) spanning the membrane and protruding from either side. The subunits are inclinated tangentially with respect to the 6-fold axis of the junctional unit.

In one configuration ("open"), the central opening outlined by the 6-subunits is about 2.0 nm. By rotational displacement, together with tilting of the subunits, the transition to the second configuration ("closed") is produced. The transition of the junctional oligomers from the open configuration to the closed one was obtained after long dialysis of the detergent extracted isolated junctions. The existence of the two quaternary states of the oligomeric junctional proteins might imply that *in vivo* the transition relies upon a cooperative control according to a model derived from the theory of allosteric enzymes [41]. That the cooperativity is an inherent consequence of the lattice organization rather than of the conformation of each individual oligomer is merely hypothetical. Although this elegant model proposes a "simple" mechanism for opening and closing the pathway through the junctional membrane, it remains to be established whether the action of the uncoupling factors (i.e. Ca^{2+} concentration and/or pH) [23, 36] operates on the lipid closed environment rather than primarily on the junctional protein-oligomer.

It is tempting to speculate that Unwin and Zampighi's model might compromise or arbitrate the two open and closed configurations and conform the pore size of the junctional channels to the possible functional needs. It has been shown that by progressively elevating the cytoplasmic Ca^{2+} concentration, the molecular size limit for junctional permeation diminishes [23, 36, 42] and each quantal down step of conductance represents a complete or partial closure of one unitary channel [36]. One might anticipate that the control mechanism of the junctional permeability could either rely upon a selective and progressive restriction in the transfer of larger molecules without hampering the transit of smaller ions by channel structure modulation, or that there exists at least two distinct types of cell-to-cell gateway [36, 43, 44]. A number of studies have shown that fluorescein failed to pass between electrically coupled embryonic cells, leading to the conclusion that the permeability of gap junctions is more stringent and selective in early embryonic tissues than in the adult [45]. Some of these results were open to doubt because of the relative insensitivity of the methods used [23, 45]. However, other interesting experiments are in agreement with the existence of more subtle properties of the junctional sieve. Unambiguous experiments of Lo and Gilula [13, 14], on junctional communication in the post-implantation mouse embryo, demonstrate that the total cell population is ionically coupled. However, restriction of the junctional path, monitored by the lack of transfer of fluorescein and lucifer yellow could be detected between electrically-coupled inner cell mass and trophoblasts [13, 14]. The hypothesis for gap junction phenotype modulation during embryonal differentiation is further corroborated by the results of Goodman and Spitzer [46] on the development of the dorsal unpaired neuroblast in the grasshopper. All cell types at early embryonic stages are electrically coupled to each other, and lucifer yellow injected into the neuroblast at day 7 spreads throughout all its progeny. At day 8, the oldest dorsal unpaired median (DUM) neuroblasts are still electrically coupled to other cells but dye-uncoupled. As the developmental pattern proceeds, the DUM neuroblast becomes electrically uncoupled from most embryonic cells, until mature DUM neurones become electrically uncoupled even to one another.

The study of channel competence in various cell phenotypes in culture, also indicates that the impairment of the dye-transfer is not necessarily associated with ionic uncoupling. On the other hand, in several hybrid cell combinations, the channel competence parallels the extent of gap junction particle aggregates [44, 47–49]. Rudimental junctional domains such as narrow and interrupted particulate rows are found in the intermediate hybrid cells with incomplete channel competence, characterized by the transfer only of small inorganic ions, but not of larger molecules [48, 49]. Furthermore other experiments clearly implicate that, in mammalian cell cultures, two distinct junctional pathways exist: one larger and highly Ca^{2+} sensitive and the other smaller and less sensitive to intracellular increase of Ca^{2+} [4, 36, 43]. It appears from these observations that true cell-to-cell communication does not operate as a simple all-or-none phenomenon, and that its competence relies on the correct combination of appropriate gene-products.

5. The assembly of gap junctions

The establishment of gap junction and metabolic cooperation, the transit of inorganic ions and of higher-molecular-weight substances are not restricted to cells of the same kind. On the contrary, a junctional channel may be found between heterologous types of cells [23] with the exception of the arthropod-derived cells [50]. However, the efficiency of the junctional domain differs markedly in heterologous cell systems. Differences may also involve the ability for a cell type either to receive or to transfer the message throughout the communicating junctions. For instance, one embryonic carcinoma cell line (PCC_4 azal) is a rather good donor but a poor recipient in heterologous metabolic coupling [15, 17]. Again, one may speculate that the stringency in the ability and in the rate of channel formation might reside in the production program of the junctional constituents. At this point we must admit that the important question of whether translation of the junctional precursor is needed for the proper assembly of gap junctions is not easily understood. In reaggregating cells, the onset of the electrical coupling indicates that the formation of a communicating pathway occurs within a rather short lapse of time – of the order of a few minutes – in homologous systems and a little longer in heterologous cell combinations [23, 24]. Even within 20 minutes after dissociation, a new contact and coupling can be restored between two opposed cell surfaces without any restriction to a particular area [24]. Hence, the cell surface is competent for junctional domain formation at any site and independently of where the original position of the junction was before the dissociation [23]. In reaggregating Novikoff hepatoma cells, the inhibition of protein synthesis for up to 12 h preceding and including the reaggregation, does not prevent gap junction assembly and cell coupling [23, 51]. Cycloheximide also had no effect on the assembly of gap and tight junctions in a trypsinized human adenocarcinoma cell line [52]. Hence, these results imply the existence of a rather stable junctional precursor pool, and that the recruitment of the junctional protein units might be regarded as a process of "self-assembly". Conversely, protein biosynthesis is needed for cell adhesion and gap junction formation during the acquisition *in vitro* of synchronous beating in embryonic heart cells [53, 54]. One more result positively suggests that transcription and translation are necessary steps in the junctional assembly, at least in a developing system. Actinomycin-D or cycloheximide, prevent the junctional assembly directed by thyroid hormone, in differentiating ependymoglial cells of hypophysectomised *Rana pipiens* [55, 56].

The varying statements concerning the necessity and extension of the protein synthesis during the junctional assembly, demonstrate the complexity of the various biochemical and structural parameters controlling cell surface domain formation. This brings to mind the question of whether the inherent features of the cell surface furnish a means of interaction and sorting out of the cell type, competent for cell contact and communication, and of facilitating the assembly in time and space of preexisting junctional constituents. It has been proposed, for instance, that the impairment of communication competence in mouse L cells in culture, could be related to changes involving abberations of carbohydrates containing membrane components, at least partly represented by the synthesis of incomplete, low-molecular-weight fucosyl glycopeptides [57]. No one has yet explored, however, whether the nascent or preexisting junctional constituents during the initiation and the precursor stage of the assembly are either uncovered or chemically and/or structurally associated with other entities exposed at the true cell surface. In the latter case, the junctional assembly could be regarded as a process involving serial steps: (a) the reciprocal and stereospecific binding of cell surface receptor(s), followed by (b) conformational and/or topographic changes of the receptor protein which in turn and(c) generate the recruitment of the membrane protein oligomers.

Several situations are known where tissue-specific cell contact and adhesion are mediated by specific recognition membrane protein and glycoprotein [58]. Since cell contact is an obvious requirement for gap junction formation, it is hard to avoid the assumption that the appropriate domain formation relies upon the stereospecific recognition and binding of component(s) present on the two adjoining cell surfaces. It is of interest that Noll et al. [59] have found that a butanol-extracted membrane protein strongly stimulates the rate of reaggregation of dissociated blastomers in sea urchin embryos. The point to be emphasized is also that the aggregation was prevented by Fab fragments obtained by immunization with purified blastomer membranes. It is also relevant in these experiments that the competence for cell aggregation could be restored by the "insertion" of butanol extracts from purified membrane from different species.

We have also reported [40] a striking effect on cell contact and junctional assembly provoked by monovalent antibodies against cell surface antigen(s) F9 which are implicated in cell recognition during early embryonal development. Treatment of mouse embryonal carcinoma cells (PCC_4) with the anti-F9 Fab-fragments disrupts cell adhesion and generates cell surface alterations which are followed by the deletion of the junctional domains, in particular of the gap junctions.

The means by which the coordinated assembly of intramembranous protein constituents is initiated by local changes of the lipid environment are more obscure. Rapid segregation of specific classes of phospholipids, neutral lipid – in particular of cholesterol – and free fatty acid, might in turn favour the clustering of specific classes of membrane protein(s). It has been reported that the differentiation of the eye lens fibers and of extensive junctional domains, correlates with remarkable changes of the membrane lipid [60, 61]. The ratio of cholesterol to phospholipid increases and the sphingomyelin fatty acid shows an increase in main chain length and mono-unsaturation or full saturation [60, 61]. On the other hand, one might speculate that, initially, the recruitment of junctional precursors could arise as a result of a freedom to move in the plane of the membrane reflecting, say, a weaker connection between intramembranous protein(s) and the constituents of the cytoskeleton. Some clues have recently emerged, implicating free fatty acids as a possible perturbant of the lipid close environment of transmembrane protein and in turn of the specific interaction between membrane protein and the cytoskeleton. This interesting and new model has been proposed by Klausner et al. [62], who have shown that when *cis*-unsaturated free fatty acids are intercalated into lymphocyte plasma membrane, the sequential process of the energy-dependent movement of the patched receptors into a cap is blocked. The alteration of the lipid environment would impair the control signal which links the receptor to the transducer – a Ca^{2+} binding protein – interacting with the cytoskeleton. It is striking that by increasing the extracellular calcium concentration, the capping inhibition induced by free fatty acids, is relieved. Positively, it is premature to derive from the inspiring study of Klausner et al., a model consistent with the molecular event underlying the junctional assembly. At present, we have little information on the chemical interaction between junctional constituents and the cytoskeletal organization. End-on attachment of cytoplasmic microfilaments, which is a common feature of the inner aspect of various other types of intracellular junctions, has been very well documented only during the internalization of gap junctions in granulosa cells [63].

6. Morphological features of gap junction assembly

This process, which has been extensively reviewed by Sheridan [24, 64] is characterized by several steps visualized on freeze-fracture replicas. The precursor stage or initiation (5′ to 30′ after reaggregation in Novikoff hepatoma cells), seems to correlate with the appearance of small regions of cell apposition, a few tenths of a micron in diameter, which have been termed "formation plaques".

The P-fracture face of these areas are void of intramembranous particles (IMP) in contrast with the surrounding domain where the heterogeneous classes of particulate entities are randomly scattered [65–70].

That the formation plaques stand for the initial segregation of the lipid junctional domain is an attractive assumption. Striking similarities in the freeze-fracture features exist among the "formation plaques" and the very initial stages of membrane fusion [71]. The formation plaques which are initiated in pairs in each apposed plasma membrane, are during the successive stages of junctional assembly (more than 30′), progressively occupied by large intramembranous particles (9–11 nm in diameter) which might be initial points of membrane attachment. At this stage, linear array or small clusters of 8 nm particles are visualized on P fracture face. Whether the smaller particulate entities are generated by the breakdown of the larger particles is not clear [72]. It is also doubtful whether the particles penetrate through the membrane leaflet and match with complementary particles on the opposite plasma membrane. As junctional assembly proceeds (maturation), more elaborated arrays and clusters of particles are detected on P fracture face and arrays and clusters of pits are visible on E fracture face. All these features are in close proximity to membrane regions where the intracellular space is abruptly reduced. The most advanced step of the junctional development (30′ to 60′) is characterized by the disappearance of the larger 11 nm particles, and by the accumulation of packed arrays of 8 nm particles. The matching pairs of 8 nm particles now span the entire width of the two plasma membranes in close apposition, and each channel being insulated from the intracellular space, may already represent preferential sites of communication. Although the morphological sequence of junctional assembly that we have depicted, displays similar

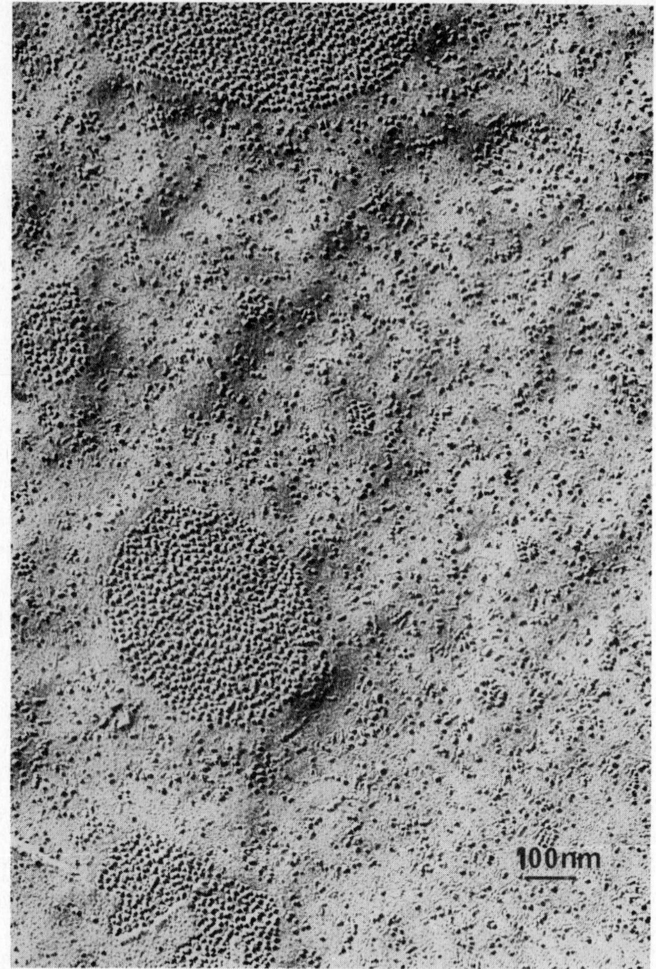

Fig. 3. Replica of freeze-fractured eye lens elongating zone. Multiple clusters of 9 nm intramembranous particles (PF) characterize the multicentric assembly of gap junctional elements.

features in various tissues (fig. 3) [64, 73], several variations of assembly pattern, which may be species specific, have been described [74–76]. These variations involve the extension of the formation plaques, the absence of larger "precursor" particles and the arrangement of the initial rows and clusters of the junctional particles [64, 74–76].

It seems relevant to add some data here about the postulated chemical nature of the gap junctions.

7. Chemical nature of the gap junctions

A striking common feature of the gap junctions isolated from different tissues is the property of being almost insoluble in detergents [28, 77].

Early studies by SDS gel electrophoresis on the gap junction-rich fraction, claimed that gap junctions also shared another common feature: a major polypeptide of about 34 000 daltons [77, 78]. Further reports however, casted some doubt on this conclusion and revealed considerable disagreement concerning the number and the molecular weight of the junctional proteins [79–83]. One pitfall could be inherent to the method of isolation of gap junctions based upon a sequential treatment of the crude plasma membrane preparation with hydrolytic enzymes, chaotropic agent and/or detergents, generating loss and degradation of junctional components, even though the overall structural organization of the isolated junction could appear unaffected. The latter criterion is seriously misleading in the absence of any other assay that may provide a better information on the chemical "integrity" of the isolated gap junctions, than SDS gel electrophoretic analysis. Protease-free isolation yielded highly enriched liver gap junction fractions characterized by one broad band with an apparent molecular weight of 47 000 and another very sharp one with an apparent molecular weight of 27 000 [83]. SDS gel electrophoretic analysis on eye lens fiber plasma membrane isolated without the use of detergents or proteases indicates that the protein profile comprises two major polypeptides, one of 34 000 daltons (MP 34) and one of 26 000 daltons (MP 26) [64, 84] (fig. 4). The 26 000 dalton component found in eye lens plasma membrane is particularly sensitive and its conversion to high-molecular-weight aggregates may easily result from overheating and unappropriate ionic strength conditions during solubilization in SDS [85]. Broekhuyse et al. [86] have called the MP 26 the "main intrinsic polypeptide" (MIP) of bovine eye lens fiber plasma membrane. These authors have also shown that this component, which is not a glycoprotein, shares with proteolipid, the feature that it can be extracted in chloroform–methanol and in butanol. The MP 26 polypeptide has been purified by preparative SDS gel electrophoresis [87]. If the amino acid composition of this lens fiber polypeptide is compared with that of MIP extracted by Broekhuyse et al. by chloroform methanol [86, 88], then it is evident that the MP 26 and MIP are identical polypeptides. A recent study of Henderson et al. [82] also indicates that a polypeptide of about 26 000 dalton is the major component of detergent isolated liver gap junctions. A minor 21 000 mol wt subunit is also detected, being probably a

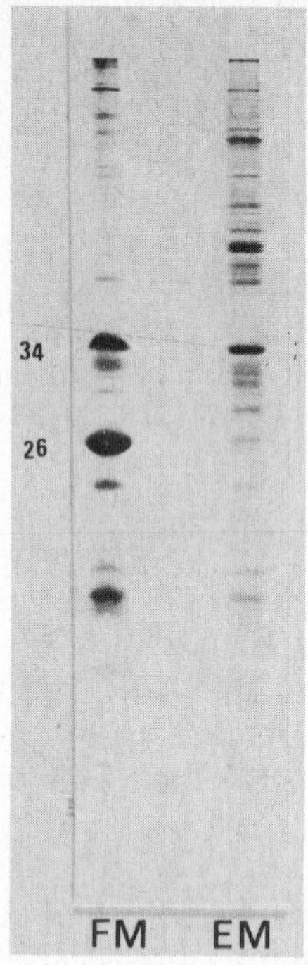

Fig. 4. SDS polyacrylamide gel electrophoresis of lens fiber membrane proteins showing the two major bands MP 34 and MP 26 (FM). For comparison, the protein pattern of lens epithelial plasma membrane (EM) is shown. Note that the MP 26 is almost absent.

degradation product of the larger 26 000 polypeptide. Consistent with the finding in eye lens fiber proteins, overheating of the samples during solubilization for SDS electrophoretic analysis, produced several higher-molecular-weight bands. Other interesting implications of the study of Henderson et al. [82], concern the amino acid composition of the junctional protein that outlines the amphipatic character of the 26 000 polypeptide and the fact that polar residues of this putative trans-membrane protein are still accessible to protease. Comparison of the amino acid analysis of the lens MP 26 component and the major junctional polypeptide from liver gap junction reported by Henderson et al. [82], indicates also that the overall polarity of the two proteins is similar. Hence, both can be defined as "intrinsic" membrane proteins.

The MP 26 component is present in lens membrane derived from different animal sources. However, the evidence for a species-specific antigenic property of this membrane protein has been provided. Antiserum directed against chick lens fiber MP 26 component precipitates the corresponding polypeptide isolated from turkey lens fiber, but not the MP 26 of bovine lens plasma membranes [89]. MP 26 is a predominant component of the eye lens fiber plasma membrane and accounts for more than 50% of the protein recovered from the membrane [88]. The question arises whether MP 26 is the major constituent of the eye lens gap junctions, in particular of the fibers that are associated by very extensive junctional domains [64]. One possibility is that MP 26 is a widespread plasma membrane component though preferentially recruited in the gap junction domains. We have already mentioned that the isolation of the lens fiber junctions can be obtained by detergent solubilization followed by equilibrium density gradient centrifugation (fig. 5). SDS gel electrophoresis applied to this detergent-insoluble fraction shows that MP 34 and MP 26 are the major protein constituents (fig. 6). It is noteworthy that both polypeptides are present in the urea-insoluble membrane fraction which also comprises mostly junctional fragments. At this time, we may usefully take the view that the lens fibers communicating junctions comprise two predominant components, and that at least one, MP 26, constitutes the transmembrane permeable oligomer. Conversely the type of association of MP 34 with the membrane backbone requires further comments. A polypeptide of approximately 34 000 mol wt found in isolated liver gap junction has been considered a contaminant component, in particular uricase [83]. We do not consider that this is the case in eye lens fiber gap junctions for the following reasons. MP 34 (about 5% on membrane protein basis) is defined by Bouman et al. [90] as an "extrinsic" lens membrane protein, different from the crystallines and bound to the membrane by calcium ions since it can be eluted from the urea-insoluble membrane fraction by EDTA-containing buffer. Surprisingly the MP 34 or "EDTA extractable protein (EEP)", though it has been called "extrinsic", is substantially urea and detergent-insoluble. Consistent with the amphipatic nature of MP 34 is also the amino acid composition [90] showing that the rough percentage of hydrophobicity, even if it is not as high as that estimated from MP 26, is nevertheless substantial. This molecular feature could reinforce the assumption that MP 34, which in our experiments is found in the protein profile of a detergent-insoluble junctional fraction, is at least partially in contact with the hydrophobic lipid core. The complexity of the MP 34 nature is also shown by the observation that this protein, extracted by EDTA-solution, contains two subunits of 32 000 and 35 000 daltons. Two-dimensional electrophoresis

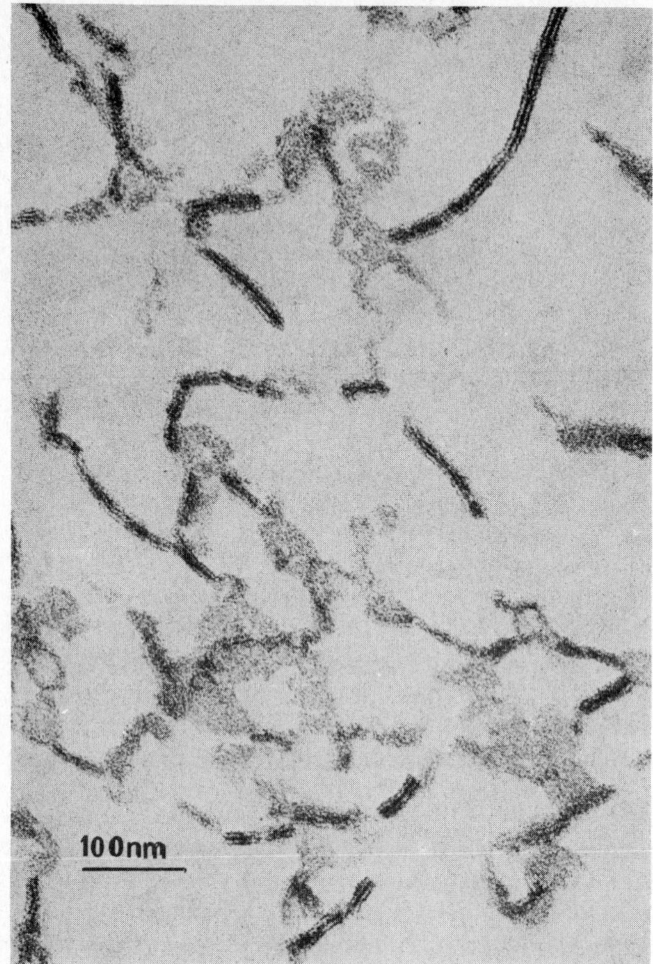

Fig. 5. Isolated lens fiber gap junctions obtained by detergent solubilization followed by equilibrium density gradient centrifugation. Thin section stained with uranyl acetate and lead citrate.

and immunoelectro-focusing, give a strong indication that the two subunits of the bovine EEP membrane component are antigenically different [90].

In the eye lens, the results obtained both on thin-sectioned material and on freeze-fracture replicas imply that the junctional complexes are present at the lateral surface of the epithelial cell, between the basal surface of the epithelial monolayer and the cortical fibers, and also in

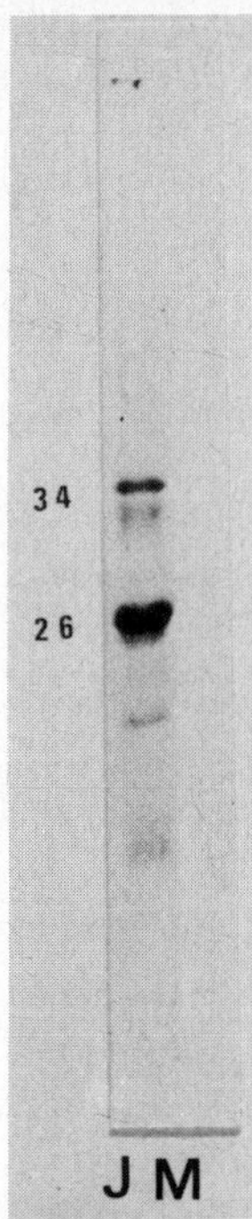

Fig. 6. SDS polyacrylamide gel electrophoresis of detergent insoluble junction-rich fraction of lens fiber plasma membrane. MP 34 and MP 26 are the major polypeptides. In the 22 region, a minor component represents a product of degradation.

deeper lens regions [64, 91]. Morphological differences exist between epithelial gap junctions and the extensive junctional domains connecting lens fibers. The latter type is more pleomorphic than the epithelial junctions which are characterized by smaller polygonally-clustered, particulate domains. It is striking that the SDS gel electrophoretic analysis of plasma membranes isolated from the lens epithelium shows the presence of MP 34 but not of MP 26 in contrast with the finding that both polypeptides are found in the junction-rich fraction isolated from lens fibers (fig. 4). Hence, qualitative and/or quantitative differences in protein composition may exist even within one presumed single type of tissue. These variations seem to be inherent markers, at least in the lens, of different stages of tissue differentiation [92].

Although studies of the lipid content of the gap junctions are relatively scarce, they indicate that the average phospholipid composition, at least in liver, is very similar to that obtained with the general plasma membrane [82, 83]. The most remarkable difference between isolated gap junctions and bulk plasma membrane concerns the neutral lipids, in particular the cholesterol to phospholipid ratio which is much higher in the isolated junctions (1.5 as compared to 0.9 according to Henderson et al.). Depending upon the choice of the detergent and the combination with chaotropic agent, more phospholipid may be extracted, but the molar content of cholesterol-per-milligram of protein remains about the same. This interesting result of Henderson et al. [82] implicates that the cholesterol strongly interact with the protein. A similar conclusion applies to the lens gap junctions [64].

8. Concluding remarks

The data reported here imply the gap junction assembly as one of the key steps of cell surface domain formation. There is a direct horizontal communication between cells in close contact, and the transfer of active metabolites, including nucleotides [93–97] may proceed unimpaired. One striking observation involves a tridimensional model of the junctional membrane. Accordingly the coupling device would consist of bimodal oligomers comprising six protein subunits [33, 34]. The oligomers, forming in the plane of the membrane a polygonal lattice, are set up tangentially tilted and a short range reversible rotation around the major axis of the unit generates two quaternary states of the oligomers: an open and closed configuration respectively. This model thus offers an explanation for a highly efficient and "simple" control of the permeable channel's pore size. If we now turn to the more specific mechanism of the junctional permeability, we must admit that the molecular event(s) triggering the structural transition *in vivo* still remains a wide-open question. A striking feature of the cell-to-cell aqueous pathway is its high sensitivity to the cytoplasmic-free, Ca^{2+} concentration [23, 36]. This concept, consistent with extensive experimental evidence, states that the permeability of the junctional sieve gradually decreased as the Ca^{2+} concentration in the cytoplasmic milieu is raised up to 5×10^{-5} M [36]. However, several other electrophysiological observations imply that the control mechanism of the junctional sieve is not exclusively an all-or-none phenomenon and that the permeable unit population is not always sensitive to Ca^{2+} regulation in equal terms [36]. Alternatively, the permeation of molecules through the junctional membrane might be selectively controlled by different classes of cell-to-cell pathways. Some restriction in the transit of the molecules would be associated with variation in the sensitivity to Ca^{2+} and hydrogen-ion concentration of the charged channels [36]. Also the use of transit probes at different molecular size indicates that there are different pathways or channels through the junctional membrane for the passage of larger and smaller molecules selectively [23, 43–49]. All these relevant experimental data reflect the existence between various animal cell types and even between the various developmental steps of a single tissue, of basic differences in the chemical and structural features of the permeable gateway. Growing biochemical evidence, though still unsatisfactory, supports the existence of a chemical diversity of the major junctional protein subunits even within a single developing type of tissue [92]. One important consequence of such a situation could well be that the appropriate and specific assembly of the junctional component is a process depending on a stringent expression of gene products. This notion has been reinforced by several interesting results on the existence of several mutant phenotypes controlling various states of junctional competence [43–49]. It is now conceivable that the incomplete channel competence described in several hybrid cell systems may reflect the alteration in the production of other chemical constituents of the cell surface that are crucial for the correct assembly of preexisting junctional polypeptides. Even though the formation of the junctional domain can be depicted as a self-assembly of repeating identical or quasi-equivalently selected protein subunits, yet the transmembrane control that brings about the junctional modulation apparently implies several parameters which are still not fully clarified. It has been proposed that the transmembrane association of fibronectin and actin is implicated in the junctional assembly [98]. Yet the putative link between the cell surface constituents, cytoskeleton elements and junctional modulation remain to be elucidated. The biogenesis of the junctional domain is characterized by a multistep process, during which transient and catalytic functions may operate within a programmed pathway. A problem of considerable current interest concerns the activation of proteases which could enhance the fitness of the two merging junctional domains. It is of great interest that Griepp and Revel [72] have described the formation of gap junction following the adhesion between synchronous beating embryonic heart cells in culture as either promoted or triggered by mild proteolysis. A number of studies have also well documented a rapid accumulation of junctional domains, in particular gap junctions in response to a variety of hormonal stimulation of normal developing or transformed growing tissues, but the experimental data do not yet answer the question of whether the hormonal sensitivity of the junctional program depends directly upon the presence of junctional receptor(s) or from a more indirect action, or by the stimulation of any of the several steps of the membrane protein topogenesis [99]. In several instances the increase of the intracellular cyclic AMP levels or of cyclic AMP derivatives, parallels the formation of gap junctions and the electrical couplings [24]. Conversely, 8-bromo cGMP has an antagonist effect on junctional assembly. Also in these experiments, several discrepancies remain to be elucidated [24]. If the apparent relationship between hormone sensitivity and the gap-junctional assembly is well substantiated, the question of the role of cyclic nucleotides as regulatory messengers of the junctional assembly still remains unanswered. The results of Decker et al. [68] that in hormonal unsensitive cells, the increase of cyclic nucleotide levels has no effect on the production of gap junctions, cast some doubts on the intimate and direct connection of the cyclic nucleotide and junctional program.

Finally, the finding that a polyribosomal fraction isolated from the cytoskeleton plasma-membrane complex in eye lens fibers directs *in vitro* the translation of MP 26 junctional protein, might implicate a new and surprising aspect of the relationship between cytoskeleton organization and junctional domain formation [100].

Acknowledgements

We wish to thank Professor Hans Bloemendal for his interesting critics and remarks on the manuscript. We would also like to express our appreciation for the secretarial assistance of Mrs. Emmanuel. This work has been supported by the following grants: DGRST No. A 650 1720 and INSERM No. A 650 5075.

References

[1] F. Jacob, Proc. R. Soc. London B 201 (1978) 249.

[2] P. Weiss, J. Embryol. Exp. Morph. 1 (1953) 181.

[3] P. Weiss, in: The Chemistry and Physiology of Growth, ed. A. Parport (Princeton Univ. Press, 1949) pp. 135–186.

[4] G. M. Edelman, in: Cellular Selection and Regulation in the Immune Response, ed. G. M. Edelman (Raven Press, New York, 1974) pp. 1–38.

[5] I. Yahara and G. Edelman, Exp. Cell Res. 91 (1975) 125.

[6] C. R. Kahn, J. Cell Biol. 70 (1976) 261.

[7] L. Wolpert, in: International Cell Biology, eds. B. M. Brinkley and K. R. Porter (The Rockfeller Univ. Press, New York, 1977) pp. 31–35.

[8] J. M. Diamond, Fed. Proc. 33 (1974) 2220.

[9] T. Ducibella and E. Anderson, Develop. Biol. 47 (1975) 45.

[10] T. Ducibella, D. F. Albertini, E. Anderson and J. Biggers, Develop. Biol. 45 (1975) 231.
[11] T. Magnuson, A. Demsey and C. W. Sackpole, Develop. Biol. 61 (1977) 252.
[12] M. H. Johnson, J. Chakraborty, A. H. Handyside, K. Willinson and P. Stern, J. Embryol. Exp. Morph. 54 (1979) 241.
[13] C. W. Lo and N. B. Gilula, Cell 18 (1979) 411.
[14] C. W. Lo and N. B. Gilula, Cell 18 (1979) 399.
[15] C. W. Lo and N. B. Gilula, Develop. Biol. 75 (1980) 112.
[16] C. W. Lo and N. B. Gilula, Develop. Biol. 75 (1980) 93.
[17] C. W. Lo and N. B. Gilula, Develop. Biol. 75 (1980) 78.
[18] N. B. Gilula, and M. L. Epstein, Soc. Exper. Biol. Symp. 30 (1976) 257.
[19] N. B. Gilula, in: Cell Interaction in Differentiation, eds. M. Karkinen-Jaaske-lainen, L. Saxen and L. Weiss (Acad. Press, New York, 1977) pp. 325–338.
[20] W. J. Larsen, Tissue Cell 9 (1977) 373.
[21] W. H. Evans, Nature 283 (1980) 521.
[22] M. V. L. Bennet and D. A. Goodenough, Neurosci. Res. Prog. Bull. 16 (1978) 377.
[23] W. R. Loewenstein, Biochim. Biophys. Acta 560 (1979) 1.
[24] J. D. Sheridan, in: Receptors and Recognition Series B. and Vol. 2. Intercellular Junctions and Synapses, eds. J. Feldman, N. B. Gilula and J. D. Pitts (Chapman and Hall, London; Wiley, New York, 1978) pp. 37–60.
[25] C. Sotelo, and H. Korn, Int. Rev. Cytol. 55 (1978) 67.
[26] J. P. Revel, and M. J. Karnovsky, J. Cell Biol. 33 (1967) C.7.
[27] E. L. Benedetti and P. Emmelot, J. Cell Biol. 26 (1965) 299.
[28] E. L. Benedetti and P. Emmelot, J. Cell Biol. 38 (1968) 15.
[29] B. H. Satir and P. Satir, in: Freeze Fracture Methods Artefacts and Interpretation, ed. J. E. Mash and C. S. Hudson (Raven Press, New York, 1979).
[30] A. J. Verkleij and P. H. J. Th. Ververgaert, Biochim. Biophys. Acta 515 (1978) 303.
[31] A. J. Verkleij, C. Mombers, J. Leunissen-Bijvelt and P. H. J. Th. Ververgaert, Nature 279 (1979) 162.
[32] D. L. D. Caspar, D. A. Goodenough, L. Makowski and W. C. Phillips, J. Cell Biol. 74 (1977) 605.
[33] G. Zampighi and P. N. T. Unwin, J. Mol. Biol. 135 (1979) 451.
[34] P. N. T. Unwin and G. Zampighi, Nature 283 (1979) 545.
[35] J. D. Sheridan, M. Hammer-Wilson, D. Preus and R. G. Johnson, J. Cell Biol. 76 (1978) 532.
[36] W. R. Loewenstein, Y. Kanno and S. J. Socolar, Fed. Proc. 37 (1978b) 2645.
[37] S. Gabella and D. Blundell, J. Cell Biol. 82 (1979) 239.
[38] C. Peracchia, Trends Biochem. Sci. 2 (1977) 26.
[39] C. Peracchia, Nature 271 (1978) 669.
[40] I. Dunia, J. F. Nicolas, H. Jakob, E. L. Bendetti and F. Jacob, Proc. Natl. Acad. Sci. USA 76 (1979) 3387.
[41] J. P. Changeux, E. L. Benedetti, J. P. Bourgeois, A. Brisson, J. Cartaud, P. Devaux, H. Grünhagen, M. Moreau, J. L. Popot, A. Sobel and M. Weber, Cold Spring Harbor Symp. Quant. Biol. XL (1975) 211.
[42] J. Deleze and W. R. Lowenstein, J. Membr. Biol. 28 (1979) 71.
[43] J. Flagg-Newton and W. R. Lowenstein, J. Membr. Biol. 50 (1979) 65.
[44] J. Flagg-Newton, I. Simpson and W. R. Loewenstein, Science 205 (1979) 404.
[45] M. V. L. Bennett, M. E. Spira and D. C. Spray, Develop. Biol. 65 (1978) 114.

[46] C. S. Goodman and N. C. Spitzer, Nature 280 (1979) 208.
[47] R. Azarnia and W. R. Loewenstein, J. Membr. Biol. 34 (1977) 1.
[48] W. J. Larsen, R. Azarnia and W. R. Loewenstein, J. Membr. Biol. 34 (1977) 34.
[49] R. Azarnia and W. J. Larsen, in: Intercellular Communication and Cancer, ed., W. C. DeMello (Plenum Press, New York, 1977) p. 145.
[50] M. L. Epstein and N. B. Gilula, J. Cell Biol. 75 (1977) 769.
[51] M. L. Epstein, J. D. Sheridan and R. G. Johnson, Exp. Cell Res. 104 (1977) 25.
[52] S. Polak-Charcon, J. Shoham and Y. Ben-Shaul, Exp. Cell Res. 116 (1978) 1.
[53] E. B. Griepp and M. R. Bernfield, Exp. Cell Res. 113 (1978) 263.
[54] E. B. Griepp, J. H. Peacock, M. R. Bernfield and J. P. Revel, Exp. Cell Res. 113 (1978) 273.
[55] R. S. Decker and D. S. Friend, J. Cell Biol. 62 (1974) 32.
[56] R. S. Decker, J. Cell Biol. 69 (1976) 669.
[57] L. A. Smets, H. Van Roy and C. Homburg, Exp. Cell Res. 123 (1979) 87.
[58] L. A. Culp, in: Current Topic in Membranes and Transport, eds. F. Bronner and A. Khinzeller, Vol. 11 (Academic Press, New York, 1978) pp. 327–396.
[59] H. Noll, V. Matranga, D. Cascino and L. Vittorelli, Proc. Natl. Acad. Sci. USA 76 (1979) 288.
[60] R. M. Broekhuyse and J. H. Veerkamp, Biochem. Biophys. Acta 152 (1968) 316.
[61] R. M. Broekhuyse and E. D. Kühlman, Exp. Cell Res. 19 (1974) 297.
[62] R. D. Klausner, D. K. Bhalla, P. Dragsten, R. L. Hoover and M. J. Karnovski, Proc. Natl. Acad. Sci. USA 77 (1980) 437.
[63] W. J. Larsen, H. N. Tung, S. A. Murray and C. A. Swenson, J. Cell Biol. 83 (1979) 576.
[64] E. L. Benedetti, I. Dunia, C. J. Bentzel, A. J. M. Vermorken, M. Kibbelaar and H. Bloemendal, Biochim. Biophys. Acta 457 (1976) 353.
[65] E. A. Johnson, M. Hammer, J. Sheridan and J. P. Revel, Proc. Natl. Acad. Sci. USA 71 (1974) 4536.
[66] M. Epstein and J. Sheridan, J. Cell Biol. 63 (1974) 95a.
[67] E. Anderson and D. F. Albertini, J. Cell Biol. 71 (1976) 680.
[68] R. S. Decker, S. T. Donta, W. J. Larsen and S. A. Murray, J. Supramol. Struct. 9 (1978) 497.
[69] R. D. Ginzberg and N. B. Gilula, Develop. Biol. 68 (1979) 110.
[70] M. Porvaznik, R. G. Johnson and J. D. Sheridan, J. Supramol. Struct. 10 (1979) 13.
[71] N. Kalderon and N. B. Gilula, J. Cell Biol. 81 (1979) 411.
[72] E. B. Griepp and J. P. Revel, in: Gap Junctions in Development, Intercellular Communication, ed. W. C. de Mello (Plenum Press, New York/London, 1977) pp. 1–32.
[73] E. L. Benedetti, I. Dunia and H. Bloemendal, Proc. Natl. Acad. Sci. USA 71 (1974) 5073.
[74] M. L. Kapsenberg and W. Leene, Exp. Cell Res. 120 (1979) 211.
[75] F. Mazet and J. Cartaud, J. Cell Sci. 22 (1976) 427.
[76] F. Mazet, Dev. Biol. 60 (1977) 139.
[77] I. Dunia, C. Sen-Ghosh, E. L. Benedetti, A. Zweers and H. Bloemendal, FEBS Lett. 45 (1974) 139.
[78] J. C. Ehrhart and J. Chauveau, FEBS Lett. 78 (1977a) 295.
[79] J. R. Duguid and J. P. Revel, Cold Spring Harbor Symp. Quant. Biol. 40 (1975) 45.
[80] W. H. Evans and J. W. Gurd, Biochem. J. 128 (1972) 691.

[81] D. A. Goodenough, Invest. Ophthalmol. Visual Sci. 18 (1979) 1104.
[82] D. Henderson, H. Eibl and K. Weber, J. Mol. Biol. 132 (1979) 193.
[83] E. L. Hertzberg and N. B. Gilula, J. Biol. Chem. 254 (1979) 2138.
[84] H. Bloemendal, A. J. M. Vermorken, M. Kibbelaar, I. Dunia and E. L. Benedetti, Exp. Eye Res. 24 (1977) 413.
[85] M. M. Wong, N. P. Robertson and J. Horwitz, Biochim. Biophys. Res. Comm. 84 (1978) 158.
[86] R. M. Broekhuyse, E. D. Kühlmann and H. J. Winkens, Exp. Eye Res. 29 (1979).
[87] M. A. Kibbelaar and H. Bloemendal, Exp. Eye Res. 29 (1979) 679.
[88] R. M. Broekhuyse, E. D. Kühlmann and A. L. H. Stols, Exp. Eye Res. 23 (1976) 365.
[89] J. Alcala and H. Maisel, Exp. Eye Res. 26 (1978) 219.
[90] A. A. Bouman, A. L. M. de Leeuw, E. F. J. Tolhuizen and R. M. Broekhuyse, Exp. Eye Res. 29 (1979) 83.
[91] E. L. Benedetti, I. Dunia, F. C. S. Ramaekers and M. A. Kibbelaar, in: Molecular Biology of Eye Lens, ed. H. Bloemendal (Wiley, New York, in press).
[92] A. J. M. Vermorken, J. M. H. C. Hilderink, I. Dunia, E. L. Benedetti and H. Bloemendal, FEBS Lett. 83 (1977) 301.
[93] J. D. Pitts and R. R. Burk, Nature 264 (1976) 762.
[94] I. Fentiman, J. Taylor-Paradimitriou and M. Stoker, Nature 264 (1976) 760.
[95] S. Cavenay, Science 199 (1978) 192.
[96] C. L. Browne, H. S. Wiley and J. N. Dumont, Science 203 (1979) 182.
[97] Th. S. Lawrence, W. H. Beers and N. B. Gilula, Nature 272 (1979) 501.
[98] I. I. Singer, Cell 16 (1979) 675.
[99] G. Blobel, Proc. Natl. Acad. Sci. USA 77 (1980) 1496.
[100] F. C. S. Ramaekers, A. M. E. Selten-Versteegen, E. L. Benedetti, I. Dunia and H. Bloemendal, Proc. Natl. Acad. Sci. USA 77 (1980) 725.

Recently, Weinbaum has proposed a mathematic model for the interpretation of the junctional particle assembly: J. Theor. Biol. 83 (1980) 63.

COURSE 7

ION TRANSPORT THROUGH LIPID BILAYER MEMBRANES*

Peter LÄUGER

Fachbereich Biologie,
Universität Konstanz,
Postfach 7733, D-7750 Konstanz,
Germany

*This course is partly based on work done in collaboration with H. Alpes, H.-J. Apell, E. Bamberg, R. Benz, K. Janko, H.-A. Kolb, and G. Stark, Department of Biology, University of Konstanz.

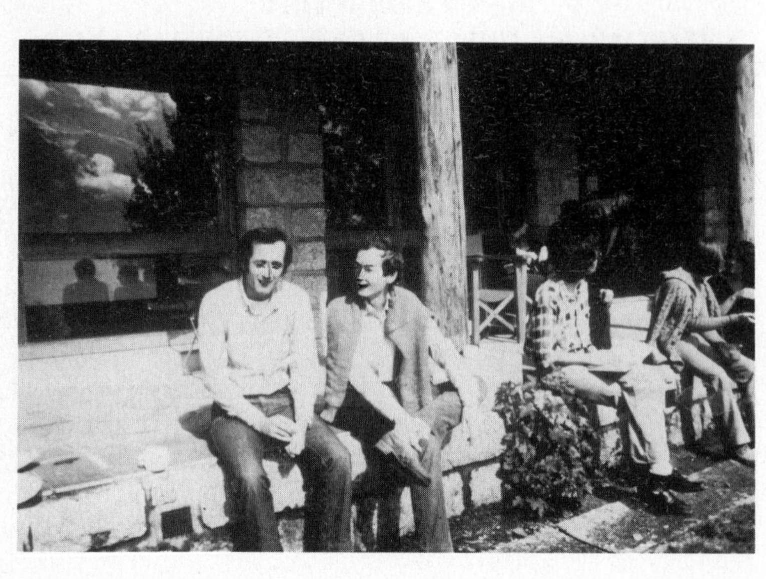

Contents

R. Balian et al., eds.
Les Houches, Session XXXIII, 1979 – Membranes et Communication Intercellulaire / Membranes and Intercellular Communication

1. Basic properties of the lipid bilayer, as related to ion transport

The interior of a lipid bilayer is a medium of low dielectric constant and therefore represents an extremely high energy barrier for the passage of small ions such as Na^+ or K^+. The ion permeability of biological membranes depends, to a large extent, on the presence of specialized membrane constituents which provide energetically favourable pathways for ion transport through the apolar core of the membrane. The following course deals with the study of such ion transport mechanisms (carrier and channel mechanisms) using artificial lipid bilayer membranes.

1.1. Dielectric properties, generalized Nernst–Planck equation

To a first approximation, the bilayer may be regarded as a dielectric film interposed between two aqueous media. The energy w required to transfer an ion of radius r and valency z from a semi-infinite aqueous phase (dielectric constant ε) into an infinitely thick membrane phase (dielectric constant ε_m) is given by Born's equation

$$w = \frac{a}{r}\left(\frac{1}{\varepsilon_m} - \frac{1}{\varepsilon}\right), \tag{1}$$

$$a \equiv \frac{z^2 e_0^2}{8\pi\varepsilon_0 kT} \simeq 28.0 \text{ nm}, \qquad (T=298 \text{ K}, z=\pm 1) \tag{2}$$

e_0 is the elementary charge, $\varepsilon_0 = 8.85 \times 10^{-12}$ CV^{-1} m^{-1} is the permittivity of free space and w is expressed in units of kT (k is Boltzmann's constant and T the absolute temperature). For an ion the size of the unhydrated potassium ion ($r \simeq 0.13$ nm) the energy w assumes the prohibitively high value of $w \simeq 100$ ($\varepsilon_m = 2.1$, $\varepsilon = 79$).

For a membrane of finite thickness, d the dielectric energy of the ion in the center of the membrane is less than the Born limit w by the amount [1]:

$$\Delta w = \frac{2a}{\varepsilon_m d}\ln\left(\frac{2\varepsilon}{\varepsilon + \varepsilon_m}\right). \tag{3}$$

In the vicinity of the interface of the two dielectric media, the ion experiences a force (the so-called image force) which tends to attract the ion towards the medium with the higher dielectric constant (water). The potential energy $w(x)$ of the ion in the membrane, therefore, has the form of a barrier with a flat peak in the center. The shape of the potential energy may be calculated by the method of the electrical images [2]; some results are represented in fig. 1. Given the shape of the energy barrier, the flux Φ of ions through the membrane may be calculated from the generalized Nernst–Planck equation (2):

$$\Phi = -D\left(\frac{\mathrm{d}C}{\mathrm{d}x} + zC\frac{\mathrm{d}\phi}{\mathrm{d}x} + C\frac{\mathrm{d}w}{\mathrm{d}x}\right), \tag{4}$$

where Φ is the ion flux referred to unit area, D the diffusion coefficient of the ion in the membrane, C the ion concentration in the membrane, and x the coordinate normal to the membrane surface; the electrical potential ϕ is expressed in units of $kT/e_0 \simeq 25$ mV:

$$\phi(x) = \frac{\psi(x)}{kT/e_0}, \tag{5}$$

where $\psi(x)$ is the electrical potential in the membrane. Equation (4) may be easily integrated for a membrane extending between $x = -s$ and

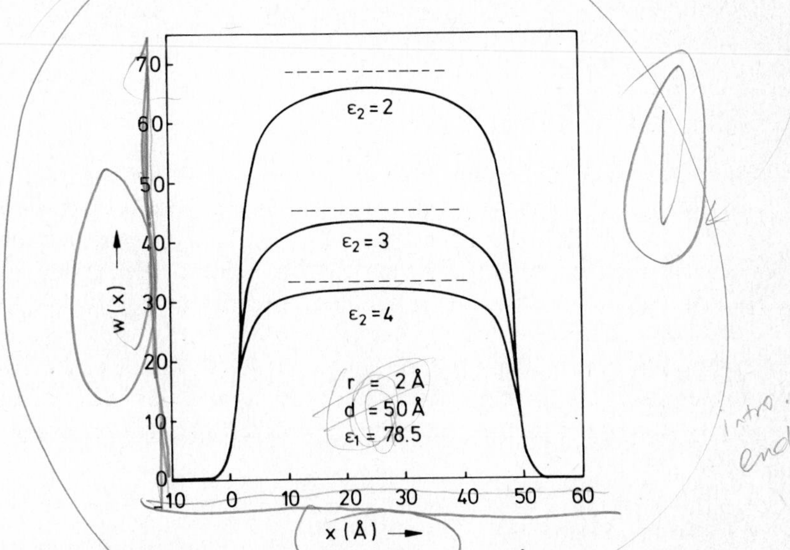

Fig. 1. Potential energy $w(x)$ of a univalent ion of radius $r = 2$ Å $= 0.2$ nm in a membrane of thickness $d = 50$ Å and dielectric constant ε_m [2]. w is expressed in units of kT. The dashed lines indicate the Born energy of the ion in the limit $d \to \infty$.

$x = s$. Using the notation

$$h(x) \equiv \exp[z\phi(x) + w(x)], \tag{6}$$

the result reads

$$\Phi = [C(-s)h(-s) - C(s)h(s)] \Big/ \int_{-s}^{s} \Big[h(x)/D(x) \Big] \, \mathrm{d}x. \tag{7}$$

This relation can be used, for instance, for the calculation of transport rates of hydrophobic ions in lipid bilayer membranes (see below). In the application of eq. (7) it is often assumed that the potential ϕ is a linear function of x (constant-field approximation) and that the diffusion coefficient D is independent of x.

1.2. *Interfacial potentials*

A drop of the electrostatic potential across the membrane–solution interface may result from fixed charges on the lipid and/or from layers of oriented dipoles [3]. If the membrane surface contains a net charge of density σ, the electrical potential ϕ_s at the membrane surface with respect to the bulk aqueous solution of a 1 : 1 electrolyte of concentration c is given by the Gouy–Chapman equation:

$$\phi_s = 2 \ln \left[\frac{\sigma}{\sigma_0} + \sqrt{\left(\frac{\sigma}{\sigma_0}\right)^2 + 1} \, \right], \tag{8}$$

$$\sigma_0 \equiv \sqrt{8\varepsilon_0 \varepsilon RTc} \,, \tag{9}$$

where R is the gas constant. For instance, if a membrane is formed from a lipid with a single net negative charge per molecule, such as phosphatidylserine, the surface charge density is about 1 elementary charge per 0.60 nm^2, or $\sigma \simeq -0.27 \ \mathrm{C\ m^{-2}}$. At an ionic concentration of $c =$ 0.1 M, eq. (8) predicts an interfacial potential of $\psi_s = (kT/e_0)\ \phi_s =$ -140 mV. The interfacial potential ϕ_s leads to an accumulation of counterions and a depletion of coions at the surface, i.e. the surface concentrations c_s^+ and c_s^- of univalent cations and anions at the surface are related to the bulk concentration c by the Boltzmann relations:

$$c_s^+ = c \cdot \exp(-\phi_s) \tag{10}$$

$$c_s^- = c \cdot \exp(\phi_s). \tag{11}$$

This means that the conductance of a cation-specific transport system can be substantially increased by a negative interfacial potential. Equations (8) and (9) further predict that the absolute magnitude of ϕ_s decreases with increasing ionic concentration. The Gouy–Chapman treatment gives only an approximate description, however, since the formation of a surface layer of adsorbed counterions (the so-called Stern layer) is neglected.

Even if the net charge at the interface is zero, a potential difference between the membrane interior and the aqueous phase may be created by layers of oriented dipoles. The overall dipolar potential may result from several contributions, such as layers of oriented water molecules on the solution side of the interface and oriented polar groups of the lipid molecules. Each of these single contributions to the total dipolar potential may be large. If N dipoles are present per unit area and if each dipole contributes with a dipolar moment μ in a direction normal to the membrane surface, the total dipolar potential ψ_D may be estimated to be

$$\psi_D = N\mu/\varepsilon_0. \tag{12}$$

For a monolayer of perfectly oriented water molecules, eq. (12) would predict $\psi_D \simeq 5$ V. Or if we assume that the positive and negative charges of the zwitterionic phosphorylcholine group in a lecithin membrane would be out of plane by only 0.01 nm, the dipolar potential would be about 0.4 V.

An interesting situation arises if the two halves of the bilayer have different lipid compositions. In this case differences in the density of net charges and/or in the dipolar potential may create an internal electrical field even in the absence of an externally applied voltage (fig. 2).

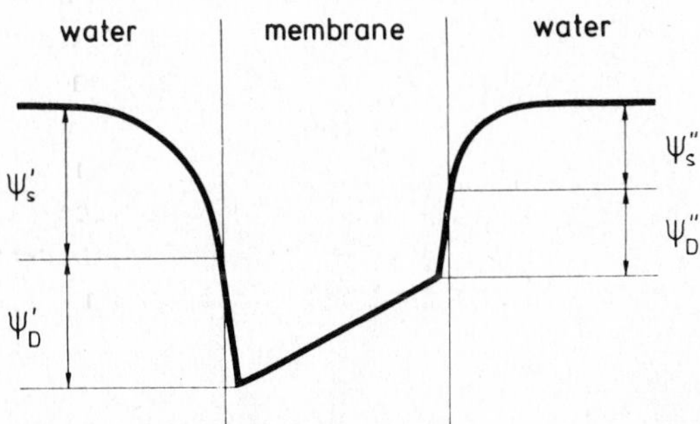

Fig. 2. Interfacial potentials of an asymmetric bilayer. ψ_s' and ψ_s'' are the contributions of net (negative) charges and ψ_D' and ψ_D'' the contributions of dipolar layers.

2. Artificial planar bilayer membranes

For the study of ion transport systems, such as carriers or channels, artificial planar bilayer membranes have been used extensively in the last years. Bilayer membranes with an area of several mm^2 may be formed from a variety of pure lipids using the technique introduced by Mueller et al. [4]. In this technique, a solution of a lipid such as dioleoyllecithin in a solvent (e.g., *n*-decane) is spread over a hole in a teflon diaphragm which is immersed in an aqueous electrolyte solution. In this way, a thin liquid film is formed which thins further and spontaneously forms an optically black membrane which covers most of the area of the hole. By measuring the electrical capacitance [5] or the light reflectance [6], the thickness of these membranes is found to be close to the value expected for a lipid bilayer. The exact value of the membrane thickness depends on the nature of the solvent used for membrane formation indicating that the membrane still contains some solvent.

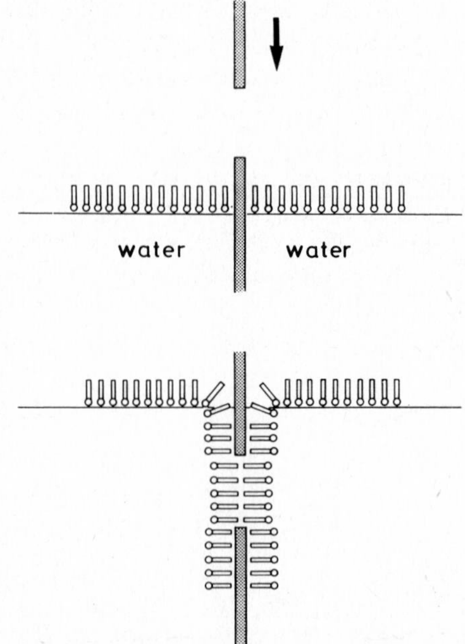

Fig. 3. Formation of planar bilayer membranes by the method of Montal and Mueller [7]. In most cases the teflon film is held fixed and the water levels are raised one after the other.

Virtually solvent-free planar bilayers may be obtained by another method [7] in which a monolayer of lipid is spread from a volatile solvent, such as *n*-hexane, on a water surface and a thin teflon film with a hole of about 0.2 mm in diameter is drawn through the monolayer (fig. 3). If such membranes are made from a series of monoglycerides with varying chain lengths, the membrane thickness, as determined from capacitance measurements, increases with an increasing number of methylene groups in the fatty acid chain of the lipid, as expected [8]. Instead of spreading the monolayer from a solvent, a suspension of single-bilayer lipid vesicles may be applied to the water surface and thereafter a planar bilayer may be formed by the Montal–Mueller technique [9].

3. Transport of hydrophobic ions

The simplest ion transport mechanism so far studied with lipid bilayer membranes is the transport of hydrophobic ions, such as tetraphenylborate or dipicrylamine [10, 11]. In this case the total interaction energy of the ion with the membrane contains two terms, one arising from the electrical image forces (as discussed above) and the second from the hydrophobic interaction (fig. 4). The superposition of both energies leads to deep energy minima at the membrane solution interface (fig. 4). Hydrophobic ions spend most of the time in these energy wells and occasionally may jump across the central barrier to the other side.

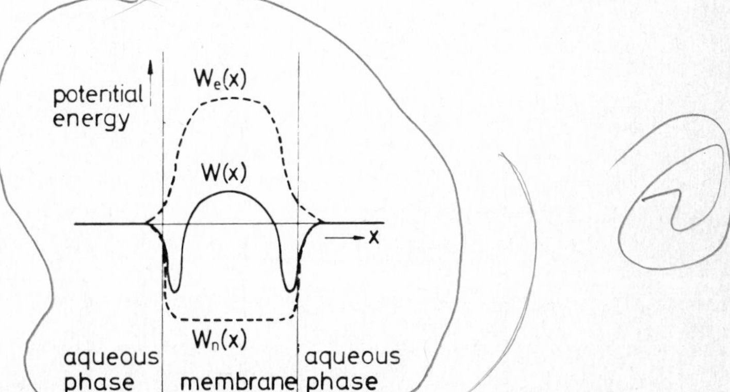

Fig. 4. Dielectric contribution w_e and hydrophobic contribution w_n to the total potential energy of a hydrophobic ion in a lipid membrane. The influence of surface potentials is omitted.

3.1. *Electrical relaxation methods for the study of ion transport processes in membranes*

The rate of transfer of hydrophobic ions across the central energy barrier in the membrane may be studied using fast electrical relaxation methods. (These methods are also used for the analysis of carrier-mediated ion transport and of channel processes). In the voltage–jump relaxation method (fig. 5) a voltage is suddenly applied to the membrane and the relaxation of the membrane current is measured [10]. In the charge–pulse method (fig. 5) which has a time-resolution of the order of 100 ns, the membrane capacitance is charged up by a brief current pulse. After the current pulse the external circuit is switched to virtually infinite resistance and the decay of the membrane voltage is measured [12].

3.2. *Analysis of relaxation experiments with hydrophobic ions*

If a voltage is suddenly applied to a bilayer membrane in the presence of hydrophobic ions, an initial current is observed which declines to a much smaller stationary current [10]. The initial current is interpreted as

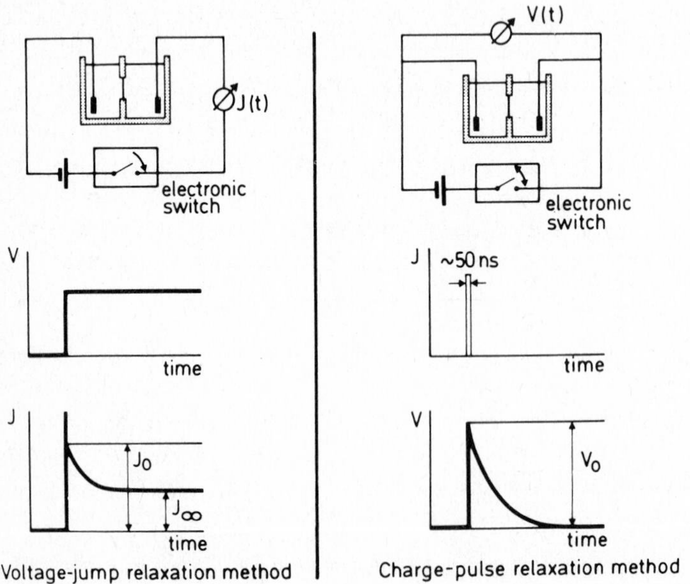

Fig. 5. Electrical relaxation methods for the study of ion transport processes in membranes.

resulting from the fast transport of ions across the central barrier, whereas the steady-state current is limited by the slow exchange of ions between the interfacial energy minima and the aqueous solutions. The current density I may be approximately described by introducing the interfacial concentrations (mol/cm^2) N' and N'' of hydrophobic ions at the left-hand and right-hand interface and the rate constants k_i' and k_i'' for the transport across the central barrier from left to right and from right to left:

$$I = zF(k_i'N' - k_i''N''). \tag{13}$$

F is the Faraday constant and z is the valency of the ion. k_i' and k_i'' are functions of the applied voltage V_m. For convenience we introduce the reduced voltage u:

$$u \equiv \frac{V_m}{RT/F} = \frac{\psi' - \psi''}{RT/F}, \tag{14}$$

(ψ' and ψ'' are the electrical potentials of the left-hand and right-hand aqueous phase). If we restrict the analysis to small voltages ($|u| \ll 1$), k_i' and k_i'' may be approximately represented by

$$k_i' \approx k_i(1 + \alpha z u/2) \qquad k_i'' \approx k_i(1 - \alpha z u/2), \tag{15, 16}$$

k_i is the value of k_i' and k_i'' at zero voltage and α is the fraction of total voltage which drops between the two energy minima (fig. 4). Equations (13), (15), and (16) may be justified on the basis of the Nernst-Planck treatment, eq. (7), in the following way. For a symmetric membrane which behaves as a linear dielectric, both $w(x)$ and $\phi(x)$ are symmetric functions with respect to the middle of the membrane ($x = 0$). We may therefore set $w(-s) = w(s) = w_m$ and $\phi(-s) = \alpha u/2$, $\phi(s) = -\alpha u/2$. The voltage drop between the two adsorption planes is then equal to αu; as the dielectric constant is a function of position, α is, in general, different from ($1-2\,s/d$). We further assume that the energy minima are deep ($-w_m \gg 1$) and that the central barrier is high ($[w(0) - w_m] \gg 1$). Under these conditions where most of the ions are located in the vicinity of $x = \pm s$, it is reasonable to introduce interfacial concentrations N' and N'' which may be set proportional to the volume concentrations at $x = \pm s$: $N' = \vartheta C(-s)$, $N'' = \vartheta C(s)$. Accordingly, the equation for the ion flux assumes the form

$$\Phi = k_i'N' - k_i''N''. \tag{17}$$

Comparing eqs. (7) and (17) it is seen that

$$k_i' = k_i e^{z\alpha u/2} f(u); \qquad k_i'' = k_i e^{-z\alpha u/2} f(u) \tag{18; 19}$$

where the function

$$f(u) = \frac{\int_{-s}^{s} \exp\{[w(x)]/[D(x)]\}\, dx}{\int_{-s}^{s} \exp\{[w(x)+z\phi(x)]/[D(x)]\}\, dx} \tag{20}$$

accounts for the shape of the central barrier, and k_i is given by:

$$k_i = \left\{ \vartheta \int_{-s}^{s} \frac{\exp[w(x)-w_m]}{D(x)}\, dx \right\}^{-1}. \tag{21}$$

We now apply eqs. (18)–(20) to the limiting case $|zu| \ll 1$, $|z\phi| \ll 1$ where the approximation $\exp(z\phi) \approx 1 + z\phi + (z\phi)^2/2$ may be used. As $\exp w(x)$ is an even function and $\phi(x)$ an odd function of x, the relation

$$\int_{-s}^{s} \phi(x) \exp[w(x)]\, dx = 0 \tag{22}$$

holds. Writing $\phi(x) = u \cdot \chi(x)$ where $\chi(x)$ is independent of u, it is easy to show that $f(u)$ has the expansion

$$f(u) \approx 1 + Bu^2, \tag{23}$$

where B is a constant. This proves eqs. (6) and (7). It is thus seen that up to terms of the order of u the rate constants k_i' and k_i'' depend only on the effective voltage αu but are independent of the detailed shape of the barrier.

3.3. Experimental results

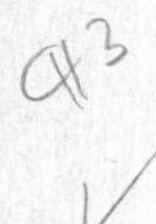

Most studies on the transport of hydrophobic ions have been carried out with dipicrylamine of tetraphenylborate [10–13]. The translocation rate constant k_i was found to be strongly dependent on the structure of the lipid used for membrane formation (table 1). k_i decreases with increasing chain length of the lipid and increases with increasing unsaturation. The chain length effect presumably results, in part, from the change in membrane thickness (change of the height of the energy barrier) and, in part, from the increased microviscosity of the film. The influence of unsaturation probably also results from an increase of membrane fluidity with increasing number of double bonds. Furthermore, the dielectric constant of the hydrocarbon increase with unsaturation which reduces the height of the energy barrier. Translocation rate constants for tetraphenylborate are considerably lower than those of

Table 1

Translocation rate constant k_i of dipicrylamine in bilayer membranes made from lecithins with different chain lengths and number of double bonds[a)]

Fatty acid	16 : 1	18 : 1	20 : 1	22 : 1	24 : 1
k_i (s^{-1})	850	430	170	90	37
Fatty acid	18 : 1	18 : 2	18 : 3		
k_i (s^{-1})	430	1500	4810		

[a)]18 : 1 denotes a lecithin with 18 carbon atoms and one double bond in the fatty-acid chain. The membranes were formed from a 1–3% solution of the lipid in *n*-decane, $T = 25°$ C. For further details, see ref. [12].

dipicrylamine. For di-(18 : 1)-lecithin (dioleoyllecithin) k_i was found to be 10 s^{-1} at 25° C [10].

4. Carrier-mediated ion transport

In recent years a number of compounds, such as valinomycin or enniatin B, have been characterized which act as mobile carriers for univalent cations [14]. In organic solvents these compounds form alkali–ion complexes with a high specificity, for instance, valinomycin discriminates between Na^+ and K^+ by more than a factor 1000. In the valinomycin/K^+ complex the central K^+ ion is surrounded by six carbonyl oxygen atoms, whereas the exterior of the complex is hydrophobic (fig. 6). When valinomycin is introduced into an artificial bilayer membrane in the presence of K^+ in the aqueous phase, the membrane becomes selectively permeable for K^+ ions. The membrane conductance is a linear function of the carrier concentration in water, suggesting that the current-carrying species is a 1 : 1 complex between K^+ and valinomycin.

A transport scheme consistent with the experimental results obtained with valinomycin and monactin is depicted in fig. 7. The transport occurs in four distinct steps: (1) formation of a complex between ion M^+ and carrier S at the interface (rate constant k_R); (2) translocation of the complex MS^+ to the opposite side (rate constant k'_{MS}); (3) release of the ion to the solution (rate constant k_D); and (4) back transport of the unloaded carrier (rate constant k_S). This transport process is purely

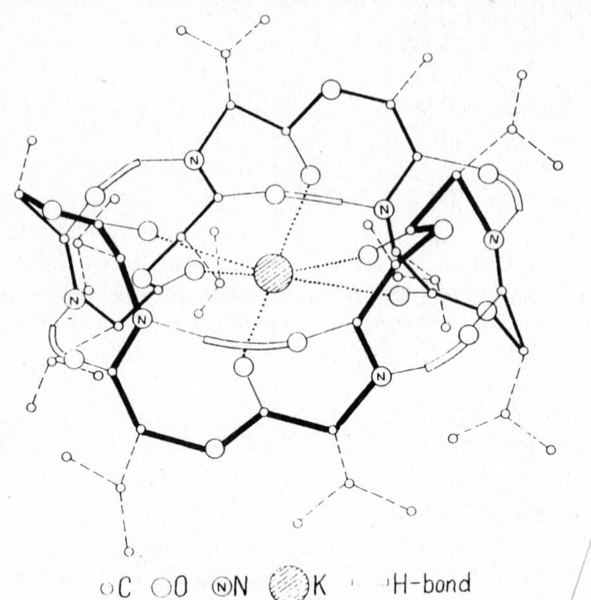

Fig. 6. Structure of the potassium–valinomycin complex [14].

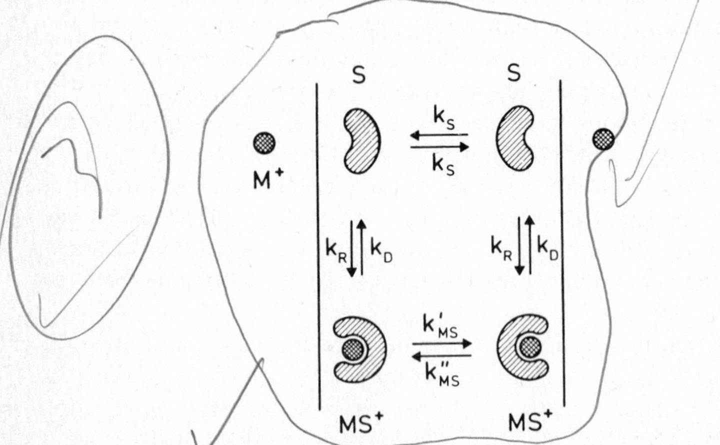

Fig. 7. Transport of cation M^+ mediated by a neutral carrier S.

passive, i.e. the transport is driven (at equal activity of M^+ on both sides) by the electric field strength in the membrane.

4.1. *Kinetic analysis with relaxation methods*

Some information on the values of the rate constants may be obtained from stationary current–voltage measurements, but steady-state data are not sufficient for a complete kinetic analysis. For this reason fast relaxation methods have been used for the study of carrier-mediated ion transport (fig. 5). For the analysis of the relaxation experiments it is usually assumed that only the translocation rate constants k'_{MS} and k''_{MS} depend on voltage and that the total voltage drops between the two potential minima for the charged complex MS^+. For small voltages, k'_{MS} and k''_{MS} are then obtained from eqs. (15) and (16) with $z=1$ and $\alpha \approx 1$:

$$k'_{MS} \approx k_{MS}(1+u/2) \qquad k''_{MS} \approx k_{MS}(1-u/2). \tag{24, 25}$$

The analysis of the carrier model represented in fig. 7 yields the following expression for the time–course of membrane voltage V in the charge–pulse experiment:

$$V(t) = V_0[a_1 \exp(-t/\tau_1) + a_2 \exp(-t/\tau_1) + a_3 \exp(-t/\tau_3)] \tag{26}$$

$$a_1 + a_2 + a_3 = 1. \tag{27}$$

V_0 is the initial voltage. The relaxation times τ_1, τ_2, τ_3, and the relaxation amplitudes a_1, a_2, a_3 are complicated functions of the rate constants [15]. Under favourable experimental conditions where all three relaxation processes can be resolved, the rate constants k_R, k_D, k_{MS}, and k_S (fig. 7) can be determined from records of $V(t)$. A similar analysis is possible for voltage-jump current-relaxation experiments [16].

Rate constants for a number of cation-carrier systems have been evaluated in the last years by these methods. As a specific example, we consider the results obtained for valinomycin/Rb^+ in a monoolein/*n*-decane membrane (25° C, 1 M RbCl) [15]:

$$k_R = 3 \times 10^5\ M^{-1}\,s^{-1} \qquad k_D = 2 \times 10^5\ s^{-1}$$

$$k_{MS} = 3 \times 10^5\ s^{-1} \qquad k_S = 4 \times 10^4\ s^{-1}.$$

At one-molar concentration of the transported ion ($c_M = 1$ M), the rate constants of association ($c_M k_R$), dissociation (k_D), and translocation of the loaded carrier (k_{MS}) are approximately equal (2–$3 \times 10^5\ s^{-1}$). The rate-determining step in this system is the back-transport of the free carrier ($k_S = 4\times 10^4\ s^{-1}$). $k_{MS} = 3\times 10^5\ s^{-1}$ is the frequency of jumps of an ion-carrier complex from one interface to the other. The reciprocal value $1/k_{MS} \simeq 3\ \mu s$ is the average time required for the translocation. This time may be compared with the diffusion time $\tau \simeq d^2/2D$ of a spherical particle of the size of the carrier (radius $\simeq 0.7$ nm) across the same distance (membrane thickness $d \simeq 5$ nm) in water (diffusion coefficient $D \simeq 3\times 10^{-6}\ cm^2\ s^{-1}$), which is about 0.04 μs. From the rate constants, another important quantity may be calculated, the maximum turnover rate f of the carrier. f is defined as the limiting transport rate which is approached under short-circuit conditions for infinite ion concentration on the *cis*-side and zero ion concentration on the *trans*-side. f may be calculated from the known values of the rate constants [17]:

$$f = \left(k_{MS}^{-1} + k_S^{-1} + 2k_D^{-1}\right)^{-1}. \tag{28}$$

In the above example, f is about $3\times 10^4\ s^{-1}$. The high efficiency of valinomycin as an ion carrier mainly results from this high turnover rate, whereas the binding constant for the ion, $k_R/k_D = 1.5\ M^{-1}$, is rather low.

4.2. *Influence of membrane structure on the rate constants*

4.2.1. *Variation in the number of double bonds*

Kinetic parameters for valinomycin-mediated Rb^+ transport in membranes made from monoglycerides with varying degree of unsaturation [18] are given in table 2. k_R and k_D are not much sensitive to a variation in the number n of double bonds. On the other hand, the translocation
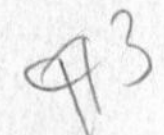
rate constant k_{MS} (and, to a lesser degree, also k_S) strongly increases with n, the change of k_{MS} being 24-fold between $n = 1$ and $n = 4$. Again, this variation of k_{MS} presumably results (at least in part) from an increased disorder and decreased microviscosity in membranes made from highly unsaturated monoglycerides. Another effect which may influence k_{MS} is the increase of dielectric constant of the membrane with increasing unsaturation.

4.2.2. *Charged head-groups*

Conductance measurements with membranes made from charged lipids are in qualitative agreement with the theoretical predictions, eqs. (8)–(11).

Table 2

Rate constants of valinomycin-mediated Rb^+-transport through membranes made from α-monoglycerides (G) differing in the number double-bonds in the fatty-acid residue (18) : oleoyl (18 : 1), lineoyl (18 : 2), linolenoyl (18 : 3), Δ^{11}-eicosenoyl (20 : 1), $\Delta^{11,14}$-eicosadienoyl (20 : 2), $\Delta^{11,14,17}$ = eicosatrienoyl (20 : 3), and arachidonoyl (20 : 4)[a)]

Lipid	$k_R/10^4\ (M^{-1})\ s^{-1}$	$k_D/10^4\ (s^{-1})$	$k_{MS}/10^4\ (s^{-1})$	$k_S/10^4\ (s^{-1})$
(18 : 1)-G	37	24	27	3.5
(18 : 2)-G	67	13	143	6.2
(18 : 3)-G	74	8	250	9.6
(20 : 1)-G	23	12	10	1.8
(20 : 2)-G	34	9	39	3.2
(20 : 3)-G	34	5	136	9.4
(20 : 4)-G	42	3	240	12

[a)]The solvent for membrane formation was *n*-decane; $T = 25°$ C.

An example is shown in fig. 8 in which the conductance of a phosphatidylethanolamine membrane in the presence of nonactin and K^+ is given as a function of ionic strength [19]. Nonactin acts as a carrier for K^+ by forming a positively charged complex $(\text{nonactin} \cdot K)^+$. The ionic strength has been varied at constant K^+ concentration by adding LiCl (Li^+ is not transported to any appreciable extent by nonactin). It is seen

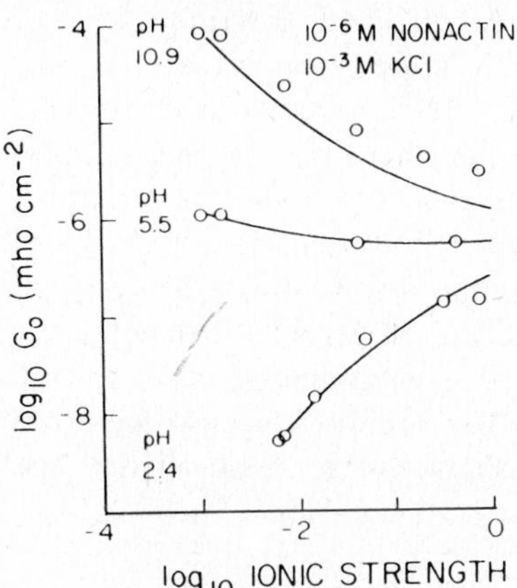

Fig. 8. Conductance of a phosphatidylethanolamine membrane in the presence of nonactin and K^+ different pH values, according to McLaughlin et al. [19]. The ionic strength was varied by adding the inert electrolyte LiCl. The solid lines are theoretical curves drawn with the following values of the surface charge density σ (e_0 is the elementary charge): $\sigma(\text{pH } 10.9) = -e_0/7\ \text{nm}^2$; $\sigma(\text{pH } 5.5) = -e_0/120\ \text{nm}^2$, $\sigma(\text{pH } 2.4) = +e_0/3.7\ \text{nm}^2$.

from fig. 8 that at pH 10.9 where phosphatidylethanolamine is negatively charged, the conductance decreases with increasing ionic strength [decreasing absolute magnitude of the surface potential ϕ_s in eq. (10)]. At pH 5.5 the lipid is mainly in the zwitterionic (electrically neutral) form, and the conductance is virtually independent of ionic strength. On the other hand, at pH 2.4 where phosphatidylethanolamine is positively charged, the conductance is an increasing function of ionic strength.

4.2.3. *Effect of oriented dipoles at the membrane-solution interface*

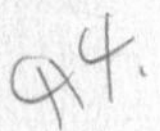

Evidence for the existence of dipolar layers at the membrane surface (subsection 1.2) comes from experiments with lipid monolayers at the air–water surface. If a lipid monolayer is spread at the surface, the electrical potential of the air phase with respect to the water phase becomes more positive by several hundred millivolts. It should be emphasized that the absolute value of the dipolar potential cannot be measured in such an experiment; furthermore results from monolayers can be extrapolated to bilayers only with great caution. Nevertheless, this experiment is consistent with the notion that the interior of a phospholipid bilayer assumes a positive potential with respect to the aqueous phase. This would mean that the lipid bilayer is intrinsically more permeable to anions than to cations. From monolayer experiments it has been proposed that the interior of a lecithin membrane is approximately 120 mV more positive than the interior of a monoolein membrane [20]. This difference would correspond to a conductance ratio of about 100, and indeed it has been found that the nonactin-mediated K^+ conductance was about 100 times higher in a monoolein membrane than in a lecithin membrane [20]. This picture is supported (at least in part) by the results of kinetic experiments. Charge–pulse relaxation studies have been carried out with membranes made from dipalmitoleoyl phosphatidylcholine [di-(16 : 1)-PC] and from glycerol-mono-palmitoleate [(16 : 1)-G] in the presence of valinomycin and Rb^+. Both lipids have identical fatty acid chains (palmitoleic acid) but different polar residues. They differ considerably in all four rate constants [18]:

	$k_R/10^4\ M^{-1}\ s^{-1}$	$k_D/10^4\ s^{-1}$	$k_{MS}/10^4\ s^{-1}$	$k_S/10^4\ s^{-1}$
di-(16 : 1)-PG	8.2	45	9.1	2.2
(16 : 1)-G	43	13	74	8.5.

The most striking difference occurs in the value of the stability constant $K_h = k_R / k_D$ of the complex, K_h being about 20 times larger in the case of the monoglyceride as compared with the phosphatidylcholine. This finding is consistent with the notion that the interior of a monoglyceride is less positive than the interior of a phosphatidylcholine membrane. It is seen, however, from the above data that also the two translocation rate constants k_{MS} and k_S differ considerably in membranes made from the two lipids.

5. Ionic channels

The extent to which nature uses carriers is not clear at the moment, but for some ion transport systems it is rather certain that mobile carriers are not involved. An example is the sodium system in nerve where about 10^7–10^8 Na^+ pass per second through the single transport unit in the activated state. This number is by about three orders of magnitude higher than the maximum transport rate of a carrier of the valinomycin type. It is therefore rather unlikely that the sodium channel is operated by a carrier mechanism. But, of course, the high transport rate could well be explained by a pore-like channel.

5.1. Gramicidin A as a model channel

The isolation and functional characterization of membrane proteins which may act as channels is still, as yet, in the beginning. However, fortunately there exists a number of simpler molecules, such as gramicidin A, that are useful for studying the mechanism of ion transport through channels.

Gramicidin A is a linear peptide consisting of 15 amino acids (fig. 9). This molecule has several characteristic properties. With the exception of glycin in position 2 it consists of strongly hydrophobic amino acids. As both end groups are blocked (by a formyl residue at the amino terminal and by an ethanolamino residue at the carboxyl terminal), the molecule is electrically neutral. Furthermore, there is a peculiar alternation in the optical configuration of the amino acids.

If gramicidin A is introduced into a biological or artificial membrane, the membrane becomes cation permeable. In this respect gramicidin is similar to the macrocyclic carriers. But it turned out that the action mechanism is quite different from the macrocyclic carriers, and that gramicidin forms channels in a lipid membrane [20].

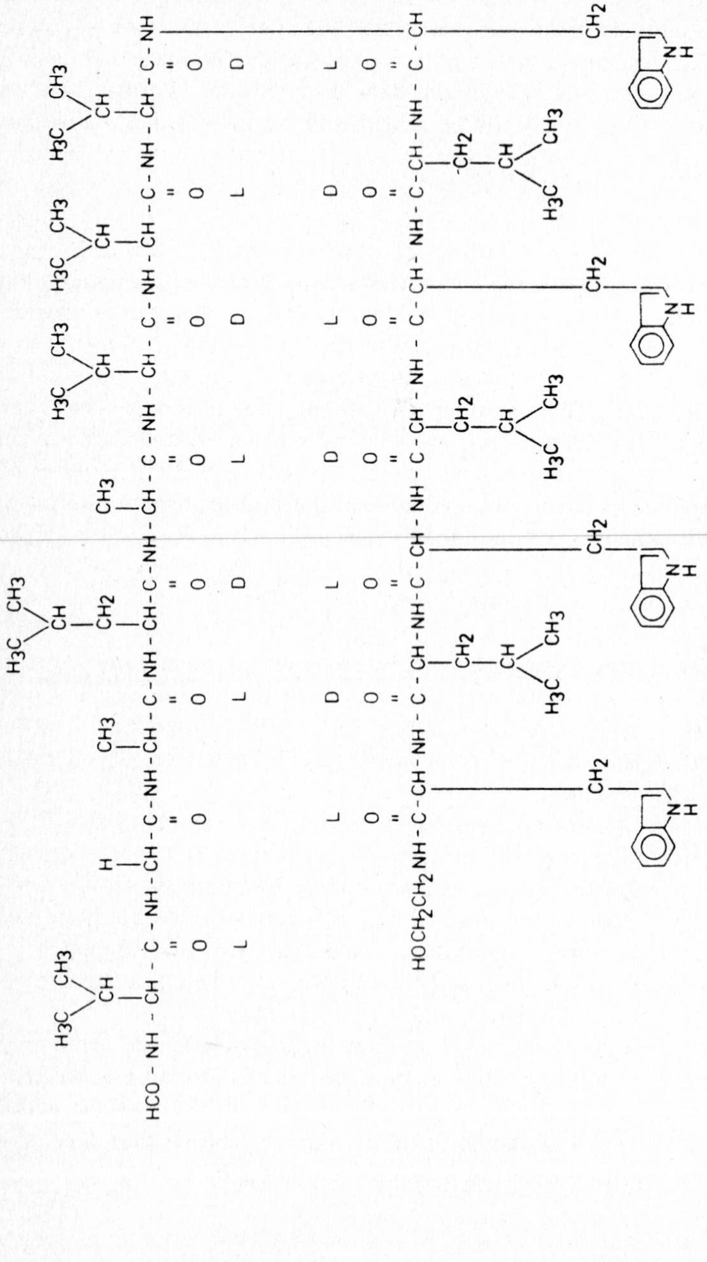

Fig. 9. Structure of valine-gramicidin A.

A detailed model of the gramicidin A channel has been proposed by Urry [21] on the basis of conformational energy considerations. The model of Urry consists of a helical dimer that is formed by head-to-head (formyl end-to-formyl end) association of two gramicidin monomers and that is stabilized by intra- and intermolecular hydrogen bonds (fig. 10). The central hole along the axis of the π^6 (L, D)-helix has a diameter of about 0.4 nm and is lined with the peptide C-O-moieties, whereas the hydrophobic residues lie on the exterior surface of the helix. The total length of that dimer is about 2.5 nm, which is the lower limit of the hydrophobic thickness of a lipid bilayer. The length of the dimer would thus be sufficient to bridge the membrane if a local thinning of the lipid structure is assumed.

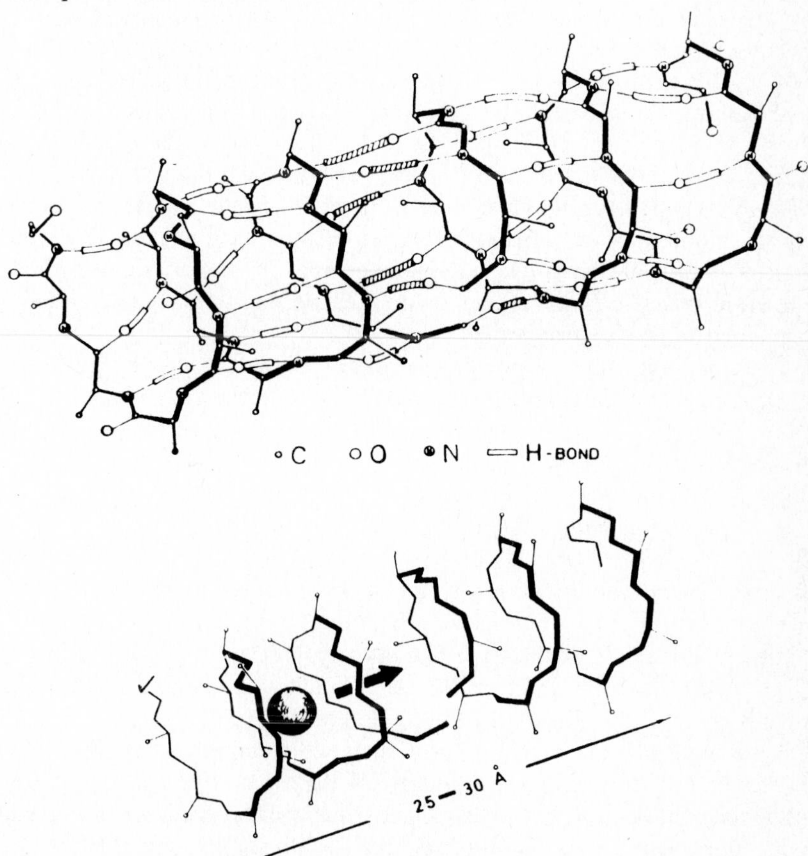

Fig. 10. Structure of the dimeric gramicidin channel [14] according to Urry [21]. The amino acid side chains are not shown.

5.1.1. Kinetics of channel formation

Many details about the nature of the gramicidin-mediated cation permeability have been revealed by studying the electrical properties of gramicidin-doped artificial bimolecular lipid films. An instructive experiment, which was first performed by Hladky and Haydon [20], consists of adding extremely small amounts of gramicidin A to the membrane and recording the time–course of the electric current at a given voltage. Under these circumstances the current shows discrete fluctuations with more or less the same amplitude (fig. 11). If increasing amounts of gramicidin are added to the membrane, more and more fluctuations build up on top of each other and eventually fuse into an average macroscopic current. This experiment can be explained by the assumption that the single current fluctuation results from the formation and the disappearance of a single channel. The conductance of the channel, which is calculated from the current fluctuations, is about 90 pS (1 pS $= 10^{-12}\ \Omega^{-1}$) in 1 M CsCl [22]. This corresponds to a transport of about 6×10^7 cesium ions per s through the single channel at a voltage of 100 mV. This value is larger by a factor of 10^3 than the turnover number of a translatory carrier such as valinomycin. The high transport rate of the single conductance unit of gramicidin A would therefore be difficult to reconcile with a carrier model but can be easily explained by a pore mechanism.

Evidence that the channel is a dimer comes from voltage-jump current-relaxation experiments as well as from measurements of membrane conductance as a function of gramicidin concentration (for a recent review see reference [22]).

5.1.2. Electrically charged derivatives of gramicidin A

An interesting modification of the channel consists of introducing electric charges at the channel mouth. A negatively charged analogue of gramicidin may be obtained by covalently binding a pyromellityl residue to the hydroxyl end of the peptide (fig. 12). *O*-pyromellitylgramicidin forms ion channels in lipid membranes in a way similar to that of gramicidin. The records of conductance fluctuations at very low peptide concentrations have qualitatively the same appearance as those obtained with gramicidin. Also the current relaxation after a voltage jump is similar for the neutral and the negatively charged peptide. In other properties, however, both compounds differ markedly.

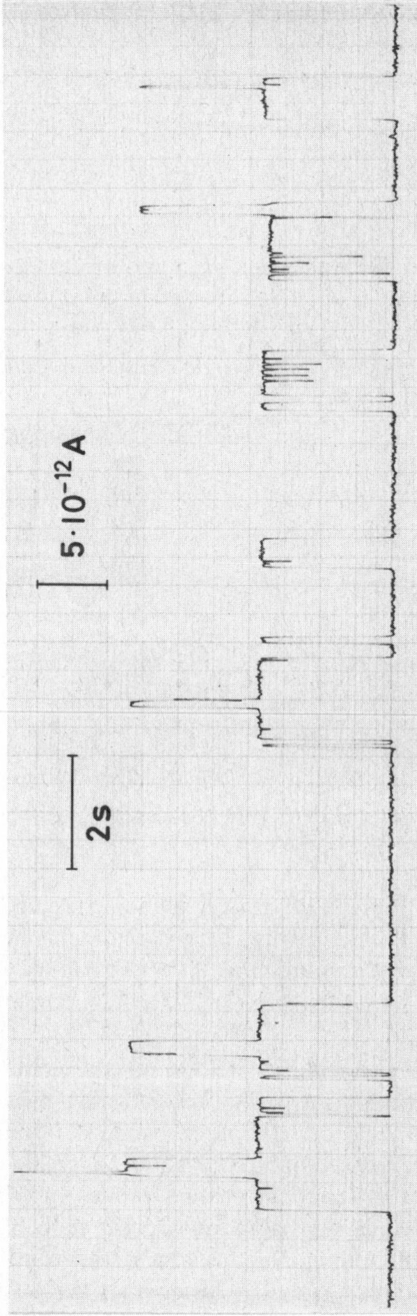

Fig. 11. Fluctuations of membrane current in the presence of small amounts of gramicidin A. 1 M CsCl, 25° C, $V_m = 100$ mV. The membrane has been formed from monoolein. The baseline corresponds to the membrane conductance in the absence of gramicidin [22].

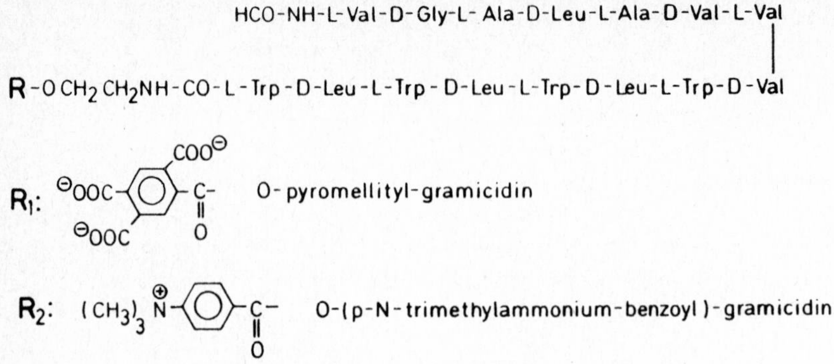

HCO-NH-L-Val-D-Gly-L-Ala-D-Leu-L-Ala-D-Val-L-Val

R-OCH_2CH_2NH-CO-L-Trp-D-Leu-L-Trp-D-Leu-L-Trp-D-Leu-L-Trp-D-Val

R_1: $^{\ominus}$OOC–C_6H_2(COO$^{\ominus}$)(COO$^{\ominus}$)–C(=O)– O-pyromellityl-gramicidin

R_2: $(CH_3)_3\overset{\oplus}{N}$–$C_6H_4$–C(=O)– O-(p-N-trimethylammonium-benzoyl)-gramicidin

Fig. 12. Positively and negatively charged derivatives of gramicidin A.

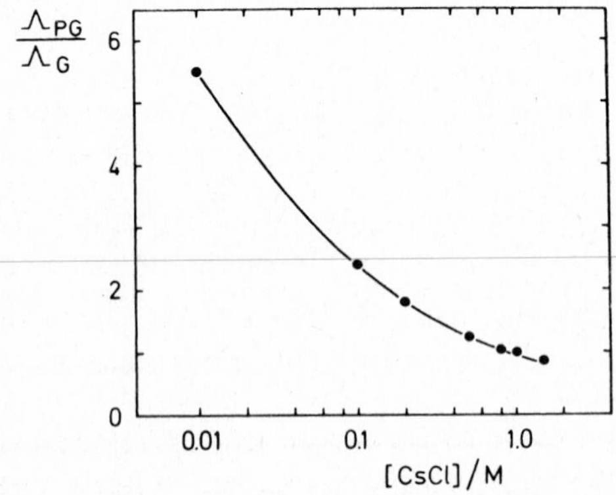

Fig. 13. Single-channel conductance Λ_{PG} of *O*-pyromellitylgramicidin divided by the single-channel conductance Λ_G of gramicidin. Monoolein-*n*-hexadecane, 25° C [23].

It may be seen from fig. 13 that at a low ionic strength (0.01 M), the conductance Λ_{PG} of the negatively charged channel is between five and six times higher than the conductance Λ_G of the neutral channel. On the other hand, at high ionic strength (>1 M), Λ_{PG} becomes equal to (or slightly less) than Λ_G.

The effect of the pyromellityl residue on the conductance of the channel may be twofold: the bulky residue may partially block the entrance of the channel; on the other hand, the negative potential created by the ionized carboxyl groups should increase the concentration of permeable cations near the channel mouth and therefore should enhance the conductance. The observation that at high ion concentrations (where the Coulombic effect is small) the conductance of the *O*-pyromellitylgramicidin channel is lower than that of the gramicidin channel may be tentatively explained by a steric blocking effect. The electrostatic effect becomes evident at low ion concentrations c where the conductance of the negative channel is enhanced 5.6-fold (at $c = 10^{-2}$ M) over that of the neutral channel (fig. 12). A rough estimate (to the order of magnitude) of the expected electrostatic modification of the single-channel conductance may be made in the following way. We represent the pyromellityl residue by a charged sphere of radius a centered at the point where the channel axis intersects the membrane surface. The electrical potential at the surface of the sphere is then approximately given by the Debye–Hückel relation:

$$\phi(a) = \frac{ze_0^2}{4\pi\varepsilon_0\varepsilon akT}\,\frac{1}{1+a/l_D} \simeq \frac{z(56\ \mathrm{nm})}{\varepsilon a}\,\frac{1}{1+a/l_D}; \tag{29}$$

$$l_D = \sqrt{[(\varepsilon_0\varepsilon kT)/(2e_0^2 c)]}, \tag{30}$$

where e_0 is the elementary charge, z the valency, ε_0 the permitivity of free space, ε the dielectric constant, k Boltzmann's constant, T the absolute temperature, c the concentration of the 1 : 1 electrolyte in water, and l_D the Debye length; the potential ϕ is expressed in units of kT/e_0. If the single-channel conductance Λ is assumed to be proportional to the ion concentration at the mouth of the channel, then $\exp(\phi)$ appears as a Boltzmann factor in the expression for Λ. The channel mouth may be represented by a hemispherical surface with radius r_0, the so-called effective capture radius. If, for the purpose of a crude estimate, we identify the capture radius of the channel with the radius a, the ratio q of the conductance Λ_c of the charged channel to the conductance Λ_u of the uncharged channel in the same electrolyte solutions is given by

$$q = \Lambda_c/\Lambda_u \simeq e^{-\phi(a)}. \tag{31}$$

In order to eliminate the steric blocking effect of the pyromellityl residue, it is convenient to consider ratios of q values determined at two different ion concentrations c_1 and c_2. The experimental results for $q(c_1)/q(c_2)$ may indeed be fitted with reasonable values of a and ε. For instance, $\varepsilon = 80$, $a = 0.6$ nm, and $z = -3$ gives $q(0.01\ \mathrm{M})/q(1\ \mathrm{M}) = 5.7$ and $q(0.1\ \mathrm{M})/q(1\ \mathrm{M}) = 2.7$ which is rather close to the experimentally observed values (fig. 13). A more exact treatment should account for the precise location of the fixed charges with respect to the channel, the discontinuity of the dielectric constant at the membrane surface, deviations from the Debye–Hückel theory at high concentration, and saturation effects in the channel. In any case, the observed variation of

Λ_{PG}/Λ_G with ion concentration at least qualitatively agrees with expected effects of fixed charges on the conductance of the channel.

A gramicidin derivative with a positive charge at the channel mouth is obtained by introducing a *p*-*n*-trimethylammonium-benzoyl residue at the hydroxyl end of the peptide (fig. 12). Experiments with black lipid films show that this compound is able to form ion channels, but in this case the conductance of the single channel is smaller by a factor of 1.6 (in 0.2 M CsCl) as compared with neutral gramicidin. When positively charged gramicidin is added to one aqueous phase and negatively charged gramicidin to the other, hybrid channels are formed with a pronounced asymmetry in the current-voltage characteristic (fig. 14). At 200 mV the conductance is about 3.5 times higher in the forward direction (current flow from the negative side to the positive side of the channel) than in the reverse direction. By estimating the number of monomers and dimers present in the membrane under the conditions of this experiment, it may be shown that the over-all surface potential of the membrane created by the fixed charges on the two gramicidin species is negligibly small (far below 1 mV); this means that the observed asymmetry in the current–voltage characteristic is an intrinsic property of the hybride channel.

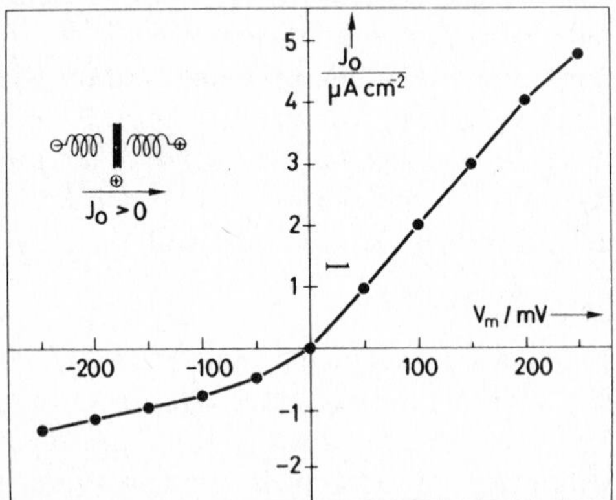

Fig. 14. Current-voltage characteristic in the presence of hybride channels formed from positively charged *O*-(*p*-*N*-trimethylammonium-benzoyl)-gramicidin and negatively charged *O*-pyromellitylgramicidin. Dioleoyllecithin/*n*-decane membrane, 5 mM CsCl, 25° C. J_0 is the initial current which is measured 1 ms after the application of a voltage pulse; in this way the current–voltage characteristic is obtained at constant channel number [23].

5.2. *Theoretical description of ion transport in channels*

5.2.1. *Barrier model of an ion channel*

An ion channel is a structural element that offers to an ion an energetically favourable pathway through the apolar core of a lipid membrane. Such a channel may be represented by a sequence of "binding sites" which are separated by activation energy barriers (fig. 15). The "binding sites" are the minima in the potential energy profile which result from interactions of the ion with one or several ligand groups of the channel. A simple situation arises when the ion concentration is low enough so that the probability of finding more than one ion at a time in the channel is vanishingly small [24]. This case in which ion–ion interactions within the channel may be neglected is treated in the following.

We assume that the membrane contains N_c channels and that the channels are permeable to a single ion species which is present in the external phases in concentrations c' and c'' (fig. 15). If N_0 is the average number of the ions (referred to total membrane area) located in the outermost energy minimum at the left-hand mouth of the channel, then $p_0 = N_0/N_c$ is the probability that, for a given channel, the outer minimum is occupied by an ion. This probability is assumed to be voltage-independent and proportional to the aqueous ion concentration; a similar statement applies to the right-hand mouth of the channel. Thus,

$$p_0 = vc', \qquad p_{n+1} = vc'', \tag{32}$$

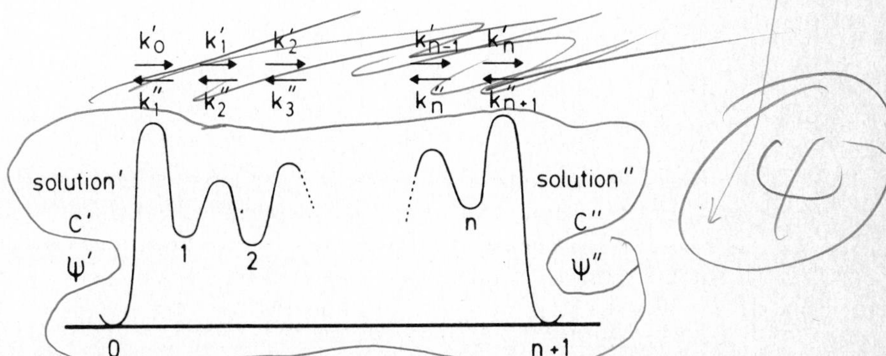

Fig. 15. Barrier model of an ion channel. The channel is represented by n ion binding sites separated by energy barriers.

where v is a proportionality constant. We denote the probability of finding the ith minimum in a given channel occupied by p_i ($p_i \ll 1$). The average net ion flux Φ_i in the single channel over the ith barrier is then given by:

$$\Phi_i = k'_{i-1} p_{i-1} - k''_i p_i \qquad (i = 1, 2, \ldots, n+1), \tag{33}$$

k'_{i-1} and k''_i are the voltage-dependent rate constants for jumps over the ith barrier from left to right and from right to left (compare fig. 15). In the equilibrium state ($\Phi_i \equiv 0$) the unidirectional fluxes over the ith barrier in either direction are equal:

$$\bar{k}'_{i-1} \bar{p}_{i-1} = \bar{k}''_i \bar{p}_i \equiv F_i \tag{34}$$

where $\bar{k}'_i$, $\bar{k}''_i$, and $\bar{p}_i$ are the equilibrium values of k'_i, k''_i, and p_i, respectively, and F_i is the unidirectional flux over the ith barrier at equilibrium. Relation (34) represents a system of $(n+1)$ equations which is easily solved, starting either with $i=1$ or $i=n+1$, to give

$$\bar{p}_i = p_0 \frac{\bar{k}'_0 \bar{k}'_1 \ldots \bar{k}'_{i-1}}{\bar{k}''_1 \bar{k}''_2 \ldots \bar{k}''_i} = p_{n+1} \frac{\bar{k}''_{i+1} \bar{k}''_{i+2} \ldots \bar{k}''_{n+1}}{\bar{k}'_i \bar{k}'_{i+1} \ldots \bar{k}'_n}. \tag{35}$$

(As the probabilities p_0 and p_{n+1} that the outer minima are occupied are assumed to be constant, we may write $\bar{p}_0 = p_0$ and $\bar{p}_{n+1} = p_{n+1}$.) Eq. (35) yields, in accordance with the principle of microscopic reversibility, the relationship

$$p_0 \bar{k}'_0 \bar{k}'_1 \ldots \bar{k}'_n = p_{n+1} \bar{k}''_1 \bar{k}''_2 \ldots \bar{k}''_{n+1} \equiv H. \tag{36}$$

The equilibrium voltage V_e of the permeable ion (valency z) is given by

$$\frac{c''}{c'} = \frac{p_{n+1}}{p_0} = \exp(z u_e), \tag{37}$$

$$u_e \equiv \frac{V_e}{kT/e_0} \equiv \frac{(\psi' - \psi''_e)_e}{kT/e_0}, \tag{38}$$

where k is the Boltzmann constant, T the absolute temperature, e_0 the elementary charge, and ψ' and ψ'' the electrical potentials in the left-hand and right-hand aqueous phase (fig. 15). Equations (36) and (37) together give

$$\frac{\bar{k}'_0 \bar{k}'_1 \ldots \bar{k}'_n}{\bar{k}''_1 \bar{k}''_2 \ldots \bar{k}''_{n+1}} = \exp(z u_e). \tag{39}$$

As any value of the equilibrium voltage u_e can be achieved by a suitable choice of c' and c'' and as the rate constants k_i', k_i'' are independent of c' and c'', a relation of the form of eq. (39) holds at arbitrary voltages $u=(\psi'-\psi'')e_0/kT$:

$$\frac{k_0'k_1' \ldots k_n'}{k_1''k_2'' \ldots k_{n+1}''} = \exp(zu). \tag{40}$$

5.2.2. *Ion permeability and electrical conductance of the channel*

We consider the stationary state of the channel where the ion fluxes over all barriers are equal ($\Phi_i \equiv \Phi$). Relation (33) then represents a system of $(n+1)$ equations for the $(n+1)$ unknown quantities Φ, $p_1, p_2, \ldots, p_n$. The solution for Φ reads [after introduction of eq. (40)]

$$\Phi = P[(zu/2)/\sinh(zu/2)][c'\exp(zu/2) - c''\exp(-zu/2)] \tag{41}$$

$$= Pzu\frac{c'\exp(zu) - c''}{\exp(zu) - 1}. \tag{42}$$

Equation (41) has the form of Goldman's flux eq. (25). P is the voltage-dependent permeability coefficient of the single channel which is given by:

$$P = \{[1-\exp(-zu)]/zu\}\left[vk_0'/\left(1+\sum_{\nu=1}^{n} S_\nu\right)\right], \tag{43}$$

$$S_\nu = \frac{k_1''k_2'' \ldots k_\nu''}{k_1'k_2' \ldots k_\nu'}. \tag{44}$$

At zero voltage, eqs. (41) and (43) reduce to

$$\phi = P(c'-c'') \qquad P = \left[v\tilde{k}_0'/1+\sum_{\nu=1}^{n}\tilde{S}_\nu\right] \equiv P_0 \tag{45, 46}$$

where $\tilde{k}_0'$ and $\tilde{S}_\nu$ are the values of k_0' and S_ν for $u=0$.

As the ions move independently through the channel, the unidirectional fluxes Φ' and Φ'' are simply obtained by applying eq. (41) to the case $c''=0$ or $c'=0$:

$$\Phi = \Phi' - \Phi'' \tag{47}$$

$$\Phi' = Pc'\frac{zu}{1-\exp(-zu)} \qquad \Phi'' = Pc''\frac{zu}{\exp(zu)-1}. \tag{48, 49}$$

Equations (48) and (49) may be used to determine the permeability coefficient P from tracer flux experiments.

According to the theory of absolute reaction rates [26], the voltage-dependence of the rate constants may be expressed by

$$k_i' = \bar{k}_i' \exp(\alpha_{i+1} zu/2) \qquad k_i'' = \bar{k}_i'' \exp(-\alpha_i zu/2), \tag{50, 51}$$

where $\bar{k}_i'$ and $\bar{k}_i''$ are the values of k_i' and k_i'' at zero voltage and α_i is the fraction of the total voltage u which drops across the ith barrier:

$$\sum_{i=1}^{n+1} \alpha_i = 1. \tag{52}$$

In order to calculate the electric conductance Λ of the single channel in the vicinity of the equilibrium voltage V_e, we assume that a small voltage increment ΔV is applied in addition to V_e:

$$V = V_e + \Delta V.$$

If $\Delta I = ze_0\Phi$ is the electric current, the single-channel conductance is defined by

$$\Lambda = \left(\frac{\Delta I}{\Delta V}\right)_{\Delta V \approx 0}. \tag{54}$$

For small values of the voltage increment ($|e_0 \Delta V/kT| \ll 1$), Λ is obtained in the form [27]:

$$\frac{1}{\Lambda} = \left(\frac{kT}{z^2 e_0^2}\right) \sum_{i=1}^{n+1} \frac{1}{F_i}. \tag{55}$$

Thus, Λ is related in a simple way to the unidirectional fluxes F_i at equilibrium. Equation (55) also shows that for a sequence of barriers with unequal heights, the barrier with the lowest F_i tends to dominate the conductance of the channel. Furthermore, it is interesting to note that Λ is independent of the coefficients α_i. Introducing eqs. (34)–(36) into eq. (55), Λ may be expressed in terms of the rate constants k_i' and k_i'':

$$\frac{1}{\Lambda} = \left(\frac{kT}{z^2 e_0^2}\right) \frac{1}{H} \sum_{i=1}^{n+1} \rho_i; \tag{56}$$

$$\rho_i = \bar{k}_1'' \bar{k}_2'' \ldots \bar{k}_{i-1}'' \bar{k}_i' \bar{k}_{i+1}' \ldots \bar{k}_n'; \tag{57}$$

$$(\rho_1 = \bar{k}_1' \bar{k}_2' \ldots \bar{k}_n'; \qquad \rho_{n+1} = \bar{k}_1'' \bar{k}_2'' \ldots \bar{k}_n'').$$

A further interesting relation may be obtained by introducing the unidirectional ion fluxes Φ' (from left to right) and Φ'' (from right to left) which may be measured using isotopes. At equilibrium Φ' and Φ''

become identical:

$$(\Phi')_{u=u_e} = (\Phi'')_{u=u_e} \equiv f_0 \tag{58}$$

The "exchange flux" f_0 may be shown to be related to the F_i and to Λ in the following way:

$$\frac{1}{f_0} = \sum_{i=1}^{n+1} \frac{1}{F_i} = \frac{z^2 e_0^2}{kT} \frac{1}{\Lambda}. \tag{59}$$

We finally apply eq. (56) to the case of symmetrical aqueous solutions ($c' = c'' = c$) where the equilibrium voltage u_e is zero. Denoting the value of Λ for $u_e = 0$ by Λ_0, one finds, after some rearrangement:

$$\Lambda_0 = \left[z^2 e_0^2 / kT \right] \left[vc\tilde{k}_0' \middle/ \left(1 + \sum_{\nu=1}^{n} \tilde{S}_\nu \right) \right]. \tag{60}$$

Comparison with eq. (46) shows that the permeability coefficient at zero voltage, P_0, and the ohmic single channel conductance Λ_0 are connected by the relation

$$P_0 = \left(\frac{kT}{z^2 e_0^2} \right) \left(\frac{\Lambda_0}{c} \right). \tag{61}$$

6. Electrical fluctuations in membranes

Lipid bilayers are inherently small systems and are therefore subjected to large fluctuations. In recent years it has been realized that detailed information on ion transport mechanisms may be obtained by analyzing electrical fluctuations (current and voltage noise) in membranes [28, 29].

6.1. Opening–closing noise of ion channels

This type of noise has been studied in detail with artificial bilayer membranes in the presence of gramicidin A [30, 31]. In a membrane doped with gramicidin (G), dimeric channels form and disappear at random according to the reaction

$$G + G \underset{k_D}{\overset{k_R}{\rightleftarrows}} G_2 \tag{62}$$

k_R and k_D are the rate constants of association and dissociation, respectively. If a voltage is applied to the membrane, the current $J(t)$

fluctuates in time t around a mean current $\bar{J}$:

$$J(t) = \bar{J} + \delta J(t). \tag{63}$$

The randomly varying function $\delta J(t)$ reflects fluctuations in the number of dimeric channels.

A straightforward way to analyze the fluctuating component $\delta J(t)$ of the membrane current is to compute the so-called autocorrelation function $C_J(\tau)$:

$$C_J(\tau) = \overline{[\delta J(0)][\delta J(\tau)]}\,. \tag{64}$$

$C_J(\tau)$ describes the average rate at which a current fluctuation decays that has occurred at time $\tau = 0$. The fluctuation–dissipation theorem states that the decay of a spontaneous fluctuation follows (on the average) the same time–law as the relaxation from a macroscopic perturbation. This means that for the dimerization reaction considered here, the autocorrelation function has the form:

$$C_J(\tau) = \overline{(\delta J)^2}\, \exp(-\tau/\tau_c), \tag{65}$$

where τ_c is the relaxation time of the channel-formation reaction (62) which is given by:

$$\frac{1}{\tau_c} = k_D + 4k_R N_1^\infty = k_D + 4\sqrt{(k_R k_D \lambda_\infty / L\Lambda)}\,. \tag{66}$$

N_1^∞ and λ_∞ are the mean monomer concentration (mol/cm^2) and specific membrane conductance in the stationary state, L is Avogadro's number and Λ the single-channel conductance.

The autocorrelation function may be computed directly from a record of $J(t)$ with the aid of suitable instruments [30, 31]. Figure 16 gives an example of current fluctuations observed with a dioleoyllecithin membrane in the presence of gramicidin A. The autocorrelation function $C(\tau)$ of the current noise (fig. 17) is found to be very nearly exponential with a single time constant τ_c. From here on the analysis proceeds in the same way as in the case of the relaxation experiments. If the correlation time τ_c is plotted as a function of the square root of the mean membrane conductance, it is found that τ_c varies linearly with $\lambda_\infty^{1/2}$. The rate constants k_R and k_D which are obtained from the $1/\tau_c$ vs $\lambda_\infty^{1/2}$ plot agree within a factor of two with the values calculated from relaxation experiments (table 3).

As the theoretical analysis shows, the mean square of the current fluctuations is related to the single-channel conductance Λ; at

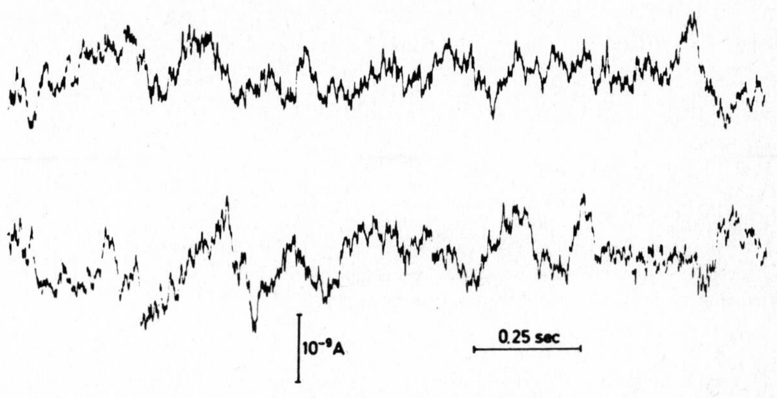

Fig. 16. Current noise from a dioleoyllecithin membrane in the presence of gramicidin A (upper traces). The mean current $\bar{J}$ was 390 nA, corresponding to a mean membrane conductance $\lambda = 3.1$ mS cm^{-2} (membrane area $A = 0.68$ mm^2, external voltage $V_m = 18.5$ mV). The aqueous phases contained 1 M NaCl. The lower trace represents a control experiment in which the noise was recorded in the same way as above but from a gramicidin-free membrane with an external resistor of 47 $k\Omega$ simulating the gramicidin-induced conductance [31].

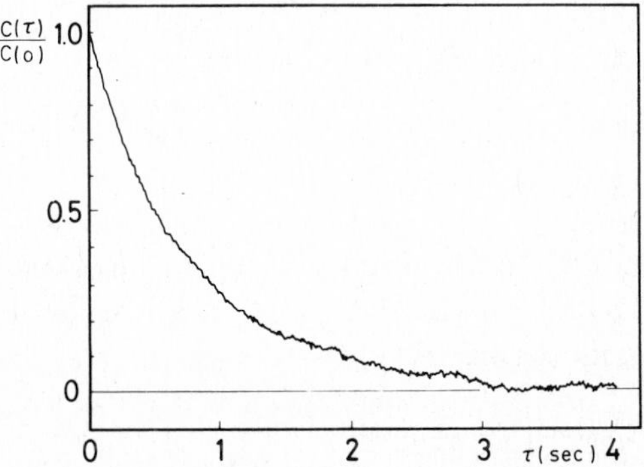

Fig. 17. Autocorrelation function $C(\tau)$ of current noise, divided by the initial value $D(0) \simeq 7.8 \times 10^{-22} A^2$. Membrane area $A = 0.70$ mm^2, external voltage $V_m = 18.5$ mV. The aqueous phase contained 1 M NaCl [31].

Table 3
Kinetic analysis of the gramicidin A channel[a)]

Method	k_R (cm^2 mol^{-1} s^{-1})	k_R (cm^2 mol^{-1} s^{-1})	k_D (s^{-1})	k_D (s^{-1})	Λ (pS)
	18.5 mV	98 mV	18.5 mV	98 mV	
Noise analysis	0.62×10^{14}	1.4×10^{14}	1.7	1.9	9
Relaxation method	1.3×10^{14}	1.5×10^{14}	–	1.6	–
Single-channel experiments	–	–	–	1.4	12

[a)]Comparison between noise analysis, relaxation method, and single-channel experiments. Dioleoyllecithin membranes, 1 M NaCl, 25° C [31].

sufficiently low values of the conductance λ_∞ the relation

$$\overline{(\delta J)^2}\,/\,(\bar{J}\,)^2 \approx \Lambda / A\lambda \tag{67}$$

holds, where A is the membrane area. Thus, from $C_J(0)=\overline{(\delta J\,)^2}$ information on Λ may be obtained. As shown in table 3, the values of Λ that are calculated from noise analysis and from single-channel experiments are in satisfactory agreement.

A second independent method for noise analysis consists of measuring the spectral intensity of the current noise. The spectral intensity $S_J(f)$ is connected with the autocorrelation function $C_J(\tau)$ through the Wiener–Khintchine theorem:

$$S_J(f) = 4\int_0^\infty C_J(\tau)\cos(2\pi f\tau)\,d\tau, \tag{68}$$

where f is the frequency. In the case considered here, $S_J(f)$ is given by

$$S_J(f) = \left[4\tau_c\,\overline{(\delta J)^2}\,\right] / \left[1 + (2\pi\tau_c f)^2\right]. \tag{69}$$

Thus, $S_J(f)$ yields the same information as $C(\tau)$, namely, the correlation time τ_c [eq. (67)] and the variance $\overline{(\delta J\,)^2}$ of the current from which the single-channel conductance may be obtained.

6.2. *Transport noise in ion channels*

In addition to opening–closing noise, ion channels are a source of an additional type of noise termed "transport noise" which occurs even in permanently open channels. Transport noise results from random fluctuations in the number of ions jumping across the individual energy barriers of the channel. Each jump may be thought to contribute a single current pulse to the total current in the external measuring circuit.

A simple situation arises if both aqueous phases have identical composition and if the voltage across the membrane is zero. In this case the system is at equilibrium and the membrane current fluctuates around zero. Under such equilibrium conditions the Nyquist theorem may be applied which relates the spectral intensity $S_J(f)$ of current noise to the complex (small signal) admittance $Y(f)$ of the transport system:

$$S_J(f) = 4\,kT\,\mathrm{Re}[\,Y(f)\,], \tag{70}$$

where Re signifies "real part of".

The theoretical analysis then reduces to the problem of calculating the frequency-dependent admittance $Y(f)$ which in turn is related to the relaxation-time spectrum of the channel. If τ_ν ($\nu = 1, 2, \ldots, n$) are the n relaxation times of a channel with n binding sites [34] (fig. 15), the spectral intensity of current noise is obtained in the form [27]:

$$S_I(f) = 4z^2e_0^2N_c\left(\sum_{\nu=1}^{n}\frac{\theta_\nu}{1+\omega^2\tau_\nu^2}+\sum_{i=1}^{n+1}\alpha_i^2F_i\right), \tag{71}$$

where $\omega = 2\pi f$ is the angular frequency. (Compare subsection 5.2 for the definition of α_i and F_i). The frequency-independent quantities θ_ν are expressions containing the parameters α_i and the rate constants $\bar{k}_i'$ and $\bar{k}_i''$. Equation (71) may be interpreted in the following way. For a channel with n internal binding sites the spectral intensity $S_I(f)$ has n dispersion regions (regions where S_I changes steeply with frequency) which are centred at angular frequencies $\omega_\nu = 1/\tau_\nu$. Both in the limit of low and high frequencies the transport noise becomes frequency-independent ("white"). For $\omega = 0$, S_I is given by

$$S_I(0) = 4z^2e_0^2N_c\left(\sum_{\nu=1}^{n}\theta_\nu+\sum_{i=1}^{n+1}\alpha_i^2F_i\right) = 4kTN_c\Lambda. \tag{72}$$

$S_I(0)$ represents the thermal noise from a conductance of magnitude $N_c\Lambda$. On the other hand, at high frequencies, correlations between fluctuations in the fluxes ϕ_i vanish so that each barrier in the channel behaves as an independent shot noise source of spectral intensity $(2ze_0\alpha_i)^2F_i$:

$$S_I(\omega) = 4z^2e_0^2N_c\sum_{i=1}^{n+1}\alpha_i^2F_i. \tag{73}$$

As mentioned above, these relations have been derived for the equilibrium state of the channel. Recently, Frehland [35] has extended the analysis to stationary non-equilibrium states of ion channels.

6.3. Current fluctuations connected with transport of hydrophobic ions and carrier-mediated ion transport

Electrical noise associated with the transport of dipicrylamine [32] and with valinomycin-mediated alkali ion transport [33] in artificial bilayer membranes has recently been analyzed. In this case again noise results from random fluctuations in the number of jumps of ions across the central energy barrier in the membrane. For the equilibrium case where the Nyquist relation [eq. (70)] can be applied, theory predicts the following form of the current-noise spectrum for a membrane in the presence of hydrophobic ions [32]:

$$S_J(f) = \frac{\omega^2\tau_i^2}{1+\omega^2\tau_i^2} S_J(\infty) \tag{74}$$

$$S_J(\infty) = 2nk_i(\alpha z e_0)^2 \qquad \tau_i = 1/2k_i \tag{75, 76}$$

n is the average number of ions adsorbed to the membrane (both surfaces); k_i and α have the same meaning as in eq. (15).

The theoretical expression given in eq. (74) predicts a spectral intensity which increases with the square of frequency at low ω and becomes independent of frequency in the limit $\omega \gg 1/\tau_i$. The experimentally observed current-noise spectra closely agree with this prediction. An example is given in fig. 18 in which the theoretical curve has been drawn according to eq. (74) with a suitable choice of the parameters $S_I(\infty)$ and τ_i. A significant deviation between the observed and the calculated spectrum is only found at low frequencies where the observed values of S_I are higher than the spectrum predicted from eq. (74). This deviation is not unexpected, since other noise sources of the system (such as noise originating from the non-zero steady-state conductance of the membrane) which are not included in the model tend to keep the measured $S_I(\omega)$ at a finite level at low frequencies, whereas the model predicts $S_I(\omega) \rightarrow 0$ for $\omega \rightarrow 0$.

In the case of carrier-mediated ion transport, the spectral intensity may be calculated on the basis of the model described in section 4 (fig. 7). This yields [33]:

$$S_J(\omega) = 4e_0^2 A N_{MS} k_{MS}\left(1 - \frac{\alpha_1}{1+\omega^2\tau_1^2} - \frac{\alpha_2}{1+\omega^2\tau_2^2}\right), \tag{77}$$

where A is the membrane area and N_{MS} the surface concentration of charged complexes MS^+ at equilibrium. The time constants τ_1, τ_2 and

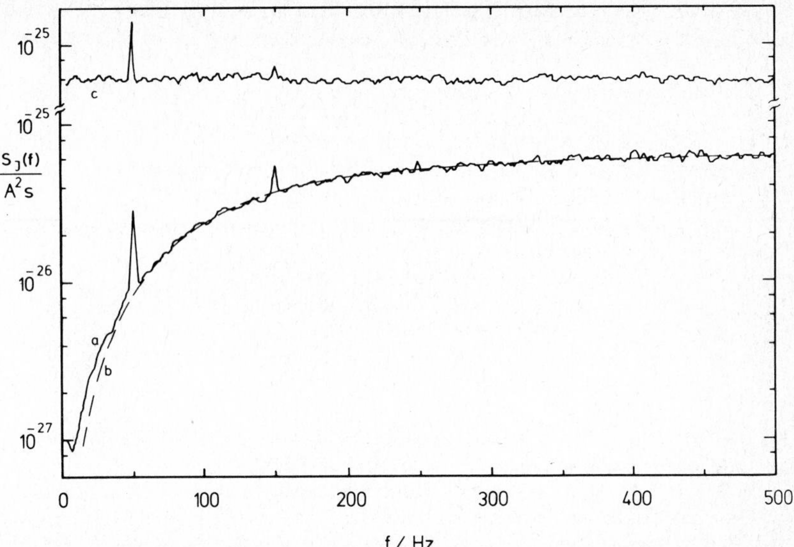

Fig. 18. Spectral intensity $S_I(f)$ of current noise from a dioleoyllecithin/n-decane membrane in the presence of 30 nM dipicrylamine and 0.1 M NaCl as a function of frequency f (curve a). The membrane area was $A=0.36$ mm^2; $T=25°$ C. Curve b is the theoretical curve which has been calculated from eq. (21) with $S_I(\infty)=5.9\times10^{-26}A^2$ s and $\tau_i=1.15$ ms. These parameter values have been determined from a least-squares fit starting at the highest frequencies down to the frequency at which $S_{exp}-S_{theor}$ exceeded the mean scatter of the trace. Curve c represents the result of a control experiment without dipicrylamine, in which the dipicrylamine-induced (high frequency) conductance has been simulated by an external resistance of 278 $k\Omega$ in parallel to the membrane [32].

the "amplitudes" α_1, α_2 are complicated functions of the rate constants [33]. The experimentally observed frequency dependence of S_J for valinomycin-mediated Rb^+-transport [33] is consistent with the predictions of eq. (77).

References

[1] A. Parsegian, Nature 221 (1969) 844.
[2] B. Neumcke and P. Läuger, Biophys. J. 9 (1969) 1150.
[3] S. McLaughlin, Electrostatic Potentials at Membrane-Solution Interfaces, in: Current Topics in Membranes and Transport, eds. F. Bronner and A. Kleinzeller, vol 9, (Academic Press, New York, 1977) pp. 71–144.
[4] P. Mueller, D. O. Rudin, H. T. Tien and W. D. Wescot, Nature 194 (1962) 979.
[5] T. Hanai, D. A. Haydon and J. Taylor, Proc. Roy. Soc. A 281 (1964) 377.
[6] C. Huang and T. E. Thompson, J. Mol. Biol. 13 (1965) 183.

[7] M. Montal and P. Mueller, Proc. Nat. Acad. Sci. USA 69 (1972) 3561.
[8] R. Benz, O. Fröhlich, P. Läuger and M. Montal, Biochim. Biophys. Acta 394 (1975) 323.
[9] H. Schindler and J. P. Rosenbusch, Proc. Natl. Acad. Sci. USA 75 (1978) 3751.
[10] B. Ketterer, B. Neumcke and P. Läuger, J. Membrane Biol. 5 (1971) 225.
[11] O. S. Andersen and M. Fuchs, Biophys. J. 15 (1975) 795.
[12] R. Benz, P. Läuger and K. Janko, Biochim. Biophys. Acta 455 (1976) 701.
[13] R. Benz and P. Läuger, Biochim. Biophys. Acta 468 (1977) 245.
[14] Yu. A. Ovchinnikov, V. T. Ivanov and A. M. Skrob, Membrane-Active Complexones (Elsevier Scientific Publishing Company, Amsterdam, 1974).
[15] R. Benz and P. Läuger, J. Membrane Biol. 27 (1976) 171.
[16] G. Stark, R. Benz, B. Ketterer and P. Läuger, Biophys. J. 11 (1971) 981.
[17] P. Läuger, Science 178 (1972) 24.
[18] R. Benz, O. Fröhlich and P. Läuger, Biochem. Biophys. Acta 46 (1977) 465.
[19] S. G. A. McLaughlin, G. Szabo, G. Eisenman and S. M. Ciani, Proc. Natl. Acad. Sci. USA 67 (1970) 1268.
[20] S. B. Hladky and D. A. Haydon, Biochim. Biophys. Acta 274 (1972) 294.
[21] D. W. Urry, Proc. Natl. Acad. Sci. USA 68 (1971) 672.
[22] E. Bamberg, H. Alpes, H.-J. Apell, R. Benz, K. Janko, H. A. Kolb, P. Läuger and E. Gross, Studies on the Gramicidin Channel, in: Biochemistry of Membrane Transport, FEBS Symposium No. 42, eds., G. Semenza and E. Carafoli (Springer Verlag, Berlin, 1977) pp. 179–201.
[23] H.-J. Apell, E. Bamberg, H. Alpes and P. Läuger, J. Membrane Biol. 31 (1977) 171.
[24] P. Läuger, Biochim. Biophys. Acta 311 (1973) 423.
[25] A. B. Hope, Ion Transport and Membranes, Section 1.4 (Butterworths, London, 1971).
[26] S. Glastone, K. J. Laidler and M. Eyring, The Theory of Rate Processes, (McGraw Hill, New York, 1941) ch. 9.
[27] P. Läuger, Biochim. Biophys. Acta 507 (1978) 337.
[28] A. A. Verveen and L. J. DeFelice, Progr. Biophys. Mol. Biol. 28 (1974) 189.
[29] E. Neher and C. F. Stevens, Ann. Rev. Biophys. Bioeng. 6 (1977) 345.
[30] H. P. Zingsheim and E. Neher, Biophys. Chem. 2 (1974) 197.
[31] H.-A. Kolb, P. Läuger and E. Bamberg, J. Membrane Biol. 20 (1975) 133.
[32] H.-A. Kolb and P. Läuger, J. Membrane Biol. 37 (1977) 321.
[33] H.-A. Kolb and P. Läuger, J. Membrane Biol. 41 (1978) 167.
[34] E. Frehland and P. Läuger, J. Theor. Biol. 47 (1974) 189.
[35] E. Frehland, Biophys. Chem. 8 (1978) 255.

SEMINAR

SURFACE CHARGES ON BIOLOGICAL MEMBRANES

Berthold NEUMCKE

I. Physiologisches Institut der Universität des Saarlandes, D-6650 Homburg / Saar, F. R. G.

1. Introduction

Almost all biological membranes bear negative fixed charges at the membrane-solution interfaces. These membrane surface charges are polar groups of proteins or lipids which are attracted towards the high dielectric aqueous phases surrounding the membrane. Many decisive membrane properties are influenced by the presence of surface charges, e.g. the ionic permeability, the profile of the electrical potential in the membrane phase, the ion concentration at the membrane surface, the temperature of phase transition, and membrane–membrane interactions. The purpose of this supplement to the lecture on membrane surface charges is to illustrate the importance of surface charges for

R. Balian et al., eds.
Les Houches, Session XXXIII, 1979 – Membranes et Communication Intercellulaire / Membranes and Intercellular Communication

various biological membranes, in particular for nerve membranes, and to suggest papers for further reading. Several reviews on surface charges at biological membranes and at artificial lipid bilayers have appeared recently [1–4].

2. Implications of membrane surface charges

2.1. Ion concentration at membrane surface

Due to the presence of negative surface charges, the concentration of cations (anions) in the aqueous phases will be higher (lower) near the membrane surface than in the bulk of the solution. These concentration changes may be very significant. To take typical values for a biological membrane we assume a surface charge density of 1 $e_0/(2\text{ nm})^2$ (e_0: elementary charge) and a bulk concentration of 100 mM for univalent ions. The cation concentration at the membrane surface is then increased 6.8-fold, whereas the anion concentration is depressed by the same factor. Still higher concentration shifts will occur for multivalent ions (e.g. Ca^{++} or La^{+++}). Since these considerations also apply to H^+ ions, the pH value at the membrane surface will be lower than the bulk pH value ($\Delta pH = 0.83$ for an increment of H^+ concentration by a factor of 6.8).

The deviations between surface and bulk ion concentrations have various biological implications. For example, the activity of the Na^+–K^+ exchange pump in cell membranes is regulated by the local concentration of Na^+ and K^+ ions which can be changed by modifying the neighbouring surface charges. This has been suggested from experiments on Purkinje cardiac muscle fibres [5]. The mitochondrial ADP-phosphorylation is influenced by the presence of negative surface charges at the inner mitochondrial membrane [6]. Thus, the inhibitory effects of biguanides and alkylguanidines on oxidative phosphorylation may be due to a decrease of negative surface charges [7]. The effectiveness of uncouplers of oxidative phosphorylation also depends on the density of mitochondrial surface charges [8]. Similarly, the photophosphorylation in the chloroplasts of green plants could be influenced by surface charges on the thylakoid membrane [9]. Finally, at the postsynaptic membrane of the endplate the binding potency of the positively charged transmitter acetylcholin and of the divalent competitive inhibitor curare seems to depend on the magnitude of negative surface charges [10].

2.2. *Ion permeability of membranes*

Since membrane surface charges influence the local ion concentration at the membrane-solution interfaces, they also affect the ion flux through the membrane. The permeability of counterions thus will be higher and that of coions smaller than the permeability of a membrane without surface charges but otherwise identical composition [11, 12]. Hence surface charges are an important factor in the discrimination between the fluxes of cations and anions through membranes. This has been demonstrated for lipid bilayer membranes containing the positively charged nonactin-K^+ carrier complex or the negatively charged poly-iodide complex [13]. More recently the effects of surface charges on the conductance of gramicidin pores in lipid bilayers could also be verified [14].

2.3. *Electric field in membrane phase*

Membrane surface charges will produce an electrical potential in the aqueous solutions adjacent to the interface. This surface potential depends on the valency, arrangement and density of surface charges and on the ionic composition of the solutions (compare with section 3, following). If an asymmetry exists between the outer and inner membrane surface, the corresponding surface potentials Ψ_o and Ψ_i will also

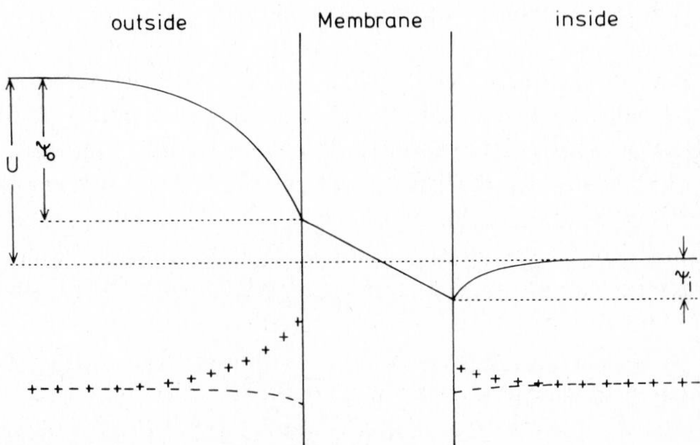

Fig. 1. Schematic profile of the electrical potential (———) and of the aqueous concentrations of cations (+) and anions (−). *U*: membrane potential as measured between the bulk solutions, Ψ_o, Ψ_i: outer and inner surface potential.

be different. In this case the drop of the electrical potential within the membrane phase will no longer be the voltage U between the bulk aqueous phases but will be equal to $U - \Psi_o + \Psi_i$ (see fig. 1). Thus the electric field strength in the membrane depends on the magnitude of surface potentials on both membrane surfaces. Therefore, the field dependent gating properties of excitable membranes can be modified by changing the ionic composition of the solutions. For example, the increase of the threshold of excitation at elevated concentrations of free calcium in the outer solution can be quantitatively explained by the creation of a less negative surface potential [15].

2.4. Lipid phase transition

At a certain temperature the membrane lipids undergo an endothermic phase transition from the gel to the liquid crystal phase [16]. The location of the phase transition temperature depends on the interactions between polar groups in the membrane surface and thus on the magnitude of surface charges. An increase of the charge density will enhance the mutual repulsion between surface groups, expand the lipid bilayer and decrease the transition temperature [17]. This prediction could be verified in experiments using lipid dispersions [18–21]. Hence, surface charges may not only modify the electrical but also the mechanical properties of membranes.

2.5. Membrane–membrane interactions

An electrostatic repulsion between equally charged surface groups will also occur between two adjacent membranes. The repulsion could be reduced by decreasing the number of negative surface groups, preferably by the addition of multivalent cations. The known action of Ca^{++} ions to facilitate the fusion of cell membranes could be due to this effect. Some evidence exists that these surface charge effects are of importance in the fusion of presynaptic vesicles with the plasma membrane [22, 23].

3. Calculation of membrane surface potential

An electrical potential near the membrane surface may be created either by fixed net charges or by electrical dipoles at the membrane–solution interface. Up till now estimates of dipole potentials have been performed for artificial lipid bilayers only [24, 25]. Therefore, we only discuss the contribution of net charges to the surface potential at biological membranes.

3.1. Screening and binding

Membrane surface charges attract counterions from the adjacent aqueous solution. These counterions either form a diffuse layer near the membrane surface or they directly bind to the surface charges. These two possibilities are denoted as "screening" or "binding", respectively. In the case of screening the counterions are still mobile and their concentration profile near the interface is entirely determined by the valency. On the other hand, bound counterions are immobile and the binding affinity depends on individual binding constants which may be different for different ions of the same valency. These criteria may be helpful to distinguish between screening and binding. For example, the voltage dependence of the steady-state potassium activation of myelinated nerve is shifted along the voltage axis by the addition of divalent cations to the extracellular solution. Ca ions produce about four times more shift than the same concentration of Mg ions [26]. Since these voltage shifts are created by a corresponding change of the outer surface potential (see section 5), Ca and Mg ions have different effects on surface charges. Hence, at least Ca ions are bound at the axon membrane.

3.2. Gouy–Chapman theory, Grahame and Stern equation

The screening of fixed membrane surface charges by diffuse counterions is normally described by the Gouy–Chapman theory. In this theory it is assumed that surface charges are homogeneously distributed on the membrane surface, that the ions in the solutions can be treated as point charges, and that the dielectric constant of the aqueous phase is constant up to the membrane surface. The appropriate equation relating the surface potential Ψ with the surface charge density and the bulk ion concentrations can be found in textbooks of physical chemistry (e.g., [27]). To give some values of Ψ we assume that the solutions contain univalent ions of concentration $c = 100$ mM. A surface charge density $\sigma = 1e_0/(2\text{ nm})^2$ then creates a surface potential $\Psi = -48$ mV (at 25° C), a four times higher density $1e_0/(1\text{ nm})^2$ would produce $\Psi = -110$ mV. Since the screening of surface charges will be more effective at higher ion concentrations, Ψ will be less negative. Thus with $c=500$ mM one arrives at $\Psi=-24$ mV and -72 mV for $\sigma=1e_0/(2\text{ nm})^2$ and $1e_0/(1\text{ nm})^2$, respectively. For $|\Psi|<25$ mV the electrical potential declines exponentially with increasing distances r from the membrane surface: $\Psi(r)=\Psi\exp(-\kappa r)$. $1/\kappa$ is the so-called Debye–Hückel length which is about 1 nm at $c=100$ mM and 0.45 nm at 500 mM. For surface potentials much higher than 25 mV the potential decays more steeply with increasing r.

Several extensions of the original Gouy–Chapman theory exist to include the effects of mixed electrolytes and the binding of counterions to surface charges. Physiological solutions normally contain a small amount of divalent cations and thus are mixed electrolytes. The surface potential then can be calculated from a formula, due to Grahame [28]. In reference [29], a more recent treatment of this topic is presented. The binding of counterions to surface charges may be formulated by a Langmuir adsorption isotherm. If this relation is combined with the Gouy–Chapman or Grahame equation one arrives at the so-called Stern equation which adequately describes the adsorption of amphipathic molecules to lipid bilayer membranes [30].

3.3. *Discrete surface charges*

In the above mentioned theories, surface charges are considered to be homogeneously distributed on the membrane surface whereas they are actually located at discrete spots. The discrete nature of surface charges affects the calculation of the surface potential if the product κb between the reciprocal of the Debye–Hückel length $1/\kappa$ and the separation b of surface charges is larger than 1 [31]. Thus for $1/\kappa=b=1$ nm almost no differences from uniform and discrete charge distributions would be obtained, whereas lower densities $b>1$ nm of uniform or discrete charges would create different surface potentials. In general, more discrete than uniformly distributed surface charges are required to obtain a given surface potential [31]. Several theoretical studies have been published recently treating different arrangements and lateral mobilities of discrete surface charges and assuming that the charges are either located at the membrane–solution interface or buried in the membrane phase [1, 32–34]. However, these results are at present of little practical value because the actual arrangement and mobility of surface charges on biological membranes are still unknown.

4. Determination of density of membrane surface charges

A direct way to determine the charge density σ at membrane surfaces would be to measure the surface potential Ψ and to calculate σ from Ψ employing the theories described above. However, since the electrical potential decays within a few nm from the interface, Ψ cannot be measured with microelectrodes. Therefore, various indirect methods have been applied to determine the magnitude of membrane surface potentials.

4.1. Electrophoresis

Vesicles with a charged membrane surface migrate in an external electric field. The velocity of electrophoresis is proportional to the so-called zeta-potential which is the potential at the plane of shear near the vesicle surface [2]. Due to a layer of fixed counterions the zeta-potential determined from electrophoresis may be smaller than the actual surface potential. This has been demonstrated for yeast cells [35]. A further limitation of the electrophoresis method is its restriction to single cells or to biological membranes which can be prepared as vesicles.

4.2. Indicator dyes

Due to the presence of surface charges the aqueous concentrations of charged substances near the interface deviate from their corresponding bulk concentrations. These concentration shifts may be used to estimate the surface potential and the density of surface charges. For example, the fluorescent quantum yield of the negatively charged 1-anilino-8-naphthalenesulfonate (ANS) is much higher in low dielectric media than in aqueous solutions. Thus the amount of ANS bound to the membrane phase can be determined and analyzed for various ionic compositions of the surrounding solutions. Changes of the ANS quantum yield then indicate corresponding shifts of the ANS surface concentration from which Ψ and σ can be calculated [36]. Similarly, a pK shift of a pH sensitive indicator bound to a membrane can be interpreted as difference between surface and bulk pH values which directly yields the surface potential [37–39]. However, this method must be applied with caution since a pK shift may already occur by the indicator binding to a neutral membrane surface [40].

4.3. Spin labels

The distribution of a charged, amphiphilic spin label between a membrane and a salt solution depends on the surface charge density of the membrane. Spin labels tumbling rapidly in aqueous solution produce a sharp line spectrum, whereas labels bound to or in the membrane contribute a broad signal. Hence the ratio between free and bound labels can be obtained from paramagnetic resonance signals, and the surface charge density then can be calculated from the Gouy–Chapman theory [41, 42].

4.4. Ion flux through membrane

The dependence of the membrane permeability on the presence of surface charges (see subsection 2.2) may be used to estimate the charge density. By comparing the net currents through lipid bilayers prepared from the neutral phosphatidylethanolamine and from the negatively charged phosphatidylserine, the density of surface charges at the latter membrane could thus be estimated [13]. This method requires that the two membranes investigated have identical properties except for surface charges.

4.5. Capacitance measurements

This method does not yield the membrane surface potential but the difference between the surface plus dipole potentials at the inner and outer membrane surfaces. It is based on a capacity measurement during ramp voltages. The displacement of the center of the resulting hysteresis figure from the origin then directly gives the asymmetry between the potentials at both membrane surfaces. Up till now this method has been applied to asymmetrical lipid bilayers only [43, 44].

4.6. Voltage shift of gating parameters

Excitable membranes contain ionic channels which are gated by the electric field strength in the membrane phase. A change of the outer or inner surface potential then will cause a displacement of the voltage dependence of gating parameters along the voltage axis. The measured voltage shift may be used to determine the corresponding change of the surface potential from which the density of surface charges can be calculated. Experimentally, the surface potential may be modified by applying solutions with various pH values or with different concentrations of multivalent cations, e.g. Ca^{++}, La^{+++}. In numerous investigations this procedure has been applied to estimate the density and pK values of surface charges on nerve membranes (see section 5), on the plasma membrane [45] and the membrane of the transverse tubuli [46] of skeletal muscle, on cardiac muscle fibres [1], on tunicate egg cell membranes [47], and on the postsynaptic membrane of the neuromuscular junction [48]. Strictly speaking the method of voltage shift gives the density of surface charges at the location of the "electric field sensor" connected to the gate under investigation. In principle, this field sensor could be separated from the gate or from the ionic channel. However, for sodium channels in myelinated nerve it has been shown that at least part of the surface potential seen by the field sensor is also acting on the entrance of the channel [49].

5. Surface charges on nerve membranes

With the method of voltage shift the density and pK value of surface charges on nerve membranes have been determined for various axons, for squid giant axons, for the nodal membrane of myelinated nerve, for crayfish axons [50–52], and for Myxicola giant axons [53, 54]. Of these only the first two preparations will be discussed.

5.1. Squid giant axon

5.1.1. Inner surface charges

Lowering the internal K^+ concentration in perfused squid giant nerve fibres depresses the resting potential but leaves the height of the action potential unchanged. This phenomenon is caused by a shift of the voltage dependencies of sodium inactivation and sodium conductance towards more positive potentials [55]. To explain this result, negative surface charges near the sodium channels of density $1 e_0/(2.7\ \text{nm})^2$ were postulated which produce a more negative internal surface potential at a lowered ionic strength of the axoplasm [56]. This was the first work in which voltage shifts have been interpreted as changes of a surface potential. The concept of surface charges has proven to be very successful and has stimulated many subsequent investigations on various biological membranes. Recently, the presence of negative internal surface charges near the potassium channels of squid giant axons was inferred from the voltage shift of the potassium conductance curve induced by a change of the internal pH [57].

5.1.2. Outer surface charges

Negative surface charges on the extracellular side of squid giant axons were detected near potassium and sodium channels. From the voltage shift of the potassium conductance [58] or of the time constant of potassium activation [59] induced by changing the concentration of divalent extracellular cations a surface charge density of $1e_0/(1.1\ \mathrm{nm})^2$ near the potassium channels was estimated. A still higher density of $1e_0/(0.8\ \mathrm{nm})^2$ near the sodium channels was inferred from the voltage shift of sodium gating parameters at varying extracellular pH [60].

5.2. Myelinated nerve

5.2.1. Outer surface charges

In myelinated nerve excitation is restricted to the nodes of Ranvier. The nodal membrane is in direct contact with the extracellular solution and thus is a suitable object to study properties of outer surface charges. Using data for the voltage shift of the sodium conductance at lowered extracellular pH [61], a surface charge density of $1e_0/(1.5\ \mathrm{nm})^2$ near sodium channels was calculated [62]. In later investigations a somewhat lower [63, 64] or higher [65] density of surface charges near the sodium channels was obtained, or a mixed population of surface charges was suggested [66]. Different types of surface charges were also postulated near the potassium channels of myelinated nerve [67–70]. Comparative studies on the voltage shifts of sodium and potassium parameters have, with one exception [65], yielded approximately the same density of negative outer surface charges near the sodium and potassium channels [63, 71, 72].

5.2.2. Inner surface charges

Myelinated nerve fibres are so thin that they cannot be perfused with solutions of controlled ionic composition. Therefore, no systematic variations of the pH value or the concentration of divalent cations in the axoplasm at the node are possible, and the density of internal surface charges cannot be determined from voltage shifts induced by changes of the internal ion concentration. However, a voltage shift of the sodium inactivation curve can be generated by UV radiation and could be due to a decrease of the number of internal negative surface charges. If this interpretation is correct, a density of $1 e_0/(3.5\ \mathrm{nm})^2$ for internal surface charges near the sodium channels may be estimated [73].

5.3. *Implications of charge asymmetry*

Although various densities of surface charges on the squid giant axon and on myelinated nerve fibres have been reported, it seems that for both preparations the density of negative charges is higher on the outer than on the inner membrane surface. This situation is illustrated in fig. 1. To be specific we take surface charge densities of $1 e_0/(2\ \mathrm{nm})^2$ and $1 e_0/(3.5\ \mathrm{nm})^2$ for the outer and inner surface of the nodal membrane. The corresponding surface potentials under physiological conditions are $\Psi_o \approx -50$ mV and $\Psi_i \approx -20$ mV, respectively. This asymmetry between outer and inner surfaces implies that under resting conditions only 40 mV potential drop occurs across the axon membrane though the resting potential between the bulk solutions is $U \approx -70$ mV. Thus a depolarization of only 40 mV would be required to have zero electric field strength in the membrane phase. Indeed, the midpoints of the steady-state sodium and potassium activation curves lie close to this depolarization indicating that the corresponding gates are then not subject to an electric field. The origin of the charge asymmetry on either sides of the axon membrane is not yet clear. It has been suggested that surface charges may not be fixed but were able to diffuse across the hydrophobic interior of the membrane toward the opposite membrane–solution interface. Since under resting conditions the axoplasm is negatively charged with respect to the extracellular solution, more internal negative surface charges would be driven to outside than outer surface charges to inside. This would explain the observed charge asymmetry in nerve membranes [74]. However, no evidence for a transmembrane motion of surface charges could be detected during 30 min depolarizations at squid giant axons [75]. Hence a "flip-flop" of surface charges does not exist or it proceeds with a time constant longer than one hour.

Acknowledgements

This work was supported by Deutsche Forschungsgemeinschaft SFB 38 "Membranforschung". I thank Professor Dr. R. Stämpfli and Dr. W. Schwarz for reading the manuscript.

References

[1] R. H. Brown, Jr., Progr. Biophys. Molec. Biol. 28 (1974) 343.
[2] D. L. Gilbert, in: Biophysics and Physiology of Excitable Membranes, ed. W. J. Adelman, Jr. (van Nostrand Reinhold, New York, 1971) pp. 359–378.
[3] S. McLaughlin, in: Current Topics of Membranes and Transport, vol. 9, eds. F. Bronnen and A. Kleinzeller (Academic Press, New York, 1977) pp. 71–144.
[4] S. Ohki, Progr. Surface Membr. Sci. 10 (1976) 117.
[5] I. Cohen, D. Noble, M. Ohba and C. Ojeda, J. Physiol. 297 (1979) 163.
[6] G. Schäfer and G. Rowohl-Quisthoudt, FEBS Lett. 59 (1975) 48.
[7] G. Schäfer and E. Rieger, Eur. J. Biochem. 46 (1974) 613.
[8] S. McLaughlin, J. Membr. Biol. 9 (1972) 361.
[9] H. T. Witt, Biochim. Biophys. Acta 505 (1979) 355.
[10] W. G. van der Kloot and I. Cohen, Science 203 (1979) 1351.
[11] B. Neumcke, Biophysik 6 (1970) 231.
[12] B. Neumcke, J. Electrochem. Soc. 123 (1976) 1331.
[13] S. G. A. McLaughlin, G. Szabo and G. Eisenman, J. Gen. Physiol. 58 (1971) 667.
[14] H. J. Apell, E. Bamberg and P. Läuger, Biochim Biophys. Acta 552 (1979) 369.
[15] B. Hille, Ann. Rev. Physiol. 38 (1976) 139.
[16] D. Chapman, Quart. Rev. Biophys. 8 (1975) 185.
[17] F. Jähnig, Biophys. Chem. 4 (1976) 309.
[18] H. Träuble and H. Eibl, Proc. Nat. Acad. Sci. USA 71 (1974) 214.
[19] H. Träuble, M. Teubner, P. Woolley and H. Eibl, Biophys. Chem. 4 (1976) 319.
[20] A. G. Lee, Biochim. Biophys. Acta 514 (1978) 95.
[21] H. Eibl and A. Blume, Biochim. Biophys. Acta 553 (1979) 476.
[22] R. U. Muller and A. Finkelstein, Proc. Nat. Acad. Sci. USA 71 (1974) 923.
[23] J. E. Hall and S. A. Simon, Biochim. Biophys. Acta 436 (1976) 613.
[24] G. Szabo, Nature 252 (1974) 47.
[25] R. Latorre and J. E. Hall, Nature 264 (1976) 361.
[26] T. Brismar and B. Frankenhaeuser, Acta Physiol. Scand. 85 (1972) 237.
[27] G. Kortüm, Lehrbuch der Elektrochemie (Verlag Chemie, Weinheim, 1966).
[28] D. C. Grahame, Chem. Rev. 41 (1947) 441.
[29] B. Abraham-Shrauner, J. Mathem. Biol. 2 (1975) 333.
[30] S. McLaughlin and H. Harary, Biochemistry 15 (1976) 1941.
[31] K. S. Cole, Biophys. J. 9 (1969) 465.
[32] A. P. Nelson and D. A. McQuarrie, J. Theoret. Biol. 55 (1975) 13.
[33] R. Y. Tsien, Biophys. J. 24 (1978) 561.
[34] D. Attwell and D. Eisner, Biophys. J. 24 (1978) 869.
[35] A. P. R. Theuvenet, Thesis (Univ. of Nijmegen, 1978) ch. VII.
[36] D. H. Haynes, J. Membr. Biol. 17 (1974) 341.
[37] J. V. Moller and U. Kragh-Hansen, Biochemistry 14 (1975) 2317.

[38] K. Kano and J. H. Fendler, Biochim. Biophys. Acta 509 (1978) 289.
[39] W. L. C. Vaz, A. Nicksch and F. Jähnig, Eur. J. Biochem. 83 (1978) 299.
[40] M. S. Fernández and P. Fromherz, J. Phys. Chem. 81 (1977) 1755.
[41] B. J. Gaffney and R. J. Mich, J. Am. Chem. Soc. 98 (1976) 3044.
[42] J. D. Castle and W. L. Hubbell, Biochemistry 15 (1976) 4818.
[43] P. Schoch and D. F. Sargent, Experientia 32 (1976) 811.
[44] P. Schoch, D. F. Sargent and R. Schwyzer, J. Membrane Biol. 46 (1979) 71.
[45] D. T. Campbell and B. Hille, J. Gen. Physiol. 67 (1976) 309.
[46] M. Dörrscheidt-Käfer, Pflügers Arch. 362 (1976) 33.
[47] H. Ohmori and M. Yoshii, J. Physiol. 267 (1977) 429.
[48] R. Sterz, F. Dreyer and K. Peper, Pflügers Arch. 377 (1978) R 44.
[49] B. Hille, J. M. Ritchie and G. R. Strichartz, J. Physiol. 250 (1975) 34P.
[50] P. Shrager, J. Gen. Physiol. 64 (1974) 666.
[51] J. S. D'Arrigo, J. Membr. Biol. 22 (1975) 255.
[52] A. Strickholm and H. R. Clark, Biophys. J. 19 (1977) 29.
[53] T. Begenisich, J. Gen. Physiol. 66 (1975) 47.
[54] C. L. Schauf, J. Physiol. 248 (1975) 613.
[55] T. Narahashi, J. Physiol. 169 (1963) 91.
[56] W. K. Chandler, A. L. Hodgkin and H. Meves, J. Physiol. 180 (1965) 821.
[57] E. Wanke, E. Carbone and P. L. Testa, Biophys. J. 26 (1979) 319.
[58] D. L. Gilbert and G. Ehrenstein, Biophys. J. 9 (1969) 447.
[59] G. Ehrenstein and D. L. Gilbert, Biophys. J. 13 (1973) 495.
[60] E. Carbone, R. Fioravanti, G. F. Prestipino and E. Wanke, J. Membr. Biol. 43 (1978) 295.
[61] B. Hille, J. Gen. Physiol. 51 (1968) 221.
[62] D. L. Gilbert and G. Ehrenstein, J. Gen. Physiol. 55 (1970) 822.
[63] T. Brismar, Acta Physiol. Scand. 87 (1973) 474.
[64] H. Drouin and B. Neumcke, Pflügers Arch. 351 (1974) 207.
[65] W. Vogel, Pflügers Arch. 350 (1974) 25.
[66] B. Hille, A. M. Woodhull and B. I. Shapiro, Phil. Trans. R. Soc. London B270 (1975) 301.
[67] G. N. Mozhayeva and A. P. Naumov, Nature 228 (1970) 164.
[68] G. N. Mozhayeva and A. P. Naumov, Biophysics 17 (1972) 429.
[69] G. N. Mozhayeva and A. P. Naumov, Biophysics 17 (1972) 644.
[70] G. N. Mozhayeva and A. P. Naumov, Biophysics 17 (1972) 839.
[71] H. Drouin, Bioelectrochem. Bioenerg. 3 (1976) 222.
[72] B. Neumcke, in: Electrical Phenomena at the Biological Membrane Level, ed. E. Roux (Elsevier, Amsterdam, 1977) pp. 257–272.
[73] W. Schwarz and J. M. Fox, J. Membr. Biol. 36 (1977) 297.
[74] S. McLaughlin and H. Harary, Biophys. J. 14 (1974) 200.
[75] G. Ehrenstein and D. L. Gilbert, Biophys. J. 15 (1975) 847.

COURSE 8

THE EXCITABLE MEMBRANE OF NERVE FIBRES

Claude BERGMAN

Laboratoire de Neurobiologie,
Ecole Normale Supérieure,
46 rue d'Ulm,
75005 Paris,
France

and

Hans MEVES

I. Physiologisches Institut,
Universität des Saarlandes,
665 Homburg-Saar,
West Germany

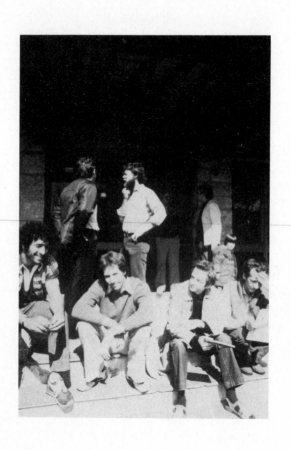

Contents

R. Balian et al., eds.
Les Houches, Session XXXIII, 1979 – Membranes et Communication Intercellulaire / Membranes and Intercellular Communication

1. Membrane potential in living cells

1.1. Some definitions

We define membrane potential as a voltage difference that can be measured between the internal and external cell compartments. When the cell is in the resting state, this potential is found to be negative inside (vs outside) and ranges between -50 and -90 mV, depending on the cell type. For a given cell, the resting potential is remarkably constant. It is therefore taken as a reference level, especially for excitable cells. Any potential variation making the interior less negative than the resting level is termed a "depolarization". Conversely, any variation leading to a more negative level than the resting potential is called a "hyperpolarization".

In most excitable cells, transient depolarizations constitute the electrical sign of physiological activity. When these depolarizations develop in an all-or-none fashion (regenerative depolarization) they are called "action potentials". The action potentials are generally propagated along the cell membrane, especially in axons, skeletal muscle fibres and heart. Trains of action potentials of constant amplitude and variable frequency constitute the nerve impulse in the central and peripheral nervous system. During each action potential, the membrane temporarily reverses its electrical polarization and can reach a positive level approaching $+50$ mV. Hence, when starting from a resting level near -70 mV, the action potential represents a brief voltage pulse of about 120 mV propagating along a cable-like structure.

1.2. Origin of the membrane potential

In the very beginning of this century the so-called "animal electricity" was first recognized as resulting from diffusion potential variations. This view remains essentially valid nowadays.

The membrane potential arises from the unequal distribution of ions on either side of the cell membrane, together with the relatively high ionic selectivity of this membrane. As long as the equilibrium potential (Nernst potential) for each ion species is kept constant, and so far as the active transport of ions (uphill fluxes requiring energy) is neglected, the membrane potential can be regarded as the e.m.f. of a compound voltage generator made of several diffusion batteries in parallel (see fig. 2 in the following subsection).

Potassium (K^+), sodium (Na^+), and chloride (Cl^-) are the main permeating ion species in biological membranes (calcium will be neglected here). Accordingly, the diffusion batteries E_K, E_{Na}, and E_{Cl} contribute to build up the membrane potential E.

The e.m.f. of each battery can be calculated on the basis of the well-known Nernst–Planck relation:

$$E_I = (RT/zF)ln([I]_0/[I]_i),$$

where E_I is the equilibrium potential for the ion species I; R, T, and F are the usual thermodynamic constants; $[I]_0$ and $[I]_i$ being the respective external and internal activities of ion I of valence z. Note that E_I is the membrane potential that would be reached if the membrane was exclusively permeable to ion species I. Note also that if $E = E_I$ the net flux of ion I through the membrane is nil.

In living cells (see fig. 1), the internal compartment is rich in K^+ and poor in Na^+ and Cl^-; electroneutrality is achieved by non-diffusing organic anions (quoted R^-). On the other side of the membrane, the extracellular fluid is poor in K^+ and rich in Na^+ and Cl^-. Figure 1 summarizes the data for a frog neuron as they can be deduced from voltage clamp experiments performed at a temperature of 20° C. As in most animal cells, E_K is more negative than the resting level (E_r). E_{Na} is the sole positive equilibrium potential and E_{Cl} is nearly equal to E_r. This latter observation might imply that, at rest, the membrane is selectively permeable to chloride. Actually, this is not the case since the membrane proves to be permeable to potassium and sodium (see below). E_K and E_{Na} represent the extreme values between which the membrane potential can vary. During activity the action potential peak approaches the equilibrium potential for sodium, thus indicating that in this particular instance the Na permeability temporarily predominates in this excitable membrane.

From the preceding remarks, it can immediately be inferred that the membrane potential E depends on the values of the equilibrium potentials for the various ions to which the membrane is permeable, and on the relative permeability of this membrane to each ion species present in

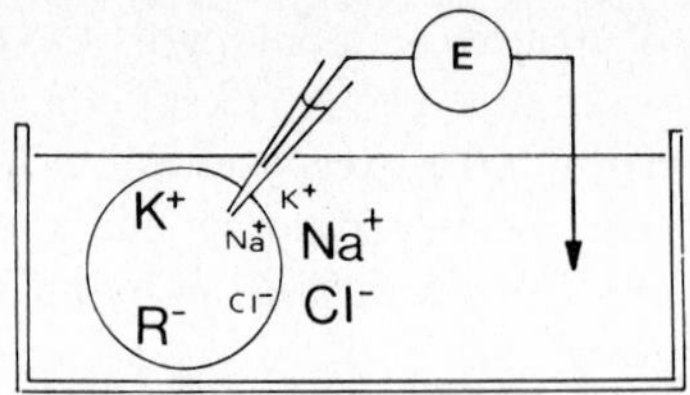

	in	out	E(mV)
K	117	2.5	−96
Na	12	114	+56
Cl	8	120	−68

(mM) (20°C)

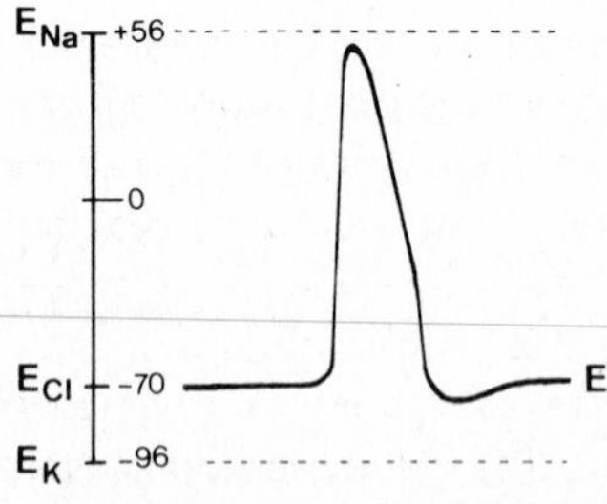

Fig. 1. Distribution of ions between internal and external cell compartments. The table gives the potassium, sodium and chloride concentrations (in mM) and the corresponding equilibrium potentials (in mV) as calculated on the basis of the Nernst equation (20° C) for a myelinated axon from the frog. The drawing in the lower part of the figure represents the membrane potential change during excitation (action potential) with respect to the equilibrium potentials for the three main permeant ions.

both cell compartments. In excitable cells the equilibrium potentials E_K, E_{Na}, and E_{Cl} can be considered as constant to a first approximation (see below). Hence the variation of E during activity essentially arises from changes of membrane permeability.

1.3. A useful expression for the resting potential

Assuming the membrane is permeable to the three ions K, Na, and Cl, and that the respective equilibrium potentials for these ions are fixed to constant values (see below), a formal model for the cell can be used as represented in fig. 2.

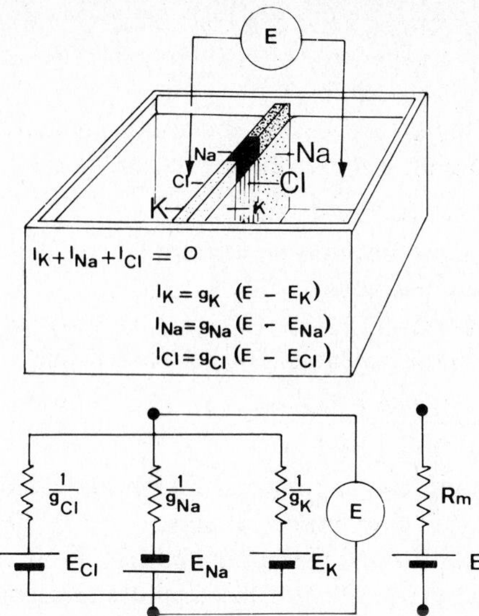

Fig. 2. A simplified model and its two equivalent electrical circuits for the cell membrane when assuming three permeant ion species: Na, K, and Cl. The membrane capacitance has not been represented. The membrane potential (E) is a mixed diffusion potential corresponding to the zero current condition.

A steady-state membrane potential (E) can be reached, which a priori differs from each specific equilibrium potential. As a consequence, three fluxes of ions flow through the membrane, and for each ion species the net flux is proportional to the potential difference $E - E_I$ (which represents the "driving force" for ion species I). Observing that the net flux of ion (J_I) is equivalent to a current (I_I) carried by ions of species I, we can write:

$$I_I = J_I zF$$

where F is the Faraday number and z the valence of ion I.

Accordingly, the ionic current can be expressed (in the terms of Ohm's law) as:

$$I_I = g_I(E - E_I)$$

where g_I is the reciprocal of a resistance, namely the membrane conductance to ion I. We can thus write the three currents:

$$I_K = g_K(E - E_K) \qquad I_{Na} = g_{Na}(E - E_{Na}) \tag{1, 2}$$

$$I_{Cl} = g_{Cl}(E - E_{Cl}). \tag{3}$$

Note that in these expressions, and provided the membrane behaves like an ohmic resistor, the specific conductances can be used as expressions for the membrane permeability.

The condition for a steady-state membrane potential is that the net flux of charges passing through the membrane is nil. In other words:

$$I_K + I_{Na} + I_{Cl} + I_C = 0 \tag{4}$$

where I_C is the membrane capacity current ($I_C = C\mathrm{d}E/\mathrm{d}t$) equal to zero under steady-state conditions.

Combining relations (1), (2), (3), and (4), an expression for the steady-state membrane potential can be worked out:

$$E = \frac{g_K E_K + g_{Na} E_{Na} + g_{Cl} E_{Cl}}{g_K + g_{Na} + g_{Cl}} \tag{5}$$

in which the denominator is the total membrane conductance equal to the reciprocal of the "membrane resistance" (R_m). Figure 2 represents the equivalent circuit for the membrane battery. Note that eq. (5) can be used as a practical expression for the membrane potential as far as the contribution of the active transport of sodium and potassium ions can be neglected (which is the case in axons). A more complete expression for E will be presented later.

It is obvious that, due to the existence of net fluxes through the membrane, the ions tend to redistribute on either side of the membrane, thus leading to a progressive change in the equilibrium potentials. In living cells, the active transport exactly compensates the passive leak of ions and continuously restores the equilibrium potentials to their original values. It follows that blocking the cell metabolism leads to an equilibrium corresponding to $E=0$ (the internal ionic concentrations become equal to the external ones).

1.4. Verifying some major assumptions

A simple way to test equation (5) might consist in changing, successively and separately, the equilibrium potentials for K^+, Na^+, and Cl^- by modifying the ionic composition of the artificial medium bathing the cell. For instance, the external concentrations can be made equal to the internal ones, thus reducing each equilibrium potential to zero. Then, measuring E under these new conditions should give an estimate of the membrane permeability to the ion species the activity of which has been modified.

Reducing the external Na concentration can be achieved by replacing a large fraction of NaCl by an equimolar amount of choline, caesium, or tetramethylammonium chloride (these three cations being almost impermeant in biological membranes). In the same way, chloride can be replaced by a non-permeant anion like methylsulphate or benzene sulfonate, which are inert in many other respects.

When $[Na]_0$ is made equal to $[Na]_i$, E_{Na} changes from +50 to 0 mV. Only a slight increase (a few mV more negative) of the resting potential can be observed. However, when $[K]_0$ is elevated by substituting potassium for sodium, E reaches a steady level equal to the predicted value for E_K. Finally, when most of the external chloride is replaced by methylsulphate, the membrane slightly depolarizes. However, it slowly returns to its initial resting level [this particular behaviour is typical for muscle fibres and has been extensively studied by Hodgkin and Horowicz (1959)].

From these observations, the following conclusions can be drawn:

(i) In the resting state, the membrane is only slightly permeable to Na and Cl. It is, however, much more permeable to potassium. This explains that under normal conditions, E_r approaches E_K without reaching this negative limit.

(ii) When the external K concentration is high, and especially when $[K]_0=[K]_i$, the membrane behaves like a selective potassium electrode thus implying that the overall membrane selectivity changes. This is essentially due to the fact (see the two following lectures) that the potassium permeability increases while the sodium permeability decreases ("sodium conductance inactivation") when the membrane is depolarized for a long time.

(iii) New steady-state levels can be reached when either K^+ or Na^+ concentrations in the external medium are altered. This indicates that both the internal K^+ and Na^+ concentrations are somehow fixed in the cell. However, since after a large change in E_{Cl} towards a positive value, the membrane first depolarizes then returns to its initial level, we can conclude that the internal Cl concentration is not fixed. In other words, Cl ions redistribute passively according to the value of E fixed by the two other ion species, K and Na, until a new equilibrium potential for Cl^- (equal to E) is reached.

1.5. Some additional comments

At rest, the membrane potential is held by only the K and the Na permeability systems. As a result, when the permeability to one of these ions is blocked, the membrane potential should reach the equilibrium potential for the other ion. More specifically, when blocking the K conductance of an axon by TEA, E should become equal to E_{Na}. In practice, only a slight depolarization is observed. Similarly, when blocking g_{Na} by TTX, only a slight hyperpolarization takes place, E remaining far (some 20 mV) from the calculated value for E_K.

The immediate and small effect of TTX is easily explained by the fact that in the resting state (at negative membrane potential) g_{Na} is much smaller than $g_K + g_{Cl^-}$. However, E should slowly tend toward E_K at a rate limited by the chloride redistribution until $E_{Cl} = E_K$. This should be the case for membranes exhibiting relatively high Cl permeability like that of muscle fibres (Hodgkin and Horowicz 1959, Adrian and Freygang 1962). It is probably the case for axons. However, in the case of this latter preparation, the chloride permeability is very low so that Cl-*re*distribution takes a very long time. This makes the variation of E insignificant within the usual duration of an *in vitro* experiment. Another reason for a smaller-than-expected, TTX-induced hyperpolarization is that it is very likely that E_K is less negative under normal conditions than the value calculated taking into account the K-concentration in the external solution. In fact, the actual $[K]_0$ at the external membrane surface is slightly higher than in the bulk solution. This arises from: (a) the presence of either unstirred layers or restricted diffusion spaces (Frankenhaeuser and Hodgkin 1956, Dubois and Bergman 1975) on one hand, and (b) the continuous leak of potassium from the internal compartment into the restricted extracellular space (where K-ions accumulate), on the other hand.

The relatively small (4–10 mV) depolarization usually produced by TEA (instead of a voltage change bringing E to E_{Na}) results from the fact that, as soon as the membrane tends to depolarize, inactivation of the sodium conductance takes place so that the Na permeability becomes smaller than the remaining chloride permeability. Hence, E_{Na} cannot be reached despite the blocking of the K-permeability by TEA. The membrane potential thus remains at a negative level near E_{Cl}. Finally, the fact that neither TTX nor TEA induce marked alterations of the resting potential could be very well accounted for by assuming that in the presence of the specific blocker the membrane remains permeable to either Na or K via a non-specific (leakage) channel.

A further point which deserves attention concerns the validity of eq. (5). The main advantage of this expression is its simplicity. However, it can only be generalized if the instantaneous conductances are independent of both E and the ionic concentrations (which is not always the case). Owing to these restrictions, Hodgkin and Katz (1949) have proposed an expression for the steady-state (zero-current) membrane potential based on Goldman's constant field theory. This equation has been proved to be applicable to a large variety of membranes though the assumptions made (the ions move independently of each other, their diffusion coefficient, as well as the electric field, are constant throughout the whole membrane) appear questionable, at present, at least for excitable membranes. Despite these reservations, the so-called Goldman–Hodgkin–Katz equation remains a useful expression, especially for determining the permeability (P) ratios under zero-current conditions. Therefore, it is given here:

$$E = \frac{RT}{F}\ln\frac{P_{\mathrm{K}}[\mathrm{K}]_0 + P_{\mathrm{Na}}[\mathrm{Na}]_0 + P_{\mathrm{Cl}}[\mathrm{Cl}]_i}{P_{\mathrm{K}}[\mathrm{K}]_i + P_{\mathrm{Na}}[\mathrm{Na}]_i + P_{\mathrm{Cl}}[\mathrm{Cl}]_0}.$$

For a discussion of these equations, see Barr (1965), Hille (1975a) and Jack (1976).

1.6. The relative stability of the equilibrium potentials

As already pointed out, the cell under normal conditions is not in thermodynamic equilibrium. Neither the resting polarization (mainly depending on E_{K}), nor the large positive value of E_{Na} can be maintained without counter-transport compensating the passive leak of Na and K. The cell, however, can tolerate transient variations of the K and Na equilibrium potentials without significant alterations of its physiological functions. These discrete variations usually occur during and after a period of activity. It follows that the notion of steady state has to be considered over a finite period of time $(t_1 - t_0)$ unless the cell is maintained in the resting state. The steady-state condition is therefore:

$$\int J_{\mathrm{K}}\mathrm{d}t = \int_{t_0}^{t_1} M_{\mathrm{K}}\mathrm{d}t \qquad \text{for } [\mathrm{K}]_i$$

and

$$\int J_{\mathrm{Na}}\mathrm{d}t = \int_{t_0}^{t_1} M_{\mathrm{Na}}\mathrm{d}t \qquad \text{for } [\mathrm{Na}]_i.$$

This does not necessarily imply that the instantaneous active (M) and passive (J) fluxes are equal and opposite at any time, although they likely are when the cell is maintained in the resting state for long periods.

The direct proof for the active transport of sodium in excitable cells was first given by Hodgkin and Keynes (1955) working on the squid axon. Further investigations on mammalian C-nerve fibres (Ritchie and Straub 1957), muscle fibres (Keynès and Swan 1959), mollusc neurones (Kerkut and Thomas 1965, Thomas 1969) tend to regard the ATP fueled pump (Caldwell et al. 1960) as very similar to that extensively studied in red blood cells [for a review, see Thomas (1972)].

The major features of the metabolic Na/K pump can be summarized as follows (fig. 3):

(a) Outward Na and inward K-active transports are coupled (Na extrusion is blocked by external K removal).

(b) The pump is "electrogenic". Under normal conditions, its stoichiometry is roughly two K ions taken in for every three Na ions pumped out, with one ATP split.

(c) Provided the external K concentration is sufficiently high (i.e. normal $[K]_0$), the rate of pumping depends on the internal Na concentration (the higher $[Na]_i$, the more active the pump).

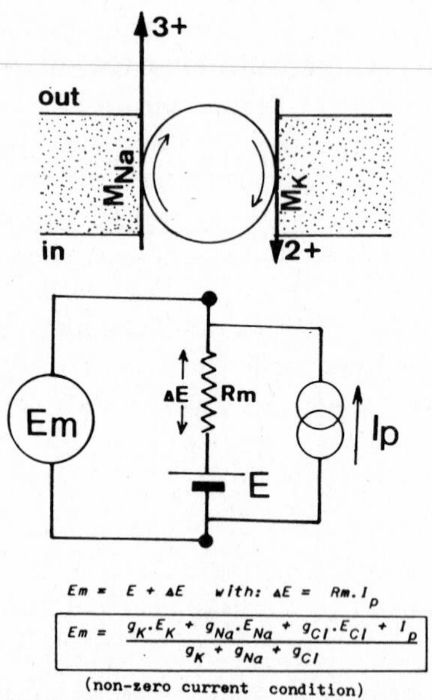

Fig. 3. The coupled Na/K transport system is represented as a current generator connected to the passive branch of the membrane equivalent circuit. When activated, the pump creates a voltage drop proportional to the pump current I_P and the membrane resistance R_m.

The latter finding is of importance to understand how the cell regulates its internal cation distribution. The automatic stimulation of the pump by slight increases in $[Na]_i$ arises from the fact that ATP splitting is catalysed by a Na-dependent ATPase. It follows that the amount of energy available for the pump is directly related to the entry of Na and, consequently, used to extrude these ions. This has been demonstrated by Thomas (1969) in snail neurones, showing in particular (fig. 4) that, as soon as the internal Na concentration becomes higher than 4–6 mM, the rate of Na extrusion increases almost linearly with increasing internal Na. Since the coupling ratio K/Na of the pump is $\frac{2}{3}$ and since the pump activity is regulated according to $[Na]_i$, one may ask how $[K]_i$ is held constant. A possible explanation is as follows. Most of the negative charges of the cytoplasmic medium are sequestred in the cell in the form of non-permeant organic anions. To satisfy electroneutrality, an equivalent amount of cations has to be present inside. Since Na is extruded by the pump while K is taken in, most of the anionic cell content is neutralized by K. In other words, there is a K concentration adjustment which is directly correlated to the Na extrusion. Since Cl is assumed to redistribute passively according to the value of E, its internal concentration is indirectly fixed by the Na pump.

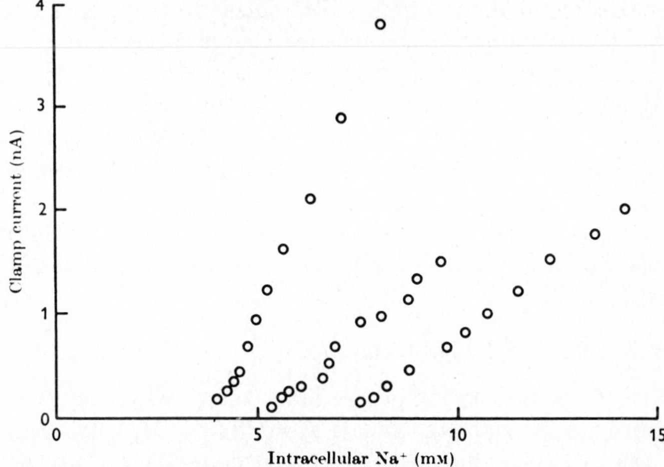

Fig. 4. Membrane current generated by the Na/K pump as a function of intracellular Na concentration, for three different snail neurones. The pump current was measured under voltage clamp conditions in response to several injections of sodium into the cell. The internal sodium concentration was measured by means of a Na-selective glass microelectrode. [From R. C. Thomas (1969).]

In summary, assuming the osmotic pressure in the internal and external fluids to be balanced, the Na-dependent ATPase, together with the pool of internal anions and a fixed value for the P_K/P_{Na} ratio are responsible for the relative constancy of the K, Na, and Cl activities. The corresponding external concentrations for their own are fixed by the various regulatory mechanisms controlling the electrolyte balance in the body fluids. However, it must be pointed out that in some tissues the tightness of the intercellular spaces represents a diffusion barrier. As previously mentioned, K ions in particular can accumulate in the immediate vicinity of the membrane after a long period of activity. It is very likely that in this case the Na/K pump contributes to restore the K concentration in the clefts to an optimum level. A transient increase in E_K can thus occur (and accordingly a membrane hyperpolarization) which is not easily distinguishable from the "electrogenic" pump contribution [see Bergman et al. (1979)].

1.7. The electrogenic character of the pump: contribution to E_m

Beyond the fact that the Na/K pump regulates the internal ion concentration, and thereby E_m, a more direct contribution to the membrane polarization results from the electrogenic character of the pump. It has been emphasized that the pump stoichiometry was estimated to be 2 K/3 Na. As a result, one net positive charge is taken out for each "pump turn", leading to a membrane hyperpolarization. The electrogenic contribution of the pump to E_m can thus be expressed as the immediate voltage drop that would result from the blocking of the Na/K pumping (for instance, by a specific pump inhibitor like ouabain).

We thus regard the Na/K pump as a current generator shunting the membrane resistance R_m. In operation, it creates a potential difference (see figs. 3 and 4):

$$\Delta E = I_p R_m = I_p/(g_K + g_{Na} + g_{Cl}) \tag{6}$$

where I_p is the pump current, proportional to the difference between the active fluxes of K and Na, that is $I_p = F(M_{Na} - M_K)$. Note that ΔE (which can be easily measured) is proportional to I_p only if R_m is independent of the potential variation created by the pump. This is not always the case in excitable cells, since g_K and g_{Na} are voltage and time dependent.

As demonstrated by Thomas (1969), an injection of sodium into a snail neuron leads to a membrane hyperpolarization (fig. 5) that can be attributed to the pump stimulation. The direct measurement of the pump current under voltage clamp conditions (Thomas 1969) confirms that the pump is electrogenic. Under physiological conditions, very similar transient hyperpolarizations can occur in some preparations after long trains of action potentials leading to a massive entry of Na. These potential changes have been called "post-tetanic hyperpolarizations". Some of them are indisputably attributable to the pump stimulation (Ritchie and Straub 1957). They are usually slow and of moderate amplitude. Increasing the membrane resistance by substituting non-permeant anions for external chloride enhances the post-tetanic hyperpolarization amplitude (Rang and Ritchie 1968), as predicted by eq. (6).

In some circumstances, it can be of importance to estimate the pump contribution to the resting potential. Measurements can be made by comparing the resting potential in the presence and in the absence of ouabain in the external medium (see fig. 5). The experiment shows that

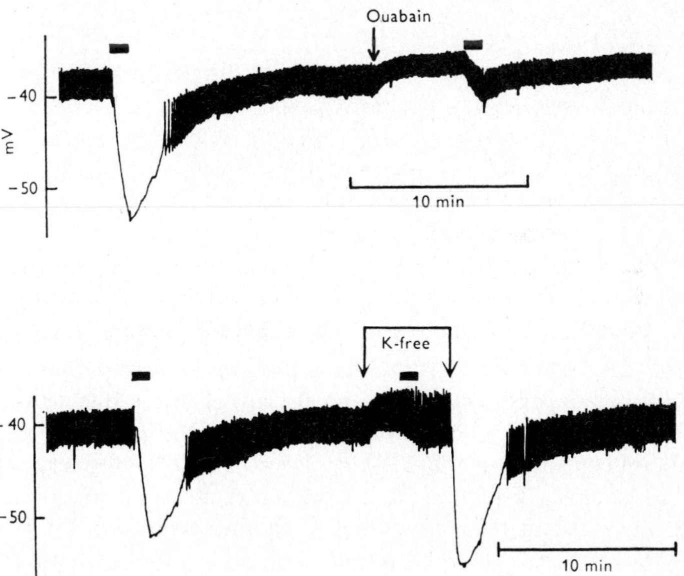

Fig. 5. Pen recordings of the membrane potential of two snail neurones. The normal resting potential is near −40 mV. An iontophoretic injection of sodium (the period of injection is indicated by solid bars) leads to a hyperpolarization of 12 mV. In the presence of either ouabain (upper trace) or K-free external solution (lower trace) the membrane slightly depolarizes (thus showing the contribution of the pump to the resting potential). Under these new conditions, the same injection of Na induces an almost negligible hyperpolarization. Note that restoration of the normal $[K]_0$ is followed by an immediate hyperpolarization (lower trace). (From R. C. Thomas 1969.)

the electrogenic pump contribution is usually very small in axons [1.4 mV for the squid axon, according to De Weer and Geduldig (1973)] larger and highly sensitive to external K concentration in neurones from the marine mollusk *Anisodoris* (Marmor and Gorman 1970). These variations are in agreement with calculations based on the following assumptions:

(a) The resting membrane potential (E_r) represents a strict steady state (zero current potential).

(b) The internal concentrations are maintained rigorously constant (i.e. the passive and active fluxes of Na and K are equal at any time).

(c) The K/Na coupling ratio of the pump is constant.

(d) Cl ions redistribute passively so that $E_{\mathrm{Cl}} = E_r$ (i.e. their contribution to E_r can be omitted).

Writing $M_{\mathrm{K}}/M_{\mathrm{Na}} = c$ (coupling ratio for the pump), observing that $I_{\mathrm{p}} = (1-c)M_{\mathrm{Na}}F = (1-c)I'_{\mathrm{Na}}$, and that $[\mathrm{Na}]_i$ remains constant at all times if $I_{\mathrm{Na}} = I'_{\mathrm{Na}}$, the zero-current condition is: $I_{\mathrm{K}} + I_{\mathrm{Na}} + I_{\mathrm{p}} = 0$, thus $g_{\mathrm{K}}(E_r - E_{\mathrm{K}}) + g_{\mathrm{Na}}(E_r - E_{\mathrm{Na}}) = (1-c)I'_{\mathrm{Na}}$. By replacing I'_{Na} by I_{Na}, the zero current equation becomes:

$$g_{\mathrm{K}}(E_r - E_{\mathrm{K}}) + cg_{\mathrm{Na}}(E_r - E_{\mathrm{Na}}) = 0$$

from which E_r can be obtained:

$$E_r = \frac{g_{\mathrm{K}}E_{\mathrm{K}} + cg_{\mathrm{Na}}E_{\mathrm{Na}}}{g_{\mathrm{K}} + cg_{\mathrm{Na}}}. \tag{7}$$

The pump contribution can be calculated by subtracting eq. (5) from (7) provided $E_{\mathrm{Cl}} = E$ in eq. (5). It is interesting to observe that the pump contribution depends on both c and the $g_{\mathrm{K}}/g_{\mathrm{Na}}$ ratio, the smaller these values, the larger the pump contribution to E_r. One can thus predict that the pump contribution will be fairly large in cells having resting potentials far from E_{K}. Equation (7) is valid under the same conditions as eq. (5). If the constant field theory holds, another expression for E_r is:

$$E_r = \frac{RT}{F}\ln\frac{P_{\mathrm{K}}[\mathrm{K}]_0 + cP_{\mathrm{Na}}[\mathrm{Na}]_0}{P_{\mathrm{K}}[\mathrm{K}]_i + cP_{\mathrm{Na}}[\mathrm{Na}]_i}. \tag{8}$$

Both eqs. (7) and (8) imply some assumptions on how the ions pass the membrane and how the specific conductances depend on the ion concentrations on either side of the membrane.

2. Voltage clamp experiments on squid giant axons

The basis of modern electrophysiology is the work of Hodgkin and Huxley (1952b). They measured the voltage clamp currents in squid giant axons and described the currents by a set of mathematical equations. From these equations they were able to reconstruct the propagated action potential and the membrane action potential.

The voltage clamp method is illustrated in fig. 6. Two electrodes are longitudinally inserted into the axon, an internal potential electrode C

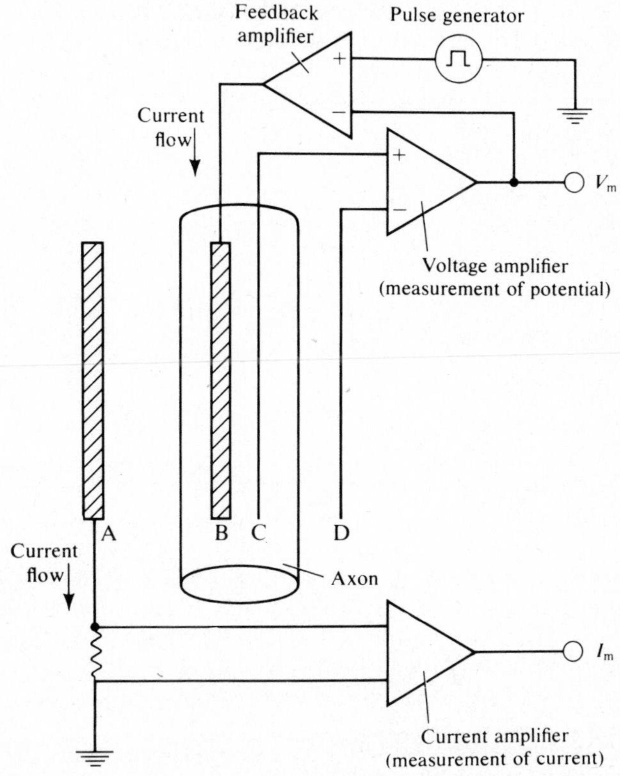

Fig. 6. Voltage clamp on a squid axon. The membrane potential V_m is measured between electrodes C and D. The feedback amplifier forces the membrane potential to a preset level by passing current through an internal electrode B, the membrane and an external electrode A to ground. The membrane current I_m is recorded as the voltage drop across a small resistor. [From Kandel (1976).]

and an internal current electrode B. The voltage amplifier measures the potential between the internal and the external potential electrode (C and D). The feedback amplifier compares the measured potential and the command potential as in fig. 6 and sends a current through the internal current electrode B, the membrane and the external current electrode A to ground. The current adjusts the potential across the membrane to the command potential and is measured by the current amplifier.

An example of a voltage clamp record is shown in fig. 7. A step change in membrane potential (from the resting potential −50 mV to +15 mV) produces a brief surge of outward current (the capacitative current I_C), a transient inward current (I_{Na}), and a delayed outward current (I_K). In Na-free external medium (containing an inert cation,

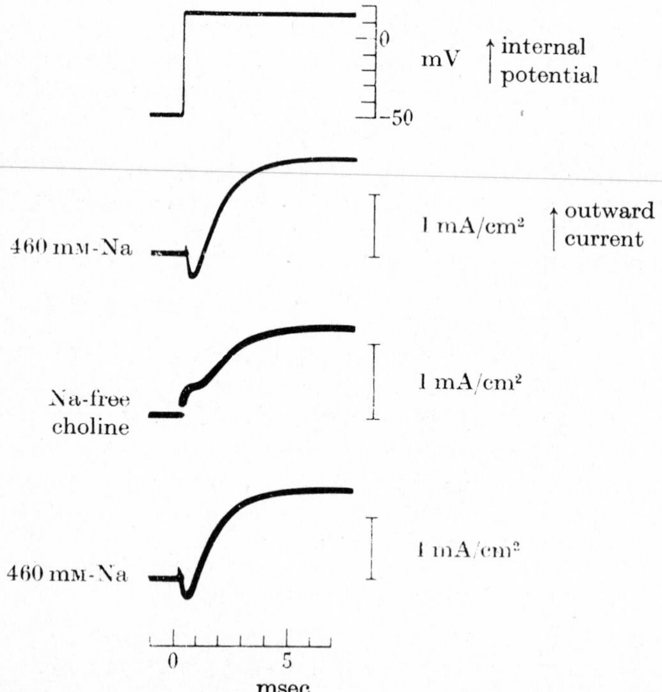

Fig. 7. Example of voltage clamp records in presence and absence of external Na. Top: step change of membrane potential from −50 mV (resting potential) to +15 mV. Lower three records: membrane current associated with the step change in membrane potential. In the presence of external Na the membrane current consists of a brief capacitative current (I_C), an early inward current (I_{Na}), and a delayed outward current (I_K). When NaCl is replaced by choline chloride, the early current is outward. [From Hodgkin (1958).]

choline, instead of Na) the transient inward current (I_{Na}) is replaced by a hump of outward current, carried by internal Na ions. The total current flowing through the membrane is given by the equation

$$I = I_C + I_{Na} + I_K + I_{leak}, \tag{9}$$

where

$$I_C = C\mathrm{d}E/\mathrm{d}t \qquad I_{Na} = g_{Na}(E - E_{Na})$$

$$I_K = g_K(E - E_K) \qquad I_{leak} = g_{leak}(E - E_{leak}).$$

In these equations, g_{Na}, g_K, g_{leak} represent conductances. The terms $(E - E_{Na})$, $(E - E_K)$, and $(E - E_{leak})$ are driving forces. The equilibrium potentials E_{Na}, E_K are defined by the Nernst equations:

$$E_{Na} = \frac{RT}{F}\ln\frac{[\mathrm{Na}]_0}{[\mathrm{Na}]_i} = +56\ \mathrm{mV}$$

$$E_K = \frac{RT}{F}\ln\frac{[\mathrm{K}]_0}{[\mathrm{K}]_i} = -93\ \mathrm{mV},$$

and E_{leak} is equal to the resting potential.

Voltage clamp currents associated with voltage pulses to different internal potentials are reproduced in fig. 8 and the current voltage relations for the early current (I_{Na}) and the delayed outward current (I_K) are given in the same figure. The early current (I_{Na}) is inward for small depolarizations; it increases with increasing pulse height to a maximum, then decreases again, reverses sign at a potential of +40 mV, and becomes outward for larger depolarizations. The delayed outward current (I_K) simply grows with increasing pulse height.

Hodgkin and Huxley (1952b) have described the voltage clamp currents by assuming that the Na conductance g_{Na} is determined by the cube of an activation variable m and by the first power of an inactivation variable h whereas the K conductance g_K is proportional to the fourth power of an activation variable n:

$$g_{Na} = \bar{g}_{Na}m^3h \qquad g_K = \bar{g}_K n^4$$

where $\bar{g}_{Na}$ and $\bar{g}_K$ are proportionality factors. The variables m, h, and n are functions of potential and time. The voltage dependence of the three variables and of their time constants.

$$\tau_m = (\alpha_m + \beta_m)^{-1} = m_\infty/\alpha_m,$$

$$\tau_h = (\alpha_h + \beta_h)^{-1} = h_\infty/\alpha_h,$$

$$\tau_n = (\alpha_n + \beta_n)^{-1} = n_\infty/\alpha_n,$$

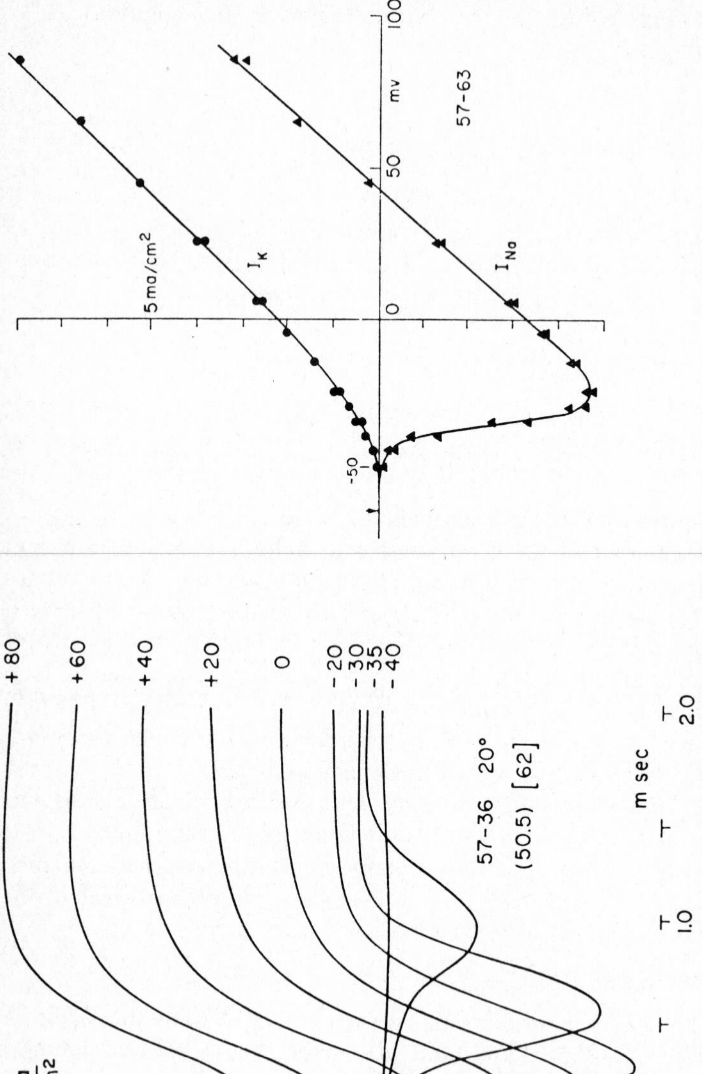

Fig. 8. Left: voltage clamp currents associated with pulses from −62 mV (resting potential) to different potentials; pulse potentials indicated at right end of traces. Right: peak of early current (I_{Na}) and steady-state current (I_K) plotted against pulse potential; resting potential indicated by arrow. [From Cole (1962).]

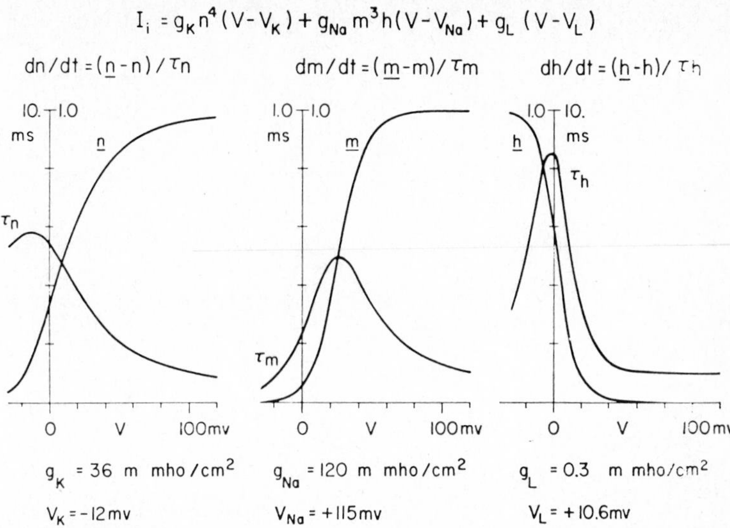

Fig. 9. Voltage dependence of potassium activation variable *n*, sodium activation variable *m*, sodium inactivation variable *h*, and of their time constants. Abscissa: V = change of membrane potential; $V=0$ represents resting potential. [From Cole (1962).]

is shown in fig. 9 where $V=0$ represents the normal resting potential of -62 mV. Note different scales for τ_m and τ_h, τ_n, respectively.

The changes in g_{Na} and g_K at various depolarizations from the resting potential are illustrated in fig. 10. The Na conductance rises rapidly to a peak (increase of *m*) and then declines (decrease of *h*). The K conductance rises slowly along an S-shaped curve to a maintained level (increase of *n*). With increasing depolarization the conductance changes become larger and faster.

The basic ideas underlying the Hodgkin and Huxley analysis were: (a) that the membrane currents are due to ions moving down their electrochemical gradients given by the driving forces $(E - E_{Na})$, $(E - E_K)$, $(E - E_{leak})$; (b) that I_{Na} and I_K are independent from each other and have a different voltage and time dependence, suggesting that Na and K ions move through different channels (dual channel hypothesis); (c) that activation (*m*) and inactivation (*h*) of the sodium conductance are parallel processes which start at the beginning of a depolarizing pulse and follow exponential time courses; and (d) that the voltage dependence of g_{Na} and g_K may be due to electrically charged molecules inside the membrane which alter their position according to the electric field, thereby opening or closing a pathway for the ions.

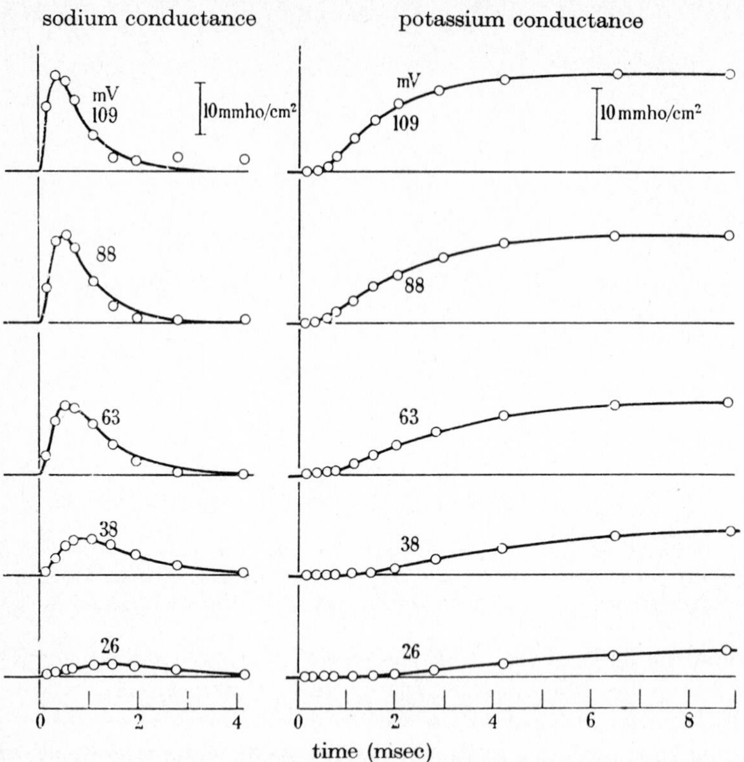

Fig. 10 Change of sodium conductance g_{Na} and potassium conductance g_K during different depolarizations. The numbers give the depolarizations from resting potential in mV. Circles are experimental values, smooth curves are solutions of the Hodgkin and Huxley equations. [From Hodgkin (1958).]

In 1961, techniques for the intracellular perfusion of squid giant axons were invented (Baker et al. 1961, Oikawa et al. 1961) The axoplasm is removed by squeezing it out of the cut end of the axon or by inserting a glass pipette longitudinally into the axon and forcing perfusion fluid through the pipette. As shown in fig. 11, the resting and action potential of a perfused axon are the same as those of an intact axon, indicating that the bulk of the axoplasm is not essential for the conduction of impulses. The perfused axon technique makes it possible to change the intracellular fluid and to apply chemical substances to the inner side of the membrane. Most of the recent results on squid giant axons have been obtained with this technique.

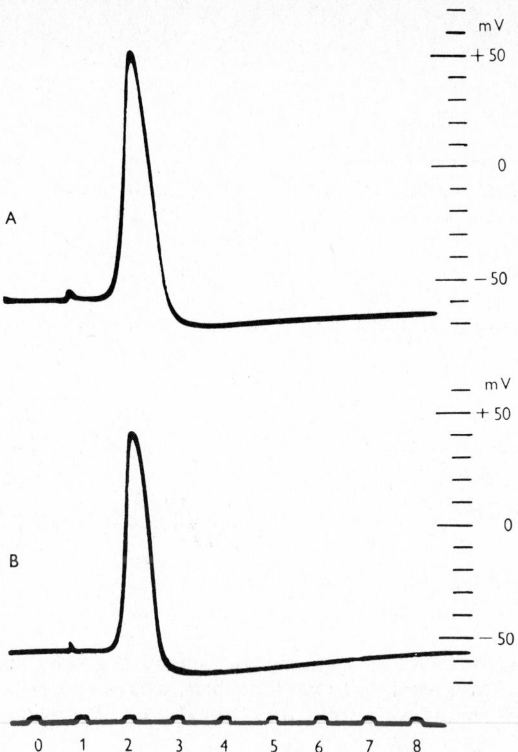

Fig. 11. Action potential from an axon perfused with K_2SO_4 solution (A) and from an intact axon (B). Temperature 16° C in A and 18° C in B. [From Hodgkin (1964).]

An important tool for electrophysiologists are drugs which selectively block either the Na or the K channels, thereby allowing one to study I_{Na} or I_K separately. The most important of these drugs are tetrodotoxin (TTX) which selectively blocks the Na channels (dissociation constant 1–10 nM) and tetraethylammonium chloride (TEA) or 4-aminopyridine (4-AP) which selectively inhibits the K currents. An example for the effect of TTX on an axon perfused with 300 mM KF + sucrose is shown in fig. 12. The drug completely inhibits the early inward current (carried by external Na ions) and the early outward current (carried by internal K ions through the Na channel, see traces labelled 97 and 130 mV in fast time base record) but does not affect the delayed outward current.

With the help of selective channel blockers and with the perfused axon technique it became possible to demonstrate that (contrary to the

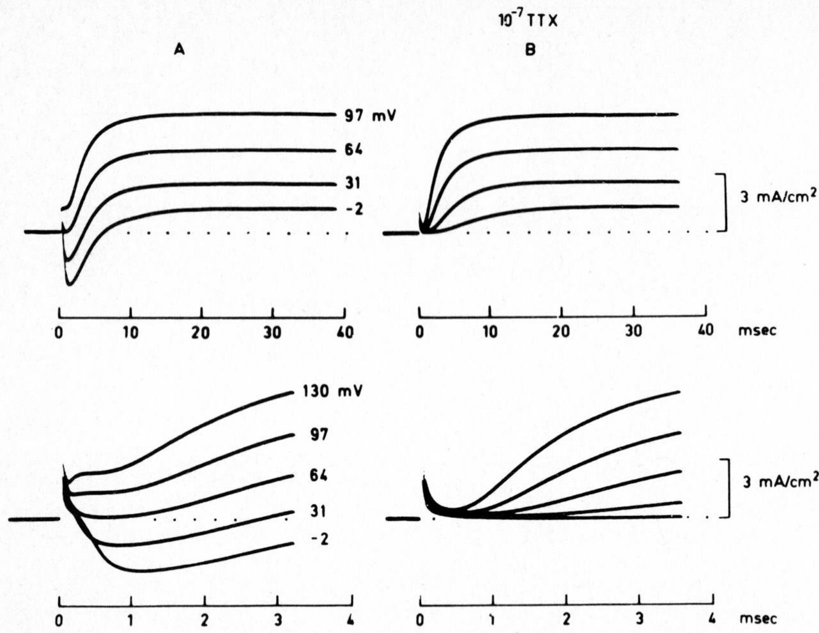

Fig. 12. Effect of tetrodotoxin on the membrane currents of an axon perfused with 300 mM KF + sucrose. Note ten times faster sweep speed in lower row. (A) Control records. (B) After external application of 10^{-7} g/ml tetrodotoxin. Temperature 2° C. [From Chandler and Meves, (1970a).]

inactivation curve shown in the right part of fig. 9) inactivation in squid giant axons is incomplete. Incomplete inactivation is most easily seen in axons perfused with NaF but is also present in intact axons. Voltage clamp currents from an axon perfused with NaF are presented in fig. 13. Small pulses produce inward currents while large pulses are associated with outward currents. Both inward and outward currents decay from a peak to a maintained level. Plotting peak current and maintained current vs voltage (right half of fig. 13) reveals that the maintained current is a small fraction of the peak current at small depolarizations but a large fraction at large depolarizations, i.e. inactivation becomes less complete for larger depolarizations. Chandler and Meves (1970b) explained this observation by assuming that the inactivation gate is closed by small depolarizations but forced open again by large depolarizations, according to the reaction scheme

$$\underset{(h_1)}{\text{open}} \rightleftharpoons \text{closed} \rightleftharpoons \underset{(h_2)}{\text{open}}\,.$$

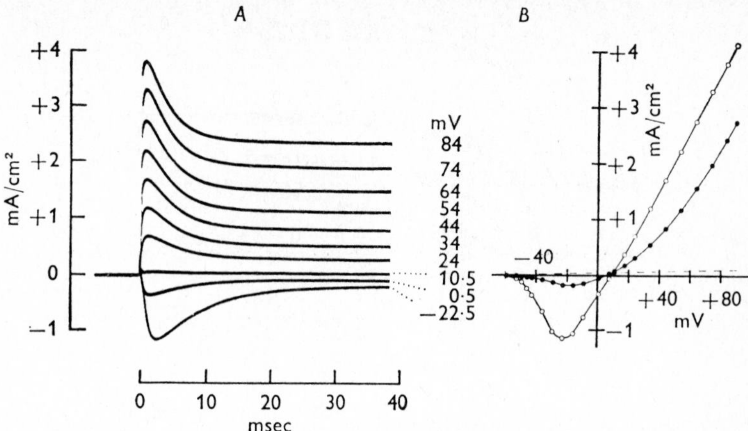

Fig. 13. Incomplete inactivation in an axon perfused with 300 mM NaF + sucrose. (A) currents associated with 39 msec pulses of different height; pulse potential indicated. (B) Peak current (○) and current at 39 ms (●) plotted against pulse potential; dashed line indicates leakage current. Holding potential −76 mV. Temperature 0° C. [From Chandler and Meves (1970a).]

3. Voltage clamp experiments on the node of Ranvier

In many respects, the ionic currents recorded from isolated myelinated axons under voltage clamp conditions resemble those obtained from squid giant axons (compare figs. 8 and 14A).

When the membrane potential of an isolated node of Ranvier is changed abruptly from its normal resting level (−70 mV) to $E=0$, a complex ionic current flows through the membrane. An early transient inward current is followed by a delayed outward current. The early current is abolished by the paralytic poison TTX or by the complete removal of external sodium. It is therefore regarded as mainly carried by sodium, and thus termed I_{Na}. The delayed current disappears on external application of TEA (the specific inhibitor of the K conductance). It becomes inward at negative potentials when all the external sodium is replaced by an equimolar amount of potassium. Under this experimental condition, the delayed current reverses its direction near $E=0$. It is therefore considered as carried by K. A leakage current component can also be demonstrated when the voltage pulses are hyperpolarizing. To a first approximation, this latter current does not depend on time. Its intensity is proportional to the membrane potential change.

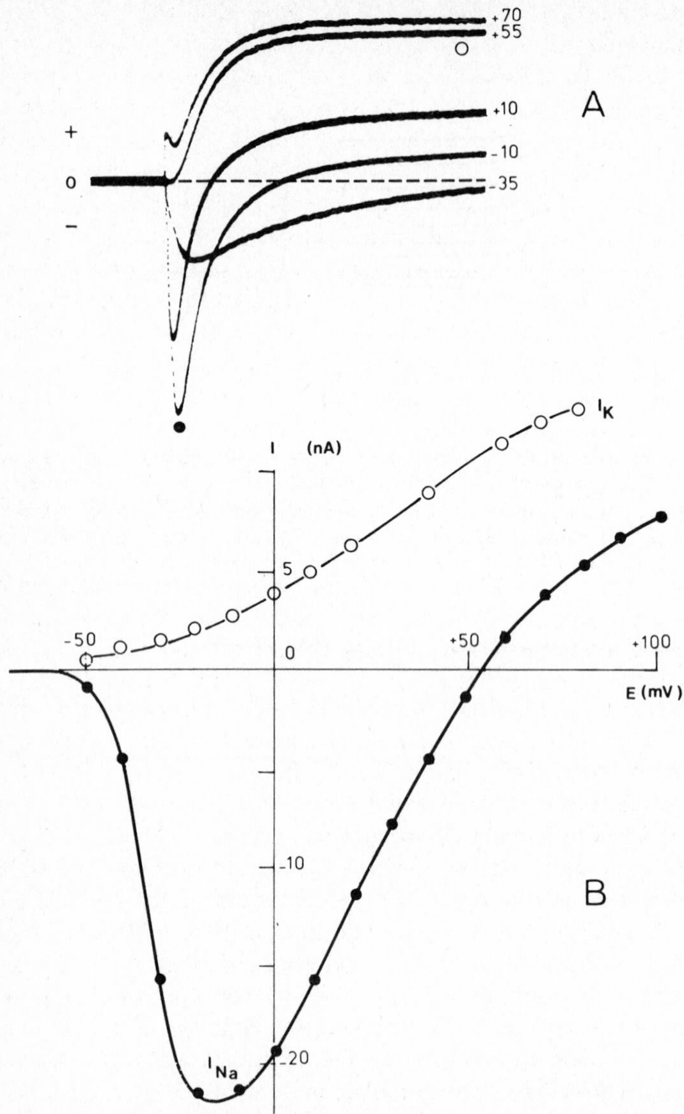

Fig. 14. (A) Membrane current recordings associated with 10 ms voltage pulses from −70 mV (resting level) to various potentials indicated at the right end of each trace. (B) Peak of the early current (I_{Na}, black points) and steady-state current (I_K, circles) plotted vs pulse potential (E). Inward current is negative (downward in the figure). Note that the early peak of current (mainly carried by sodium) reverses its direction at $E = +55$ mV. This value is therefore taken as the equilibrium potential (E_{Na}) for sodium. Sensory myelinated nerve fibre from the frog *R. esculenta*. Temperature: 15° C.

The I_{Na} and I_K voltage curves resemble those obtained from voltage clamp experiments in squid axons (fig. 14B). However, a closer inspection reveals that, at positive potentials, the Ranvier node current–voltage relationships are not linear like those of the squid axon. For instance, a curvature appears in the $I_{Na}(E)$ curve, especially at membrane potentials more positive than E_{Na}. In fact, the Na current increases less than expected from an ohmic conductor. It follows that a Ranvier node conductance curve calculated on the basis of the usual relation $g_{Na} = I_{Na}/(E - E_{Na})$ does not show a plateau but a maximum (fig. 15). The Na-conductance increases first with moderate depolarization, reaches a maximum near $E = 0$, then decreases. This particular behaviour is due to the instantaneous rectifying properties of the nodal membrane, which can be demonstrated by measuring the current responses to instantaneous variations of the driving force $E - E_{Na}$.

Two kinds of instantaneous current measurements can be performed (see fig. 16A and B):

(a) Starting from a negative holding potential, the membrane is depolarized to a given level by a voltage step of constant amplitude and duration. When the Na current elicited by this pulse reaches its peak value, the membrane is suddenly repolarized to various levels (fig. 16A), thereby inducing instantaneous changes in current. The purpose of the experiment is to activate the Na-permeability system to a certain level,

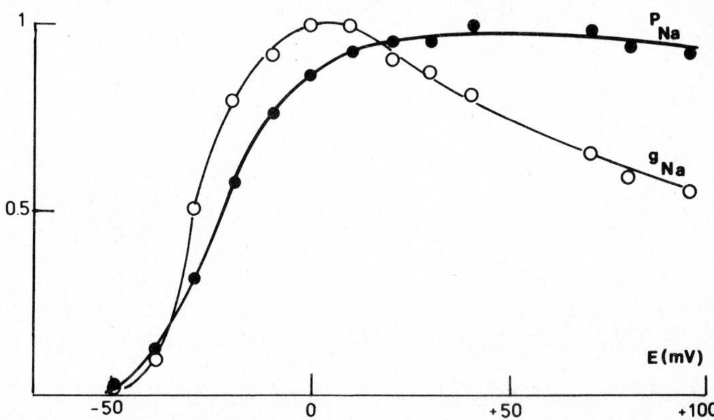

Fig. 15. Na conductance (circles) and Na permeability (black points) as a function of membrane potential (E) for the same nerve fibre. To facilitate comparison the maximum values of g_{Na} and P_{Na} have been normalized to 1. g_{Na} was calculated as $I_{Na}/(E - E_{Na})$. P_{Na} was obtained from the constant field equation (see text). In both cases, I_{Na} was the peak of early current measured at the various values of E. The reversal potential of the early current was taken as E_{Na} from which the internal Na concentration was calculated using the Nernst relation.

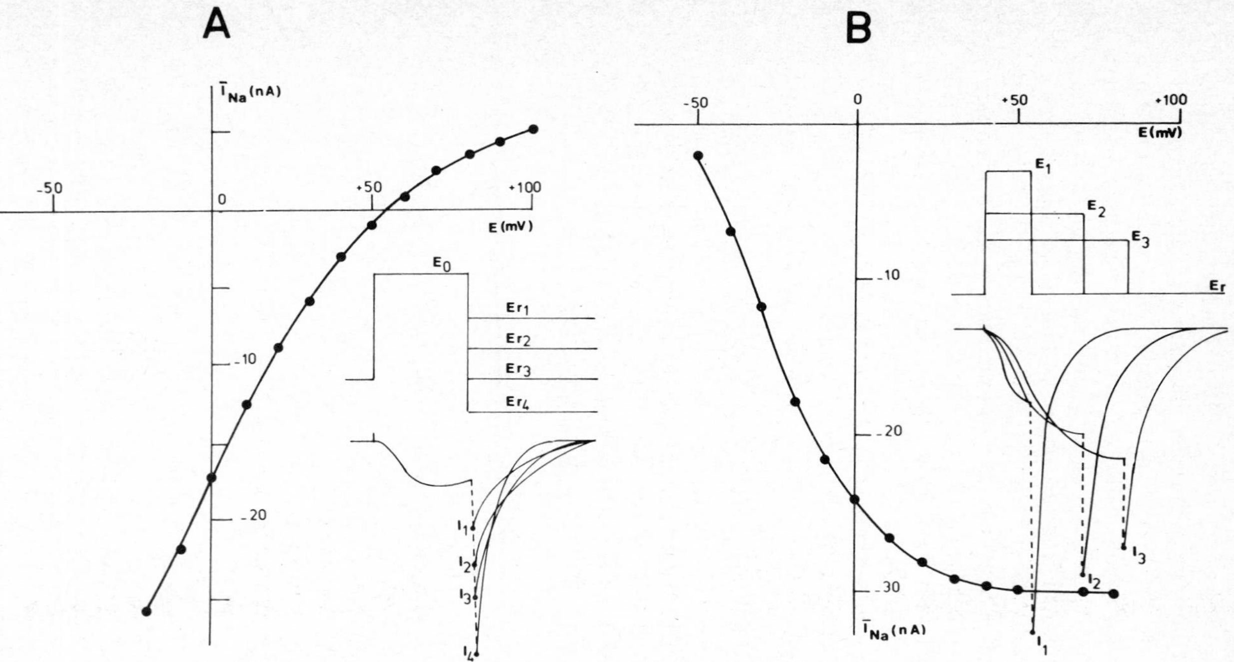

Fig. 16. Instantaneous sodium current (I_{Na}) as a function of membrane potential (E). (A) I_{Na} was measured at various repolarization levels (E) following a depolarizing pulse of constant amplitude (130 mV) and duration (500 μs) from a holding level of −90 mV. The experimental procedure described in the text has been schematically represented in the right part of the figure. (B) I_{Na} was measured at a constant repolarization level (E_r) of −70 mV and has been plotted as a function of the membrane potential (E) during voltage pulses of variable amplitude. These pulses were interrupted as soon as the peak of early current was reached. Note that this curve can be regarded as the mirror image of a P_{Na} voltage relationship (see fig. 15). The experimental procedure described in the text has been schematically represented in the right part of the figure.

then to suddenly alter the driving force. If the membrane would behave like an ohmic conductor, the current measured at the very time of repolarization ("instantaneous current") should vary linearly with $E - E_{Na}$, with a slope $I_{Na}/(E - E_{Na})$ equal to the conductance at the end of the depolarizing voltage pulse. In the node of Ranvier, the instantaneous current–voltage curve is not linear (fig. 16A), thus indicating that the membrane conductance varies instantaneously with the membrane potential independently of the permeability. As a result, the electrochemical expression of Ohm's law cannot be used to describe the variation of the membrane permeability with the potential unless another measurement procedure is developed (see below).

(b) This experiment differs from the preceding one in that the repolarization level remains constant (i.e. the driving force and the potential at which the instantaneous current is measured are kept constant) while the depolarizing voltage pulse is changed in amplitude and duration to bring the Na-permeability system to various degrees of activation. The instantaneous current measured at the very moment of repolarization under these new conditions has to be directly proportional to the sodium permeability at the end of each depolarizing pulse. If the various depolarizing pulses are interrupted when the current reaches its peak value (fig. 16B) the instantaneous Na current–voltage curve thus obtained has to reflect the sodium permeability change with potential (for comparison, see fig. 15).

The instantaneous rectification of the nodal membrane was first observed by Dodge and Frankenhaeuser (1958) and explained in terms of the constant field theory developed by Goldman (1943).

The constant field theory applies to thin homogeneous membranes in which the ions are assumed to move with a constant mobility or diffusion coefficient while subjected to a constant electric field. The instantaneous conductance changes arise from variations in ion concentration within the membrane. Assuming a constant permeability coefficient to an ion species which is present in different concentrations on either side of the membrane, the instantaneous ion concentration in the membrane increases when the potential difference moves the ions down their concentration gradient, thus leading to a rise in conductance. Conversely, the conductance decreases when the potential difference moves the ions in the opposite direction, from the low to the high concentration. This instantaneous rectification, predicted by the Goldman theory, is superimposed on the voltage and time-dependent permeability changes arising from the opening of the channels. The absolute value of the permeability (P_I) for a given ion I can be calculated from the current (I_I) by the constant field equation:

$$I_I = P_I E \frac{zF^2}{RT} \frac{[I]_0 - [I]_i \exp(zFE/RT)}{1-\exp(zFE/RT)}, \tag{10}$$

where $[I]_0$ and $[I]_i$ are the external and internal concentrations, z is the valence of the ion I, E the membrane potential, and R, T, and F are the usual thermodynamic constants. The permeability coefficient is defined as

$$P_I = \mu_I \beta_I (RT/\varepsilon F)$$

where μ_I is the ion mobility within the membrane, β_I the partition coefficient between the aqueous solution and the membrane phase, and ε the membrane thickness. Note that relationship (10) becomes linear only when $[I]_0 = [I]_i$. In this case

$$I_I = P_I E(zF^2/RT)[I]_0.$$

The main assumptions made in the constant field theory seem now to be unrealistic, particularly in view of the fact that the ions most probably move through very asymmetrical narrow channels influenced by mobile dipolar structures or charges which certainly affect the local electric field in the membrane. Not withstanding this, the predictions of the constant field equation are generally in satisfactory agreement with the experimental observations.

The reason why the constant field equation seems to apply to the myelinated axon and not to the squid axon in artificial sea water is not clear. Frankenhaeuser (1960a) has proposed an explanation first suggested by Hodgkin. It is assumed that the electric field in the nerve membrane is modified by the presence of surface charges fixed on one side of the membrane. These charges introduce a potential step at the membrane boundary δE leading to a redistribution of ions in the immediate vicinity of the channels. For instance, the actual sodium concentration $[\mathrm{Na}]'_0$ at the outer boundary of the membrane would differ from the sodium concentration in the bulk solution ($[\mathrm{Na}]_0$) according to:

$$[\mathrm{Na}]'_0 = [\mathrm{Na}]_0 \exp(-\delta EF/RT).$$

The constant field theory predicts that the instantaneous rectification vanishes when the internal and the external concentrations are equal, i.e. $E_{\mathrm{Na}} = 0$. The same result can be obtained, in the case of an asymmetrical distribution of Na, if $E - E_{\mathrm{Na}} = 0$, in other words if the surface charge density is such that $[Na]'_0=[Na]_i$. Another possibility is that the fixed charge density on the inner side of the membrane is such that $[Na]_0=[Na]'_i$. Eventually, a third possibility is that the internal and external charges in the squid axon are just of the right density and of the right charge to abolish the concentration gradient within the membrane. This may sound like ad hoc hypotheses. However, the Frankenhaeuser–Hodgkin interpretation is well supported by the finding that the squid axon membrane shows instantaneous rectification when $[Na]_0$ is changed (Hodgkin and Huxley 1952a).

The validity of the constant field equation has been recently questioned by Hille (1975a), especially for the Na-permeability system of the node of Ranvier. The author shows that at various external Na concentrations deviations occur in the I_{Na} voltage curves between the measured currents and the predictions of the constant field theory (or the independence principle). Hille explains the deviations by assuming the presence of saturable binding sites and of four energy barriers within the sodium channel. His model, based upon the rate diffusion theory (Eyring and Eyring 1963), accounts for instantaneous rectification and fits the experimental measurements better than the free-diffusion model.

According to Frankenhaeuser (1962a), the potassium permeability system of the Ranvier node also shows instantaneous rectification (abolished in isotonic KCl solution) in the direction predicted by the constant field equation. However, Frankenhaeuser (1962b) pointed out that the potassium permeability, as calculated from the constant field equation, was different at low and high external K concentrations. This result is obviously inconsistent with the assumption made in Goldman's hypothesis (the permeability coefficient is independent of the concentration of permeant ion). More recent analyses (Dubois and Bergman 1975 and 1977b), performed in the presence of tetrodotoxin to suppress any possible Na-current contamination, have shown that in spite of marked asymmetry in the K concentration on both sides of the membrane no rectification can be demonstrated (fig. 17). It has also been shown that a marked change in the equilibrium potential for potassium (E_K) takes place at low $[K]_0$ (fig. 17) and arises from an accumulation of K ions in the perinodal space during large depolarizing voltage pulses. This introduces considerable errors in the calculation of both the absolute value and the time course of g_K. Dubois and Bergman (1977b) also found that the K conductance of the nodal membrane at constant voltage markedly depends on $[K]_0$. The conductance increases with

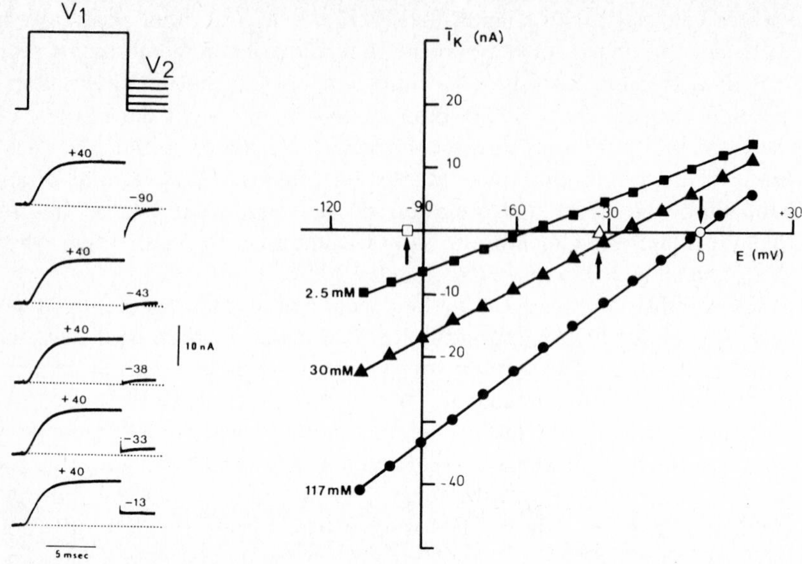

Fig. 17. Instantaneous potassium current (I_K) as a function of membrane potential (E) in the presence of three different K concentrations (2.5, 30, 117 mM) in the external Ringer solution. The left part of the figure shows the pulse program and a family of K-current recordings in the presence of 2.5 mM K + tetrodotoxin. I_K was measured at the instant of repolarization (beginning of pulse V_2 to potential E) following a conditioning pulse (V_1) of constant amplitude and duration. Note that the current–voltage relationships are linear and that the slope (i.e. the chord conductance) increases with the K concentration. The open symbols (arrows) on the voltage axis are the equilibrium potentials for K, calculated on the basis of the Nernst equation assuming $[K]_i = 117$ mM and $[K]_o = 2.5$ mM (square), 30 mM (triangle), and 117 mM (circle). The reversal potential for I_K clearly differs from the calculated values for E_K in 2.5 and 30 mM. This is due to the fact that during the conditioning pulse V_1, K ions accumulate in the perinodal space so that the actual K concentration in the vicinity of the membrane is higher than in the solution.

increasing external K concentration, then saturates, following a hyperbolic function (Michaëlis–Menten kinetics). This prompted the authors to assume that the K conductance of the nodal membrane was not only controlled by a voltage dependent gating mechanism but also by a saturable binding site for K. They have, therefore, proposed that the K flux is determined by a double transition in the K channel:

$$\underset{\text{(closed)}}{S_c} \overset{(a)}{\rightleftharpoons} \underset{\text{(activated)}}{S_a} + K \overset{(b)}{\rightleftharpoons} \underset{\text{(conducting)}}{S_aK}$$

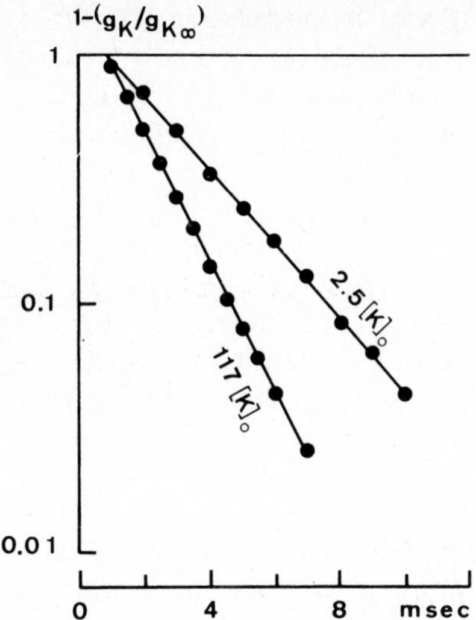

Fig. 18. Semilogarithmic plot of $1-(g_K/g_{K\infty})$ as a function of time in response to an abrupt voltage change from $E=-90$ mV to $E=-20$ mV, in the presence of two different external K concentrations. g_K was calculated taking into account the continuous change in E_K accompanying the outward current in low $[K]_0$. Note that the time-course of the conductance change can be described as a single exponential preceded by a short delay (see text). Note also that the K-conductance activation is faster in 117 mM than in 2.5 mM K solution. The delay, however, remains unaltered.

Transition (a) is purely voltage dependent and obeys a first order (H–H like) kinetics. It lowers a barrier which allows K to bind the site (S) in the activated (S_a) state. Transition (b) can be accounted for in terms of the rate diffusion theory. It is therefore voltage-dependent. The S_aK complex corresponds to the conducting state of the channel, whereas S_c represents the non-conducting (closed) state of the potassium channel. It is assumed that the binding reaction stabilizes the channel in the open configuration. It is clear that increasing $[K]_0$ displaces the equilibrium towards the right and therefore contributes to activate the potassium conductance. It also follows that the kinetics of the channel activation has to depend on $[K]_0$, a prediction which has been recently confirmed by Dubois (fig. 18).

4. Kinetics of the P_{Na} and P_K changes in the node of Ranvier

Frankenhaeuser (1959, 1960b, 1963) has extensively studied the sodium permeability of the node of Ranvier in terms of the Hodgkin–Huxley model. He found that Na inactivation follows a single-exponential function of time while the activation time course can be accounted for by an exponential function raised to the second power. The author, therefore, proposed the following basic equation to describe the Na-permeability change:

$$P_{Na} = \bar{P}_{Na} m^2 h$$

where m and h are dimensionless parameters varying between 0 and 1 with potential and time, as for the squid axon. Frankenhaeuser also observed that the potassium permeability decreases when the membrane is maintained depolarized for a long time. He proposed the following equation for the K system:

$$P_K = \bar{P}_K n^2 k$$

where n is the activation variable (as in squid axon) and k the inactivation variable making P_K decline exponentially with time. The voltage and time dependence of variable k has been studied by Schwarz and Vogel (1971). They found time constants of the order of 2–3 s, thus making unlikely the contribution of K inactivation to the normal excitation process. $\bar{P}_K$ and $\bar{P}_{Na}$ are the maximum permeability constants calculated on the basis of the constant field equation from currents I_K and I_{Na} recorded at large positive potentials when all the channels are assumed to be activated (m, n, h, and k being assumed to be at their maximum 1).

Indisputably, the m^2 and n^2 H–H kinetics (note the difference from m^3 and n^4 in squid axon) account, to a first approximation, for the permeability changes in the nodal membrane. It is worth noting, however, that recent analyses making use of improved voltage clamp techniques, together with selective pharmacological inhibitors like TTX, reveal deviations of the current kinetics from the H–H model predictions. Chiu (1977) has found that the Na-inactivation process is better described in terms of second order kinetics. Neumcke et al. (1976) found that m^2 kinetics represent only an approximation and do not account for the time course of I_{Na} at all membrane potentials. Using m^3 instead of m^2 does not improve the fitting of the experimental measurements to the H–H model predictions. In the case of the K-permeability system, similar deviations are observed when corrections are introduced for the progressive change in E_K during a depolarizing pulse. In this latter case, the best description for the K-conductance activation (fig. 18) is an exponential rise, preceded by a short delay between the onset of the depolarization and that of the conductance change:

$$g_K = g_{K\infty}\left[1 - \exp\frac{-(t-\Delta t)}{\tau}\right],$$

where $g_{K\infty}$ is the steady-state conductance reached at the end of a voltage step, Δt is the time lag and τ the time constant. The experiment shows that τ depends on E and $[K]_0$ whereas Δt depends on the membrane potential just before the abrupt depolarization inducing the conductance change (i.e. Δt depends on the holding potential). The meaning of this delay is unclear at the moment.

5. Ionic selectivity of excitable membranes

Assuming that the Hodgkin–Huxley model is adequate for describing the voltage- and time-dependent events underlying excitation, the question arises what are the molecular mechanisms responsible for the membrane selectivity? More precisely: what do the ionic pathways consist of? Are they pores or carriers? Are the ion pathways the same for all the accepted ion species or are there separate specific channels for Na and K ions?

5.1. Pore or carrier

In the absence of direct evidence, several kinetic arguments support the view that the ion pathways (the "ionic channels") are more likely pores than carrier molecules.

(a) When the Na or K conductances are fully activated by a depolarizing voltage pulse, a further abrupt change in driving force (a sudden repolarization for instance) can lead to an instantaneous change in current direction; this would not be expected if a carrier molecule first had to be displaced from one side of the membrane to the other.

(b) Recent estimates of the individual channel conductances based upon voltage and current fluctuation measurements (see Conti et al. 1975 and 1976, Begenisich and Stevens 1975) have led to figures of the order of 5 to 10×10^{-12} mho, thus allowing us to calculate that one discrete membrane pathway could transfer several millions of ions per second. On the basis of our knowledge at the moment, the turnover rate of identified carriers would be 10^2–10^6 times too slow to account for such enormous elementary conductances (see Stark et al. 1971, Ellory and Keynes 1969).

(c) In some instances, the K pathway can be asymmetrically blocked by foreign cations introduced in the intracellular medium (Bergman 1970, Bezanilla and Armstrong 1972). Under these conditions the membrane behaves like an instantaneous voltage-dependent rectifier (Bezanilla and Armstrong 1972, Dubois and Bergman 1977b) the properties of which are accounted for by the rate diffusion theory developed by Hille (1975). The fact that tetraethylammonium derivatives block the K conductance of the squid axon from inside only has been regarded (Armstrong 1971) as an argument against mobile carriers.

5.2. "Single channel" or "dual channel" hypothesis

Restricting the discussion to the sodium and the potassium pathways in axonal membranes, it is worth noting that, although the H–H model treats the Na- and K-conductance kinetics as separate entities, the same set of equations can be used for a single pore that would undergo transitions leading to a change in selectivity.

The "single channel" hypothesis was proposed by Mullins (1959). Although this hypothesis has not stood the test of time, it served to stimulate important experimental work. The idea of Mullins was based on the observation that the kinetics of Na inactivation are very similar to those of the K activation. Furthermore, the fact that the maximum Na and K conductances of the squid axon can reach similar magnitudes when fully activated by large depolarizing pulses suggested that K and Na could utilize the same channels. The latter idea was reinforced by the fact that, in any case, the total membrane conductance ($g_K + g_{Na}$) could be found higher than either $\bar{g}_K$ or $\bar{g}_{Na}$, the maximum conductances for a single (Na or K) ion species (Mullins 1968).

In substance, Mullins proposed that during a depolarization the individual pore behaves like the whole membrane. At the beginning of the depolarization, the pore first favours Na by exactly matching the ion diameter in a partially dehydrated form. As a consequence of its progressive increase in diameter, the pore then ceases to accept Na and becomes more permeable to K. A very important idea was introduced in the model: while entering the channel, the ion sheds part of its water shell and replaces it by some polar groups of the pore wall. It was assumed that during the transition the pore radius varies from 3.65 to 4.05 Å and that the ions are accepted with only one layer of water molecules. The variation of the energy barriers encountered by the ions at the level of flexible filtering structures could serve as voltage and time dependent gates obeying the Hodgkin–Huxley kinetics.

The model of Mullins has been regarded as plausible until it was shown that two very different molecules like tetrodotoxin (TTX) and tetraethylammonium (TEA) could abolish the Na conductance (fig. 19) and the K conductance, respectively, with a very high specificity. Mullins argued that a TTX molecule, either bound to the channel or to a distant site, could affect the affinity of the flexible "single channel" for Na ions, whereas TEA could block this channel in the K-permeable state. The argument was of interest because it prompted the supporters of the dual-channel hypothesis to search for more convincing evidence than pharmacologically-induced conductance blocks. On the other hand, it explicitly suggested that the TEA binding site could constitute a strategic part of the potassium-permeable pathway.

The decisive proof that Na and K ions utilize separate channels was suggested first by Mullins (1968) and produced five years later by Armstrong et al. (1973). These authors succeeded in almost selectively destroying the mechanism underlying Na inactivation by perfusing squid axons with pronase (a proteolytic enzyme mixture). Under this new condition, the Na conductance can be maintained as long as the membrane is depolarized (see fig. 33, section 7). Despite the complete destruction of Na inactivation (without significant alteration of the Na-activation kinetics) the K conductance increases in a normal fashion. Hence, it was demonstrated that the membrane can conduct Na while g_K is fully activated, thereby making the single channel hypothesis no longer tenable.

Several other arguments strongly support the dual channel hypothesis. They are essentially based upon the differential influence of physical or pharmacological agents on the Na and K conductances. Most of the

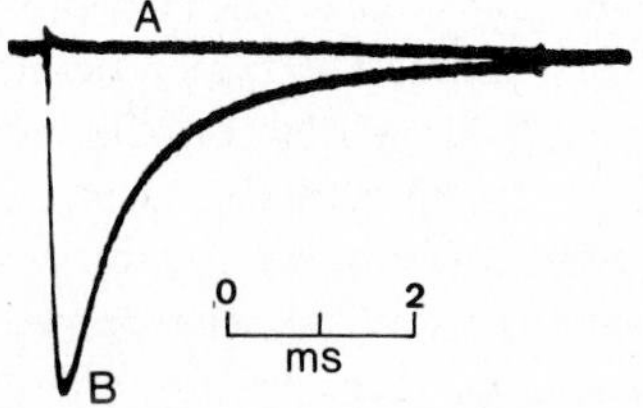

Fig. 19. The effect of tetrodotoxin (TTX) on the sodium current of a myelinated axon from the frog. Trace A represents the Na current recorded in a Ringer solution containing 5 mM of tetraethylammonium (TEA) and associated with a voltage pulse from −90 mV to +10 mV. The outward potassium current is abolished by TEA (compare with fig. 14A). Trace B was obtained a few seconds after TTX was added to the external solution. The Na current is fully abolished; only a very small leakage current can be detected in response to the same voltage pulse.

so-called "local anaesthetics" (see Narahashi 1974) belong to this class of chemical agents. Ultraviolet light irradiation of the nodal membrane of myelinated nerve fibres destroys the Na system while leaving the K system almost unaffected (Fox 1974). Changes of pH and Ca concentration in the external medium produce different shifts of the voltage-dependent conductance curves for Na and K, thus suggesting that the negative charge density at the external mouth of Na and K channels is different (Hille 1968a).

There seems to be no doubt that axonal membranes contain separate and independent channels for K and Na. This notion has been extended to calcium and leakage channels, not only for axons but for many other excitable structures. It is worth noting that the concept of Na or K specific channels does not imply that all the Na or K channels are the same in the various natural membranes. This notion can be illustrated by the finding that in molluscan neurones three classes of K channels can be found in the same membrane, differing by their voltage sensitivity, their inactivation mechanism and the fact that one class of K channels exhibits a Ca-mediated activation.

5.3. *The movement of ions through the selective channel*

Although a great deal of progress has been made concerning the selectivity and the gating mechanism of the ionic channels, little is known how the ions once accepted in an open channel move through the channel. Advances in this particular field are mainly due to extensive investigations in artificial membranes (see Läuger 1973 and 1979, Eisenman et al. 1978). In natural membranes, there is now good evidence that the ions move through long and narrow pores in files or packets of more than two ions. This was first proposed by Hodgkin and Keynes (1955) in a very important paper dealing with unidirectional K-flux measurements in giant axons. Similar pieces of evidence have been recently obtained from current measurements in voltage-clamped, myelinated axons (see Hille 1975a, b). It emerges from these investigations that the ionic channels can be regarded as narrow tunnels lined with successive binding sites separated by energy barriers over which the ions jump. This discontinuous diffusion can be accounted for by the rate–diffusion theory (Eyring and Eyring 1963) in which the electrostatic potential of the ion within the membrane electric field is added to the field-independent energy barriers of the pore (Hille 1979). It results that the rate constants of the binding reactions between the ion and the considered site in the channel depend on the fraction of voltage felt by the ion while reaching the transition state. Based on this theory, Hille (1975b) has recently proposed a model with four successive barriers and three internal sites for the Na channel of myelinated axons. A recent experimental analysis provides some qualitative support for the idea that the channel is a charged pore. Flux measurements of positively charged and neutral molecules (of the same size and shape) through Na channels from neuroblastoma cells (Huang et al. 1979) show that: (a) non-charged molecules can enter the channel and diffuse through it and (b) a positively charged molecule (guanidinium) is far more permeant than neutral ones (urea and formamide).

5.4. *The usefulness of selective channel blockers*

Many investigators have sought to understand the mechanisms by which the channels discriminate between similar alkaline cations like K and Na. Progress in this field had to wait upon the introduction of specific blocking agents for each type of ion channel (figs. 12 and 19).

5.4.1. *Sodium channel*

Two highly selective and reversible blockers are available for the Na channel: tetrodotoxin (TTX) and saxitoxin (STX). The properties of these paralytic natural poisons have been extensively studied (for review, see Evans 1972). As pharmacological tools, their properties can be summarized as follows. The two toxins have a very high affinity for the voltage sensitive Na channels in axonal membranes (but not necessarily for all kinds of Na channels). The equilibrium dissociation constant at normal pH is near 3×10^{-9} M. At this concentration, TTX (or STX) does not influence the K channels. Both toxins are strictly ineffective on either K or Na channels when applied internally. This reveals the asymmetrical structure of Na channels. When applied externally, the dose-reponse curves at equilibrium show that one toxin molecule blocks one channel (Hille 1968b). This property, together with the high affinity of the molecule, has been employed for estimating the Na-channel density (Moore et al. 1967, Keynes et al. 1971, Colquhoun et al. 1972) and isolating solubilized membrane components assumed to represent at least part of the Na channels (Henderson and Wang 1972). Figures of the order of 100 channels per μm^2 have thus been obtained (for details, see Ulbricht 1974).

Both the TTX and the STX molecule have a guanidinium (one group for TTX, two group for STX). It is assumed that the positively charged (at physiological pH) guanidinium enters the external mouth of the channel where the bulky part of the molecule sticks, thereby plugging the channel. However, the guanidinium group which is known to enter the Na channels (Hille 1971) cannot be regarded as the functional binding site of the molecule. If this were the case, other molecules bearing one guanidinium (like amiloride) would act like TTX or STX. Therefore, it is assumed that the high affinity arises from some stereo-specificity of the channel mouth for the rest of the molecule (Hille 1975c). As far as the TTX receptor represents an important part of the channel, indirect information on the channel itself can be obtained from careful analysis of the toxin–receptor binding and unbinding kinetics (Schwarz et al. 1973), as well as from possible competition with other cations (Wagner and Ulbricht 1974). It emerges from recent investigations that TTX (or STX) binding is opposed by protons as well as by a variety of cations such as Na, Li, or choline. It is thus tempting to deduce that the toxin binding site and the selectivity filter are part of the same structure (Hille 1975c). It should not be concluded, however, that the presence of a TTX–STX membrane receptor is a necessary condition for a highly selective sodium filter. As an illustration, let us recall that some of the Na channels are TTX-insensitive. Moreover, a recent investigation (Huang et al. 1979) has shown that two kinds of voltage-sensitive Na channels, exhibiting very different TTX sensitivity, show exactly the same cation selectivity.

5.4.2. Potassium channel

The two major blockers for the potassium channel are TEA (see fig. 19) and 4-amino-pyridine (4-AP). Unfortunately, their efficiency is not as high as that of TTX or STX for the Na channel. Here again not all K channels are blocked by the two inhibitors. Apparently the Ca-activated class of K channels is not blocked by TEA. In the squid axon, TEA blocks the channel from inside only whereas it inhibits the K conductance of the myelinated axon when applied either internally or externally. Moreover, in squid axon, internal TEA blocks the outward K current but not the inward current. In both preparations, the TEA blocking is fully reversible. The equilibrium dissociation constant for the external TEA receptor of the myelinated fibre has been estimated to be 0.4 mM, one TEA ion blocking one K channel (Hille, 1967). When applied externally at moderate concentrations, the activation kinetics of the remaining conductance are unaffected in the node of Ranvier (Koppenhöfer 1967, Hille 1967). It has been proposed that TEA plugs the external mouth of the channel without interfering with the K-gating mechanism. However, when applied internally, either in squid axon or in myelinated axons, the blocking of the outward current is time-dependent and resembles inactivation (see Armstrong and Binstock 1965, Armstrong and Hille 1972). It is therefore assumed that external and internal TEA receptors are different. The external receptor does not exist in the squid axon membrane. In both the squid axon and the myelinated fibre, the inner mouth of the K channel is supposed to resemble a funnel. When the channel gates open, outward moving K ions as well as TEA rush into the funnel. As soon as TEA reaches the channel restriction where it sticks, the outward moving file of K ions is blocked (this accounts for the inactivation-like time course of the internal TEA blocking). Accordingly, inward moving K ions knock TEA from its internal receptor, thereby accounting for the unblocking of the inward going flux of K (Armstrong 1971).

4-AP has been more recently discovered as a K-conductance inhibitor. It selectively blocks the K channel of the squid axon from the inside and outside (Meves and Pichon 1977) and probably from inside when externally applied to the myelinated axon (Ulbricht and Wagner 1976). It seems, therefore, that 4-AP diffuses through the membrane before blocking the channels, thus making its action almost irreversible. Another interesting peculiarity is that the 4-AP induced blocking is voltage- and time-dependent and can be removed by repetitive or long-lasting depolarizations. It has been suggested that the 4-AP binding site cannot be reached when the K-channel gates are closed at rest. It is interesting to mention that in the node of Ranvier there is a class of slow K channels (Dubois unpublished results) which are activated only by long lasting depolarizing pulses or a repetition of short pulses. These channels, at variance with the "classical" ones, are insensitive to 4-AP (fig. 20).

5.5. The selectivity filter of the Na and K channels

Several hypotheses have been advanced to account for the ionic selectivity of excitable membranes (for review see Hille 1975a). The most elaborated and satisfactory model is that of Hille. His hypothesis is based on the work of Conway, Mullins and Eisenman and on his own

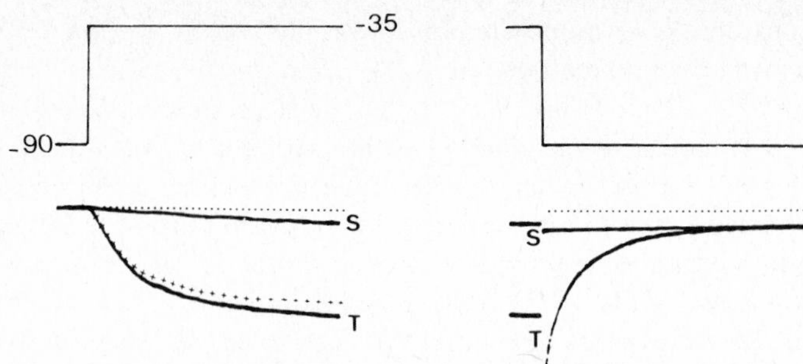

Fig. 20. The effect of 4-aminopyridine (4-AP) on the K current. Inward potassium currents recorded from a node of Ranvier in isotonic KCl solution. The recordings on the left represent the currents produced by responses to a potential change from −90 to −35 mV. The recordings in the right part of the figure are the ("tail currents" associated with repolarization to the initial (−90 mV) level. *T* is the total current under "normal" conditions, *S* is the slow current component (corresponding to a second class of K channels) remaining after exposure to 4-AP (1 mM). The dotted line represents the zero current level while crosses represent the difference between *T* and the 4-AP insensitive (*S*) fraction of K current.

experimental measurements of the relative permeability of a single class of channels to a large variety of cations.

Chandler and Meves (1965) succeeded in measuring ionic currents carried by cations other than sodium through the Na channels, thus proving that the Na channel is not exclusively permeable to Na. A very important finding was that K ions could generate a current activating and inactivating with exactly the same kinetics as the Na current, thus suggesting that the selectivity filter and the channel gating mechanism are separate entities, contrary to what was implicitly assumed in the Mullins model (1959).

Chandler and Meves estimated the relative permeability of the Na channel to the five alkali–metal cations (in fact, the permeability of K, Li, Rb, and Cs relative to that of Na). Based upon the Goldman–Hodgkin–Katz zero-current equation (see subsection 1.5), the relative permeabilities were determined from experimental measurements of the reversal potential for the current passing through the Na channel only. This particular zero-current potential (E_e) is defined as (for instance):

$$E_e = \frac{RT}{F}\ln\frac{P_{Na}[\mathrm{Na}]_0}{P_K[\mathrm{K}]_i}, \tag{11}$$

Table 1
Ionic channels in nerve membranes

Property	Alkaline cations (I)				
	Li	Na	K	Rb	Cs
Hydration energies (Kcal × mole $^{-1}$)	–	−98	−81	–	−67
Dehydrated diameter = cristal radius ×2(Å)	1.20	1.90	2.66	2.98	3.34
Relative permeability in sodium channel: P_I/P_{Na}					
Squid axon[a)]	1.1	1	0.083	0.025	0.016
Ranvier node[b)]	0.93	1	0.086	0.012	0.013
BTX-treated R node[c)]	–	1	0.45	0.25	0.15
Relative permeability in potassium channel: (P_I/P_K)					
Ranvier node[b)]	0.018	0.010	1	0.91	0.07

Organic cations (I')[d)]	Van der Waals (size in Å)	Relative permeabilities Na channel $(P_{I'}/P_{Na})$	K channel $(P_{I'}/P_K)$
NH_4	3.5×3.9	0.16 0.27[e)]	0.13
$NH_3{-}OH$	4.2×2.2	0.94	<0.025
$NH_3{-}NH_2$	4.2×2.3	0.59	<0.029
$NH_3{-}CH_3$	4.2×2.3	0.00	<0.02
$NH_2{-}NH_2{=}NH_2$	5.9×3.7	0.13	<0.013
$NH_2{-}NH_2{=}NH_2$ in BTX-treated R node		0.40[c)]	

a) Chandler and Meves (1965).
b) Hille (1971, 1972, 1973).
c) Khodorov (1978).
d) Most of these data taken from Hille (1971, 1972, 1973).
e) Binstock and Lecar (1969).

where Na is the only cation outside and K the only cation inside the (perfused) axon. Knowing $[Na]_0$ and $[K]_i$, the ratio P_K/P_{Na} can be easily obtained. Note that, in this equation, (11), E_e is regarded as the Nernst equilibrium potential for a hypothetical ion, the activities of which would be modulated by two factors, different for inside and outside.

Among other results (see table 1) Chandler and Meves found that the Na channel was about 12 times less permeable to K than to Na. The complete perm-selectivity sequence determined experimentally was found to be Li > Na > K > Rb > Cs. The authors pointed out that this permeability sequence follows the progressive increase in crystal radius of the five alkali cations, but also the sequence predicted by Eisenman (1962) for selective glass electrodes, in which the strength of coulombic binding between negative sites in the glass wall and the cations in the solution is the predominant factor that governs selectivity. Very similar results (see table 1) were obtained by Hille (1972) from myelinated axons. These observations support the view that the ions enter the channel in a partially dehydrated state.

Considering that the hydration energy of sodium is near −100 kcal/mole, it is clear that a tremendous energy difference has to be supplied by the membrane if the ions have to cross the channel in a fully dehydrated state. Moreover, if dehydration was the sole necessary condition for an ion to enter the channel, Cs and even Rb or K ions should be more permeant than Na in the sodium channel since the hydration energy depends on the crystal radius (the larger the crystal radius of the ion, the lower the hydration energy).

It was, therefore, assumed by Hille that three main parameters govern the selectivity sequence determined experimentally in axonal membranes: (a) the respective diameters of the pore and the ion (i.e. an ion which is larger than the pore cannot cross it); (b) the ion hydration energy (which determines the ease with which an ion can be removed from the aqueous solution to enter the channel); and (c) the negative charge density at the level of the pore (which provides coulombic energy to dehydrate, at least partially, the cations).

Hille determined the permeability sequence for a large variety of organic cations differing in size and in ability to form hydrogen bonds. Of the permeant organic cations, the largest was amino guanidine (a planar molecule of 3.7 × 5.9 × 7.6 Å) which should a priori give an upper estimate of 3.7 × 5.9 Å for the channel opening if the van der Waals size only had to be considered. This, however, could not explain why the Na channel does not accept Cs (a spheric ion of 3.34 Å in crystal diameter with the lowest hydration energy among the alkali cations). Hille (1971) found the solution in the comparison of the permeability coefficients for three small cations of similar size and shape, namely hydrazine, hydroxylamine, and methylamine. The three cations are smaller than aminoguanidine; however, both hydroxylamine and hydrazine are permeant, whereas methylamine is not. Of these three cations, only the third is incapable of forming hydrogen bonds due to its methyl group. Observing that all methylated cations were impermeant, Hille proposed that the ability of large cations to form hydrogen to oxygen bonds determines their permeability. The main reason for this is that, while forming a hydrogen bond, the donor (–OH or –NH) and the acceptor (–O) may overlap by up to 0.9 Å. Therefore, the molecule appears smaller than its usual van der Waals size if it interacts with oxygen atoms. Accordingly, if the pore is lined with oxygen atoms amino and hydroxyl groups would be reduced to about 3.0 Å in diameter whereas

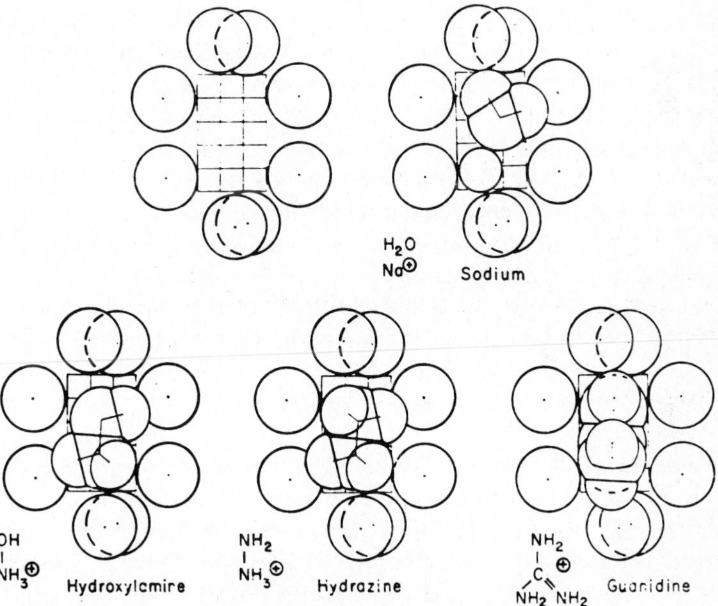

Fig. 21. Planar representation of the hypothetical model proposed by Hille (1971) for the selectivity filter of the Na channel. The left frame in the upper part of the figure represents the "mouth" of an empty pore lined with oxygen atoms. Each circle represents an oxygen atom. The grid inside is scaled to 3 Å by 5 Å. The upper right frame represents the same pore containing one Na ion (small circle) with one accompanying water molecule. The successive lower frames show the pore with three different permeating organic cations (hydroxylamine, hydrazine, and guanidine). Hydrogen bonds are formed wherever the hydrogens belonging either to the water or to the permeating molecules overlap with oxygen atoms forming the pore wall. [From Hille (1971).]

methyl groups would keep their van der Waals size of 3.8 Å. Under this condition, a pore accepting aminoguanidine (the largest permeant cation) would have an opening of only 3.1×5.1 Å. This led Hille to propose that the restricted part of the channel was formed by a ring of 6 oxygen atoms (fig. 21). In this pore, one Na ion would enter with 3 to 4 water molecules, the oxygen of the pore replacing the shedded water molecules normally surrounding the ion in an aqueous solution. Incorporating in his hypothesis the theory of Eisenman (1962) which invokes electrostatic forces between the cation and the negative sites in the pore, Hille was thus able to account for the permeability sequence of the alkali cations. It is worth noting that the guanidinium group of TTX exactly fits the mouth of Hille's selectivity filter.

Based on a similar series of experiments, Hille (1973) has postulated a selectivity filter for the K channel which would be lined by 5 oxygen atoms thereby forming a restricted opening of 3.0×3.5 Å. This pore accepts one K ion with only two water molecules and also Rb, but excludes Cs (which is too large) and cations smaller than K (like Na and Li). In this latter case, the discriminating ability does not arise from the geometry of the pore entry but rather from the fact that these ions have a much higher hydration energy. It is, therefore, necessary to postulate that the strong selectivity against small cations arises from a low surface charge density. In contrast to the selectivity filter of the Na channel, the K channel would be a "low field strength" pore.

5.6. *Selectivity filter and gating mechanism*

If the permeability changes observed in the whole membrane do not result from a selectivity change at the level of each individual channel, but from the voltage and time dependent opening of two distinct channel populations, it is necessary to postulate that each individual channel (either for K or Na) is equipped with a voltage dependent gating mechanism controlling the movement of ions accepted by a voltage insensitive filter. This is equivalent to saying that the gating mechanism and the selective filter are two separate structures in series within the pore.

Experimental evidence supporting this view should essentially show that: (a) the filter selectivity does not depend on the membrane voltage; (b) experimental alterations of the gating mechanism do not influence the channel selectivity; and (c) modifying the amount of energy exchanged at the level of the filter does not affect the channel gating (i.e.

the time course of the current is the same, whatever the nature of the permeant ion in the channel).

Convincing experimental proofs that the selectivity filter is voltage insensitive are very rare and difficult to obtain, simply because the ion selectivity is determined from zero-current measurements. Chandler and Meves (1965) were able to show, in perfused giant axons, that the P_{Na}/P_K ratio of the Na channel was not changed by voltage prepulses modifying the inactivation state of the Na channel. However, it must be pointed out that the inactivated channels are closed and thus escape investigation, while those which are still conducting are probably not yet influenced by the prepulse. Hille (1971, 1972) has studied the time-course of currents carried through the Na channel by different ions in the node of Ranvier. A change in the kinetics of these currents might arise from a variation of the relative permeability of the channel to the ion species carrying the current, since their respective driving forces are necessarily different. The author indeed observed slightly altered kinetics, especially when external Na was replaced by K. These variations are accounted for by a voltage shift of some 8–10 mV of the activation parameters (m), without significant changes in inactivation (h). This probably arises from a surface potential change and does not necessarily reveal interactions between the selectivity filter and the gating mechanism. Hence, here again, the experimental results are not conclusive. Another kind of argument has sometimes been advanced. Assuming the binding sites for specific blockers to be strategic parts of the selectivity filter, and observing that the binding of TTX (or that of TEA in the Ranvier node) is not voltage-dependent and does not affect the opening and the closing of the channels, it has been inferred that the selectivity filter is superficial and distinct from the gating mechanism. However, the information obtained under these conditions from the conductance kinetics may refer only to those channels which are not influenced by the drug at the time when they are conducting. The fact that the binding of cationic channel blockers is voltage-independent most likely reveals that the receptor is superficial.

Probably more convincing are experiments showing that agents altering the gating mechanism do not affect the channel selectivity. There is a large variety of such agents. Actually, all those which do not affect the apparent reversal potential for either the Na or K current should be considered as belonging to this class. Among these agents, the most spectacular is veratridine (Ulbricht 1969). This alkaloid considerably slows down the Na activation. Moreover, the treated channels fail to inactivate even after extremely long depolarizations. The relative permeability for Li and Na is, however, not altered and the channels remain extremely sensitive to TTX. It is, therefore, tempting to assume separate structures for filtering the ions and gating the channel. But both structures are necessarily located very close to each other in the pore wall. Therefore, it is hardly suprising that agents like batrachotoxin (see Khodorov 1978, Huang et al. 1979) alter both channel functions. In this case, the Na channel becomes measurably permeable to ions which are normally excluded (like Cs). The K permeability is enhanced by a factor of five and becomes nearly half that of Na. Interestingly, TTX remains a powerful inhibitor of the BTX treated channel. This important observation draws attention to the fact that the selectivity filter cannot be regarded as a single superficial structure, but rather represents a succession of energy barriers, not necessarily located at the same depth in the channel for all the ions competing for the transfer. As an example, it is well known that both Na and Cs do not permeate through the potassium channel of the myelinated nerve fibre. External sodium does not influence the inward K current whereas external caesium, at the same concentration, dramatically reduces the K influx. The block of K conductance arises from the fact that Cs enters a long way into the channel before reaching a receptor where it sticks (Dubois and Bergman 1977b). The Cs-induced blocking is instantaneous and markedly voltage dependent. Calculations based upon the rate diffusion theory lead to an estimate of the blocking site location at 60% of the membrane depth (external surface taken as reference). The sodium ions which neither cross the channel nor impede the K influx are readily excluded at the level of a very superficial structure (low field strength) representing an energy barrier over which Cs can easily jump.

Therefore, it seems justified to assume that the channel consists of a selectivity filter in series with the gating mechanism. This assumption, however, should not be taken too literally when thinking in terms of molecular structure.

6. Gating currents

The voltage-dependent permeability changes, i.e. the opening and closing of the gates in the ionic channels, are probably due to orientational changes of electrically charged molecules inside the membrane under the influence of the electric field (intramembrane-charge movement). This idea was expressed by Hodgkin and Huxley (1952), Johnson et al.

(1954), Goldman (1964) and others. Following the discovery of intramembrane charge movement in muscle fibres Schneider and Chandler (1973) and Armstrong and Bezanilla (1973) published the first records of "gating currents" from intracellularly perfused squid axons. Keynes and Rojas (1974) and Meves (1974) also studied gating currents in squid axons. Similar currents were found in myelinated nerve fibres (Nonner et al. 1975), *Myxicola* axons (Rudy 1976) and molluscan neurones (Adams and Gage 1976, Kostyuk et al. 1977). The literature about gating currents has been reviewed by Almers (1978), Armstrong and Bezanilla (1975), Keynes (1975), Meves (1978) and Neumcke et al. (1978).

The gating currents are much smaller than the ionic currents. To record gating currents the ionic currents I_{Na} and I_K must be blocked by tetrodotoxin, tetraethylammonium or Cs. Signal averaging is used to improve the signal to noise ratio. To remove the fast capacitative current and the symmetrical part of the leakage current equal numbers of positive and negative pulses of exactly the same amplitude are applied and the currents produced by the negative pulses are subtracted from the currents produced by the positive pulses.

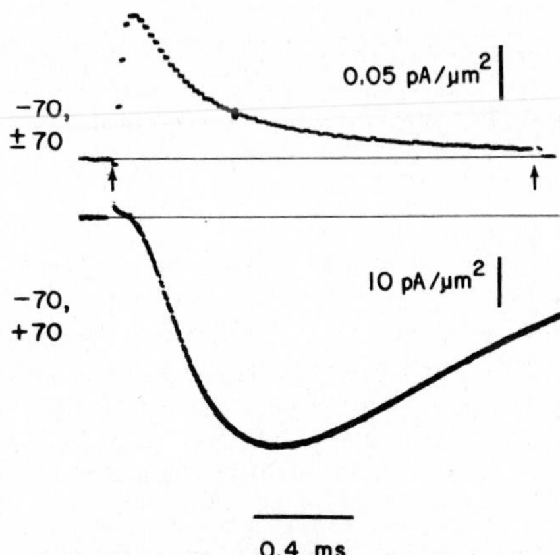

Fig. 22. Gating current (upper record) and Na current (lower record) of a squid giant axon. Upper record: axon in Na-free tris sea water, internally perfused with 550 mM CsF, averaged current from 2000 positive and 2000 negative pulses of 70 mV amplitude from a holding potential of −70 mV. Lower record: same axon in Na sea water, internally perfused with 275 mM KF + 400 mM sucrose, current associated with a depolarizing pulse of 70 mV from a holding potential of −70 mV. Calibration in pA/μm² = 0.1 mA/cm². Temperature 3.5° C. [From Armstrong and Bezanilla (1973).]

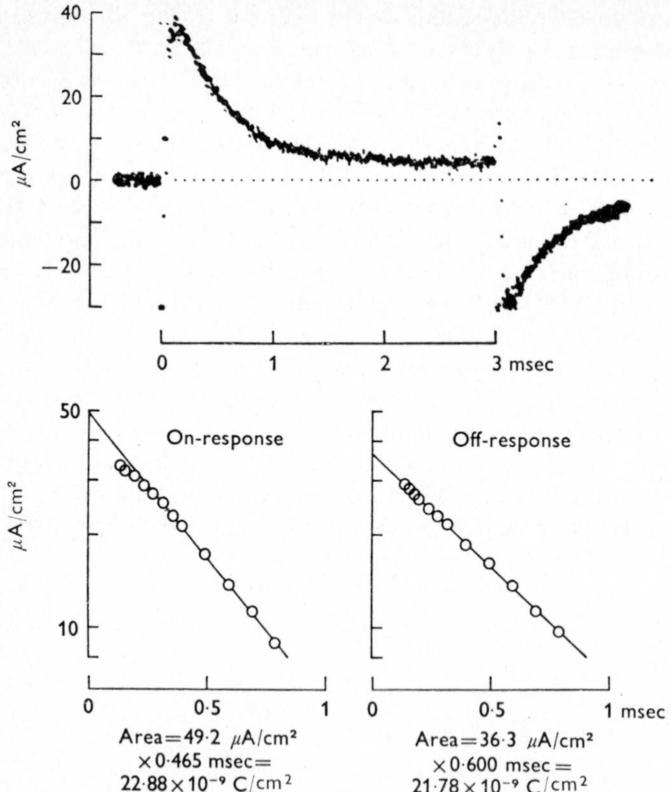

Fig. 23. Gating current of a squid giant axon. Upper half: current obtained by averaging the membrane currents associated with 32 positive and 32 negative pulses of 110 mV amplitude superimposed on a holding potential of −88 mV; axon in Na-free tris sea water, internally perfused with 275 mM RbF + 50 mM tetraethylammonium chloride + sucrose; temperature 1° C. Lower half: the transient outward current at the beginning of the pulses (on-response) and the inward current at the end of the pulses (off-response) are plotted on a logarithmic scale against time. The area under the on- and off-response is calculated from the current at zero time and the time constant. [From Meves (1974).]

Figure 22 shows the gating current (upper record) together with the Na current (lower record) of a squid axon (Armstrong and Bezanilla 1973). At the beginning of the pulse the gating current rises almost immediately to a peak and then decays exponentially as the intramembrane charges approach their new position. The peak of the gating current clearly precedes the peak of the Na inward current. At the end of the pulse a gating current of reversed polarity occurs (not shown), reflecting the return of the intramembrane charges into the resting position.

Two other examples of gating current are illustrated in figs. 23 and 24, one again from the squid axon and the other from a myelinated nerve fibre. In each case the signal consists of a transient outward current at the beginning of the pulse (on-response) and a transient inward current at the end of the pulses (off-response). The on-response decays to a small sustained current (outward in fig. 23 and inward in fig. 24) which represents the asymmetrical part of the leakage current (leakage rectification). In the lower part of each figure the on-response (after subtracting the sustained current) and the off-response are plotted on a logarithmic scale against time. Both responses follow an exponential time-course, apart from a deviation at the beginning of the on-response in fig. 23. (More recent experiments showed, however, that the responses can be more accurately described as the sum of two or more exponentials.) The areas under the on- and off-response were obtained from the extrapolated current at zero time and the time constant and

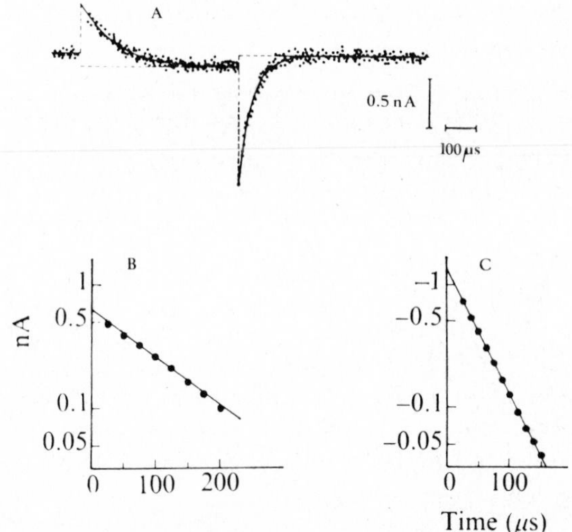

Fig. 24. Gating current of a myelinated nerve fibre. Record obtained by averaging the currents produced by 15 positive and 15 negative pulses of 100 mV amplitude superimposed on a holding potential of − 100 mV. Delayed K current blocked by external tetraethylammonium chloride and internal Cs. Temperature 12° C. The graphs show on-response and off-response plotted on a semi-logarithmic scale against time. Time constants $\tau_{on} = 113$ μs, $\tau_{off} = 42$ μs; charges $Q_{on} = 71$ fC, $Q_{off} = 55$ fC. [From Dubois and Bergman, (1977a).]

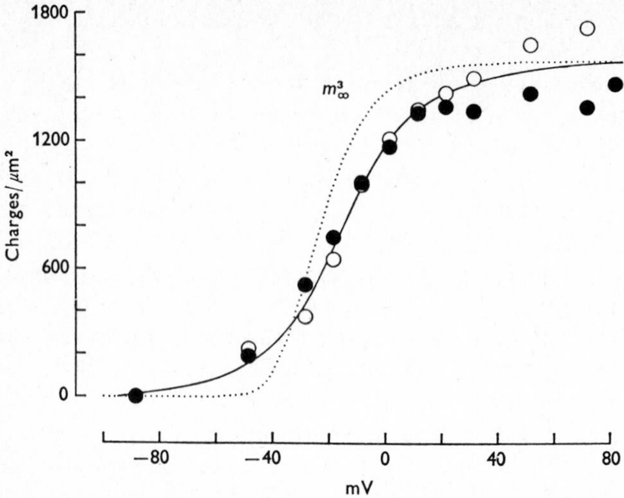

Fig. 25. $Q(E)$ curve of a squid giant axon. Q_{on} (open circles) and Q_{off} (solid circles) plotted against membrane potential during the positive pulses. Same experiment as in fig. 23. The continuous curve was obtained from eq. (12) with $\mu = 840$ debyes, $1 = 7$ nm, and $E' = -16$ mV. The dotted curve represents m^3_∞ calculated from Hodgkin and Huxley (1952b). [From Meves (1974).]

represent the amount of charge movement during the gating current. The figures given in fig. 23 and in the legend of fig. 24 show that the charge movement during the off-response (Q_{off}) is the same as the charge movement during the on-response (Q_{on}) or somewhat smaller. The approximate equality suggests that the charges are an integral part of the membrane.

The areas under the on- and off-response (Q_{on} and Q_{off}) depend on the height of the clamp pulses. With increasing pulse height the areas Q_{on} and Q_{off} increase until a maximum is reached at very large pulse heights. This is illustrated for the squid axon in fig. 25 and for the myelinated nerve fibre in fig. 26 (upper part). Mathematically, a sigmoid $Q(E)$ curve with a half potential E' can be described by the Langevin–Debye equation

$$Q = \coth - 1/x \tag{12}$$

(where $x = \mu\Delta E/kTL$, $\mu =$ dipole moment, $\Delta E/1 =$ electric field, and $\Delta E = E - E'$) or by the flip-flop equation

$$Q = \frac{Q_{max}}{1 + \exp\left(\frac{-z'e}{kT}\Delta E\right)}, \tag{13}$$

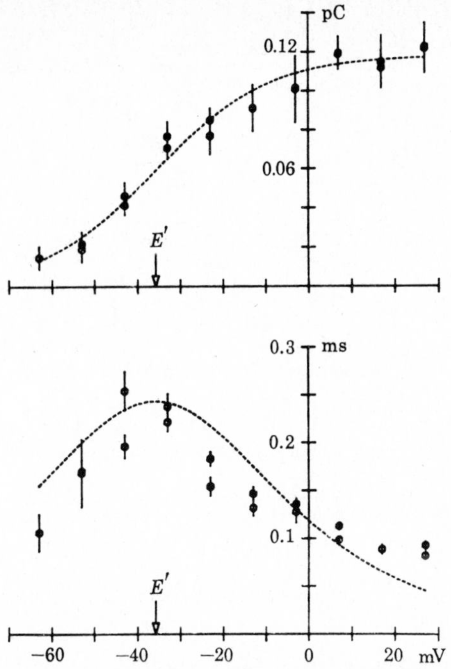

Fig. 26. Upper graph: $Q(E)$ curve of a myelinated nerve fibre; curve calculated from eq. (13) with $z'=1.85$, $E'=-35.8$ mV, $Q_{max}=118$ fC. Lower graph: time constant τ_{on}. Holding potential -113 mV, temperature 6° C. [From Nonner et al. (1975).]

where z' is the effective valency of the intramembrane charges. The continuous curves in figs. 25 and 26 (upper half) have been calculated from equations (12) and (13), respectively.

In fig. 25 the m_{∞}^3 curve (which is a measure for the Na conductance) is plotted as a dotted curve for comparison with the $Q(E)$ curve. The latter is clearly much less steep whereas E' is similar for both curves. The ratio slope of the m_{∞}^3 curve to slope of the $Q(E)$ curve is between 2 and 3, depending on the preparation.

Figure 26 (lower part) shows the time constant of the on-response of the gating current (τ_{on}) as a function of membrane potential. The points follow a bell-shaped curve, reminiscent of the bell-shaped voltage dependence of τ_m, the time constant of Na activation (fig. 9). Closer inspection (see fig. 27) shows, however, that the time course of Na activation (+) lags behind the time-course of charge movement (■) as if other processes (conformational changes?) are interposed between charge movement and opening of the Na channels. The unequality τ of

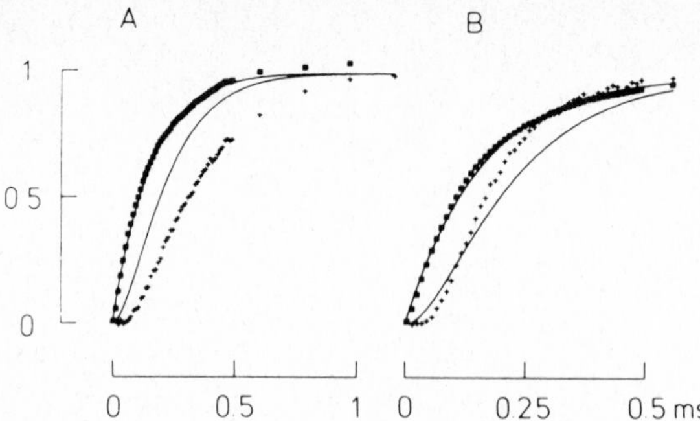

Fig. 27. Time course of charge movement (■) and sodium activation m^2 (+) in a myelinated nerve fibre. Holding potential −28 mV, potential during depolarizing pulses 40 mV in A, 64 mV in B; all potentials are referred to the resting potential. Temperature 10° C. In both graphs, the left curve was fitted to the charge points assuming an exponential time-course and the right curve gives the second power of the left curve. [From Neumcke et al. (1978).]

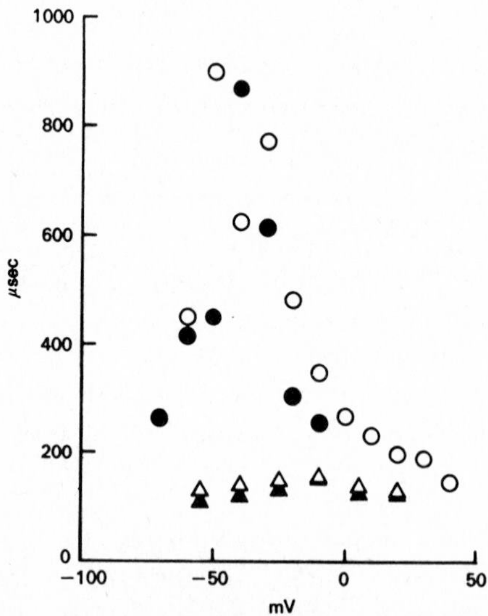

Fig. 28. Time constant of sodium activation and time constant of gating current as function of membrane potential in a squid giant axon. Circles: time constant of sodium activation (τ_m) from measurements of the turning-on (○) and the turning-off (●) of the sodium conductance. Triangles: time constant of gating current, τ_{on}(△) and τ_{off}(▲). Holding potential −100 mV. Temperature 6.3° C. (From Keynes and Kimura 1978.)

charge movement (triangles) $<\tau$ of Na activation (circles) is again demonstrated in fig. 28.

A characteristic property of the Na conductance is its inactivation which is the basis of refractoriness. The intramembrane charge movement also inactivates, presumably due to immobilization or neutralization of the charges. Inactivation of the gating current is most easily demonstrated by increasing the pulse duration. This leads to a decrease of Q_{off} so that the ratio Q_{off}/Q_{on} (which is close to unity for short pulses) becomes smaller and smaller. The immobilized charges return so slowly to the resting position that their movement escapes detection. Examples illustrating the decrease of Q_{off}/Q_{on} with increasing pulse duration are given in figs. 29 and 30. As can be seen from the latter figure, other parameters which characterize the size of the off-response decay as well. Originally, it was reported that inactivation of the gating current follows the same voltage and time dependence as inactivation of the Na conductance (Armstrong and Bezanilla 1977), but more recent publications indicate that the time-course of charge immobilization is slower than that of Na inactivation (Meves and Vogel 1977, Bullock and Schauf 1979).

Gating current cannot only be blocked by a depolarizing pulse of sufficient strength and duration but is also totally or partially abolished by Zn, glutaraldehyde, local anaesthetics, and ultraviolet light.

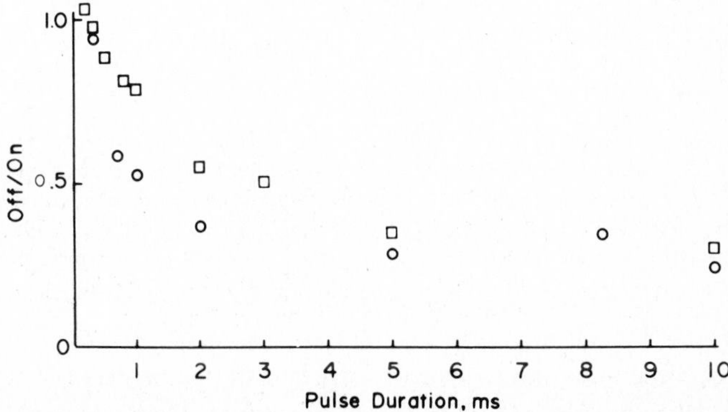

Fig. 29. Q_{off}/Q_{on} ratio as function of pulse duration in a squid giant axon. The charge movement during the on-response (Q_{on}) and during the off-response (Q_{off}) was determined by integrating the gating current record. Two different experiments, both at 8° C:□, test pulses from −70 mV to 10 mV; ○, test pulses from −70 to 50 mV. [From Armstrong and Bezanilla, (1977).]

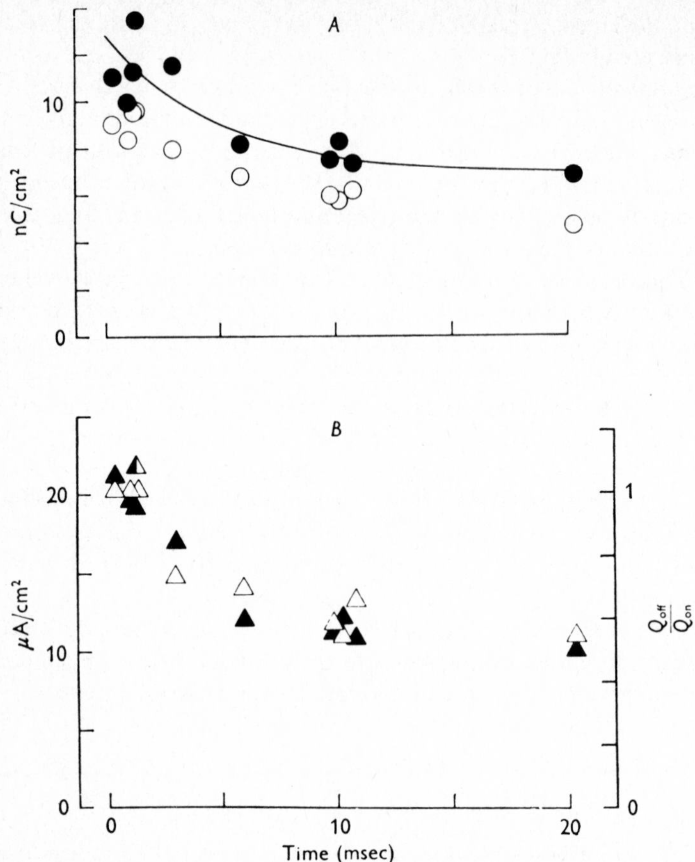

Fig. 30. Effect of pulse duration on the off-response of the gating current in a squid giant axon. Abscissa: pulse duration. Ordinate in A: ●, area under off-response; ○, area under early part of off-response (67–558 μs after pulse end). Ordinates in B: △, amplitude of off-response at a given time (223 μs) after pulse end (left scale); ▲, ratio area off-response to area on-response (right scale). Test pulses from −70 to 20 mV, temperature 8.5° C. Curve through points ● drawn with a time constant of 5 ms. [From Meves and Vogel (1977).]

The observations can be summarized with the statement that th relation between gating current and activation or inactivation of the N conductance is complex. It is conceivable that unknown electricall silent processes are interposed between charge movement and openin or closing of the channels. It seems also possible that only part of th charge movement is related to the function of the Na channels. However, the evidence at present available supports the view that charge movement and Na conductance are in some way connected. The evidence can be summarized in the following four points: (a) the voltage dependence of the intramembrane charge movement which turns on steeply at a potential close to the threshold of the action potential, (b) the time-course of the charge movement (characterized by the time constants τ_{on} and τ_{off}) which is similar (but not identical) to the time-course of the Na activation variable m, (c) the inactivation of the charge movement during a long depolarization which qualitatively (but not quantitatively) resembles the inactivation of the Na conductance, and (d) the simultaneous blockage of gating current and Na current by Zn, glutaraldehyde, local anaesthetics, and ultraviolet light.

7. Independent or coupled kinetics of activation and inactivation

Hodgkin and Huxley (1952b) in their analysis of the membrane currents in the squid giant axon discussed two types of mechanisms underlying inactivation: "One might explain the transient nature of the rise in sodium conductance by supposing that the activating particles undergo a chemical change after moving from the position which they occupy when the membrane potential is high. An alternative is to attribute the decline of sodium conductance to the relatively slow movement of another particle which blocks the flow of sodium ions when it reaches a certain position in the membrane". Two different mathematical approaches correspond to these two alternatives: "First, we might assume that the sodium conductance is determined by a variable which obeys a second order differential equation. Secondly, we might suppose that it is determined by two variables, each of which obeys a first-order equation." Hodgkin and Huxley chose the second alternative "since it was simpler to apply to the experimental results".

A simple model which illustrates the independent operation of two charged particles (activation gate A and inactivation gate I) is shown in fig. 31. The other extreme is the sequential mode in fig. 32; here the inactivated state can only be reached through the activated and the conducting state, i.e. activation is a prerequisite for inactivation. Other models with weaker coupling between activation and inactivation can be imagined: activation and inactivation could interact to some degree, e.g. by electrostatic repulsion of attraction of electrically charged activating and inactivating particles.

There are in principle two possibilities to distinguish between independent and coupled models for activation and inactivation, the pharmacological approach and the kinetic approach. The first approach

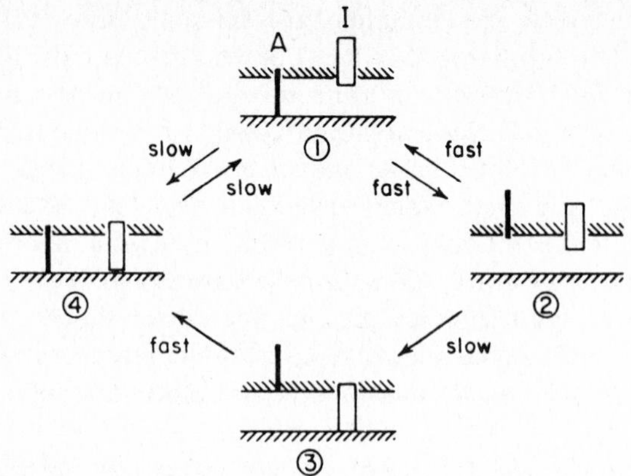

Fig. 31. Schematic drawing of the Na channel with two independent gates, the fast acting A gate (activation process) and the slow acting I gate (inactivation process). (1) At resting potential; (2) depolarized for a short time, e.g. 0.5 ms; (3) depolarized for a long time, e.g. 5 ms; (4) returned to the resting potential after a long-lasting depolarization. [From Dodge (1963).]

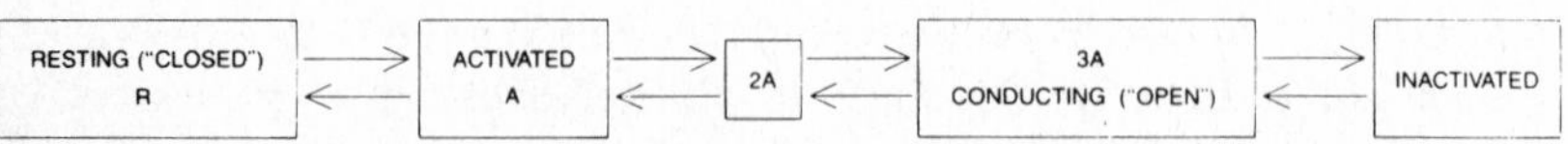

Fig. 32. Sequential model of the sodium channel. The transition from resting (closed) to conducting (open) occurs in three steps (movement of gating charges followed by two electrically silent conformational changes). The inactivated state is reached through the conducting state. [From Keynes (1979).]

looks for chemical substances which affect one process (e.g. activation) but not the other (e.g. inactivation). The second is concerned with the time-course of inactivation; intuitively a sigmoid time-course (i.e. an initial delay in the development of inactivation) would argue in favour of a sequential model while an exponential time-course would suggest independent kinetics.

However, neither of the two approaches gives a definite answer. Goldman (1976) pointed out that pharmacological separability of activation and inactivation does not necessarily indicate independence. As explained by Hoyt (1968), the absence of an initial delay (i.e. a strictly exponential time-course of inactivation) would not prove that activation and inactivation are independent processes. On the other hand, Hille (1976) stated that a sigmoid time course of inactivation does not necessarily prove coupling; all it shows is that inactivation is not a simple first-order process. Nevertheless, both approaches have led to interesting discoveries which must be taken into account by any future model of the Na channel.

Two examples for the pharmacological approach are pronase and scorpion venom from the species *Centruroides sculpturatus*. Armstrong et al. (1973) observed that 6–12 min perfusion with a solution containing 1 or 2 mg/ml pronase completely eliminates Na inactivation in internally perfused squid axons; Na activation and K activation are not affected (fig. 33). This observation is important because it shows that a protein which is accessible from the inner side of the membrane is an essential part of the inactivation mechanism; it also demonstrates that activation and inactivation of the Na channels are separate processes, and that Na channels are distinct from K channels (see subsection 5.2).

In nodes of Ranvier treated with *Centruroides sculpturatus* venom, Cahalan (1975) observed a Na inward current developing with normal h kinetics after the termination of a depolarizing pulse (fig. 34). According to Cahalan, the venom shifts the activation curve of some Na channels by 40–50 mV in the hyperpolarizing direction, i.e. Na current flows at the resting potential. The Na inward current developing at the end of a depolarizing pulse reflects the removal of inactivation which has occurred during the pulse. The observation that the Na inward current follows normal h kinetics argues against coupled models in which the rate constants α_h and β_h depend on the value of m.

The time-course of inactivation has been studied by various authors, and the results are contradictory. The pulse programme always consists of a constant test pulse preceded by a prepulse of varying length Δt. The two pulses are either separated by an interval or follow each other directly.

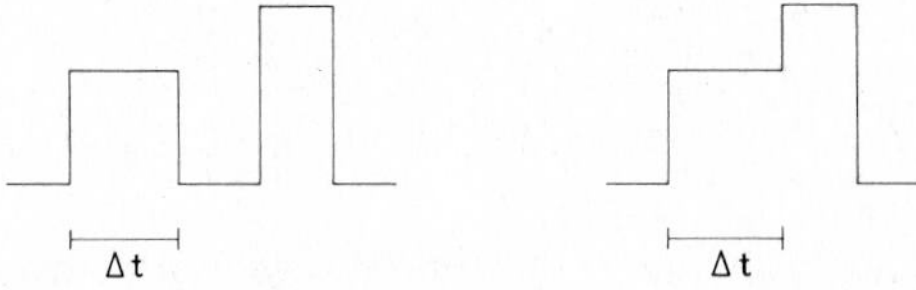

An interval which is large compared with τ_m ensures that m at the beginning of the test pulse is always the same, but it also allows h to recover partly. The first who investigated the time-course of inactivation in detail were Dodge (1963) on nodes of Ranvier, and Chandler et al. (1965) on perfused squid axons. Neither detected an initial delay. A clear delay was seen in the experiments of Goldman and Schauf (1972)

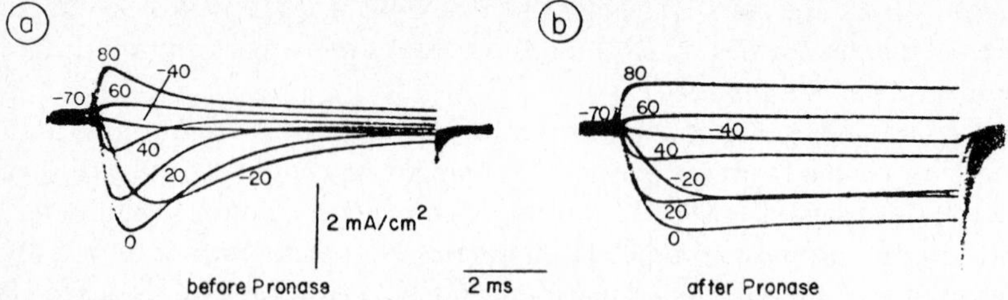

Fig. 33. Removal of Na inactivation by internally applied pronase in a perfused squid giant axon. (a) Before pronase application. (b) After 6 min perfusion with 2 mg/ml pronase. Potential during clamp pulses indicated. Internal solution: 275 mM K + 50 mM Na + 15 mM tetraethylammonium. Temperature 3° C. [From Armstrong et al. (1973).]

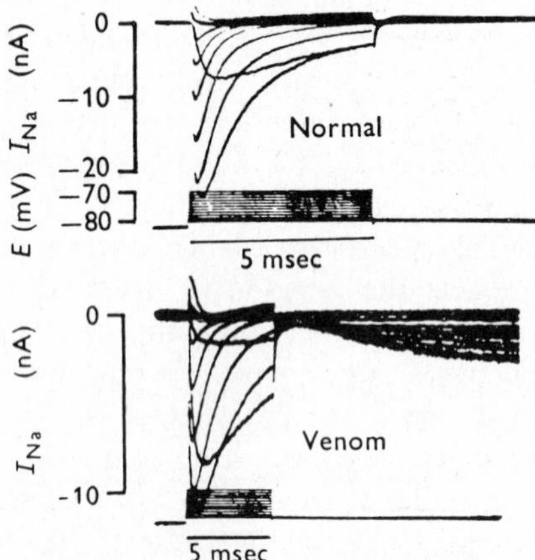

Fig. 34. Effect of *Centruroides sculpturatus* venom on the Na currents of a myelinated nerve fibre. Top: normal; bottom: after treatment with 1 μg/ml Centruroides venom for 1 min. K currents blocked, leakage currents subtracted. Note Na inward current developing after end of pulses in bottom records. [From Cahalan (1975).]

on *Myxicola* axons (fig. 35) and in those of Bezanilla and Armstrong (1977) on perfused squid axons (fig. 36). In fig. 35 the Na current I_{Na} (expressed as a fraction of I_{Na0}, the Na current without prepulse) is plotted against prepulse duration; it is clear that the experimental curve is not exponential but has some sort of shoulder at times between 0 and 1 ms. Figure 36 shows three families of records with prepulses to −20, −30, and −35 mV, respectively. In all three families, the prepulse duration was varied as indicated in the upper family. The time course of inactivation is given by the envelope of the current peaks associated with the test pulses; the time course is definitely sigmoïd, showing an initial lag before the most rapid rate of change.

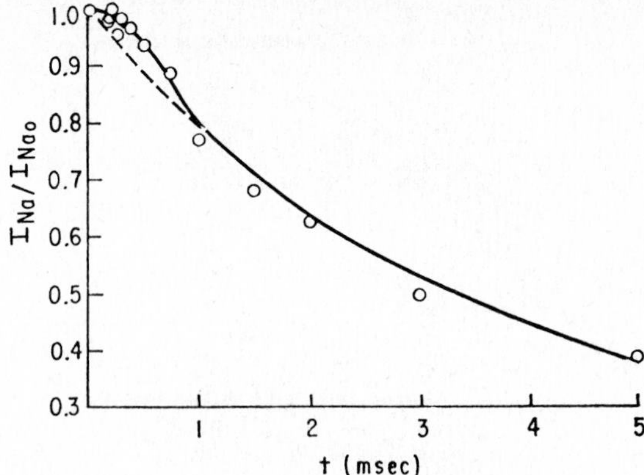

Fig. 35. Development of inactivation with a delay. *Myxicola* axon at 5° C. Pulse program (see inset) consists of a conditioning pulse and a test pulse to −20. 5 mV, separated by a 5 ms interval. The duration of the conditioning pulse is varied and plotted on the abscissa. The ordinate shows I_{Na} (elicited by test pulse) relative to I_{Na} without conditioning pulse (I_{Na0}). Continuous curve drawn through points by eye. Broken curve calculated from the equation $I_{Na}/I_{Na0}=0.167+0.833\exp(-t/3.64)$. Note the difference between the two curves in the first millisecond; later the two curves are identical. [From Goldman and Schauf (1972).]

More recent work (Gillespie and Meves 1980) is concerned with possible systematic errors which may falsify the measurement of the time-course of inactivation. Kniffki et al. (1978) pointed out that measurements with a prepulse followed directly by the test pulse can lead to an apparent initial delay, a phenomenon predicted by the equations of Hodgkin and Huxley (1952b). The delay is due to the increase of m during the conditioning pulse: when the test pulse begins m is already increased and therefore reaches its final value earlier, i.e. the time to peak is shorter and consequently $I_{Na\ peak}$ less inactivated, resulting in an increase of $I_{Na\ peak}$ which obscures any decrease of $I_{Na\ peak}$ due to inactivation. Figure 37 compares measurements with a 5 ms interval between conditioning pulse and test pulse (A, B) and measurements without an interval (C, D). In all four graphs $I_{Na\ peak}$ (elicited by the test pulse) is plotted on a logarithmic scale against prepulse duration, using an expanded time scale in B and D. It is clear that in A, B the points follow an exponential time course whereas in C, D there is an apparent delay of 200–300 μs in the development of inactivation. The earliest point in B (which is for a prepulse duration of 100 μs) is fitted by the straight line drawn through the later points, suggesting that any real delay in the development of inactivation is

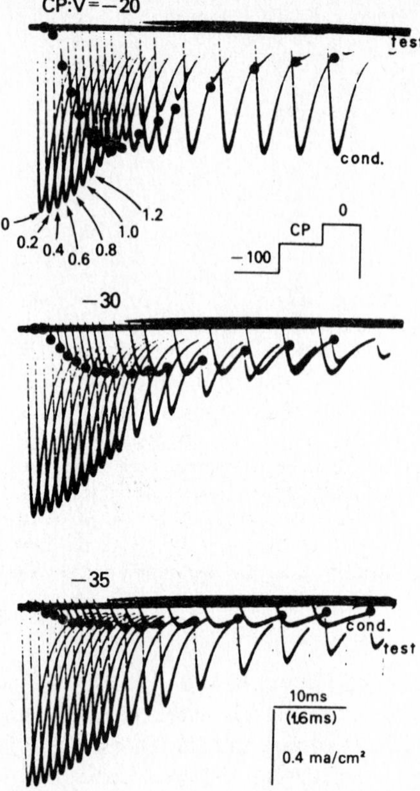

Fig. 36. Development of inactivation with a delay. Intact squid axon (injected with tetraethylammonium chloride) at 9° C. Holding potential −100 mV. Pulse program (see inset) consists of a conditioning pulse to −20, −30, or −35 mV, directly followed by a test pulse to 0 mV. Duration of conditioning pulse varied and indicated in upper family. Current during conditioning pulse and current during test pulse recorded; current at the end of conditioning pulse marked by heavy dot. The envelope of the test peaks gives the time course of inactivation and has a clearly sigmoid shape. [From Bezanilla and Armstrong (1977).]

shorter than 100 μs. In other experiments with shorter prepulse durations the time course of inactivation was exponential after the first 50 μs. The value 50–100 μs is an upper limit for an initial delay in the development of inactivation: the true duration of an initial delay may be anywhere between 0 and 100 μs.

As illustrated by fig. 37, the time course of inactivation is exponential, provided there is an interval between conditioning pulse and test pulse

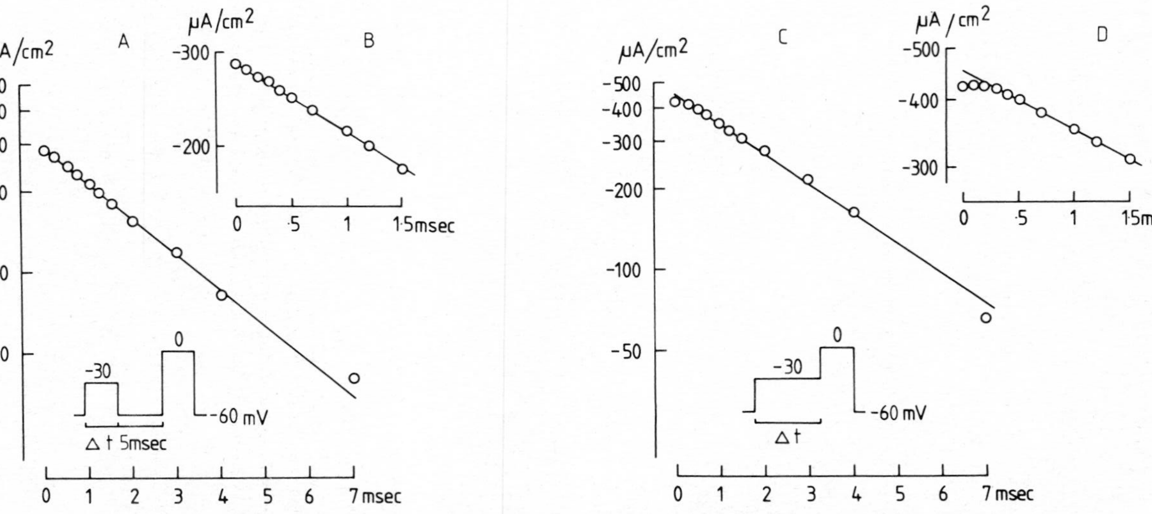

Fig. 37. Effect of conditioning pulses of varying duration Δt on the Na inward current associated with a test pulse to 0 mV. Different pulse programs (see inset) in A, B (5 ms interval), and in C, D (no interval between conditioning pulse and test pulse). Ordinate: $I_{\mathrm{Na\ peak}} - I_{\infty}$; I_{∞} is the peak Na current measured with $\Delta t = 25$ ms. Abscissa: $\Delta t =$ duration of conditioning pulse. Note expanded ordinate and abscissa scale in B and D. Straight lines fitted by eye with $\tau = 3.28$ ms (A, B) and 3.90 ms (C, D). Intact squid axon in full Na sea water with 15 mM 4-aminopyridine to block K currents. Temperature 5.4° C. [From Gillespie and Meves (1980).]

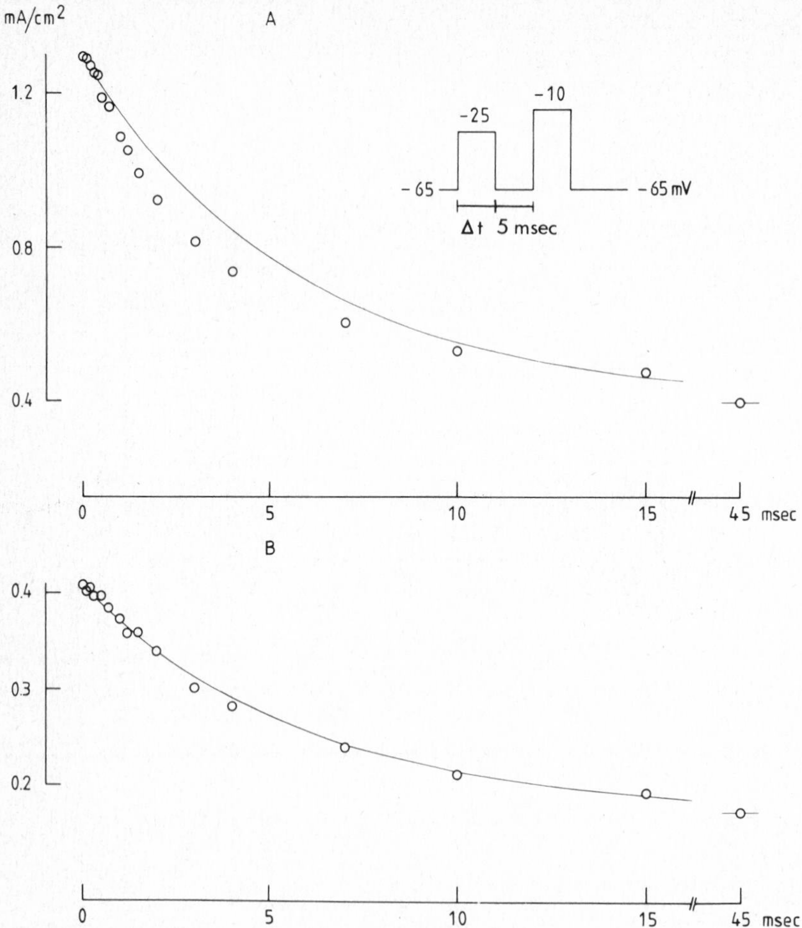

Fig. 38. Measurement of the time-course of inactivation in full external Na (A) and in $\frac{1}{3}$ Na (B) on the same axon. Pulse program see inset in A; interval between conditioning pulses and test pulse 5 ms. Ordinate: $I_{\mathrm{Na\ peak}}$ (elicited by test pulse) on a linear scale. Abscissa: Δt = duration of conditioning pulse. The points in B were fitted by the equation $I = (0.409 - 0.173)\exp(-\Delta t/5.75) + 0.173$ [mA/cm²]. In A, the equation $I = (1.294 - 0.397)\exp(-\Delta t/5.75) + 0.397$ [mA/cm²] fits only the points at $\Delta t = 0 - 0.5$ ms and at $\Delta t = 15$–45 ms. Axon perfused with 218 mM KF + 54 mM tetraethylammonium chloride + sucrose. Temperature 3.8° C. [From Gillespie and Meves (1980).]

which allows the activation variable m to return to its resting value. However, this statement must be qualified: when the Na currents are large a clear deviation from the exponential time course is seen even with intervals of 5 ms or greater. Figure 38 shows an experiment of Gillespie and Meves (1980) with full external Na (A) and $\frac{1}{3}$ Na (B) on the same fibre. The points in B are well fitted by an exponential equation whereas the points in A are not. The points in A appear to follow a time-course which consists of an initial shoulder and a subsequent faster decay. It seems likely that the non-exponential time course in full Na is an artifact due to the resistance in series with the membrane. Gillespie and Meves (1980) showed that the conditioning pulse is followed by a slow tail of inward current; the voltage drop of this inward current across the series resistance will shift the h_∞ curve to more negative internal potentials (cf shift of m_∞ curve in fig. 13 of Chandler and Meves 1970c) so that $I_{\text{Na peak}}$ (elicited by the test pulse) becomes smaller. This explanation is supported by calculations from the Hodgkin and Huxley equations which give an exponential time course of Na inactivation for a small series resistance and a small Na current, but a sigmoid time course for a large series resistance and a large Na current.

Gillespie and Meves (1980) concluded that after the first 50–100 μs of a depolarizing voltage step the time course of inactivation is exponential. The value of 50–100 μs (which is an upper limit for an initial delay in the development of inactivation) can now be related to the time course of the Na activation variable m. At 0° C and 15 mV the time constant of m (τ_m) is 0.45 ms (Kimura and Meves 1979). If m increases exponentially from 0 to 1 with $\tau_m = 0.45$ ms, it has reached the value 0.20 at 100 μs, i.e. inactivation starts long before full activation has taken place, or in other words, full activation is not a prerequisite of inactivation. This sets a limit to sequential models of the excitation process which are based on the scheme resting⟶active⟶inactive. The observations would, however, be compatible with a scheme in which the reaction resting⟶active consists of several steps and the first few of these steps are necessary for inactivation to start.

References

Adams, D. J. and P. W. Gage (1976) Science 192, 783.

Adrian, R. H. and W. H. Freygang (1962) J. Physiol. 163, 61.

Almers, W. (1978) Rev. Physiol. Biochem. Pharmacol. 82, 96.

Armstrong, C. M. (1971) J. Gen. Physiol. 58, 413.

Armstrong, C. M. and F. Bezanilla (1973) Nature London 242, 459.
Armstrong, C. M. and F. Bezanilla (1975) Ann. N. Y. Acad. Sci. 264, 265.
Armstrong, C. M. and F. Bezanilla (1977) J. Gen. Physiol. 70, 567.
Armstrong, C. M., F. Bezanilla and E. Rojas (1973) J. Gen. Physiol. 62, 375.
Armstrong, C. M. and L. Binstock (1965) J. Gen. Physiol. 48, 859.
Armstrong, C. M. and B. Hille (1972) J. Gen. Physiol. 59, 388.
Baker, P. F., A. L. Hodgkin and T. I. Shaw (1961) Nature London 190, 885.
Barr, L. (1965) J. Theoret. Biol. 9, 351.
Begenisich, T. and C. F. Stevens (1975) Biophys. J. 15, 843.
Bergman, C. (1970) Pflügers Arch. 317, 287.
Bergman, J., J. M. Dubois and C. Bergman (1979) Ann. N. Y. Acad. Sci. (in press).
Bezanilla, F. and C. M. Armstrong (1972) J. Gen. Physiol. 60, 588.
Bezanilla, F. and C. M. Armstrong (1977) J. Gen. Physiol. 70, 549.
Binstock, L. and H. Lecar (1969) J. Gen. Physiol. 53, 342.
Bullock, J. O. and C. L. Schauf (1979) J. Physiol. 286, 157.
Cahalan, M. D. (1975) J. Physiol. London 244, 511.
Caldwell, P. C., A. L. Hodgkin, R. D. Keynes and T. I. Shaw (1960) J. Physiol. London 152, 561.
Chandler, W. K. and H. Meves (1965) J. Physiol. 180, 788.
Chandler, W. K. and H. Meves (1970a) J. Physiol. 211, 623.
Chandler, W. K. and H. Meves (1970b) J. Physiol. 211, 653.
Chandler, W. K. and H. Meves (1970c) J. Physiol. 211, 679.
Chandler, W. K., A. L. Hodgkin and H. Meves (1965) J. Physiol. 180, 821.
Chiu, S. Y. (1977) J. Physiol. 273, 573.
Cole, K. S. (1962) Biophys. J. 2, pt. 2, suppl., 101.
Colquhoun, D., R. Henderson and J. M. Ritchie (1972) J. Physiol. 273, 573.
Conti, F., L. J. de Felice and E. Wanke (1975) J. Physiol. 248, 45.
Conti, F., B. Hille, B. Neumcke, W. Nonner and R. Stämpfli (1976) J. Physiol. 262, 699.
De Weer, P. and D. Geduldig (1973) Science 179, 1326.
Dodge, F. A. (1963) A Study of Ionic Permeability Changes Underlying Excitation in Myelinated Nerve Fibres of the Frog, Thesis, The Rockefeller University (University Microfilms, Inc., Ann Arbor) no. 64-7333.
Dodge, F. A. and B. Frankenhaeuser (1958) J. Physiol. 143, 76.
Dubois, J. M. and C. Bergman (1975) Pflügers Arch. 358, 111.
Dubois, J. M. and C. Bergman (1977a) Nature London 266, 741.
Dubois, J. M. and C. Bergman (1977b) Pflügers Arch. 370, 185.
Eisenman, G. (1962) Biophys. J. 2 suppl, 259.
Eisenman, G., J. P. Sandblom and E. Neher (1978) Biophys. J. 22, 307.
Ellory, J. C. and R. D. Keynes (1969) Nature London 221, 776.
Eyring, H. and E. M. Eyring (1963) Modern Chemical Kinetics. (Reinhold Publishing Co., New York) Ch. 4.
Evans, M. H. (1972) Intern. Rev. Neurobiol. 15, 83.
Fox, J. M. (1974) Pflügers Arch. 351, 287.
Frankenhaeuser, B. (1960a) J. Physiol. 152, 159.
Frankenhaeuser, B. (1960b) J. Physiol. 151, 491.
Frankenhaeuser, B. (1959) J. Physiol. 148, 671.
Frankenhaeuser, B. (1962a) J. Physiol. 160, 46.

Frankenhaeuser, B. (1962b) J. Physiol. 160, 54.
Frankenhaeuser, B. (1963) J. Physiol. 169, 445.
Frankenhaeuser, B. and A. L. Hodgkin (1956) J. Physiol. 131, 341.
Gillespie, J. I. and H. Meves (1980) J. Physiol. 299, 289.
Goldman, D. E. (1943) J. Gen. Physiol. 27, 37.
Goldman, D. E. (1964) Biophys. J. 4, 167.
Goldman, L. (1976) Q. Rev. Biophys. 9, 491.
Goldman, L. and C. L. Schauf (1972) J. Gen. Physiol. 59, 659.
Henderson, R. and J. H. Wang (1972) Biochemistry 11, 4565.
Hille, B. (1967) J. Gen. Physiol. 50, 1287.
Hille, B. (1968a) J. Gen. Physiol. 51, 221.
Hille, B. (1968b) J. Gen. Physiol. 51, 199.
Hille, B. (1971) J. Gen. Physiol. 58, 599.
Hille, B. (1972) J. Gen. Physiol. 59, 637.
Hille, B. (1973) J. Gen. Physiol. 61, 669.
Hille, B. (1975a) Ionic Selectivity of Na and K Channels of Nerve Membranes, in: Membranes, vol. 3, ed. G. Eisenman (M. Dekker Inc., New York) pp. 255–323.
Hille, B. (1975b) J. Gen. Physiol. 66, 535.
Hille, B. (1975c) Federation Proc. 34, 1318.
Hille, B. (1976) A. Rev. Physiol. 38, 139.
Hille, B. (1979) Rate Theory Models for Ion Flow in Ionic Channels of Nerve and Muscle, in: Membrane Transport Processes, vol. 3, eds. C. F. Stevens and R. W. Tsien (Raven Press, New York) pp. 5–16.
Hodgkin, A. L. (1958) Proc. R. Soc. London B 148, 1.
Hodgkin, A. L. (1964) The Conduction of the Nervous Impulse (Liverpool University Press, Liverpool).
Hodgkin, A. L. and P. Horowicz (1959) J. Physiol. 148, 127.
Hodgkin, A. L. and A. F. Huxley (1952a) J. Physiol. 116, 473.
Hodgkin, A. L. and A. F. Huxley (1952b) J. Physiol. 117, 500.
Hodgkin, A. L. and B. Katz (1949) J. Physiol. 108, 37.
Hodgkin, A. L. and R. D. Keynes (1955) J. Physiol. 128, 28.
Hodgkin, A. L. and R. D. Keynes (1955) J. Physiol. 128, 61.
Hoyt, R. C. (1968) Biophys. J. 8, 1074.
Huang, L. Y. M., W. A. Catteral and G. Ehrenstein (1979) J. Gen. Physiol. 73, 839.
Jack, J. J. B. (1976) Electrophysiological Properties of Peripheral Nerve, in: The Peripheral Nerve, ed. D. N. Landon (Chapman and Hall, England) ch. 14, pp. 740–818.
Johnson, F. H., H. Eyring and M. J. Polissar (1954), The Kinetic Basis of Molecular Biology (Wiley, New York).
Kandel, E. R. (1976) Cellular Basis of Behaviour (W. H. Freeman and Co., San Francisco).
Kerkut, G. and R. C. Thomas (1965) Comp. Biochem. Physiol. 14, 167.
Keynes, R. D. (1975) Organization of the Ionic Channels in Nerve Membranes, in: The Nervous System, vol. 1, ed. D. B. Tower (Raven Press, New York) pp. 165–175.
Keynes, R. D. (1979) Sci. Am. 240, 98.
Keynes, R. D. and J. E. Kimura (1978) J. Physiol. 284, 140 P.
Keynes, R. D., J. M. Ritchie and E. Rojas (1971) J. Physical. 213, 235.
Keynes, R. D. and E. Rojas (1974) J. Physiol. 239, 393.

Keynes, R. D. and R. C. Swan (1959) J. Physiol. 147, 626.
Khodorov, B. I. (1978) Chemicals as Tools to Study Nerve Fibre Sodium Channels: Effects of Batrachotoxin and Some Local Anaesthetics, in: Membrane Transport Processes vol. 2, eds. D. C. Tosteson, Y. A. Ovchinnikov and R. Lattore (Raven Press, New York) pp. 153–174.
Kimura, J. E. and H. Meves (1979) J. Physiol. 289, 479.
Kniffki, K. D., D. Siemen and W. Vogel (1978) J. Physiol. 284, 92 P.
Koppenhöfer, E. (1967) Pflügers Arch. 293, 34.
Kostyuk, P. G., O. A. Krishtal and V. I. Pidoplichko (1977) Nature London 267, 70.
Läuger, P. (1973) Biochem. Biophys. Acta 311, 423.
Läuger, P. (1979) Transport of Non-Interacting Ions Through Channels, in: Membrane Transport Processes, vol. 3, eds. C. F. Stevens and R. W. Tsien (Raven Press, New York) pp. 17–29.
Marmor, M. F. and A. L. F. Gorman (1970) Science 167, 65.
Meves, H. (1974) J. Physiol. 243, 847.
Meves, H. (1978) Intramembrane Charge Movement in Squid Giant Nerve Fibres, in: Ions in Macromolecular and Biological Systems, eds. D. H. Everett and B. Vincent (Scientechnica, Bristol) Colston paper No. 29.
Meves, H. and Y. Pichon (1977) J. Physiol. 268, 511.
Meves, H. and W. Vogel (1977) J. Physiol. 267, 377.
Moore, J. W., T. Narahashi and T. I. Shaw (1967) J. Physiol. 188, 99.
Mullins, L. J. (1959) J. Gen. Physiol. 42, 1013.
Mullins, L. J. (1968) J. Gen. Physiol. 52, 550.
Narahashi, T. (1974) Physiol. Rev. 54, 813.
Neumcke, B., W. Nonner and R. Stämpfli (1976) Pflügers Arch. 363, 193.
Neumcke, B., W. Nonner and R. Stämpfli (1978) Gating Currents in Excitable Membranes, in: International Review of Biochemistry, vol. 19, ed. J. C. Metcalfe (University Park Press, Baltimore).
Nonner, W., E. Rojas and R. Stämpfli (1975) Phil. Trans. R. Soc. London B 270, 483.
Oikawa, T., C. S. Spyropoulos, I. Tasaki and T. Teorell (1961) Acta Physiol. Scand. 52, 195.
Rang, H. P. and J. M. Ritchie (1968) J. Physiol. 196, 223.
Ritchie, J. M. and R. W. Straub (1957) J. Physiol. 136, 80.
Rudy, B. (1976) Proc. R. Soc. London B 193, 469.
Schneider, M. F. and W. K. Chandler (1973) Nature London 242, 244.
Schwarz, J. R., W. Ulbricht and H. H. Wagner (1973) J. Physiol. 233, 167.
Schwarz, J. R. and W. Vogel (1971) Pflügers Arch. 330, 61.
Stark, G., B. Ketterer, R. Benz and P. Läuger (1971) Biophys. J. 11, 981.
Thomas, R. C. (1969) J. Physiol. 201, 495.
Thomas, R. C. (1972) Physiol. Rev. 52, 563.
Ulbricht, W. (1969) Rev. Physiol. Biochem. Pharmacol. (Ergeb. Physiol.) 61, 18.
Ulbricht, W. (1974) Selective Blocking of Channels, in: Electrical Phenomena at the Biological Membrane Level (Elsevier, Amsterdam) pp. 203–217.
Ulbricht, W. and H. H. Wagner (1976) Pflügers Arch. 367, 77.
Wagner, H. H. and W. Ulbricht (1974) Pflügers Arch. 347, R34.

SEMINAR

THE CATION PUMPS IN NERVE AND MUSCLE CELLS

Yves DUPONT

Laboratoire de Biophysique Moléculaire et Cellulaire,
D.R.F. / G., CEA,C.E.N.G. 85 X 38041 Grenoble,
France

1. Definition

In their lectures, Bergman and Meves have shown that the resting potential and action potential in nerve and muscle are dependent on the unequal distribution of cations, mainly K^+ and Na^+, on both sides of the membrane. K^+ and Na^+ exchange during excitation and after a prolonged activity the ionic gradient would disappear if the cell were not able to pump back K^+ and to extrude the accumulated Na^+. This work is performed by the Na^+–K^+ ATPase. The cations being transported uphill against a concentration gradient. This process requires metabolic energy, which is given by the clivage of ATP molecules.

Another well documented example is the Ca^{++}-pump. Inside a relaxed muscle fiber the free calcium concentration is lower than 10^{-8} M, most of the calcium is sequestered in the internal space of a very

R. Balian et al., eds.
Les Houches, Session XXXIII, 1979 – Membranes et Communication Intercellulaire / Membranes and Intercellular Communication

specialized organelle: the Sarcoplasmic Reticulum (S. R.). When the muscle is activated Ca^{++} ions are released in the Sarcoplasm* triggering the acto-myosin system. This is the excitation–contraction phase immediately followed by a relaxation period where the Ca^{++} ions are pumped back into the S. R. This is the job of the Ca^{++} pump again fueled by ATP.

These two cases are selected examples but it is likely that ionic pumps are present in virtually all cells where they are involved in vital cellular processes like the maintenance of internal ionic composition, pH, volume and also in the control and regulation of the membrane potential.

2. Preparation and purification

For a long time the ionic pumps were viewed as black boxes and this can be compared with the present state of the ionic channels. The studies were restricted to measurement of ionic fluxes across the membranes of intact cells (red cells, axons, muscle fibers, etc.) and to the characterization with specific inhibitors (ouabain). Since the last 10–15 years, however, important progresses have been made after the isolation and purification of Na^+–K^+ ATPase [1–3] and Ca^{++} pump [4–5], first in enriched microsomal fraction, then in soluble form in the presence of detergent.

The Ca^{++} pump is isolated by a relatively simple procedure from rabbit muscles. It is possible to obtain closed vesicles which are able to transport calcium in the presence of ATP and 70–80% of the protein attached to the membrane are the Ca^{++} pump.

The Na^+–K^+ ATPase has also been obtained in very pure form from specialized tissues like: kidney, electric organ of fishes, gills, etc. (for a review see ref. [6]).

It has also been possible to extract other ionic pumps from other tissues but they have received less effort. A good example is the H^+–K^+ ATPase from gastic membrane [7].

3. Structural aspects

Little is known about the molecular structure of the ionic pumps. The biggest difficulty is that they are all intrinsic membrane proteins. They

*The way by which the external excitable membrane and the internal Sarcoplasmic system communicate, as well as the mecanism of Ca^{++} release are not yet elucidated. Some references on these problems can be found in [49–52].

are not soluble in water and are denatured if the hydrophobic part of the protein is not incorporated in a membrane or in a medium which mimics the apolar environment of the membrane. For these reasons none of the ionic pumps have been crystallized and the view we have of their structure is very poor. The only structural information comes from: (a) electron microscopy of vesicles [8,–11] and (b) X-ray diffraction of vesicles stacked by very fast centrifugation [12].

Both techniques suggest a marked asymmetry of the protein with a globular part in contact with the cytoplasm of the cell and a hydrophobic tail embedded in the membrane. This asymmetry is certainly related to the vectorial activity of the pump and the globular part of the protein facing the side where residues the metabolic energy certainly contains the main machinery of the pump.

For Na^+–K^+, Ca^+, or H^+–K^+ ATPases the main catalytic chain has a mol wt of $\simeq$ 100 000 Daltons, additional lighter glycopeptidic chains $Na^+ - K^+$ are found in association with the Na–K and H^+–K^+ ATPase, their role is unknown.

4. Ion movements

The transport of ions is tightly coupled to the ATPase activity of the pump and in optimal conditions this is given by the equations *:

$$Na^+\text{–}K^+ \rightarrow 3\,Na^+_{cyt} + 2\,K^+_{ext} + ATP \rightleftharpoons 3\,Na^+_{ext} + 2\,K^+_{cyt} + ADP + Pi$$

$$Ca^{++} \rightarrow 2\,Ca^{++}_{cyt} + ATP \rightleftharpoons 2\,Ca^{++}_{int} ADP + Pi.$$

The Na^+–K^+ ATPase catalyzes an exchange between Na^+ and K^+ while an inverse transport has never been demonstrated for the Ca^{++} pump (if any, candidates are K^+ or Mg^{++}).

The reactions are reversible and both systems are able to convert osmotic into chemical energy leading to the synthesis of ATP at the expense of an ionic gradient [13–15].

The ratio ion transported/ATP hydrolyzed does not appear to be rigidly fixed and a variable gearing has been proposed which could provide a very sophisticated way to adapt the work of the pump to the energy demand. This has been demonstrated for the Ca^{++} pump where the coupling ratio Ca/ATP is variable [16].

Various coupling ratios have also been proposed for the Na^+–K^+ ATPase [17, 18]. The relation Na/K/ATP = 3/2/1 is now accepted for

* $_{cyt}$ = cytoplasmic side of the membrane, $_{ext}$ = extra cellular space, and $_{int}$ = interior of the Sarcoplasmic Reticulum for the S. R. Ca^{++} pump.

red cells and axons in optimal Na^+, K^+, and ATP concentrations [25–27].

5. Reaction scheme

The enzymology of a membrane protein is relatively complicated by the large number of effectors involved but also because one has to control the events on both sides of the membrane, this is not always possible. Nevertheless the investigation methods are not very different from that used for soluble enzymes.

Two kinds of conditions are used:

(a) Steady-state experiments where enough substrate is given to the system. The product inhibition is limited by an appropriate choice of substrate concentration or by buffering of the products. For the Ca^{++} pump, steady-state experiments are made in the presence of oxalate to prevent the inhibition by the accumulated calcium; the membrane is permeable to oxalate ions and (Ca^{++}. Ox^{--}) precipitates inside the vesicles thus reducing the internal activity of Ca^{++}. If steady-state conditions are fulfilled, the activity of the pump can be followed over minutes and the turnover rate, the regulation of the activity and the effect of substrates measured.

(b) Rapid mixing – in contrast to the precedent method a rapid mixing experiment is only concerned with the transient events during the first few turnovers of the enzyme after rapid mixing with the substrates. This has been one of the most powerful methods during the last few years and we start to understand now the major part of the reaction scheme of the Na^+–K^+ and Ca^{++} ATPase [19–22].*

Conformational changes – a satisfactory model of the pump mechanism cannot be based on the structure since the information is at present, too limited to give a reasonable understanding of the mechanism. The study of the protein conformation by other indirect methods is then an obligatory way and the methods used so far for the identification of enzymatic states are:

(a) The measurement of the reactivity of specific groups (SH) [30, 31].

(b) The measurement of the susceptibility to proteolysis [28, 29].

(c) The use of intrinsic or extrinsic probes [32–36].

One of the most fascinating results of these studies is the remarkable analogy between the two systems so far extensively studied. Also, the

*Good sources of references on the reaction mechanism can be found in recent reviews [23, 24].

image which emerges now is that they are two main states of the catalytic chain:

$$E_1 \rightleftharpoons E_2^{**}.$$

The two states differ by the affinity for ATP and cations and what is more important by a modification of the sidedness of the cations sites. In E_1 the cation sites are accessible from the cytoplasmic side of the membrane; in E_2 from the other side. In this sense, the transition between these two states is certainly the precise location of the cation translocation.

In the two conformations the enzyme is phosphorylable but the phosphoenzyme has different properties:

E_1P exchanges his phosphate with ADP

$$E_1P + ADP \rightleftharpoons E_1 + ATP$$

E_2P exchanges his phosphate with water

$$E_2P + H_2O \rightleftharpoons E_2 + Pi.$$

During one turnover there is a sequential transformation between the two conformations and the energy to drive the cycle is given by the hydrolysis of ATP.

		ATP_{cyt} ADP_{cyt}			
cyt	E_1	$\longrightarrow$	E_1P	cyt	cyt
$K^+ \updownarrow$	$\downarrow\uparrow$		$\uparrow\downarrow$	$\updownarrow Ca^{++}$	$\updownarrow Na^+$
ext	E_2	$\longleftarrow$	E_2P	in	ext.
		Pi_{cyt} H_2O			

This scheme however is certainly oversimplified, there are some indications that the catalytic chains are associated in dimer and that each part of the dimer are describing this cycle out of phase. This mechanism termed flip-flop has been proposed by Repke et al. [37] but never proved. It is a very attractive hypothesis which could explain some properties and regulations of the transport ATPases.

**The studies of Ca^{++} and Na–K ATPases were made independantly therefore the denomination of the states are different. E_1 and E_2 is adopted for Na–K ATPase, authors working on the Ca^{++} ATPhase have preferred E and E*.

6. Electrogenic transport

The hypothesis that part of the membrane potential of nervous cells is due to the activity of an electrogenic ion pump is relatively old [38] and this is a very important aspect of the mechanism of the ionic pump.

The unequality of the active movement of K^+ and Na^+ for each turnover of the Na^+–K^+ ATPase is a fact which is now accepted and which implies that this pump is electrically active. Another proof of the electrogenic activity is the ouabain sensitive hyperpolarization observed in various excitable tissues or muscle fibers when the Na^+–K^+ ATPase is activated by an increase of internal Na^+ (by repeated stimulation or Na^+ injection) [39–41].

The electrogenicity of the Ca^{++} pump is still an open question since intact S.R. in muscle or fractionated in vesicles is too small to allow direct measurement with electrodes. Since the last few years, however some measurement have been performed with potential sensitive dyes, this is presently the unique mean of detecting potential changes across the membrane vesicles. Cyanine dyes have been used successfully for other vesicular material and the mechanism of the optical response is described by Sims et al. [42].

The experiments are not unambiguous since the response of the dye is dependent on many other factors like local charge of the membrane, ionic strength, pH etc . . . The dye called DiS-C_3-(5) (3,3′-dipropylthiodicarbocyanine) exhibits an important fluorescence change during the activity of the Ca^{++} pump.

The direction of the intensity change corresponds to an increase of potential inside the vesicles. This is in favor of an electrogenic activity of the pump [43] and the same interpretation was given by other authors [44–46]. This conclusion however is not always accepted: Beeler et al. [47, 48] have attributed the fluorescence or absorbtion changes to an interaction between the protein and the dye.

The question is then awaiting a definite answer and in any case the problem of an inverse transport (neutralizing completely or not the charges of Ca^{++}) remains to be solved.

References

[1] J. C. Skou, Biochim. Biophys. Acta 23 (1957) 394.
[2] L. E. Hokin, Ann. N.Y. Acc. Sci. 242 (1974) 12.
[3] P. L. Jorgensen, Ann. N. Y. Acc. Sci. 242 (1974) 36.

[4] W. Hasselbach and M. Makinose, Biochem. Z. 339 (1963) 94.
[5] D. H. Mc Lennan, P. Seeman, G. H. Iles and C. C. Yip, J. Biol. Chem. 246 (1971) 2702.
[6] P. L. Jorgensen, Meth. Enzymol. 32 (b) (1974) 277.
[7] G. Sachs, Hsuan Hung Chang, E. Rabon, R. Schackman, M. Lewin and G. Saccomani, J. Biol. Chem. 251 (1976) 7690.
[8] N. Deguchi, P. L. Jorgensen and A. B. Maunbach, J. Cell. Biol. 75 (1977) 619.
[9] W. B. Van Winkle, L. K. Lane and A. Schwartz, Exp. Cell. Res. 100 (1976) 291.
[10] W. Hasselbach and L. G. Elfvin, J. Ultra. Res. 17 (1967) 598.
[11] D. W. Deamer and R. J. Baskin, J. Cell. Biol. 42 (1969) 296.
[12] Y. Dupont, S. C. Harrison and W. Hasselbach, Nature 244 (1973) 555.
[13] I. M. Glynn and V. L. Lew, J. Physiol. London 207 (1970) 393.
[14] V. L. Lew, I. M. Glynn and J. C. Ellory, Nature 225 (1970) 865.
[15] W. Hasselbach, Biochim. Biophys. Acta 515 (1978) 23.
[16] B. Rossi, F. De Assis Leone, C. Gache and M. Lazdunski, J. Biol. Chem. 254 (1979) 2302.
[17] S. B. Cross, R. D. Keynes and R. Rybova, J. Physiol. London 181 (1965) 865.
[18] F. J. Brinley and L. J. Mullins, Ann. N. Y. Acc. Sci. 242 (1974) 406.
[19] T. Kanazawa, M. Saito and Y. Tonomura, J. Biochem. Tokyo 67 (1970) 693.
[20] S. Mårdh and S. Lindahl, J. Biol. Chem. 252 (1977) 8058.
[21] J. P. Froehlich and E. W. Taylor, J. Biol. Chem. 250 (1975) 2013.
[22] J. P. Froehlich and E. W. Taylor, J. Biol. Chem. 251 (1976) 2307.
[23] W. Hasselbach, Enzyme 10 (1975) 431.
[24] I. M. Glynn and S. J. D. Karlish, Ann. Rev. Physiol. 37 (1975) 13.
[25] P. J. Garrahan and I. M. Glynn, J. Physiol. London 192 (1967) 217.
[26] A. K. Sen and R. L. Post, J. Biol. Chem. 239 (1964) 345.
[27] P. F. Baker, J. Physiol. London 200 (1969) 459.
[28] G. Saccomani, D. W. Dailey and G. Sachs, J. Biol. Chem. 254 (1979) 2821.
[29] P. L. Jorgensen, Biochem. Biophys. Acta 401 (1975) 399.
[30] A. J. Murphy, Biochemistry 15 (1976) 4492.
[31] S. Yamada and N. Ikemoto, J. Biol. Chem. 252 (1978) 6801.
[32] S. J. D. Karlish and D. W. Yates, Biochim. Biophys. Acta 527 (1978) 115.
[33] Y. Dupont, Biochem. Biophys. Res. Commun. 71 (1976) 544.
[34] Y. Dupont and J. Barrington Leigh, Nature 273 (1978) 396.
[35] Y. Dupont, Biochem. Biophys. Res. Commun. 82 (1978) 893.
[36] P. Champeil, S. Buschlen, Boucly, F. Bastide and C. Gary-Bobo, J. Biol. Chem. 253 (1978) 1179.
[37] K. R. H. Repke, R. Schon, W. Henke, W. Schonfeld, B. Streckenbach and F. Dittrich, Ann. NY Acad. Sci. 242 (1974) 203.
[38] A. L. Hodgkin, Biol. Rev. 26 (1951) 339–409.
[39] A. L. Hodgkin and R. D. Keynes, J. Physiol. London 131 (1956) 592.
[40] R. P. Kernan, Nature 193 (1962) 986.
[41] R. C. Thomas, Physiol. Rev. 52 (1972) 563.
[42] P. J. Sims, A. S. Waggoner, A. S. Chao-Huei-Wang and J. F. Hoffman, Biochemistry 13 (1974) 3315.
[43] Y. Dupont, in: Cation Flux Across Biomembranes, eds. Mukuhata and Packer (Academic Press, N. Y. 1979) pp. 141–160.

[44] K. E. O. Åkerman and C. H. J. Wolff, FEBS Lett. 100 (1979) 291.
[45] P. Zimniak and E. Racker, J. Biol. Chem. 253 (1978) 4631.
[46] T. Ueno and T. Sekine, J. Biochem. Tokyo 84 (1978) 787.
[47] T. Beeler, J. T. Russel and A. Martonosi, Eur. J. Biochem. 95 (1979) 579.
[48] J. T. Russel, T. Beeler and A. Martonosi, J. Biol. Chem. 254 (1979) 2040.
[49] Y. Nakajima and M Endo, Nature N. B. 246 (1973) 216.
[50] C. Caputo, Ann. Rev. Biophys. Bioeng. 7 (1978) 63.
[51] R. H. Adrian, Ann. Rev. Biophys. Bioeng. 7 (1978) 85.
[52] M. F. Schneider and W. K. Chandler, Nature 242 (1973) 244.

COURSE 9

IONIC PERMEABILITY CHANGES PRODUCED BY SYNAPTIC TRANSMITTERS

Philippe ASCHER

Laboratoire de Neurobiologie, Ecole Normale Supérieure
46 rue d'Ulm, Paris 75005,
France

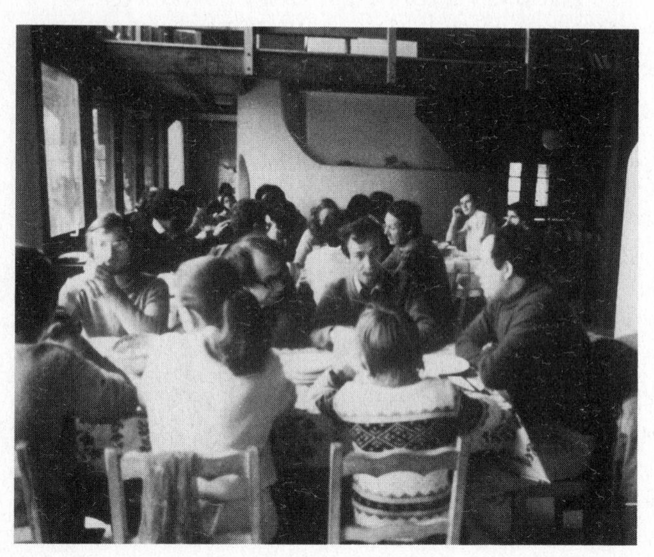

Contents

R. Balian et al., eds.
Les Houches, Session XXXIII, 1979 – Membranes et Communication Intercellulaire / Membranes and Intercellular Communication

0. Introduction

About thirty years ago Hodgkin and Huxley established that the squid axon nerve impulse could be explained by the interplay of two "voltage-dependent" conductances, the Na^+ conductance and the K^+ conductance. These two systems were then found in a host of other "electrically excitable" cells, and in each case their properties appear remarkably similar. Other voltage-dependent conductances are known – Ca^{2+} conductances and K^+ conductances in particular – and again each of them presents similar properties in very distinct cells, and appears very early in development (see Hagiwara and Jaffe 1979).

In the following review, I shall consider the situation in the case of "transmitter-controlled" conductances. At first sight, these conductances appear to be far less homogeneous than the voltage-dependent ones. However, like voltage-sensitive conductances, transmitter-controlled conductances are likely to involve two types of elements: the "gates" and the "selectivity filters". The variety found in the case of transmitter-controlled systems must result in part from the fact that their gating systems imply a large number of different transmitter–receptor interactions, and does not imply that the "selectivity filters" are different for the different cases. Therefore, I shall review what is known on these filters (or channels) in an attempt to establish if they really can be reduced to a limited number of basic types.

I shall assume that the reader has a basic knowledge of the functioning of synapses (Katz 1966, Ginsborg 1973).

1. Increases in ionic permeability leading to inhibition of the target cell

Excitation is usually the result of a depolarization leading to the generation of action potentials and/or Ca^{2+} entry. The best known inhibitory mechanisms are those in which an increase in ionic permeability (to K^+ or to Cl^-) opposes depolarizing effects by bringing the membrane potential towards a potential (E_K, E_{Cl}) situated below (more negative than) the threshold for excitation.

1.1. The reversal potential of inhibitory responses. K^+ and Cl^- conductance changes

1.1.1. Effects of acetylcholine on the sino-atrial cells of frog heart. Increase in K^+ conductance

Acetylcholine (ACh) is the transmitter liberated by the parasympathetic neurones which provide inhibitory innervation to the vertebrate heart. The observation that stimulation of these neurones can slow the heart was the first demonstration of the existence of inhibition in physiology (Volkmann 1838; see Hutter 1957; Noble 1975). Already at the end of the 19th century it was observed that inhibition was associated with an increase in membrane potential (hyperpolarization) and with an efflux of potassium. Later, the use of radioactive K^+ confirmed this efflux, and indicated that ACh increased K^+ permeability. But it was on the basis of electrophysiological data that the conclusion was drawn that the hyperpolarization produced by ACh (and responsible for the slowing of the rhythm) was entirely (exclusively) due to an increase in K^+ permeability.

The evidence leading to this conclusion is (a) the effect of ACh (which can be measured by a change in membrane potential or by a current) changes sign when the membrane potential is artificially increased and (b) the reversal potential of the ACh response (i.e., the potential at which the inversion occurs) is equal to the K^+ equilibrium potential (E_K) (calculated from measurement of internal and external K^+) and remains equal to E_K when the extracellular potassium concentration is altered.

These observations justify the use of an equivalent circuit in which the effect of the transmitter is to add a parallel pathway selective for K^+ to the elements usually considered in defining the membrane potential. If ACh simultaneously altered another ionic permeability, the "combined" reversal would not occur at E_K. Indeed, alterations in the other ionic gradients do not alter the reversal potential.*

*As will be described in subsection 3.2, ACh has another effect on heart cells, decreasing a voltage-sensitive calcium conductance. However, this effect does not occur in the membrane potential range where one finds E_K in normal (physiological) solution, and therefore in this range the permeability change can be considered completely specific.

1.1.2. Effect of gamma-amino-butyric acid (GABA) on crayfish muscle. Increase in Cl-conductance

GABA is the transmitter liberated by the inhibitory nerves of arthropod exoskeletal muscle. The ionic mechanisms of the inhibition were first elucidated in crayfish muscle. In that muscle, the resting potential is usually little affected by an application of GABA. However, in a fibre that has been artificially depolarized by a current injection, GABA produces a hyperpolarization, and on a fibre that has been hyperpolarized, GABA produces a depolarization. The situation thus resembles that found for ACh in heart muscle, except for the fact that the reversal potential is usually close to the resting potential. This does not make the inhibition less effective, as GABA "clamps" the potential

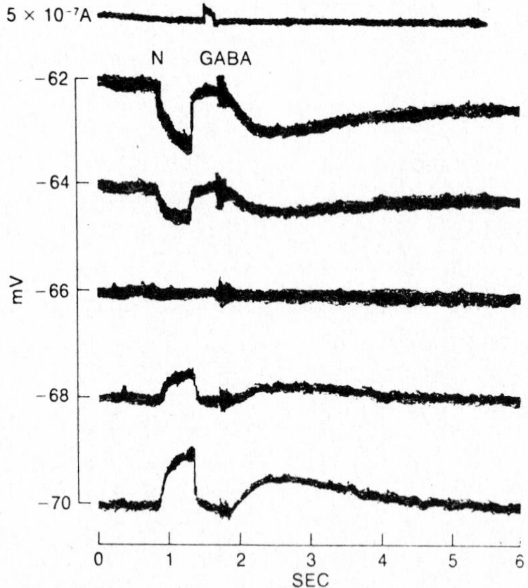

Fig. 1. Reversal of inhibitory responses resulting from an increased ionic conductance. The records were taken in crayfish muscle. The membrane potential (recorded with a KCl filled microelectrode) was set to the values indicated on the left of each record (by passing current through a second microelectrode). Two inhibitory responses were compared: the response to a brief train of stimulations applied to the inhibitory nerve (*N*) and the response to ionophoretically applied gamma-amino-butyric acid (GABA), the presumed transmitter. The synaptic potential and the GABA potentials reversed at the same level, near −66 mV. The top trace indicates the current applied through the GABA-filled pipette. [From Takeuchi and Takeuchi (1965).]

close to the resting potential, thus opposing the effects of depolarizing synaptic potentials.

A major difference between the action of ACh on heart and GABA on crayfish muscle is detected, however, when the reversal potentials of these responses are studied after varying the ionic electrochemical gradients. In the case of crayfish muscle, the reversal potential of the inhibition is identical to the chloride equilibrium potential. The same arguments used in the preceding subsection thus lead to the conclusion that the effect of GABA is a selective increase in Cl^- permeability (see Boistel and Fatt 1958, Takeuchi and Takeuchi 1967).

1.1.3. Generalization

The two types of permeability changes described above have been found in a large number of neurons and muscles (for a review see Ginsborg 1973).

1.1.4. Are there synaptic channels permeable to both Cl^- and K^+?

The idea that synaptic channels could be permeable to both Cl^- and K^+ was often considered a few years ago (e.g., see Eccles 1966), but has lost support in view of two series of observations. (a) In some cells, a given transmitter can activate both Cl^- and K^+ conductances – but these two conductances can be shown to be independent. This has been particularly well demonstrated in molluscan neurones, where the two conductance changes show marked kinetic differences, and can be separately studied by using selective agonists and antagonists (Kehoe 1972, see also Ascher and Kehoe 1975). Therefore, it appears possible that in those cases where the study of reversal potentials has suggested the simultaneous involvement of K^+ and Cl^- conductance changes, further studies would reveal that these two conductance changes involve separate ionic channels. (b) The Cl^- equilibrium potential can be altered by changes in the extracellular K^+ concentration. Such Cl^- redistribution is well known in cells which have a high "resting" Cl^- permeability (e.g., the skeletal muscle of frog), but it also occurs in neurones which have, at rest, a low Cl^- permeability, but which receive synaptic terminals controlling Cl^- channels. An increase in the extracellular K^+ concentration depolarizes these terminals and releases the transmitter, leading to a high Cl^- permeability and to redistribution of Cl^-.

A good example of such a situation is that of the stretch receptor of Crustacean muscle, where early data suggested that the inhibitory action of GABA involved K^+ and Cl^-, and where it was later shown that the conductance change was selective for Cl^- (Ozawa and Tsuda 1973, Meyer 1976) (see also Motokizawa et al. 1969 for the case of lobster muscle, Ascher et al. 1976 for the case of Aplysia neurones).

1.1.5. Are there inhibitory synaptic channels permeable to K^+ (Cl^-) and Na^+?

In molluscan neurones, a single transmitter can activate K^+, Cl^-, and excitatory "cationic" channels (see subsection 2.1) on the same neurone (see Ascher and Kehoe 1975). Similar situations have been found in vertebrate neurones (see, e.g., Hartzell et al. 1977, Kuba and Koketsu 1978). In the best known cases, pharmacological analysis has allowed the separation of these "mixed" effects into individual, selective ones. A working hypothesis is that in all cases where "non-selective" ionic permeability changes have been reported to underly inhibition, one may suspect a combination of a "pure" inhibitory effect (a Cl^- or a K^+ permeability increase) with another effect.

1.2. Potassium channels

In addition to the cholinergic inhibition of vertebrate heart, two cholinergic inhibitions involving an increase in K^+ permeability have been studied in some detail: in Aplysia ganglion cells (Kehoe 1972) and in the heart parasympathetic ganglion of the mudpuppy (Hartzell et al. 1977). Among the non-cholinergic K^+ inhibitions, an interesting example is that induced by dopamine on cockroach salivary glands (Ginsborg et al. 1974). Although transmitter-induced increases in K^+ permeability have been observed in a great number of cells (see subsection 1.2.4., and Putney 1979), those mentioned above are among the few which have been subjected to a sufficiently systematic study to establish that one was dealing with a pure K^+ permeability change.

1.2.1. Selectivity of the K^+ channels

In the systems considered above, in normal physiological saline, there is an excellent agreement between the reversal potential of the inhibitory response and the K^+ equilibrium potential. When "foreign" cations are added to the extracellular solution, the reversal potential is modified only by Rb^+ and Tl^+, indicating that those ions are able to cross the "K^+" channel. In solutions containing a mixture of Rb^+ andd K^+ (or Tl^+ and K^+) the reversal potential was shown (in Aplysia neurones) to follow the relation

$$E_{rev} = \frac{RT}{F} \ln \frac{P_K K_0 + P_{Rb} Rb_0}{P_K K_i}$$

where P_K and P_{Rb} are the K and Rb permeabilities, and K_0, Rb_0, K_i the extracellular and intracellular concentrations of K and Rb. The values obtained indicated that the sequence of permeabilities was

$$P_{Tl} : P_K : P_{Rb} \qquad 2:1:0.5$$

(Kehoe 1972, Ascher unpublished observations); i.e., the same sequence as found in squid axon K^+ channels.

1.2.2. Voltage dependence of the K^+ conductance

The voltage dependence of the transmitter controlled K^+ conductance is not always the same from one system to another, even when the same transmitter is involved (e.g., ACh).

In Aplysia neurones, the "instantaneous" I–V curve shows "outward" rectification: for a given driving force the net flux is larger when it is directed from the high concentration compartment (intracellular solution) to the low concentration one (Ginsborg and Kado 1975). In sino-atrial cells of the rabbit heart, the instantaneous I–V curve is linear (Noma and Trautwein 1979), and in frog atrial cells, the "quasi-instantaneous" I–V curve shows "inward" rectification (Garnier et al. 1978).

The picture is further complicated by the existence of slow relaxations both in Aplysia neurones and in heart cells (Marty and Ascher 1978, Noma and Trautwein 1978, 1979, Noma et al. 1979). If a voltage jump is applied after an ACh induced current has reached a steady level, the "instantaneous" current change is followed by a slow exponential relaxation which brings the current towards a new steady-state level. The relaxations have time constants of a few hundred ms. Their direction indicates an increased conductance after a hyperpolarizing jump presumably due to an increased lifetime of the channels (see subsection 2.4).

These slow relaxations explain the marked differences between the instantaneous and the steady-state I–V curves. In Aplysia neurones, where the instantaneous I–V curve shows outward rectification, the steady-state I–V relation can be nearly linear – after a hyperpolarization, the increased lifetime of the channels compensates for their reduced conductance (Marty and Ascher 1978). In rabbit cardiac (sino-atrial) cells, the instantaneous I–V relation is linear, but the steady-state relation shows inward rectification (Noma and Trautwein 1979, Noma et al. 1979).

1.2.3. Noise analysis of the K^+ channels

This analysis has until now only been done in heart cells (Noma and Trautwein 1978). The duration of the "elementary event" was found to be a few hundred ms – as expected from the time constants of the voltage jump induced relaxations. The elementary conductance was close to 4 pS. According to Noma and Trautwein (1978), the data can be fitted by a kinetic model similar to the one used at the frog endplate (Anderson and Stevens 1973). This does not account, however, for the slow rise time of the response to a brief ACh application (e.g., see Hartzell et al. 1977, Marty and Ascher 1978) and other kinetic models may have to be tested (see Kehoe and Marty 1980).

1.2.4. The role of Ca^{2+} in the opening of K^+ channels

In many cells an increase of the intracellular Ca^{2+} concentration triggers an increase in K^+ permeability. This effect, first observed in red cells, then in neurones, has been the subject of many studies in recent years (see Meech 1978) and it has been suggested that it was involved in transmitter- (and hormone-) induced K^+ permeability changes. In some cases, it was proposed that the transmitter primary effect was an increased Ca^{2+} permeability – the resulting entry of Ca^{2+} triggering an increased K^+ permeability. In other cases, the transmitter was supposed to trigger release of intracellular Ca^{2+} from an intracellular pool. Putney (1979) has recently reviewed the impressive series of arguments in favor of the general hypothesis than in secretory cells (salivary glands, liver, pancreas) and in smooth muscle, an increase of the intracellular calcium concentration is a necessary intermediate for the transmitter-induced K^+ permeability increase.

A generalization of this hypothesis appears, however, premature. Some transmitter-induced K^+ permeability increases disappear in Ca-free solutions (e.g., Bülbring and Tomita 1977), but some others persist – in particular the ACh-induced ones in Aplysia ganglion cells (Kehoe

1972). In this last case, it has been further shown that the ACh-induced K^+ permeability increase also persists after an intracellular injection of EGTA (a Ca^{2+} complexant) thus excluding also the possibility that the K^+ permeability increase be controlled by an intracellular release of Ca^{2+} (see Kehoe and Marty 1980). It therefore appears probable that there are two types of transmitter-induced K^+ permeability increases: those mediated by an increase of the intracellular Ca^{2+} concentration, and those independent of such an increase.

1.3. Chloride channels. Studies from crayfish muscle

1.3.1. Permeability sequences and conductance sequences

The GABA induced conductance in crayfish muscle is, in physiological solution, a strict Cl^- conductance. When foreign anions are introduced, they can be easily separated into those which can substitute for Cl^- (e.g., Br^-, NO_3^-) and those which are "impermeant" (e.g., pyroglutamate, sulfate, etc.). These observations, made at the crustacean neuromuscular junction but also in many vertebrate and invertebrate neurones, suggested to early observers that one of the mechanisms accounting for the channel selectivity was the relationship between the diameter of the "pore" and that of the (hydrated) ion (see Eccles 1966). On this basis alone, however, K^+ should be permeant. To explain that it is not, one has to make an additional assumption. Boistel and Fatt (1958) suggested that the anion–cation distinction resulted from the presence of a positive charge inside the channel.

A complete model of the "Cl" channel will have to account not only for the discrimination between permeant and impermeant ions, but also for the relative ease with which permeant ions cross the open channel, and for their interactions. These interactions have been the subject of a few studies, in particular by Takeuchi and Takeuchi (1971a,b). These authors analyzed the effects of GABA in solutions in which the external Cl^- had been replaced by another permeant ion (Br^-, NO_3^-, I^-, CNS^-). In one type of experiment, they measured the shift of the reversal potential when the extracellular Cl^- was replaced by anion A^-. If we designate by P_{Cl} and P_A the permeabilities to Cl^- and to A^-, the shift in the reversal potential, ΔE_{rev}, is given by:

$$\Delta E_{rev} = \frac{RT}{F}\left[\ln \frac{P_A A_0}{P_{Cl} Cl_i} - \ln \frac{Cl_0}{Cl_i}\right]$$

and one can therefore calculate P_A/P_{Cl}.

In a second series of experiments, Takeuchi and Takeuchi measured the conductance increase produced by a given dose of GABA, first with Cl^- as the external anion, then after Cl^- had been replaced by a foreign anion. From these experiments it was possible to evaluate the ratio g_{Cl}/g_A of the GABA activated conductance.

The most striking result obtained was that the permeability sequence did not match the conductance sequence. When the study was done in the presence of relatively large GABA concentrations (Takeuchi and Takeuchi 1971a), the permeability sequence was

$$CNS^- > I^- > NO_3^- > Br^- > Cl^-$$

while the conductance sequence was

$$BR^- > Cl^- > CNS^- > I^- > NO_3^- .$$

Furthermore, both sequences could be altered by varying the GABA concentrations (Takeuchi and Takeuchi 1971b).

A similar discrepancy between permeability and conductance sequences was observed for the anionic "resting" conductance of a crustacean muscle by Hagiwara et al. (1971), and interpreted by a model which may be valid for the GABA activated channels. Hagiwara et al. assumed, as previous authors had done, that the Cl^- channels were positively charged and they treated the system as an ion-exchange one. In such a case, the permeability ratio is given by

$$P_A/P_{Cl} = (U_A/U_{Cl})K_{Cl}^A,$$

where U_A/U_{Cl} is the mobility ratio, and K_{Cl}^A represents the ion-exchange equilibrium constant of the pore site for A^- and Cl^-. The ratio of the conductances (measured in a solution containing A^- and in a solution containing Cl^-) will be

$$g_A/g_{Cl} = \frac{\ln(U_{Cl}/U_A)}{(U_{Cl}/U_A)-1} .$$

The conductance sequence will therefore depend only on the mobility ratio (U_{Cl}/U_A), whereas the permeability sequence will depend also on the value of K_{Cl}^A. The two sequences can be different, as an ion with low mobility may have a high affinity for the channel site.

There are other possible complications in the case studied by Takeuchi and Takeuchi since the measured conductances depend not only on the elementary conductance of the Cl^- channels, but also on the number of open channels. The number of open channels depends on the GABA concentration, but probably also on the ion present in the solution, as shown by the variations in the decay time of the synaptic current (see subsection 1.3.3.). The availability of noise analysis for this system (Dudel et al. 1978) should now allow the study of the variations of both the elementary conductance and of the mean open time in the presence of foreign anions – as has been done at excitatory ACh synapses (see subsections 2.3 and 2.4).

Already, however, one can say that the data of Takeuchi and Takeuchi reinforce the hypothesis that the selectivity of the anion channel cannot be explained solely by the diameter of the pore, and that there is probably a binding step in the permeation process.

1.3.2. Voltage dependence of the elementary conductance

The peak of the inhibitory synaptic current does not vary linearly with voltage: the conductance decreases when the cell is hyperpolarized below the inversion potential (Dudel 1977, Onodera and Takeuchi 1979). This rectification is in the direction predicted by the "constant field" theory, i.e., for equal but opposite driving forces, the conductance is larger when the current flows from the compartment where the ionic concentration is higher (the outside solution in the case of Cl^-). Dudel (1977) was indeed able to fit his data with the Goldman current equation, assuming a constant permeability coefficient. The data of Onodera and Takeuchi (1979) on the other hand suggest that the rectification is larger than predicted by the Goldman equation. Both studies used the synaptic current as a measure of the conductance, and therefore the voltage dependence of the elementary conductance could have been influenced by the possible voltage dependence of opening (and perhaps closing) rates. The noise studies which are under way (Dudel et al. 1978) should help to clarify this point. They have already indicated that the elementary conductance is indeed voltage dependent, decreasing from about 14 to 9 pS when the membrane potential is increased from -60 to -100 mV.

1.3.3. Open time of the Cl^- channels

The decay of the inhibitory synaptic current in crayfish muscle is exponential, and its time constant decreases when the cell is hyperpolarized (Dudel 1977, Onodera and Takeuchi 1979). That this decay is controlled by the mean open time of the channel, as in frog muscle (see subsection 2.4) is quite likely, as similar time constants are obtained from noise analysis (Dudel et al. 1978) and from voltage jump studies (Dudel 1978).

It is not known if the voltage dependence of the open time is linked with a peculiarity of the receptor–transmitter interaction, or with a channel property.

The open time appears to depend on the ion present in the solution. It increases when Cl^- is replaced by Br^- or I^-, the degree of prolongation being in the order $I^- > Br^- > Cl^-$ (Onodera and Takeuchi 1979). This, combined with the data (subsection 1.3.1.) indicating binding of the permeant ions inside the channel, could indicate that, as suggested for another system (see subsection 2.4, Marchais and Marty 1979), the open time of the channel is controlled by the binding of ions inside the channel.

1.3.4. Receptor–channel interaction

As for all other systems (see in particular subsection 2.3) the question is open concerning how the parameters of the elementary event (elementary conductance, lifetime) depend on the agonist–receptor interaction. Observations which may help to settle this point in the case of Cl^- channels are those of Barker and McBurney (1979) on the Cl^- currents produced by GABA and glycine on mouse spinal neurones studied in culture. These authors were able to analyse the noise associated with the currents and observed that the parameters of the elementary event (measured in the same neurone) were different: the elementary conductance was about 15 pS for GABA, about 30 pS for glycine; the channel mean open time was about 27 ms for GABA, and only 5 ms for glycine.

GABA and glycine responses show "cross-desensitization" (a prolonged GABA application reduces the glycine response, and inversely), and this rules out entirely independent receptor–channel complexes for GABA and glycine. Among various other possible interpretations, the authors favor the one in which distinct GABA and glycine receptors can share a common channel. The elementary conductance and the open time would not be intrinsic properties of the channel, but would depend on the receptor through which the channel has been opened.

2. Increases in ionic permeability leading to excitation of the target cell

2.1. The reversal potential. "Cationic" channels

The best known excitatory chemical synapse is the frog neuromuscular junction where the transmitter, ACh, produces an increase in ionic permeability. Many other excitatory synapses appear to operate in a similar way (see Ginsborg 1975).

The measurement of a reversal potential for excitatory synaptic responses, e.g. at the frog neuromuscular junction (del Castillo and Katz 1954), has been more difficult than for inhibitory synaptic responses, because the reversal potential is above the threshold for action potential generation, i.e. in a membrane potential range where the conductance is high, the potential difficult to control, and where, in muscle, contraction is likely to occur. The observation of an inversion potential has been made progressively easier with the introduction of voltage clamp, and of methods suppressing depolarization-contraction coupling in muscle.

The observation of an inversion for an excitatory response allows one to describe the conductance change by an equivalent circuit similar to those used for inhibitory responses in the preceding section, with the only difference being that E_{rev} is now "above" the threshold for excitation (action potential threshold and/or activation of a Ca^{2+} conductance) (fig. 2).

In most cases where the reversal potential has been measured for an excitatory response, the value obtained was between -20 and $+20$ mV. There are a few reports of higher or lower values, but in most of those cases, the difference could be due to experimental difficulties.*

A reversal potential between -20 and $+20$ mV cannot be equated to the equilibrium potential of a single ion: in physiological solutions E_K is usually between -80 and -100 mV; E_{Cl} varies from cell to cell but lies between -30 and -90 mV; E_{Na} is usually above $+50$ mV; and E_{Ca} is still higher. It was thus soon recognized that the excitatory conductance changes involved more than one ion species. As discussed below, this has been amply confirmed and in many systems, the conductance increase has been shown to involve Na^+, K^+, Ca^{2+}, and Mg^{2+}, but not anions (Takeuchi and Takeuchi 1960).

At one point, it was considered possible that the various ionic species could cross the membrane through independent (private) channels. This has been ruled out, in particular after noise analysis at the frog neuromuscular junction showed that the ACh induced noise disappeared completely at the reversal potential (Dionne and Ruff 1977).

*Among these difficulties I shall mention (a) the distance between the site at which currents are recorded; (b) the possible activation, by a single transmitter, of excitatory and inhibitory conductances (see subsection 1.1.5); and (c) the voltage-dependence of the channel open-time, which precludes extrapolation of I–V curves for the evaluation of the inversion potential (see Dionne and Stevens 1975).

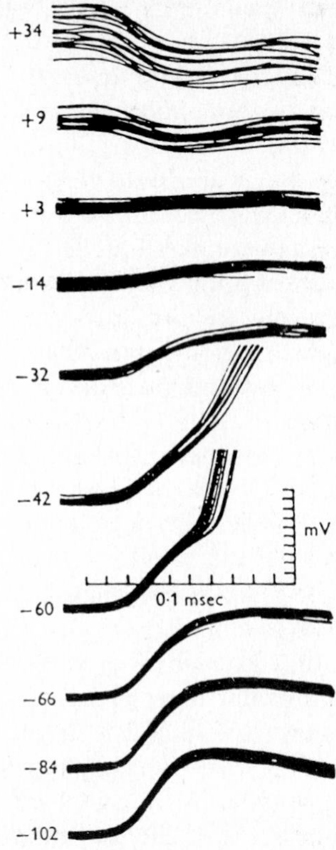

Fig. 2. Reversal of an excitatory synaptic response resulting from an increased conductance. The records were taken in Cat motoneurones. The membrane potential was set at the values indicated to the left at each set of records by passing current through one barrel of a double-barrelled intracellular microelectrode – the other barrel being used to record the membrane potential. The traces at −42 and −60 mV show action potentials starting on top of the synaptic potentials. At −66 mV and below the synaptic response does not reach the spike threshold; at −32 mV, the spike mechanism is inactivated by the prolonged depolarization. [From Coombs et al. (1955).]

2.2. Selectivity of the ionic conductance change

Many cations can replace Na^+ in carrying current across the channels opened by ACh at the frog end-plate: Li^+, K^+, Cs^+, as well as Ca^{2+}, Mg^{2+}, Sr^{2+}, and a number of organic cations. In a recent study, Maeno, Edwards and Aranku (1977) have tested the permeability to a series of organic cations of increasing size and have concluded that the data could be interpreted by assuming a channel diameter of 6.4 Å. Although the permeability data were based on rather indirect measurements, they probably give a good indication of the size of the channel, and are to be contrasted to similar, more refined studies on Na^+ and K^+ axon channels, which have led to smaller diameters (see Bergman and Meves this volume).

Another approach to the study of the selectivity of the channels opened by the excitatory transmitters has been to analyse the effects on the reversal potential of variations in the extracellular cation concentrations. In the case of the frog end-plate, the results (summarized by Lewis 1979) clearly show that the channel is permeant to Na^+, K^+, Mg^{2+}, Ca^{2+}, as well as to larger molecules like Tris(tris(hydroxymethyl) aminomethane) or glucosamine. An attempt was then made of a quantitative interpretation, and it was found that a number of theories could account satisfactorily for the data. Among these theories was the "constant field" theory (Goldman 1943, Hodgkin and Katz 1949). As shown by Lewis (1979) this theory can account for the variations observed, provided that to its original assumptions (constant field, independence of ionic fluxes) one adds the assumptions that divalent cations are charge carriers and that there is an adequate density of negative surface charges on the external side of the membrane. These are very plausible assumptions. However, they do not validate the theory used. An equally good fit of the data can be obtained from another model, derived from the Eyring rate theory, in which the channel is assumed to contain a single energy barrier over which permeant ions have to hop. Futhermore, analysis of a different set of data (concerning the elementary conductance, see subsection 2.3) strongly suggests that the hypothesis of independence of the ionic fluxes is not valid.

This latter result suggests that it may not be worth attempting to describe in too much detail the variations of the reversal potential in various ionic media, as these variations do not constitute a very sensitive test of the mechanisms of the ionic transfer. The data obtained thus far in frog and in many other preparations (electroplaque, insect muscle, ganglion cells) remain interesting – in particular because they show a remarkable similarity, suggesting that in all these systems the ionic transfer obeys similar rules.

2.3. Single channel conductance

The current carried through a single ACh induced channel at the frog end-plate ("elementary current") was first deduced from noise analysis

(Katz and Miledi 1972, Anderson and Stevens 1973), then from single channel recording (Neher and Sakmann 1976). The value is close to 2×10^{-12} Å at a membrane potential of -80 mV (E_m). Assuming a reversal potential of 0 mV, the elementary (chord) conductance, γ, is therefore 25×10^{-12} S.

A current of 2×10^{-12} Å corresponds to a net ionic flow of a few thousand ions per millisecond – a very strong suggestion that the permeation does occur through a channel and not through a carrier, for which it would imply prohibitive speeds.

In other excitatory synapses where the elementary conductance has been measured, the values obtained were usually quite close to those obtained in frog, sometimes slightly lower (e.g., in Aplysia, although our initial low value has had to be revised upward –Ascher et al. 1978a) sometimes clearly higher (100 – 200×10^{-12} S in locust muscle; Anderson et al. 1978, Patlak et al. 1979). All of these values appear higher than the corresponding ones found for the axon Na^+ and K^+ channels (see Neher and Stevens 1976) in agreement with the data indicating that the synaptic excitatory channel has a lower selectivity than the axon channels (see also subsections 1.2 and 1.3).

Systematic studies of the variations of the elementary current as a function of membrane potential, temperature, pH, composition of the extracellular solution are under way. At the frog neuromuscular junction, Lewis (1979) measured the ACh induced elementary current in solutions where the extracellular NaCl had been partially replaced by sucrose, and where the extracellular Ca^{2+} concentration was altered from 1–80 mM/L. As already mentioned (see subsection 2.2) the variations of the reversal potential in these solutions could be explained in the frame of the "constant field" theory, provided one took into account the permeability to divalent cations and assumed an adequate density of external surface charges (about 0.002 electronic charges $Å^2$). When this same approach was applied to the data on the elementary conductance, it described approximately correctly the variations observed when replacing NaCl with sucrose, but failed completely to account for the effects of variations of the extracellular concentrations of Ca^{2+}, $(Ca)_0$. In particular, the Goldman approach predicts that adding Ca^{2+} to a 75% Na^+ Ringer solution should increase γ, whereas in effect a decrease of γ was observed.

To interpret these results, Lewis and Stevens (1979) have proposed a model in which the permeant ions bind to anionic sites inside the channel. Competition for binding to these sites accounts for the observed effects of changes in $(Ca)_0$. Assuming a single binding site with an energy barrier on each side, and making a series of additional assumptions (that the energy barriers are different for each type of ion; that the barrier heights are not changed by the presence of the other ions in the bathing solution; that the binding site must be empty before it can be occupied by an ion) the authors could satisfactorily account for the experimental results. As they noted, however, the theory does not provide a unique set of values for all the parameters, and a way will have to be devised for further refinement. One possibility may be offered by the simultaneous analysis of another "single channel" parameter – the mean open time of the channel, as described in subsection 2.4.

2.4. *Channel open time*

At the frog neuromuscular junction, the mean open time of the ACh-controlled channels has been measured by a variety of methods (noise analysis, voltage-jump induced relaxations, analysis of the decay of the synaptic current, single channel recording) which all lead to similar values of a few milliseconds (see Steinbach and Stevens 1976, Neher and Sakmann 1976). The exact value of the mean open time depends on the frog species, on temperature, on pH, on the ionic composition of the extracellular solution, etc. Values in the same range have been found at other excitatory synapses operating by an increased cationic permeability, whether cholinergic or not (see Neher and Stevens 1977).

In many of the cases studied thus far – particularly in all cases where ACh is excitatory – the mean open time increases when the cell is hyperpolarized. The origin of this effect remains the subject of conflicting interpretations:

Kordås (1969) and Adams (1976) suggested that ACh binding was increased by cell hyperpolarization.

Magleby and Stevens (1972) suggested that the ACh receptor bears a net dipole moment, and that changes in the orientation of the dipole also control the changes in the mean open time.

Ascher et al. (1978a) suggested that binding of permeant cations inside the channel (see subsection 2.3) prevented the channel closure – an hypothesis which has recently received additional support from the observations of Marchais and Marty (1979). These authors have analyzed, in Aplysia neurones, the variations of the elementary current and of the mean open time when the composition of the extracellular solution was altered. They observed that the open time was decreased when divalent cations were absent, and was further reduced if NaCl was replaced by sucrose. They were able to interpret the data using a model of the channel quite similar to one of those used by Lewis and Stevens (1979) (see subsection 2.3) – two energy barriers separated by a well, the external barrier lower than the internal one – but with the additional hypothesis that the channels cannot close with a bound ion inside. The scheme can be written

$$R \rightleftharpoons R^* \overset{I}{\rightleftharpoons} R^*I,$$

where R is the closed state and R^* and R^*I the open channel without and with a bound ion, respectively. The probabilities of transition between R and R^* were assumed to be independent of the channel energy profile. The probabilities of transition between R^* and R^*I were assumed to depend on this profile, which itself depends on the ionic species, I. The first reaction (the conformation change) is assumed to be much slower than the second (binding and dissociation of the permeant ion).

The data of Marchais and Marty can be accounted for by this model. As in the case of Lewis and Stevens' model, the agreement does not imply a unique solution, and more stringent tests will have to be devised. For the model to be adequate for describing the frog end-plate, it will be necessary to account for the finding (in frog) that the channel open time is reduced when Ca^{2+} replaces Na^+ outside (Bregestovski et al. 1979), a result opposite to that obtained from Aplysia neurones (Marchais and Marty 1979).

2.5. Channel block

The data presented in the preceding sections suggest that the channels opened by excitatory transmitters are (a) relatively wide and (b) bear a negative charge. Additional support for this view comes from studies of compounds that appear to enter the mouth of a channel, but as they are unable to cross it, they "plug" it, thus acting as "channel blockers".

This type of effect, first documented by studies of Armstrong on K^+ channels in squid axon (see Armstrong 1975) has recently been found to account for the effects of a number of pharmacological agents acting at synapses – local anaesthetics, barbiturates, but also compounds which were assumed to compete with ACh at the receptor level (see Adams

1976b, Ascher et al. 1978b, Neher and Steinbach 1978). In the case of local anaesthetics, the early studies of Steinbach on the frog end-plate had already indicated that the change of shape of the synaptic potential in the presence of lidocaine derivatives could be interpreted by assuming that the blocking action of the antagonist occurred after the channels had opened ("sequential model"). After the introduction of new methods of analysis – noise analysis, voltage-jump induced relaxations – it became possible to go a step further, and to show that when the channels were blocked by the antagonists, they were completely occluded (an hypothesis that Steinbach could not test, since he had no access to the measurement of elementary current). Both the sequential mechanism of action and the all-or-none block of the channels were confirmed by the work of Neher and Steinbach (1978). These authors recorded the current flowing through single channels in the presence of ACh and of local anaesthetic derivatives, and showed that the square pulses normally observed in the presence of ACh were replaced by "bursts" of shorter pulses. The detailed analysis of these bursts showed that they corresponded to the "chopping" of the elementary event in a series of shorter ones, due to the repetitive blocking and unblocking of the channel by the local anaesthetic. The reaction scheme could be written (see Marty 1978):

$$R \rightleftharpoons R^* \overset{B}{\rightleftharpoons} R^*B,$$

where R is the closed state, R^* the open state, and R^*B the "blocked" state.

The analogy of this scheme with that presented in subsection 2.4 can be pursued by analyzing the effects of changes in membrane potential. The blockade produced by a given concentration of local anaesthetic increases when the cell is hyperpolarized, and this can be quantitatively explained by assuming that the "channel blocking" compound enters the channel and plugs it by binding to a deep site.

The behaviour of local anaesthetics is shared by a surprisingly large number of compounds, including ACh antagonists (like tubocurarine) which were for a long time considered to bind exclusively to the ACh receptor (see, e.g. Ascher et al. 1978b). There is a good possibility that the site at which all these compounds bind is the site that presumably binds the permeant ions.

These data are interesting inasmuch as they complete the description of the channel that has been deduced from other studies. But they also have important implications for the interpretation of pharmacological effects. In particular, channel-block is a frequency dependent block; i.e. the intensity of the block increases with the frequency of stimulation. This may lead to a reappraisal of the mode of action of a number of drugs for which the frequency dependence of their blocking action had suggested an alteration in presynaptic function.

3. Transmitter control of voltage dependent Ca^{2+} channels

In some of the cases considered in the preceding sections, the properties of the channels opened by the transmitter may be sensitive to change in membrane potential, but in the absence of the transmitter the channels cannot be opened by a change in membrane potential. We shall now consider cases where the transmitter affects channels which can be opened, in its absence, by depolarization. The best understood of these effects concerns Ca^{2+} channels which are opened by depolarization but where the transmitter can modify the number of channels opened by a given depolarization.

3.1. Ca^{2+} channels

Ca^{2+} channels opened by depolarization are ubiquitous. The Ca^{2+} entry which follows the depolarization triggers contraction (in muscle), liberation of transmitter (at nerve terminals) and secretory activity (in gland cells) and it possibly controls other cellular functions.

The Ca^{2+} channels found in various cells appear remarkably similar throughout the animal kingdom and from cell to cell. They have been found in egg cells, Paramecium, leucocytes, etc. Failure to detect them in a few cases may have been linked to the fact that they can be masked by the presence of fluoride in the solutions used for internal perfusion (Kostyuk et al. 1975) but also by a rise in the intracellular concentration of Ca^{2+}, values as low as 10^{-6} M being apparently sufficient to produce a substantial block (Kostyuk and Krishtal 1977, Takahashi and Yoshii 1978, Tillotson 1979).

The Ca^{2+} channels are permeable to Sr^{2+} and Ba^{2+}; they are blocked by La^{3+}, Co^{2+}, Mn^{2+}, Ni^{2+}, and Mg^{2+}. They usually start opening when the membrane is depolarized above -40 mV. The kinetics of activation are relatively well understood. Inactivation is still the matter of some dispute, probably due to difficulties encountered in studying currents while maintaining constant Ca_i^{2+}. Although the currents carried through the Ca^{2+} channels are usually much smaller than the currents crossing Na^+ and K^+ channels, the "resting" intracellular Ca^{2+} concentration is so low (usually $<10^{-7}$ M) that even weak currents may be able to change it substantially. Very powerful buffering structures exist in the cytoplasm, but they may not be able to control the Ca^{2+} concentration just below the membrane. Thus, even in those cases where it has been possible to monitor the Ca^{2+} concentration in the whole cell (e.g., with aequorin or arsenazo III or by using Ca^{2+} microelectrodes) it is still possible that local concentrations below the membrane could follow a different evolution from that followed by concentrations measured at a deeper level.

The Ca^{2+} currents can be visualized with particular clarity if other voltage dependent conductances are absent or have been reduced by pharmacological means. Under such conditions, they can lead to a regenerative depolarization, and thus to a "Ca^{2+} spike". Ca^{2+} spikes were first observed in crustacean muscles (see Hagiwara 1975). In 1969, Katz and Miledi showed that they could be produced in squid axon terminals treated with tetrodotoxin (to block voltage-dependent Na^+ channels) and tetraethylammonium (to block voltage-dependent K^+ channels). Since then, they have been observed in an increasing number of cells.

As described below, transmitters can modify the voltage-dependent Ca^{2+} conductances, either by decreasing or by increasing the number of channels opened at a given membrane potential. The demonstration of this type of effect is most easily done by showing that the transmitter shortens, or prolongs, a Ca^{2+} action potential. Although the complete analysis of the mechanisms of these effects requires voltage clamp studies, these are not likely to be easy to perform in many cases, and studies of "Ca^{2+} action potentials" are likely to remain important.

3.2. *Transmitter blockade of Ca^{2+} currents*

One of the best known cases where a transmitter reduces the voltage-dependent Ca^{2+} conductance is that of the effect of ACh on the heart action potential. The key observation of a shortening of the action potential was made quite early, but not immediately understood. In 1956, Hutter and Trautwein recorded the membrane potential in the tortoise heart (sinus venosus) and noticed that the hyperpolarizing action of ACh (see subsection 1.1) was accompanied by a marked shortening of the action potentials produced by direct electrical stimulation of the cells. This could have been due to a shunting effect resulting from the increased conductance; however, the shortening persisted after the hyperpolarization had subsided. At that time it was not known that the long duration of heart cell action potentials was due to the presence of an important voltage-sensitive Ca^{2+} conductance, and it is not therefore surprising that the observed effect could not be fully explained.

That the shortening of the action potentials was the result of an altered Ca^{2+} conductance was suggested by a number of authors in the early seventies. The complete demonstration, however, had to await the voltage clamp studies of Ikemoto and Goto (1975, 1977), Giles and Tsien (1975), and Giles and Noble (1976). These authors showed that

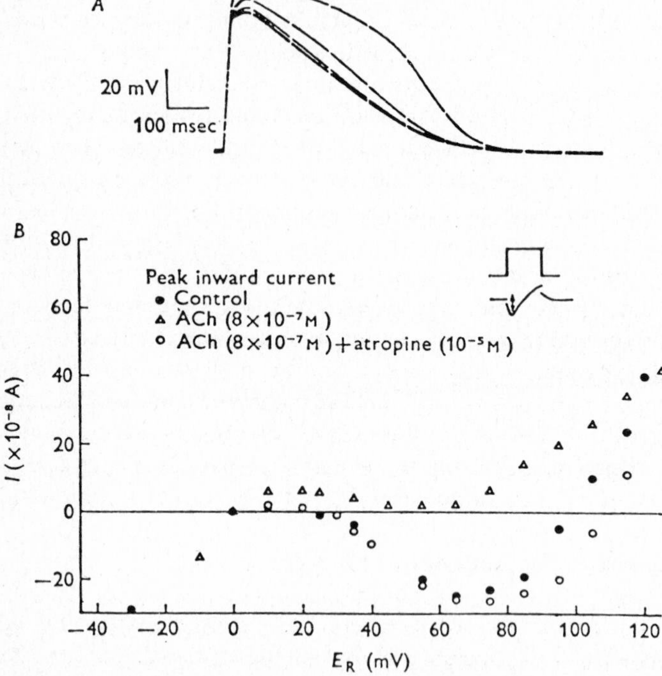

Fig. 3. Effects of acetylcholine on heart action potentials. (A) Action potentials were recorded in the atrium of the frog's heart bathed in a physiological solution containing tetrodotoxin. The highest action potential was recorded before exposure to ACh (8×10^{-7} M). Progressively lower and briefer action potentials were recorded 2, 4, and 8 min after ACh application. (B) Voltage-clamp analysis. Currents (ordinate) were recorded in the presence of tetrodotoxin, before and after step voltage changes from a holding potential of −75 mV to a variable potential (abscissa) ACh reduces the inward current produced by depolarization. The effect of ACh is blocked by atropine. [From Giles and Tsien (1975).]

the shortening was caused by a decrease in the Ca^{2+} current, and not by an increase of the voltage-dependent K^+ current (fig. 3).

The shortening of the heart action potential by ACh accounts for the "negative inotropic" effect of ACh: by reducing the entry of Ca^{2+} at each beat, ACh reduces the force of each contraction without changing the heart rhythm. The "negative chronotropic" effect of ACh (slowing of the rhythm) is, on the other hand, probably controlled primarily by the increase in K^+ permeability studied in subsection 1.1. The two affects of ACh coexist in different proportions in different heart regions, thus allowing a subtle control of the two parameters regulating blood ejection: rhythm and pressure.

Phenomena similar to those described above have been recently found in increasing numbers not only in muscle but also in neurones [see the review of Kehoe and Marty (1980)]. In most cases, the experiments involved the study of an action potential in which the duration of the plateau phase had been first increased by pharmacological means, then shown to be markedly reduced by application of a presumed transmitter. These preliminary studies are currently being followed up by voltage clamp experiments which indicate that in these instances as well the transmitter acts by reducing the voltage-dependent Ca^{2+} conductance.

Although most of the experiments on neurones have been performed on cell bodies, the effects observed appear particularly well suited for explaining the phenomenon of *presynaptic inhibition*. This is a process by which one neurone (A) can control the release of transmitter from another neurone (B) through a synapse which usually occurs between the terminals of neurones A and B. How liberation of the transmitter by neurone A inhibits liberation of transmitter from neurone B has long been a matter of speculation. Hyperpolarization of the terminals of neurone B has not appeared to be an adequate hypothetical mechanism, since in many cells such hyperpolarization increases the height of the action potential, which would thus lead to increased release. Depolarization of the terminals has also been considered as a possible alternative mechanism, but such an action would be expected to lead to continuous release rather than inhibition if the effect is too intense. In contrast, modulation of the voltage-dependent Ca^{2+} conductance would permit the modification of the release mechanism without a concomitant modification of the membrane potential of the "resting terminal".

The fact that a transmitter is able to reduce the Ca^{2+} conductance may have other functional consequences than that of reducing secretory or contractile activity. Ca^{2+} enters the cell bodies of neurones when these are invaded by action potentials. The functional role of this Ca^{2+} entry is not known, but can be expected to be modulated by those transmitters which regulate the Ca^{2+} conductance.

3.3. Transmitter-controlled increase of the Ca^{2+} current

The classical example of a transmitter induced increase in the voltage-dependent Ca^{2+} conductance is that seen in heart cells in the presence of adrenaline. This transmitter causes a marked prolongation of the plateau phase of the action potential. Voltage clamp studies have shown that the plateau phase is primarily due to the activation of voltage-dependent Ca^{2+} channels, and that adrenaline increases the number of open channels in the potential range where the plateau occurs. There is no change in the selectivity of the Ca^{2+} channels, and there is no change in the kinetics of opening and closing of these channels. The effect of adrenaline thus corresponds to an increase in the number of "available" channels (see Vassort et al. 1969, Reuter and Scholz 1977, Brown et al. 1979).

(This "primary" effect of adrenaline on Ca^{2+} conductance is associated with effects on K^+ conductances which are different according to the type of cardiac cells considered, and which will not be described in detail. I shall just mention that some of these K^+ conductance changes are secondary to an increased Ca^{2+} entry – probably via the Meech effect described in subsection 1.2.4. – while others imply direct control of voltage dependent K^+ conductances involved in determining the rhythm of the heart, as described hereafter in subsection 4.3.)

Potentiating effects of a transmitter on Ca^{2+} currents are also very likely to occur in nerve endings. In molluscan neurones, Klein and Kandel (1978) have observed a spectacular prolongation of a Ca^{2+} action potential by serotonin. This effect was observed in the soma of neurones known to be under the control of a serotonin containing neurone. Such a change in voltage dependent Ca^{2+} conductance at the level of the terminals would readily account for the increased transmitter release observed in response to activation of the presynaptic serotoninergic neurone or when serotonin was applied directly on the terminals by ionophoresis from a microelectrode (see Shimahara and Tauc 1977). Voltage clamp studies remain to be done to specify in this case the relative roles of Ca^{2+} and K^+ conductance changes.

In both heart cells and molluscan neurones the potentiation of the Ca^{2+} conductance by the transmitter is strongly correlated with an increase in cyclic AMP, suggesting a causal relation between the two phenomena (see Tsien 1977, Klein and Kandel 1978). One possibility is that "non-functional" Ca^{2+} channels present in the membrane are transformed into "functional" channels after being phosphorylated via the cyclic AMP system (see Tsien 1977, Reuter and Scholz 1977).

The functional value of an increased Ca^{2+} conductance is obvious in the case of muscle cells, gland cells, and presynaptic terminals. In the case of heart, the increased Ca^{2+} entry accounts for the well-known increase in the force of the contraction produced by adrenaline. In the case of presynaptic terminals, the increased Ca^{2+} entry probably accounts for the effects which had been previously described as "presynaptic facilitation" (some produced by neuronal interaction, others by blood borne compounds). At some neuromuscular synapses, it appears possible that the same compound acts both presynaptically (increasing transmitter release) and postsynaptically (increasing muscle contraction) (see, e.g. Weiss et al. 1978). Finally, inasmuch as the increase in Ca^{2+} entry also occurs at the level of the cell body, it is likely that it has some functional effects at that level as well.

4. Atypical transmitter-induced potential changes

4.1. Excitatory potentials resulting from a decrease in ionic permeability

Some slow depolarizing potentials (produced either by a synaptic transmitter or by a compound presumed to be a synaptic transmitter) differ strikingly from the frog end-plate potential in that, when analysed at various membrane potentials, they decrease when the cell is hyperpolarized, and eventually invert at a potential situated well below the threshold for excitation.

This behavior can be explained by an equivalent circuit in which the transmitter reduces an ionic conductance. The ionic selectivity of this conductance decrease has been analyzed in only a few cases. In two studies on molluscan neurones, the reversal potential has been shown to be equal to E_K (Gerschenfeld and Paupardin-Tritsch 1974, Kehoe 1975) and therefore the responses can be attributed to a selective decrease in K^+ conductance (fig. 4). In other cases (Weight 1974), the reversal potential may not be exactly equal to E_K, and a reduction of K^+ permeability may be superimposed on another event.

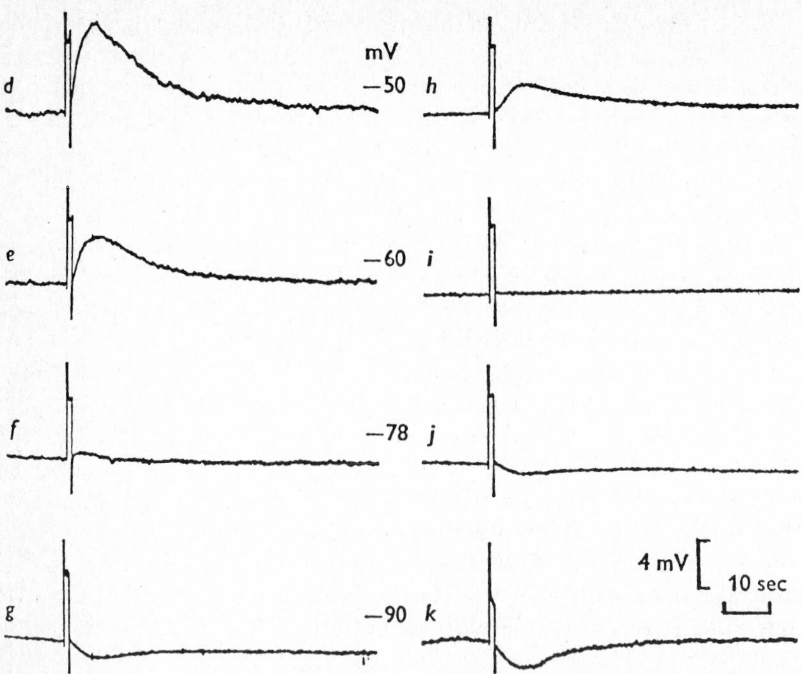

Fig. 4. Reversal of an excitatory response resulting from a decrease in ionic permeability. Snail neurone excited by serotonin. Before application of serotonin, the membrane potential was set at the values indicated in the central column by passing current through one barrel of a double-barrelled microelectrode. Serotonin was then applied by a brief ionophoretic pulse. Left: in the "physiological" solution containing 5 mM/L of K^+, the response inverts at −78 mV. Right: when the K^+ concentration in the extracellular solution was doubled the reversal potential shifted by 18 mV which is the predicted shift of the K^+ equilibrium potential. Thus, in this neurone, serotonin produces a decrease in K^+ permeability. [From Gerschenfeld and Paupardin-Tritsch (1974).]

Excitation mediated by a conductance decrease has some important functional differences with the type of excitation found at the end-plate. In particular, the fact that there is a decrease in the "input" conductance of the cell increases the depolarizing effect of other excitatory inputs (Weight 1974, Carew and Kandel 1976), whereas, when excitation is mediated by a conductance increase, other excitatory responses are likely to be reduced by a shunting effect. More generally, excitatory effects mediated by a conductance decrease appear well adapted to the production of a long-lasting series of action potentials.

4.2. *Inhibitory potentials resulting from a decrease in ionic permeability*

Contrary to the hyperpolarizing inhibitory potentials described in section 1, some inhibitory potentials decrease in amplitude when the cell is depolarized, and eventually inverted. This behavior indicates a decrease in ionic conductance. The conductance present before transmitter application produces a "resting" inward current; the suppression of this inward current induces a hyperpolarization.

This type of response has been observed in sympathetic ganglion cells (see Weight 1974, Kuba and Koketsu 1978) and in molluscan neurones (e.g., Gerschenfeld and Paupardin-Tritsch 1974). The selectivity of the channels which are closed by the transmitter action is a matter of discussion. In the case of molluscan neurones inhibited by serotonin, the channels are permeable to Na^+ and K^+ (Gerschenfeld and Paupardin-Tritsch 1974). Later studies have suggested also the involvement of Ca^{2+} (Pellmar and Wilson 1978). These observations have to be related to those described in subsection 4.3, suggesting that a transmitter can increase a inward current (Na^+/Ca^{2+}) controlling the burst pattern. More generally, this type of transmitter action presents similarities with the effects described in section 3 in that the transmitter modulates a preexisting permeability.

4.3. *Transmitter control of pacemaker and bursting cells*

Pacemaker cells emit action potentials at a regular frequency. The best known are those controlling the heart rhythm, but many neurones exhibit similar regular rhythmic activity.

Bursting cells are also rhythmic cells but they produce trains of action potentials separated by silent intervals. A classical example is found in smooth muscle cells of the digestive tract, but bursting patterns are found in many neurones.

The permeability changes underlying both pacemaker and bursting activity patterns do not appear to be of a single kind. Even in a given organ like the heart, the pacemaker currents of one region (sinus) may be different from those of another (e.g., Purkinje fibres). In many systems, a precise analysis of the conductance involved in setting the rhythm remains to be done [for recent reviews see two recent symposia published in Fed. Proc. 37 (1978) J. Exp. Biol. (August 1979) see also Noble (1975), Bolton (1979)]. The mechanisms by which transmitters can modify the rhythms of pacemakers or bursters is even less well understood. Four examples will indicate the variety of mechanisms which have been encountered:

(a) In the atrial cardiac cells adrenaline induces an acceleration which appears to result partly from a mechanism similar to that described in subsection 3.3 (i.e., an increase in the Ca^{2+} conductance activated by depolarization), and partly from a change in another voltage-sensitive current called i_f (Brown et al. 1979), activated between −90 and −60 mV and probably carried by K^+. Adrenaline increases and speeds up the hyperpolarization induced inactivation of i_f, and in so doing speeds the depolarization of the cell following a sudden repolarization at the end of a spike.

(b) In the Purkinje fibres of the heart, adrenaline also accelerates the pacemaker activity, but the mechanism is different from the one found in atrial cells. The pacemaker depolarization (the depolarization which leads to a new action potential after the preceding one has subsided) is mainly controlled by the suppression (by hyperpolarization) of a K^+ current (i_{K_2}) activated between −90 and −60 mV resembling i_f of the atrial cells. But the acceleration produced by adrenaline is explained by a shift along the potential axis of the activation curve of i_{K_2} (see Noble 1975). In this case, therefore, the transmitter does not open or close channels – nor does it modify the number of "available" channels. Rather, it changes the range of potentials over which a given set of channels open and close.

(c) In molluscan neurones presenting a bursting pattern, recent voltage clamp studies indicate that the pattern is controlled by a slow wave which resembles an action potential in its basic organization: depolarization opens a conductance leading to an inward current, which in turn increases the depolarization. The depolarization is then interrupted by the activation of a K^+ conductance. The ions carrying the inward current have not been entirely identified but are either Na^+ and/or Ca^{2+}.

Modulation of the burst pattern is produced by a variety of transmitters and hormones. The recent review of Kehoe and Marty (1980) lists some of these cases. In most of them the pattern of the effect suggests a mechanism similar to that described in section 3; i.e., a primary effect on the voltage-dependent conductance controlling the inward current. However, additional effects could imply alterations of the K^+ conductance, either by opening new K^+ channels or by interfering with those implied in the hyperpolarizing phase of the slow wave.

(d) In the case of the crayfish stretch receptor, it was shown that, at certain frequencies, repetitive stimulation of the inhibitory nerve can produce a paradoxical effect on a regular discharge produced by stretching the muscle: increasing the frequency of the inhibitory train can lead to acceleration of the discharge on the receptor axon (Perkel et al. 1964). This is explained by a "beating" between the regular inhibitory input and the regularly firing neurone. It is not certain that this phenomenon is of great functional importance, but it certainly is an example of the difficulties which separate the observation of a specific conductance change (in this case, a Cl^- conductance increase) and the prediction of the functional result.

4.4. *Transmitter-induced activation of the Na^+–K^+ pump*

The Na^+–K^+ pump is electrogenic (at each cycle, it expels more Na^+ ions than the K^+ ions it takes in), and an increase in its rate gives rise to a hyperpolarization. Contrary to hyperpolarizations resulting from conductance changes, the hyperpolarization produced by an increased pumping does not show a reversal potential, and the pump current is quite independent of the membrane potential (see Thomas 1972).

A number of authors, having observed inhibitory synaptic potentials which were not inverted by hyperpolarization or depolarization, have proposed that they could result from the activation by the transmitter of the Na^+–K^+ pump. In many cases, this appears only as one of many possible interpretations, and failure to observe an inversion may have been due to experimental problems, and particularly to the difficulty of controlling the membrane potential in remote (dendritic, axonic) branches where the transmitter may be acting. However, there are some examples where the arguments in favor of an activation of the pump are quite strong. In particular, this is the case for effects of adrenaline on skeletal muscle (see Clausen and Flatman 1977, Kuba and Koketsu 1978) and for effects of dopamine on molluscan neurones described recently by Kazachenko et al. (1979). These authors described dopamine-induced hyperpolarizations which were blocked by strophantidin (a Na^+–K^+ pump inhibitor). Under voltage clamp, dopamine produced an outward current, the amplitude of which did not change between -80 and -130 mV. As these observations were made on isolated cell bodies (without axonal or dendritic branches) the objections assuming inadequate control of a remote region cannot be held, and it appears

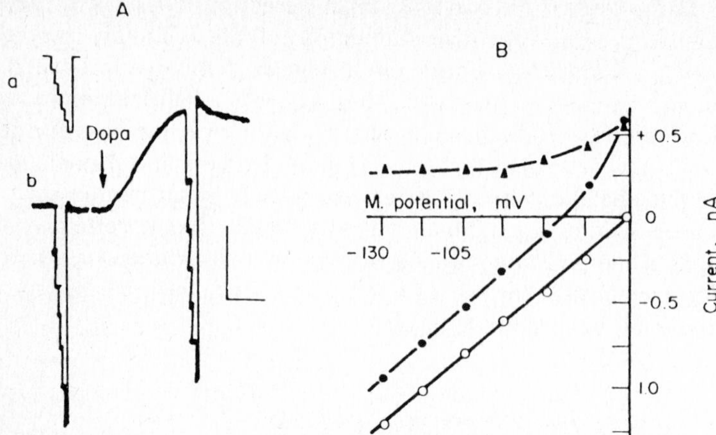

Fig. 5. An inhibitory response which cannot be interpreted by a simple change in ionic permeability. Molluscan neurone hyperpolarized by dopamine. Voltage clamp analysis. (A) The membrane potential was varied between −55 and −130 mV by steps of 12.5 mV first before, than after exposure to dopamine (10^{-5} M) (Dopa). (a) illustrates the voltage records and (b) the current records. At −55 mV, dopamine produced an outward current which accounts for the hyperpolarization observed in the absence of voltage clamp. (B) The dopamine induced outward current has been calculated (▲ – filled triangles) as the difference between the current needed to bring the membrane potential at a given value before (○) and after (●) exposure to dopamine). Calibration for A, B: 0.5 nA, 30 s. (From Kazachenko et al. 1979).

therefore quite possible that the outward current produced by dopamine results from the activation of the Na^+–K^+ pump (fig. 5).

5. Conclusion

Synaptic permeability changes appear to involve two types of mechanisms: the opening of specific channels, and the control of channels which already exist and function in the absence of the transmitter. The specific channels appear to be of three basic types: Cl^-, K^+ and cationic channels. The similarities between members of each group (e.g., between the different synaptic K^+ channels) may suggest a common structure, but may only be apparent with the differences as yet undetected due to the limited number of studies yet performed for characterizing them. Among the transmitter-modulated channels that are functioning prior to transmitter application, the Ca^+ ones are the best understood, but a large number of other types appear to be involved (particularly in rhythmic cells) about which little is known.

New data should be rapidly coming, in view of the recent progress made in both the theoretical and the experimental approach to synaptic function. Among the most promising developments one may mention the application to neuronal cell bodies of the internal perfusion techniques (Kostyuk et al. 1975) which have been so successful in the study of the squid axon channels, and which should allow the control of intracellular ionic concentrations. It is clear, however, that we are still far from the "molecular" understanding of the structure and function of any channel, and that formidable problems remain to be solved. Most synapses occur on tiny neuronal ramifications and use unknown transmitters. For many years our knowledge of the ionic mechanisms involved in synaptic function will probably remain based on a few examples selected for their experimental advantages, and the generality of the findings will have to be made with caution.

Summary

(1) Synaptic excitation and synaptic inhibition are generated by many different mechanisms. The best known processes are those which involve an ionic permeability increase and those in which the transmitter modifies a voltage activated conductance.

(2) The cases where a transmitter opens ionic channels appear to involve only three basic types of channels: K^+ channels, Cl^- channels and "cationic channels" discriminating against anions but showing little specificity for cations. New methods of analysis – in particular the study of conductance fluctuations and the obtention of "single channel recordings" – have allowed a detailed characterization of the channels in a few systems.

(3) The best studied cases where transmitters modify voltage-activated conductances are those of Ca^{++} channels. The transmitter action appears to consist in an alteration of the number of available channels – with no detectable effect on the properties of individual channels.

(4) The less-well understood synaptic potentials are those which involve transmitter-induced closure of open channels, and those where the absence of voltage dependence suggests the intervention of an electrogenic pump.

References

Adams, P. R. (1976) J. Physiol. 260, 531.

Adams, P. R. (1977) J. Physiol. 268, 291.

Anderson, C. R., S. G. Cull-Candy and R. Miledi (1978) J. Physiol. 282, 219.

Anderson, C. R. and C. F. Stevens (1973) J. Physiol. 235, 655.

Armstrong, C. M. (1975) in: Membranes, ed. G. Eisenman, vol. 3 (Dekker, New York) pp. 325–358.

Ascher, P. and J. S. Kehoe (1975) in: Handbook of Psychopharmacology, eds. L. L. Iversen, S. D. Iversen and S. Snyder, vol. 6 (Plenum Press, New York) pp. 265–310.
Ascher, P., D. Kunze and T. O. Neild (1976) J. Physiol. 256, 441.
Ascher, P., A. Marty and T. O. Neild (1978a) J. Physiol. 278, 177.
Ascher, P., A. Marty and T. O. Neild (1978b) J. Physiol. 278, 207.
Barker, J. L. and R. N. McBurney (1979) Nature 277, 234.
Boistel, J. and P. Fatt (1958) J. Physiol. 144, 176.
Bolton, T. B. (1979) Physiol. Rev. 59, 606.
Bregestovski, P. D., and R. Miledi and I. Parker (1979) Nature 279, 638.
Brown, H. F., D. di Francesco and S. Noble (1979) Nature 280, 235.
Bülbring, E. and T. Tomita (1977) Proc. R. Soc. B. 197, 271.
Carew, T. J. and E. R. Kandel (1976) Science 192, 150.
Clausen, T. and J. A. Flatman (1977) J. Physiol. 270, 383.
Coombs, J. S., J. C. Eccles and P. Fatt (1955) J. Physiol. 130, 374.
del Castillo, J. and B. Katz (1954) J. Physiol. 125, 546.
Dionne, V. E. and R. L. Ruff (1977) Nature 266, 263.
Dionne, V. E. and C. F. Stevens (1975) J. Physiol. 251, 245.
Dudel, J. (1977) Pflügers Arch. 371, 167.
Dudel, J. (1978) Pflügers Arch. 376, 151.
Dudel, J., W. Finger and H. Stettmeier (1977) Neurosci. Lett. 6 203.
Eccles, J. C. (1966). Ann. NY Acad. Sci. 137, 473.
Garnier, D., J. Nargeot, C. Ojeda and O. Rougier (1978) J. Physiol. 274, 381.
Ger, B. A. , A. N. Katchman and E. V. Zeimal (1979) Brain Res. 171, 355.
Gerschenfeld, H. M. and D. Paupardin-Tritsch (1974) J. Physiol. 243, 427.
Giles, W. and S. J. Noble (1976) J. Physiol. 261, 103.
Giles, W. and R. Tsien (1975) J. Physiol 246, 64 P
Ginsborg, B. (1967) Pharmacol. Rev. 19, 289.
Ginsborg, B. L. (1973) Biochem. Biophys. Acta 300, 289.
Ginsborg, B. L., C. R. House and E. M. Silinsky (1974) J. Physiol. 236, 723.
Ginsborg, B. L. and R. T. Kado (1975) J. Physiol. 245, 713.
Goldman, D. E. (1943) J. Gen. Physiol. 27, 37.
Greengard, P. (1976) Nature 260, 101.
Hagiwara, S. (1975) in: Membranes, ed. G. Eisenman, vol. 3 (Dekker, New York) pp. 359–380.
Hagiwara, S. and L. A. Jaffe (1979) Ann. Rev. Biophys. Bioeng. 8, 385.
Hagiwara, S., K. Toyama and H. Hayashi (1971) J. Gen. Physiol. 57, 408.
Hartzell, H. C., S. W. Kuffler, E. Stickgold and D. Yoshikami (1977) J. Physiol. 271, 817.
Hille, B. (1975) in: Membranes, ed. G. Eisenman, vol. 3 (Dekker, New York) pp. 255–323.
Hodgkin, A. L. and B. Katz (1949) J. Physiol. 108, 37.
Hutter, O. F. (1957) Brit. Med. Bull. 13, 176.
Hutter, O. F. and W. Trautwein (1956) J. Gen. Physiol. 39, 715.
Ikemoto, Y. and M. Goto (1975) Proc. Jpn. Acad. 51, 501.
Ikemoto, Y. and M. Goto (1977) J. Mol. Cell. Cardiol. 9, 313.
Katz, B. (1966) Nerve, Muscle and Synapse (McGraw Hill, New York).
Katz, B. and R. Miledi (1969) J. Physiol. 203, 459, 487.
Katz, B. and R. Miledi (1972) J. Physiol. 224, 665.

Kazachenko, V. N., V. S. Musienko, E. N. Gakhova and B. N. Veprintsev (1979) Comp. Biochem. Physiol. 63C, 67.
Kehoe, J. S. (1972) J. Physiol. 225, 85.
Kehoe, J. S. (1975) J. Physiol. 244, 23 P.
Kehoe, J. S. and P. Ascher (1970) Nature 225, 820.
Kehoe, J. S. and A. Marty (1980) Ann. Rev. Biophys. Bioeng., in press.
Klein, M. and E. R. Kandel (1978) Proc. Nat. Acad. Sci. 75, 3512.
Kordaš, M. (1969) J. Physiol. 2 and 4, 493.
Kostyuk, P. G. and O.A. Krishtal (1977) J. Physiol. 270, 569.
Kostyuk, P. G., O. A. Krishtal and V. I. Pidoplichko (1975) Nature 257, 691.
Kuba, K. and K. Koketsu (1978) Progr. Neurobiol. 11, 77.
Lewis, C. (1979) J. Physiol. 286, 417.
Lewis, C. A. and C. F. Stevens (1979) in: Membrane Transport Processes, eds. C. F. Stevens and R. W. Tsien, vol. 3 (Raven Press, New York) pp. 133–151.
Maeno, T., C. Edwards and M. Anraku (1977) J. Neurobiol. 8, 173.
Magleby, K. L. and C. F. Stevens (1972) J. Physiol. 223, 173.
Marchais, D. and A. Marty (1979) J. Physiol. 297, 9.
Marty, A. (1978) J. Physiol. 278, 237.
Marty, A. and P. Ascher (1978) Nature, 274, 494.
Meech, R. W. (1978) Ann. Rev. Biophys. Bioeng. 7, 1.
Meyer, H. (1976) J. Exp. Biol. 64, 477.
Motokizawa, F., J. P. Reuben and H. Grundfest (1969) J. Gen. Physiol. 54, 437.
Neher, E. and B. Sakmann (1976) Nature 260, 799.
Neher, E. and J. H. Steinbach (1978) J. Physiol. 277, 153.
Neher, E. and C. F. Stevens (1977) Ann. Rev. Biophys. Bioeng. 6, 345.
Noble, D. (1975) The Initiation of the Heartbeat (Clarendon Press, Oxford).
Noma, A., K. Peper and W. Trautwein (1979) Pflügers Arch. 381, 255.
Noma, A. and W. Trautwein (1978) J. Physiol. 284, 97.
Onodera, K. and A. Takeuchi (1979) J. Physiol. 286, 265.
Ozawa, S. and K. Tsuda (1973) J. Neurophysiol. 36, 805.
Patlak, J. B., K. A. F. Gration and P. N. R. Usherwood (1979) Nature 278, 643.
Pellmar, T. C. and W. A. Wilson (1977) Nature 269, 76.
Perkel, D. H., J. H. Schulman, T. H. Bullock, G. P. Moore and J. P. Segundo (1964) Science NY 145, 61.
Putney, J. W., Jr. (1979) Pharmacol. Rev. 30, 209.
Reuter, H. (1974) J. Physiol. 242, 429.
Reuter, H. and H. Scholz (1977) J. Physiol. 264, 49.
Shimahara, T. and L. Tauc (1977) Brain Res. 127, 168.
Steinbach, J. H. and C. F. Stevens (1976) in: Neurobiology of the Frog, eds. R. Llinas and W. Precht, (Springer, Berlin) pp. 33–92.
Takahashi, K. and M. Yoshii (1978) J. Physiol. 279, 519.
Takeuchi, A. and N. Takeuchi (1960) J. Physiol. 154, 52.
Takeuchi, A. and N. Takeuchi (1965) J. Physiol. 177, 225.
Takeuchi, A. and N. Takeuchi (1967) J. Physiol. 191, 575.
Takeuchi, A. and N. Takeuchi (1971a) J. Physiol. 212, 337.
Takeuchi, A. and N. Takeuchi (1971b) J. Physiol. 271, 341.
Thomas, R. C. (1972) Physiol. Rev. 52, 563.

Tillotson, D. (1979) Proc. Nat. Acad. Sci. 76, 1497.

Tsien, R. W. (1977) in: Advances in Cyclic Research, eds. P. Greengard and G. A. Robison, vol. 8 (Raven Press, New York) pp. 363–420.

Vassort, G., O. Rougier, D. Garnier, M. P. Sauviat, E. Coraboeuf and Y. M. Gargouïl (1969) Pflügers Arch. 309, 70.

Weight, F. F. (1974) in: The Neurosciences Third Study Program eds. F. O. Schmitt and F. G. Worden (MIT Press, Cambridge, Mass.) p. 929.

Weiss, K. R., J. L. Cohen and I. Kupfermann (1978) J. Neurophysiol. 41, 181.

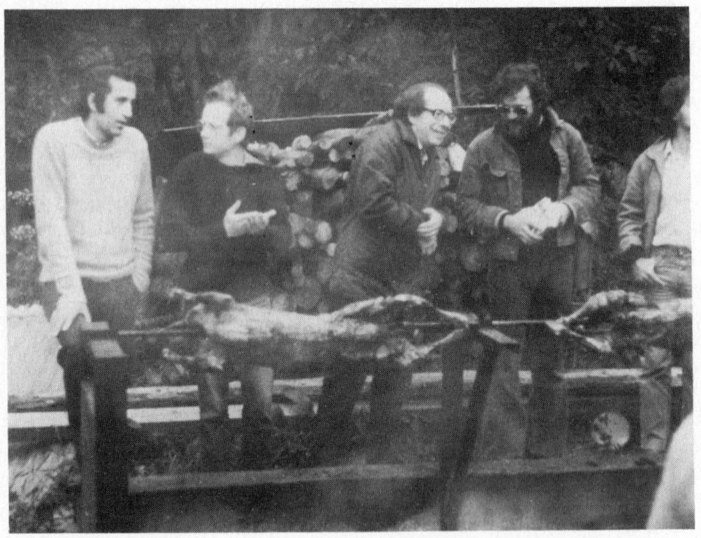

SEMINAR

FROM FUNCTION TO STRUCTURE: THE CHOLINERGIC RECEPTOR *IN VITRO*

Jean-Luc POPOT

Institut Pasteur
Laboratoire Associé au C.N.R.S.,
25 rue du Dr. Roux,
75015 Paris, France
and
Collège de France,
Paris, France

The field of cholinergic receptor biochemistry has become so large during the past ten years that covering it in detail within a few lectures cannot be envisaged. Besides, reviews are now appearing almost every year, which there is no need to duplicate (see, e.g. references [30, 41, 42, 54, 69, 76, 87, 95, 114, 142, 172, 174, 220]. After pondering each of them to compensate for the emphasis placed on the particular works and theories of their authors, the interested student will get a more detailed, up-to-date (and presumably also somewhat confused) view of our present knowledge on the subject. The only purpose of this short text, rather, is to provide one with some guide lines and references for further reading.

R. Balian et al., eds.
Les Houches, Session XXXIII, 1979 – Membranes et Communication Intercellulaire / Membranes and Intercellular Communication

Abbreviations

ACh	acetylcholine
AChR	cholinergic receptor
cmc	critical micellar concentration
DNS-C_6-Cho	[1-(5-dimethylaminonaphthalene)sulfonamido]*n*-hexanoic acid β-(*N*-trimethylammonium bromide) ethyl ester
DTT	dithiotreitol
ESR	electron spin resonance
H_{12}-HTX	perhydrohistrionicotoxin
HTX	histrionicotoxin
L.A.	local anesthetic
MPTA	4-(*N*-maleimido)phenyltrimethylammonium
Mr	molecular weight estimated by reference to standards in SDS electrophoresis
mol wt	molecular weight
NMR	nuclear magnetic resonance
SDS	sodium dodecylsulphate.

0. Introduction

The success of biochemical studies on the cholinergic receptor can be for a great part traced back to the existence of two exceptionally favorable circumstances, the peculiar physiology of fish electric organs and the high specificity of polypeptidic toxins with which evolution endowed certain species of snakes. Both of them will first be described in summary. It could be noted however from the very beginning that these special circumstances also make the approach of the cholinergic receptor a bad model for the study of other receptors where such a favorable situation does not exist. On the other hand, the knowledge of this particular receptor that was gained through this approach might undoubtedly be of use to "receptorologists" working on other systems.

The notion that there exists, at the neuromuscular junction, a particular substance to which acetylcholine binds was put forward as a result of the observation that the inhibitory effect of curare (see fig. 1) on the action of nicotine at this level could be reversed by increasing the concentration of nicotine [86]. This competition suggested that both compounds bound to the same site of action, with different physiological effects, in a mutually exclusive manner. Nachmansohn, in the 1950s, remarked that the specificity of recognition of acetylcholine by its receptor resembled that of the catalytic center of enzymes, and therefore that the receptor might be a protein, and pointed out the exceptional richness in cholinergic synapses of the electric organ of certain fish (see

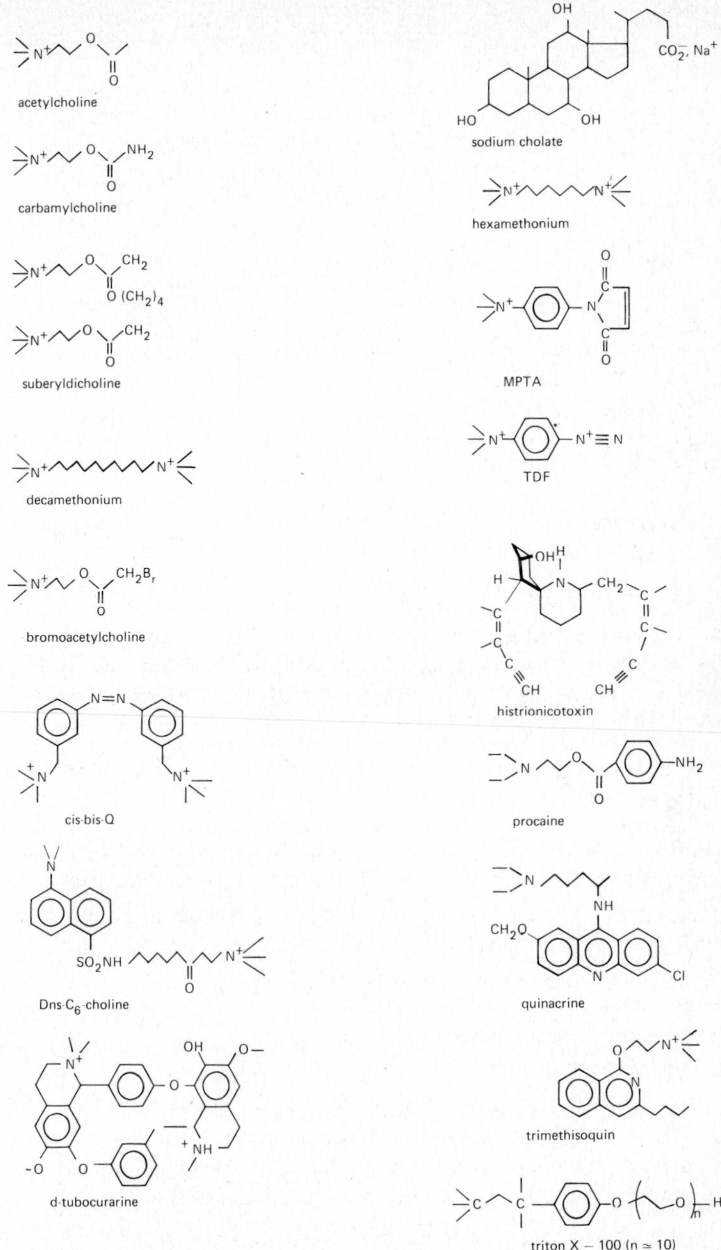

Fig. 1. Some of the compounds currently employed in the biochemical study of the receptor. (See text.)

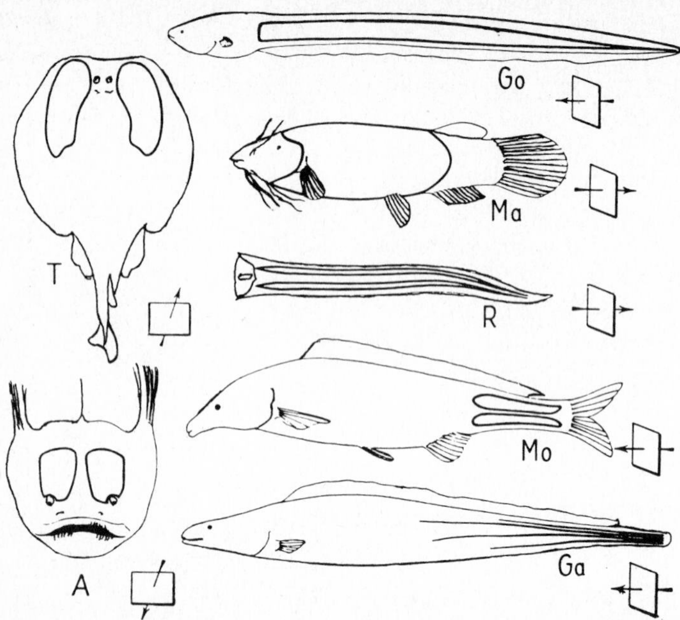

Fig. 2. The seven main kinds of electric fish, with the schematic indication of the localization of their organs (thick lines): T: *Torpedo*; A: *Astrocopus* (head only); Go: *Electrophorus* (electric eel); Ma: *Malapterurus*; R: *Raja* (tail only); Mo: *Mormyrus*; and Ga: *Gymnarchos*. Arrows indicate the direction of current flow through the organ; the planes refer to that of the electroplaques. The various species are not drawn to scale; usual specimen of electric eel are 1–1.50 m long, those of *T. marmorata* ca. 20–40 cm wide. About the physiological use of the organs, see e.g. refs. [15, 29, 89]: (From Fessard 1958.)

[157, 158]). In the case of the two most widely used species, *Electrophorus electricus* and *Torpedo* (fig. 2), the cells constituting these organs (electroplaques) are derived from embryonic muscle cells which have lost their contractile apparatus [80, 120] and specialised in the production of electrical discharges (see refs. [41, 78, 89]). They are flat syncitia a few millimeters large, packed in prisms like piled plates, one face of which receives a dense innervation covering 2% (*Electrophorus* [25, 27]) or nearly 100% of its surface (*Torpedo* [36]). The rest of the area of the innervated face in *Electrophorus* is electrically excitable and amplifies the post-synaptic potential into an action potential similar to that of the axon, while *Torpedo* electroplaques are not electrically excitable, the whole of the discharge (up to 1200 W for *T. nobiliana*) being due to the synaptic current. The pharmacology of the acetylcholine receptor is typically nicotinic and nearly identical to that of skeletal muscle

[41, 174]. Most importantly, the innervation of the electric organs is purely cholinergic and provides the biochemist with an homogeneous starting material. Up to now the electrophysiology of *Torpedo* receptors has been studied only on the top cell of dissected prisms [16, 156], while individual *Electrophorus* electroplaques can be isolated, voltage-clamped, and studied in as much detail as the frog neuromuscular junction [62, 122, 133–136, 183, 194]. This has been an important asset, in particular because it permitted an easy test of the physiological action of the numerous treatments and compounds involved in biochemical studies [107, 116, 148, 191, 192].

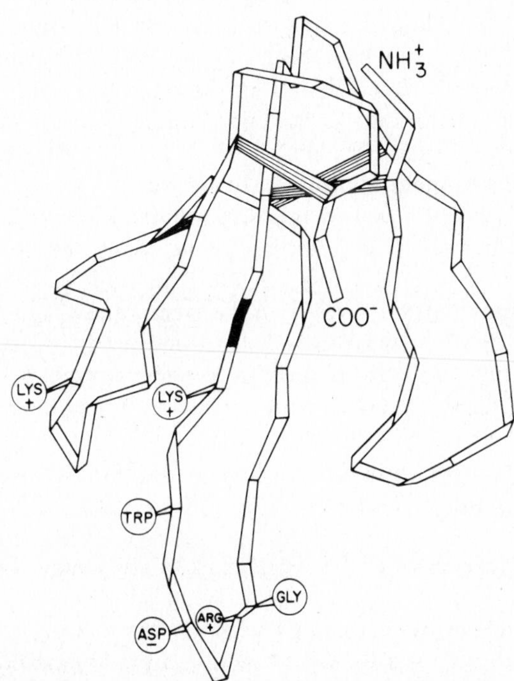

Fig. 3. Tri-dimensional structure of an α-toxin. Perspective ribbon drawing of the folding of the polypeptide chain in α-toxins a and b of *Laticauda semifasciata* determined at 2.5 Å resolution by X-ray diffraction. Folds in the ribbon occur at α-carbon positions. Viewed from this direction, the molecule is about 40 Å long and about 30 Å wide, but only about 15 Å thick. The residues believed involved in neurotoxic action are labelled; disulfide bridges are stripped. (The blackened segment represents his in α-toxin b, and Asn in α-toxin a, the rest of the 62 amino acids being identical.) (From Tsernoglou and Petsko (1977); see also ref. [141].)

The first attempts towards the purification of the acetylcholine receptor were indeed conducted on homogenates of *Electrophorus* electric organ, with a radioactive analogue of curare as ligand [37]. They were however hampered by an overwhelming non-specific binding, and the decisive impetus came 15 years later from the description by Lee and his co-workers of a class of paralysing toxins found in the venom of various snakes ([47, 128]; see refs. [126, 127, 207]). These so-called α-toxins are small basic polypeptides (60–70 amino acids) (fig. 3) which bind tightly (for most of them quasi-irreversibly) to the acetylcholine binding site, with an extremely good specificity; for instance, when a whole *Electrophorus* electroplaque is saturated with *Naja nigricollis* α-toxin, only 25% of the toxin is non-specifically bound, the binding of the remaining 75% being competitively blocked by acetylcholine analogues [26]. The α-toxins have been put to a wide variety of uses. They can be radioactively labelled by various procedures [11, 58, 129, 146], which permits to determine the cellular localization and surface density of the receptor sites ([2, 11, 25, 77, 151, 169, 170, 186]; see also [132]), to follow them during tissue fractionation and purification [48, 123, 150, 190, 199] and to measure indirectly, through competition experiments, their affinity towards cholinergic ligands (see hereafter). The toxins can be fluorescently tagged, which allows dynamic studies on the distribution of the receptor in the membrane of muscle or electric cells ([4, 5, 9, 10, 162]; see also refs. [28, 206]), and covalently linked to activated supports in view of affinity chromatography (e.g. [65, 147]). Finally, they can be activated themselves so that they bind covalently to peptidic residues in the vicinity of the acetylcholine receptor site [218], or they can be covalently cross-linked to the receptor by bifunctional reagents [110, 216].

1. Functional properties of the receptor in its membrane environment

The purification of the cholinergic receptor raises a particular problem as compared to that of a soluble protein or a membrane-bound enzyme. The receptor's function is not only to recognize and bind acetylcholine, but also to transduce this information into a permeability response, the opening of the cationic channel (described in this course by Philippe Ascher), and this response can only be measured between two topological compartments. Although historically the purification of the receptor was first achieved by solubilization of electric organ fractions and separation on affinity columns, we will, therefore, consider a more progressive approach which leads to the obtention of purified membrane fragments, in which the receptor is still embedded in its native environment [56, 67, 79, 199]. These fragments form spontaneously closed vesicles, whose permeability can be measured with the help of radioactive inorganic ions.

The technique was first established by Kasai and Changeux for homogenates of *Electrophorus* electric organ ([117]; see also [102–104] and a recent improvement in [105]) and has been later applied to highly purified *Torpedo* membrane fragments ([94, 167, 168]; see also refs. [7, 17, 152, 203]). After a series of fractionations on sucrose gradients, the receptor-rich membranes (described hereafter) are incubated for a few days with $^{22}Na^+$, which equilibrates between the inner and outer compartment. When the membranes are diluted into a cold medium, the trapped $^{22}Na^+$ equilibrates back with the mainly non-radioactive external sodium at a rate that depends on the membrane permeability to this ion. This rate can be measured by filtering at intervals aliquots of the diluted vesicles on Millipore filters and counting the radioactivity retained. Addition of acetylcholine or one of its analogues (agonists) to the external medium results in a dramatic increase in permeability (fig. 4), which is cation-specific and is blocked by competitive antagonists like curare, non-competitive blockers like the local anesthetics (see hereafter) and α-toxins [168]. In other words, it can be demonstrated that this acellular system has preserved the main physiological properties observed on the live cell. It constitutes however a much more favorable material for a number of biochemical and biophysical techniques, as the very high concentrations in acetylcholine binding sites which can be attained (over 10^{-5} M) have made feasible the use of X-ray diffraction [68, 73, 178], fluorescence spectroscopy [12–14, 20, 22, 53, 55, 90–92, 96, 97, 111, 144, 171, 182, 188, 189, 209,], ESR [18, 33, 143, 180, 181, 212, 214], and recently NMR [153] to study the structure or dynamics of the receptor and its membrane environment. Binding studies with cholinergic ligands can be conducted over an extended range of concentrations (from less than 10^{-9} M to more than 10^{-5} M) by some of these techniques or by equilibrium dialysis of radioactive derivatives. Interestingly, the rate of *Naja nigricollis* α-toxin binding to the acetylcholine receptor site is directly proportional to the unliganded fraction of these sites, which permits an indirect but relatively rapid method of determination of the receptor's occupancy [210].

Comparison of the dose-response curves for receptor occupancy and permeability response as a function of agonist concentration revealed a

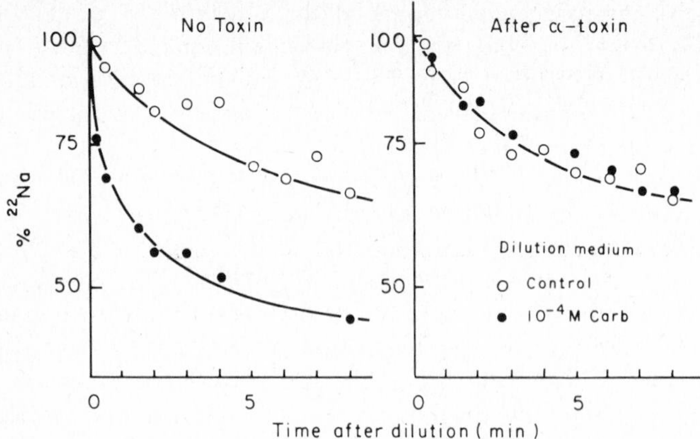

Fig. 4. Permeability increase induced *in vitro* by the agonist carbamylcholine and its blocking by α-toxin. Two 5-ml portions of a diluted suspension of membrane fragments (1.8 nM in α-toxin binding sites) were incubated for 7 min at room temperature with (b) or without (a) a stoichiometric amount of α-toxin. After centrifugation and resuspension, each fraction was incubated overnight with ^{22}NaCl, and aliquots diluted at $t=0$ into a cold medium supplemented (●) or not (○) with 0.1 mM carbamylcholine. Samples were filtered on Millipore filters at the indicated times and counted for the retention of $^{22}Na^+$. (From Popot et al., 1976.)

puzzling discrepancy (see Columns I & II of table 1) between the concentrations of agonist needed to occupy, after equilibration, half of the receptor sites (e.g. 24 nM for acetylcholine) and those at which half of the permeability increase was induced (2 μM in this case). In other words, a concentration of agonist which saturates over 90% of the binding sites induces only a barely detectable permeability increase; the permeability response develops in an upper concentration range, over which the binding of agonist appears not to increase significantly. This phenomenon has been encountered for all the agonists tested, while the discrepancy between the concentrations at which competitive antagonists block agonist binding and permeability response is smaller [168]. Since *in vitro* permeability measurements and *in vivo* depolarization dose-response curves [156] cannot be easily compared, the relatively good accordance between both sets of data, (see ref. [168]) should only with caution be considered as an indication that the low affinities measured in the flux experiments are the physiological ones. Another argument, however, strongly suggests that the affinities observed in the equilibrium binding studies are too high to be involved in the physiological process of activation: assuming a maximal, diffusion-limited rate

Table 1[a)]

Effect of the addition of agonists and competitive antagonists to receptor-rich membrane fragments on (I) cationic permeability and (II–IV) toxin-binding site occupancy after (II) or before (III) equilibration

	I[b)] $^{22}Na^{+}$-permeability change (K_{app} or K_I) (μM)	II[c)] Protection against α-Toxin (K_p) After 30′ (μM)	III[c)] After 10″ (μM)	IV[d)] K_1/K_3
Agonists:				
Acetylcholine	2	0.024	0.6	269
Carbamylcholine	46	0.48	15	341
Phenyltrimethyl-ammonium	70	1.6	35	267
Suberyldicholine	–	0.004	0.13	325
Antagonists:				
d-tubocurarine	2	0.38	0.31	~1
Gallamine (=Flaxedil)	37	1.1	0.98	~1

a) Data taken from Popot et al. (1976) (I), and from Weiland and Taylor (1979) (II–IV).

b) I = concentrations of agonists inducing an half-maximal $^{22}Na^{+}$-permeability increase (Kapp) or K_I of competitive antagonists.

c) II and III = dissociation constants calculated from the protection of the receptor site against binding of [^{125}I]-monoiodotyrosyl cobra α-toxin 30 min (II) or 10 s (III) after mixing receptor-rich membrane fragments with the ligand.

d) IV = ratio of the dissociation constants for the low affinity [R] and high affinity [D] states of scheme 2 calculated from protection experiments. The protection constant $K_p^{10''}$ (III) is taken as an evaluation of K_1, and $K_p^{30'}$ (II) as a measure of K_{eq} (defined in table 2). The ratio K_1/K_3 of the microscopic dissociation constants is greater than the ratio of the apparent dissociation constants K_1/K_{eq} (see formulae in table 2).

of binding of acetylcholine to its receptor ($k_{on} \simeq 10^9\ M^{-1}\ s^{-1}$) and a simple bimolecular association-dissociation scheme, an equilibrium dissociation constant of 20 nM corresponds to a maximal rate of dissociation $k_{off} \simeq 20\ s^{-1}$; the corresponding mean occupancy time (35 ms) is much longer than both the actual activation response (1–2 ms) and the minimum interval between two maximal responses (a few ms). An obvious interpretation of these results, which is difficult to rule out directly, would be that a majority of the receptor sites are in a high-affinity, non-functional state, while the permeability increase is due to a small number of low-affinity, functional sites that remain undetected in the binding assay. The reality however is more complex and less trivial.

The binding of agonists and competitive antagonists to the ACh binding site can be followed either directly, using radioactive, fluorescent, or spin-labelled ligands (or even by proton NMR), or, as already mentioned, indirectly by observing the rate of quasi-irreversible association of a radioactive α-toxin with the receptor site (see refs. [57, 130, 211, 214]). This rate is proportional to the concentration of unliganded site:

$$\mathrm{RL} \underset{K_\mathrm{D}}{\overset{\mathrm{L}}{\leftrightarrows}} \mathrm{R} \underset{k}{\overset{\mathrm{T}}{\rightarrow}} \mathrm{RT}$$

$$\frac{\mathrm{d}[\mathrm{RT}]}{\mathrm{d}t} = k[\mathrm{R}][\mathrm{T}] = k[\mathrm{R}_0][\mathrm{T}]\frac{1}{1+[\mathrm{L}]/\mathrm{K}_\mathrm{D}} \tag{1}$$

where [L] is the concentration of acetylcholine or a competitive analogue, [T] that of the toxin, and [R], [RL], and [RT], respectively the concentrations of free, reversibly liganded and toxin-blocked receptor sites, $[\mathrm{R}_0]$ standing for [R] + [RL], the total concentration of unblocked receptor. The free radioactive toxin can be conveniently separated from that bound to the membrane fragments on Millipore filters. This relatively rapid assay (a few tens of seconds), whose results have been subsequently developed by direct fast-mixing techniques [50, 96, 97], permitted to investigate the evolution of agonist binding in the same time-range (seconds to minutes) as the $^{22}\mathrm{Na}^+$-flux assay.

Conversely, the effects of the preincubation with the cholinergic analogues, inherent to equilibrium binding studies, on the permeability response were investigated, and it was demonstrated that the increase in cationic permeability induced by agonist was only transient [167, 203]: if the agonist is not rapidly removed (seconds or minutes), the vesicle's permeability falls back to its control level with a kinetics that depend on the agonist's nature and concentration, temperature, ionic composition of the buffer, namely the very factors that are known to *in vivo* affect the phenomenon of desensitization first analysed at the neuromuscular junction by Katz and Thesleff (1957). In both cases, the receptor reverts to its resting state upon removal of the agonist. Parallel dynamic binding studies show that immediately upon mixing of the membrane preparation and the agonist, only a small (10–15%) fraction of the receptors bind the agonist with the high affinity characteristic of the equilibrium situation, most of them exhibiting a much lower (ca. 30-fold) affinity constant. However, during prolonged incubation the low-affinity sites progressively disappear to be replaced by an equivalent number of high-affinity ones [50, 57, 130, 210, 212, 214, 215]. This phenomenon was indeed postulated by Katz and Thesleff and other electrophysiologists [119, 175–177; see 142] to account for certain kinetic properties of desensitization and its reversal. In phenomenological terms, the postulated events can (and must) be presented as a cycle in which the agonist [L] drives slowly the receptor from an "activatable" state R to a "desensitized" state D, able to bind it with a high affinity but without giving rise to a permeability increase [202, 203]. The cycle must be reversible for thermodynamic consistency:

$$\begin{array}{ccc} R + L & \overset{\text{fast}}{\rightleftharpoons} & RL \\ \text{slow} \upharpoonleft\downharpoonright & & \upharpoonleft\downharpoonright \text{slow} \\ D + L & \underset{\text{fast}}{\rightleftharpoons} & DL \end{array} \quad . \tag{2}$$

In biochemical terms, the functional states are conceived as conformational states of the receptor protein (or proteic complex), in equilibrium one with another, agonists and antagonists displacing the equilibrium according to their preferential affinities. The validity and kinetic constants of scheme 2 have been studied (a) by using spin-labelled [212, 214], fluorescent [96, 97], or radioactive [50] cholinergic analogues, monitoring their binding by spectroscopy or by a method of rapid filtration; (b) by observing the fluorescence of non-agonistic markers of various pharmacological properties [90–92, 171, 188, 189]; (c) by direct recording of the fluorescence of the membrane proteins [12, 13, 22]. Methods b and c are intended to report on conformational rather than binding states. Table 2 groups three sets of independent determinations obtained by method a (set I and II) and c (set III). Although the three sets of constants agree reasonably well, other authors [171] have been unable to fit their data (obtained by method b) to a mechanism involving preexisting conformational states.

Although convenient to fit kinetic data, scheme 2 is obviously an over-simplification. In particular, the step written as $R+L \rightleftharpoons RL$ must be more complex, as the actual mechanism involves an active conformational state in which the receptor protein induces the rise in cationic permeability. A more reasonable scheme should include this active state

Table 2

Rate and equilibrium constants for the two-state model of the receptor (scheme 2) determined from rapid-mixing experiments[a)]

$$L+R \underset{k_{-1}}{\overset{k_{+1}}{\rightleftharpoons}} LR \qquad K_1=\frac{L\,R}{LR}=\frac{k_{-1}}{k_{+1}}; \qquad K_2=\frac{LR}{LD}=\frac{k_{-2}}{k_{+2}}$$

$$k_{+4} \upharpoonleft\downharpoonright \qquad k_{-2} \upharpoonleft\downharpoonright k_{+2} \qquad K_3=\frac{L\,D}{LD}=\frac{k_{-3}}{k_{+3}}; \qquad K_4=\frac{R}{D}=\frac{k_{-4}}{k_{+4}}$$

$$D+R \underset{k_{-3}}{\overset{k_{+3}}{\rightleftharpoons}} DR \qquad K_{eq}=\frac{L[R+D]}{LR+LD}= \quad K_3\frac{1+K_4}{1+K_2}$$

Method	I: Rapid [^{3}H]-ACh binding	II: Fluorescence of bound agonist	III: Intrinsic fluorescence of proteins
Agonist	[^{3}H]-ACh	DNS-C_6-Cho	Suberyldicholine
Ref. no.	[50]	[96]	[13]
K_{eq}	1.5×10^{-8} M	1.5×10^{-8} M[b)]	~6.10^{-9} M[b)]
K_1	10^{-6} M	8.10^{-7} M	10^{-6} M[b)]
K_3	2.4×10^{-9} M	3×10^{-9} M	~2×10^{-9} M
K_2	0.013	0.015[b)]	0.004[b)]
K_4	5.6	4[b)]	2.1[b)]
k_{+1}		3.5×10^5 M^{-1} s^{-1}	9.8×10^6 M^{-1} s^{-1}
k_{-1}		0.29 s^{-1}	10.2 s^{-1}
k_{+2}	0.18 s^{-1}	0.18 s^{-1}	1.5 s^{-1}
k_{-2}	0.0024 s^{-1}	0.0027 s^{-1}	0.006 s^{-1}
k_{+3}	7×10^7 M^{-1} s^{-1} (1)	9.5×10^7 M^{-1} s^{-1}	6×10^7 M^{-1} s^{-1} (2)
k_{-3}	0.15 s^{-1} (1)	0.30 s^{-1}	0.12 s^{-1}
k_{+4}	5×10^{-4} s^{-1}	9×10^{-3} s^{-1}	8×10^{-3} s^{-1}
k_{-4}	2.8×10^{-3} s^{-1}	3.6×10^{-2} s^{-1}	1.7×10^{-2} s^{-1}
K_1/K_3	~400[b)]	~300[b)]	~500[b)]

a) Data taken from Cohen and Boyd (1980), Heidmann and Changeux (1979) and Barrantes (1978). Note that the agonists employed were different, as well as the temperature (4° C for I, except (1) 23° C; 20° C for II and III); membrane fragments for *Torpedo marmorata* except (1) *T. californica*; set III is not fully independent, one constant (2) having been taken from an earlier determination of set II.

b) Values calculated from the published data.

A, each of the three states being able to bind cholinergic ligands with various affinities:

$$\begin{array}{ccccc} & & \text{fast} \ (<\text{ms}) & & \\ & R & \rightleftharpoons & A & \\ \text{slow} \ (\sim\text{s}) & \nwarrow\!\searrow & & \swarrow\!\nearrow & \text{slow} \ (\sim\text{s}). \\ & & D & & \end{array} \tag{3}$$

Classical competitive antagonists would stabilize mostly the resting state R, metaphilic (desensitizing) antagonists [177], state D, while agonists would induce a shift to A followed by the slow conversion to D ([43, 91, 202]; see [95]). Under particular observational limitations (kinetic limitation, absence of fluorescence changes associated to some transitions), scheme 3 reduces to scheme 2, and there is yet, in addition to its physiological necessity, only indirect indications of the actual existence of state A [13, 90, 91, 97].

2. Non-competitive blocking agents

The competitive antagonists (often referred to simply as antagonists) mentioned thus far displace acetylcholine from its site and can be displaced by it; α-toxins enter in the same group of compounds as, although their action is generally quasi-irreversible and therefore seems superficially non-competitive, their binding and that of acetylcholine present the same character of mutual exclusion. This class of agents depresses and eventually blocks the post-synaptic potential by diminishing the number of receptors available to ACh, without alteration of the elementary response which becomes only less probable.

Another important (and heterogeneous) class of drugs acts in a quite different manner; as many of these non-competitive antagonists were originally characterized by their blocking action on another excitatory process, the propagation along the axon of the action potential, the whole class is often loosely referred to as that of "local anesthetics" (L.A.s). In addition to local anesthetics *sensu stricto*, it encompasses compounds like the fluorescent antimalarial agent quinacrine [1, 3, 90, 204] or the potent alkaloid toxin of the columbian frog *Deudrobates histrionicus*, *histrionicotoxin* (HTX; [3, 59, 71, 118, 145], see fig. 1). Structurally irrelated amphiphilic compounds like neutral or negatively charged detergents or free fatty acids [7, 8, 21, 31, 32, 93, 206] exert a local anesthetic-like blocking effect. The blocking action of these compounds is characterized by: (a) its non-competitivity and (b) a profound distortion of the elementary response (and therefore of the "noise" spectrum and the shape of the end-plate potential), which is generally a function of the membrane potential. On these grounds, electrophysiologists have proposed, at least for some of them, a site of action near, or in, the cation-selective channel (ionophore) itself (see presentation by Ascher).

The non-competitivity can be demonstrated biochemically, as schematically illustrated in fig. 5, by the $^{22}Na^{+}$-flux and [^{3}H]–ACh-binding assays. For the binding assay, membrane fragments are incubated with a concentration of [^{3}H]–ACh sufficient to saturate (at equilibrium) about half of the ACh-binding sites, and the effect of the blocking agent on the amount of bound ACh is studied as a function of concentration. As expected, competitive antagonists decrease this amount by competing with ACh for the receptor sites. By contrast, at the approximate concentration at which they block the permeability response, local anesthetics do not displace ACh; on the contrary, they favor its binding, and it is only at higher concentrations that they start to bind themselves to the ACh-binding site (this can be checked by measuring the diminution of rate of α-toxin binding). The increase in affinity for ACh induced by local anesthetics should be placed in parallel with their enhancing effect on desensitization observed as well *in vitro* as *in vivo*,

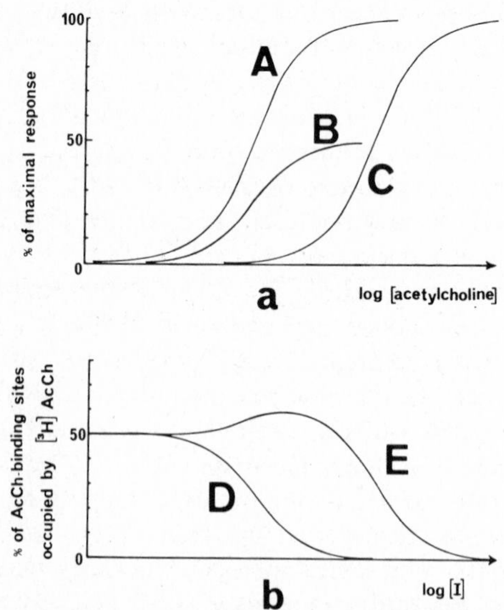

Fig. 5. Schematic representation of the effects of competitive and non-competitive blocking agents on (a) the permeability increase induced by acetylcholine (A: control; B: + L.A.; C: + competitive antagonist) and (b) the equilibrium binding of [^{3}H]-acetylcholine to its receptor site (membrane fragments are incubated in the presence of a concentration of the [^{3}H]-ACh equal to its K_D, i.e. sufficient to saturate 50% of its binding sites, and of increasing concentrations of one of the blocking agents; the bound [^{3}H]-ACh is determined by dialysis; D: I = competitive antagonist; E: I = L.A.).

and it can indeed be directly demonstrated that L.A.s shift the R⇌D equilibrium towards the D state [97]. L.A.s therefore bind to (at least) one class of sites distinct from, but closely coupled to the ACh-binding sites. It would be of interest to characterize these sites, particularly since they are suspected to be part of the cholinergic ionophore.

It is only very recently that direct studies on the binding of radioactively labelled L.A. have become possible, the major difficulty stemming from the usually low affinity of these compounds (typically 10^{-5} to 10^{-4} M) which, coupled to their amphiphilic nature (see fig. 1) results in overwhelming non-specific binding to the membrane fragments and to the experimental vessels. An idea of the difficulties encountered is given by this excerpt of a paper by Krodel et al. (1979):

> "Meproadifen interacts strongly with cellulose nitrate centrifuge tubes, and that interaction is superficially analogous to a specific binding process in that high concentrations of non-radioactive ligand reduce retention on the tube walls. Even at the high ionic strength characteristic of *Torpedo* physiological saline, at 2 μM [^{14}C]-meproadifen 20% of the ligand was adsorbed on the sides of the tube, and that adsorption was reduced by 80% in the presence of 100 μM non-radioactive meproadifen. To make matters worse, amines such as proadifen and carbamylcholine, as well as α-neurotoxin, also reduced the amount of adsorbed radioactivity."

Progresses have been achieved through the use of particularly active compounds like HTX, meproadifen itself, or trimethisoquin, but, as the L.A. concentration is raised, the binding experiments remain difficult, and this may be at the origin of discrepancies between the results of different laboratories. Cohen and his collaborators [125, 160] studied the binding of [^{14}C]–meproadifen, in the presence of 30 μM carbamylcholine (an agonist, fig. 1) in order to occupy the ACh-binding sites and found 0.25 meproadifen-binding site per α-toxin binding sites ($K_D \simeq 5 \times 10^{-7}$ M), taking the displacement by HTX, procain or cold meproadifen as the criterium of specificity (fig. 6). This high-affinity binding to a small number of sites gives place, in the absence of carbamylcholine, to a low-affinity binding to a larger number of sites (Kd$\simeq$4.4 μM, 0.9$\pm$0.2 sites per α-toxin site). The new binding curve can be interpreted as a superposition of low-affinity binding to the sites observed in the presence of carbamylcholine and to the ACh-binding sites, but more complex explanations are possible. Sobel et al. [197], using [^{3}H]–trimethisoquin, found a somewhat more complicated situation; however, again taking the displacement by HTX as the criterium of specific binding, one goes back to a similar situation with a clear

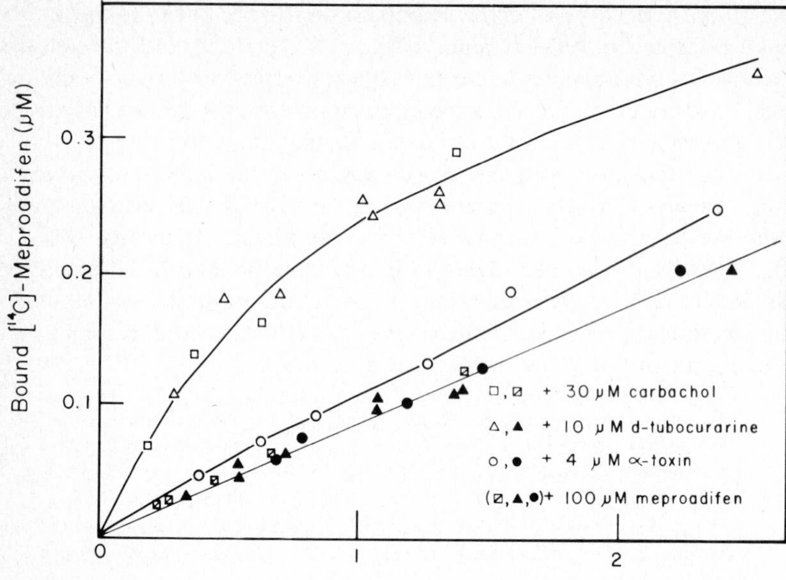

Fig. 6. Equilibrium binding of the local anesthetic [^{14}C]–meproadifen to *Torpedo* receptor-rich membranes in the presence of cholinergic ligands. A membrane suspension (0.8 μM *Naja* α-toxin sites, 0.4 g of protein per liter) in *Torpedo*, physiological saline was divided into three portions. An ultracentrifugation assay was used to measure the binding of [^{14}C]-meproadifen to suspensions containing 30 μM carbamylcholine (□, ⊠), 10 μM tubocurarine (△, ▲), or 4 μM α-bungarotoxin (○, ●). Non-specific interaction of [^{14}C]-meproadifen was determined by the inclusion of 100 μM non-radioactive meproadifen (⊠, ▲, ●). (From Krodel et al. 1979.)

demonstration that carbamylcholine changes the number of high-affinity sites. In its presence, this number appears higher than for meproadifen, ca. 0.8 site per α-toxin binding site ($K_D \simeq 2.1$ μM). Here again, the binding curves cannot be followed to much lower affinities because of non-specific binding. Elliott and Raftery [73, 74] report one site for [^{3}H]–H_{12}-HTX (perhydrohistrionicotoxin) for four α-toxin sites, with only a small effect of carbamylcholine on the affinity, not the number of sites ($K_D = 0.6$ μM without and 0.3 μM in the presence of carbamylcholine) and, conversely, a small effect of H_{12}-HTX on carbamylcholine binding. This is not incompatible with the calculated ratio of affinities for the desensitized vs resting states, which is much higher for trimethisoquin (~40) than for HTX (~3) [97]. Finally, Eldefrawi and co-workers [70, 72] report, for [^{3}H]–H_{12}-HTX also, a similar affinity (0.1–0.4 μM) but a much higher number of sites (1.4 ± 0.5 per ACh-binding site) (the ratio of α-toxin to ACh sites is variously reported as being 1:1 [61, 159, 201, 210] or 2:1 [73, 188] without obvious reason for this discrepancy).

Despite these discrepancies, several groups have now demonstrated the occurrence of a discrete number of L.A.-binding sites, which are, as expected, distinct from but functionally coupled to the ACh-binding sites. Whether these sites are indeed the ionophore itself remain a standing problem, particularly so as it is far from demonstrated that desensitization and channel blockade involve the building of L. A. to the same class of sites.

Having characterized *in vitro* the ACh-binding site, the ionophoric activity, the L.A.-binding site and their interplays, we can turn to the problem of their biochemical support: the protein(s) that carry these properties.

3. Identification of the protein(s) responsible for the functional properties

The identification of the molecules that carry the properties of acetylcholine recognition, of formation and control of a cationic channel, and of local anesthetic binding, present different problems. The easiest target is the ACh-binding site, for which numerous well-characterized ligands are available, some of them are being to bind covalently to the polypeptide chain. Local anesthetic binding, which has become only recently feasible, presents the above-mentioned difficulties which are reinforced in the presence of detergents by the amphiphilic nature of L.A.s, and the development and characterization of sufficiently specific covalent derivatives is still in progress in several laboratories. The characterization of the structure that forms the cholinergic channel raises the worst difficulties, as this property cannot yet be easily quantified in terms of number of sites and can obviously not be studied on solubilized material without first reinserting the would-be channel into a membrane system. As the only presumably intrinsic property of the channel that can be studied without electrical measurements, its cationic selectivity, is not a very discriminative criterium, only a complete reconstitution including recovery of regulation by cholinergic drugs and L.A.s can be practically considered as sufficiently safe. As will be shortly described below, the achievement of an entirely satisfying method of reconstitution has been a particularly difficult task.

The receptor-rich membrane fragments from *Torpedo* electric organ, which maintain *in vitro* the three sets of functional properties, can be purified up to a point where they contain only very few different polypeptide chains. Their appearance in electron-microscopy is shown in fig. 7: they appear densely and nearly uniformly covered by ring-like particles ("rosettes"), with a hydrophilic center that takes up uranyl

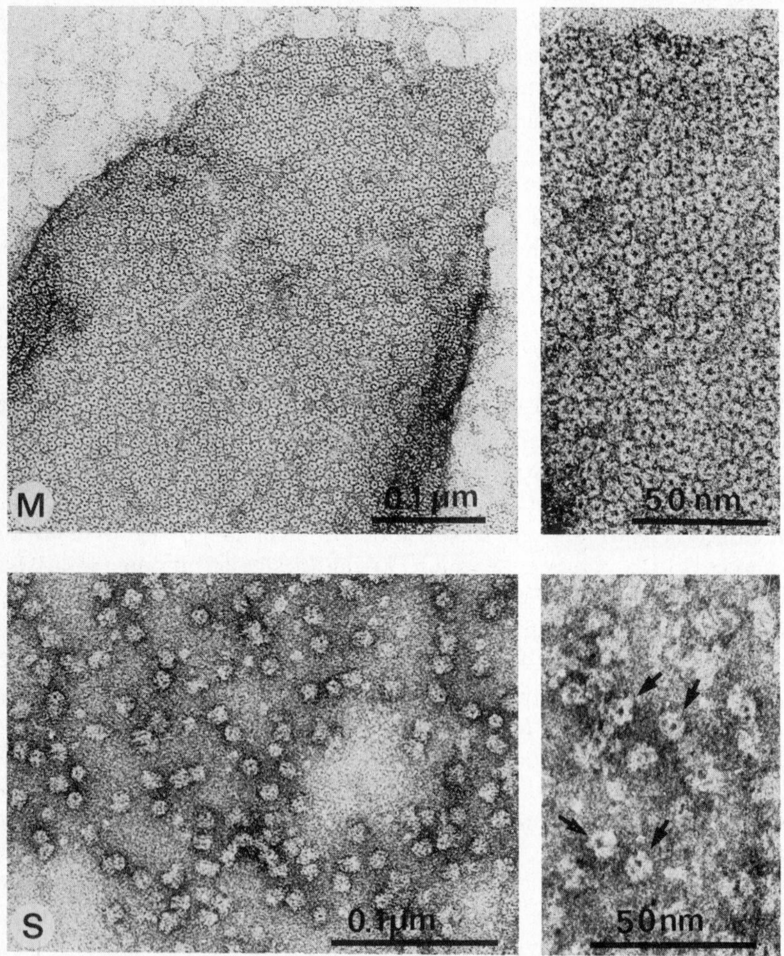

Fig. 7. Electron-micrographs of negatively stained preparations of cholinergic receptor from *Torpedo marmorata* (uranyl formate). M: parts of a receptor-rich vesicle showing the close packing of receptor rosettes (left: ×200 000; right: ×500 000). S: dispersed rosettes (arrows) of solubilized receptor (left: ×300 000; right: ×600 000). (Courtesy of J. Cartaud, see refs. [34], [36].)

formate during negative staining; the diameter of each rosette is about 80–90 Å and there is roughly 10 000–15 000 rosettes/μm^2; they often appear arranged into rows or disrupted lattices, the exact geometry and relevance of whose is still a matter of discussion (see refs. [34–36, 40 68, 73, 106, 121, 161, 178]). There is only about 0.5–0.7 g of lipids per gram of protein [166, 187], with a composition characterized by the prominence of cholesterol and long chain polyunsaturated fatty acid residues [166]; this large proteic content explains the high density of the membrane fragments (1.17), which renders possible their purification on sucrose gradients.

The polypeptide chain composition of highly purified membranes can be studied by polyacrylamide gel electrophoresis in the presence of sodium dodecylsulphate (SDS), a procedure that separates the individual polypeptides according, in first analysis, to their molecular weight. Coomassie brilliant blue or amidoblack staining reveals two major bands with apparent molecular weights (Mr) of 40 000 and 43 000 Daltons, and a few minor ones with Mr = 50 000, 65 000, 95 000, and sometimes 60 000 (fig. 8). If the denaturation by SDS is made in the absence of reducing agent and appropriate precautions taken during the purification of the membranes, the 65-K chain appears as

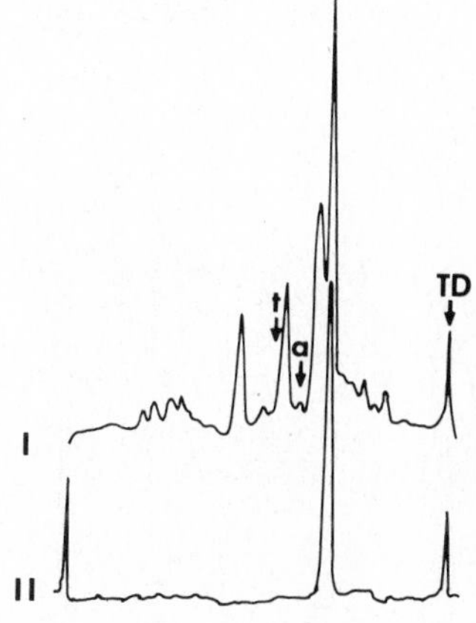

Fig. 8. Polyacrylamide gel electrophoresis, in the presence of SDS, of receptor-rich membrane fragments identification of the chain labelled with [^{3}H]-MPTA. Membrane fragments were labelled with [^{3}H]-MPTA in the absence or presence of an excess of α-toxin and 20 μg protein submitted to electrophoresis according to Anderson and Gesteland (1972). I = Scan of the Coomassie brilliant blue-stained gel; the four major bands have apparent mol wt Mr = 40 000 ± 1 000; 43 000 ± 1 000; 50 000 ± 2 000; and 66 000 ± 2 000 (from right to left); a and t, location of actin and tubulin when added to the sample; T.D. = tracking dye. II and III = Scans of the films obtained after fluorography (Bonner and Laskey 1974) of the gels obtained with membrane fragments labelled with [^{3}H]-MPTA in the absence (II) or presence (III) of α-toxin to protect the ACh-binding site. (From Sobel et al. 1977.)

a dimer of Mr$\simeq$130 000 which can be cleaved to 65 K by dithiotreitol (DTT). The stoichiometry of the minor bands with respect to the 40 K one is variously reported as constant or variable (cf. figs. 8 and 9) by different groups and is one of the most controversial subjects of receptor biochemistry (see below, and refs. [20, 30, 63, 109, 110, 114, 172, 182, 184, 196, 197, 199, 208] (*Torpedo*); [38, 115, 148, 163] (*Electrophorus*); [24, 83–85, 137, 138, 140, 147, 195] (muscle).

There is extremely strong evidence that the 40-K chain (or chains) bears the ACh-binding site. This was first shown using a labelling procedure developed by Karlin and his co-workers [60, 112, 113, 155, 196, 199] in which a disulfide bridge is first reduced by DTT (inducing a slight change in pharmacology of the still active receptor) and then alkylated with radioactive 4-(*N*-maleimido)phenyltrimethylammonium (MPTA; fig. 1). The rate of reaction of the maleimide double band with one of the new sulphydril groups is enhanced by three orders of magnitude by the phenyltrimethylammonium moiety of the molecule which directs it towards the ACh-binding site, achieving a kinetically specific affinity labelling which can even be conducted on whole electroplaques. The covalent thio–ester linkage resists denaturation of the protein, which would not be the case if α-toxins were used as markers. Analysis of the SDS-electrophoresis gels by autoradiography indicates that all of the radioactivity is associated with the 40-K band (fig. 8). The same conclusion was reached with different affinity labels like bromoacetylcholine [60, 155, 196], *p*-(trimethylammonium)benzenediazonium fluoroborate

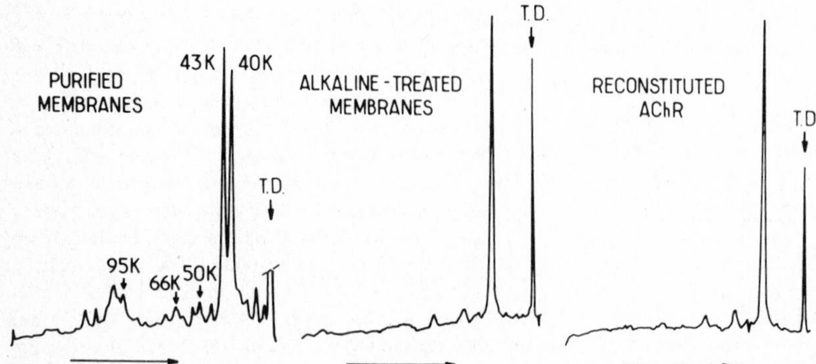

Fig. 9. Polyacrylamide gel electrophoresis, in the presence of SDS, of receptor-rich membranes, alkraline-treated membranes and purified (solubilized and reconstituted) receptor. T.D., tracking dye. (From Sobel et al. 1980.)

(TDF) [49, 213, 218], or even by cross-linking α-toxins to the surrounding polypeptides [65, 108, 110, 216]. During bi-dimensional gel analysis of the polypeptide chains (isoelectric focusing in one direction, SDS-electrophoresis in the other), the 40-K chain forms several spots in the pH_i direction, each of them labelled with MPTA [184]. This heterogeneity however does not reflect the existence of entirely distinct chains with the same Mr, but rather minor modifications of the same polypeptide, as sequencing reveals only one type of residue for each of the first 20 NH_2-terminal amino acids [64].

The search for the L.A.-binding site is not in such an advanced stage. As long as reliable covalent labelling is not available, the only way towards identification goes through further fractionation. Solubilization of the membrane fragments with non-denaturing detergents like sodium cholate, Triton X-100, Emulphogen, etc., liberates into solution an oligomeric protein of mol wt$\simeq$250 000 which still binds acetylcholine and α-toxins, the soluble receptor [46b, 47, 150]. The soluble receptor can exist mainly under two forms, a light form L (mol wt$\simeq$250 000, s$\simeq$9 S) and a heavy form H (mol wt$\simeq$500 000, s$\simeq$12 S); reduction of H with DTT yields L [114, 147b, 170b, 172, 173b, 177b, 187b]. There is about 2–3 α-toxin binding sites per L form (specific activity around 10 000 nmoles per mg protein [138b, 147b, 199, 207b, 216]. The polypeptidic composition of the soluble receptor (which does not vary much if further purification, such as by affinity chromatography, is attempted) is nearly identical to that of the most purified receptor-rich membranes, except for the disappearance of the major 43-K chain (fig. 9). The characterization of the soluble receptor is substantiated by its morphological appearance in electromicroscopy ("rosettes" identical to those observed in subsynaptic membranes) ([35]; see fig. 7) and on immunological grounds: animals injected with it produce antibodies which block postsynaptically the neuromuscular junction [164, 200] and develop an autoimmune disease directed against their own receptors (see refs. [66, 76, 85, 100, 131, 139, 140, 221, 222]).

Although the soluble receptor still binds ACh, agonists, competitive antagonists and α-toxins, it does so with profoundly affected characteristics; namely (in the particular case of *Torpedo* receptor), its affinity for agonists is roughly two orders of magnitude lower than in the membrane-bound state, the increase in affinity during incubation with an agonist, correlated with desensitization, disappears, and the binding of agonists is not affected by L.A.s anymore [31, 82, 98, 201, 210]. These alterations suggested that during solubilization part of the receptor's "functional unit" had been damaged or lost. This in turn could explain the limited success of the reconstitution experiments (see below).

Under appropriate conditions of solubilization, the 43-K protein can be recovered in virtually pure form as an insoluble aggregate. Fluorescence experiments showed that an interaction (presumably a competition) between two L.A.s, histrionicotoxin and the fluorescent L.A. quinacrine, could be demonstrated at the level of the membrane fragments and of the aggregated 43 K, but not on the soluble receptor (even after removal of the detergent), which suggested that the L.A.-binding site could be carried by the 43 K [198]. Similarly, covalent reaction of the membrane fragments with a photosensitive derivative of the L.A. procaine labels primarily the 43-K and 40-K chains (the last binding affecting probably the ACh-binding site as it is prevented by agonists), leading to the same conclusion [19]. This hypothesis could, however, be dismissed after the description [125, 154, 197] of an alkaline treatment of the membrane fragments that removes selectively the 43-K protein without affecting the number of L.A.-binding sites nor the effect of L.A.s on agonist binding. The L.A.-binding site has therefore to be carried by the polypeptide chains present in the soluble receptor, but is somehow damaged during the classical procedures of solubilization.

4. Reconstitution of a functional system after solubilization

Attempts at reconstitution started as early as the receptor could be solubilized without loss of the toxin-binding activity [45, 46, 75, 94, 115, 149, 187, 219] and met with considerable difficulties. Although the interaction of solubilized receptor with planar bilayers (black films) has been pursued for more than five years in several laboratories (for reviews, see [30, 124, 193]), only poorly satisfying results have been yet obtained and the method cannot presently be used as a test for the identification of active fractions nor for the study of the receptor's electrical properties in a completely defined environment. The reassociation of the solubilized receptor into a lipidic membrane has generally been achieved by the more traditional way of co-aggregation during detergent dialysis. In initial experiments, physical reassociation and permeability control by ACh were the only parameters followed, and the poor reproducibility indicated that some critical factors were not under control [94, 149]. Permeability control is the ultimate rather than the best criterium for reconstitution, as it presents some severe drawbacks: one of them is that, if partial reconstitution is achieved (which can give important clues as to the critical factors involved) without the reconstituted system being able to generate a permeability change, such partially successful experiments will not be distinguished from completely negative ones; another, and even more severe, disadvantage is that permeability changes cannot presently be quantified in terms of an absolute number of active ionophores, so that a reconstitution successful according to the $^{22}Na^{+}$-flux studies can in fact concern only a small minority of functional receptors, the rest of them being denaturated. It is of course in itself important to know whether one's procedure preserves 100% or 5% of the preparation's initial activity, but it becomes critical as soon as a comparison must be made with the yields in polypeptides, lipids, or binding sites. The recovery of the allosteric binding properties, which was a likely perquisite to a full reconstitution, has therefore the additional advantage to be easily quantified. Following this path, Changeux and co-workers have progressively defined conditions of detergent addition and removal leading to a quantitative recovery of low-affinity binding to the ACh site, agonist-driven affinity increase and local anesthetic sensitivity [31, 98, 201]. The importance of detergent concentration has also been stressed by Chang and Bock [39], who have shown that beyond a critical degree of delipidation the ACh-binding properties became irreversibly altered, and by Epstein and Racker [75], who also introduced the complex phospholipid mixture asolectin as a good lipidic medium for the formation of functional vesicles. Controlled recovery of permeability control [75, 187] has now been achieved in several laboratories, the reconstituted vesicles being obtained during elimination of the detergent from a receptor/lipid/detergent mixture, either by dialysis [45, 75, 165, 219] or by column chromatography [99, 165, 187]. The description of a "reconstitution cycle" by Changeux and co-workers [45, 197] includes a study of polypeptide composition, morphology, local anesthetic binding [197], phospholipid yield, equilibrium and kinetic studies of agonist binding [99] and pharmacology, ionic specificity, and desensitization of the permeability response [165]. The critical importance of a proper balance of detergent and lipids is demonstrated, which provides a satisfactory explanation for the previous partial successes or failures. Reconstitution should now play its role of a tool in the study of questions like the effect of the lipidic environment on the functioning of the receptor or its minimal polypeptidic composition, and in particular the identification of the elusive cationic channel to the 40-K chain or to one of the larger ones. Although the ratio of L.A.-binding sites to

ACh-binding sites suggests that both sets of sites could indeed be carried by the 40-K chains, no direct demonstration is yet available. The eventual role of the minor chains, the exact composition and geometry of the cholinergic receptor and the nature of the cationic channel are far from being established. The role of the 43-K protein also remains mysterious; its removal from the cytoplasmic side of the membrane where it is located [217] brings about a marked increase in the sensitivity of the ACh-receptor to heat denaturation [185], a disorganisation of the pattern of rosettes on the receptor-rich membrane fragments [179, 197] and the apparition of a rotational freedom [179] of the otherwise immobilized [9, 10, 26, 27, 81, 162, 180] receptor. Therefore, it might be involved in the structural stabilisation of the synapse (see presentation by Changeux).

The field of receptor biochemistry has become so large that such a short introduction to it must necessarily remain incomplete; among the important domains that have only been mentioned are precisely those of the purification, biochemistry, metabolism, and lateral motility of the cholinergic receptor of skelettal muscle (see ref. in [42, 44, 76, 100, 140]) and the immunological studies, which have stemmed from the description of the autoimmune disease induced by the immunological reaction to purified receptor, in many ways similar to the very grave (and rare) human disease called *myasthenia gravis* (see [66, 76, 88, 100, 131, 139, 221, 222]). This last case constitutes a perfect example of the unexpected medical repercussions of a purely fundamental research.

References

[1] P. R. Adams and A. Feltz, Nature 269 (1977) 609.

[2] E. X. Albuquerque, E. A. Barnard, C. W. Porter and J. E. Warnick, Proc. Nat. Acad. Sci. USA 71 (1974) 2818.

[3] E. X. Albuquerque and A. C. Oliveira, in: Advances in Cytopharmacology, vol. 3 eds. B. Ceccarelli and F. Clementi (Raven Press, New York, 1979) pp. 197–211.

[4] M. J. Anderson and M. W. Cohen, J. Physiol. 237 (1974) 385.

[5] M. J. Anderson and M. W. Cohen, J. Physiol. 268 (1977) 757.

[6] C. W. Anderson and R. F. Gesteland, J. Virol. 9 (1972) 758.

[7] T. J. Andreasen, D. R. Doerge and M. G. McNamee, Arch. Biochem. Biophys. 194 (1979) 468.

[8] T. J. Andreasen and M. G. NcNamee, Biochem. Biophys. Res. Comm. 79 (1977) 958.

[9] D. Axelrod, P. Ravdin, D. E. Koppel, J. Schlessinger, W. W. Webb, E. L. Elson and T. R. Podleski, Proc. Nat. Acad. Sci. USA 73 (1976) 4594.

[10] D. Axelrod, P. M. Ravdin and T. R. Podleski, Biochim. Biophys. Acta 511 (1978) 23.
[11] E. A. Barnard, J. Wieckowski and T. H. Chiu, Nature 234 (1971) 207.
[12] F. J. Barrantes, Biochem. Biophys. Res. Comm. 72 (1976) 479.
[13] F. J. Barrantes, J. Mol. Biol. 124 (1978) 1.
[14] F. J. Barrantes, B. Sakmann, R. Bonner, H. Eibl and T. M. Jovin, Proc. Nat. Acad. Sci. USA 72 (1975) 3097.
[15] P. Belbenoit and Z. Bauer, Mar. Biol. 17 (1972) 93.
[16] M. V. L. Bennett, M. Wurtzel and H. Grundfest, J. Gen. Physiol. 44 (1961) 757.
[17] J. Bernhardt and E. Neumann, Proc. Nat. Acad. Sci. USA 75 (1978) 3756.
[18] A. Bienvenüe, A. Rousselet, G. Kato and P. F. Devaux, Biochemistry 16 (1977) 841.
[19] S. Blanchard and M. A. Raftery, Proc. Nat. Acad. Sci. USA 76 (1979) 81.
[20] J. Bode, T. Moody, M. Schimerlik and M. A. Raftery, Biochemistry 18 (1979) 1855.
[21] C. Bon, J.-P. Changeux, T. W. Jeng and H. Fraenkel-Conradt, Eur. J. Biochem. 99 (1979) 471.
[22] R. Bonner, F. J. Barrantes and T. M. Jovin, Nature 263 (1976) 429.
[23] W. M. Bonner and R. A. Laskey, Eur. J. Biochem. 46 (1974) 83.
[24] J. Boulter and J. Patrick, Biochemistry 16 (1977) 4900.
[25] J.-P. Bourgeois, A. Ryter, P. Menez, P. Fromageot, P. Boquet and J.-P. Changeux, FEBS Lett. 25 (1972) 127.
[26] J.-P. Bourgeois, J.-L. Popot, A. Ryter and J.-P. Changeux, Brain Res. 62 (1973) 557.
[27] J.-P. Bourgeois, J.-L. Popot, A. Ryter and J.-P. Changeux, J. Cell Biol. 79 (1978) 200.
[28] J.-P. Bourgeois, S. Tsuji, P. Boquet, J. Pillot, A. Ryter and J.-P. Changeux, FEBS Lett. 16 (1971) 92.
[29] R. N. Bray and M. A. Hixon, Science 200 (1978) 333.
[30] M. Briley and J.-P. Changeux, Int. Rev. Neurobiol. 20 (1977) 31.
[31] M. Briley and J.-P. Changeux, Eur. J. Biochem. 84 (1978) 429.
[32] A. Brisson, P. F. Devaux and J.-P. Changeux, C. R. Hebd. Séances Acad. Sci., Sér. D, Sci. Nat. Paris 280 (1975) 2153.
[33] A. Brisson, C. J. Scandella, A. Bienvenüe, P. Devaux, J. B. Cohen and J.-P. Changeux, Proc. Nat. Acad. Sci. USA 72 (1975) 1087.
[34] J. Cartaud, in: Ontogenesis and Functional Mechanism of Peripheral Synapses, ed. J. Taxi, (Elsevier, Amsterdam, 1980) in press.
[35] J. Cartaud, L. Benedetti, J. B. Cohen, J.-C. Meunier and J.-P. Changeux, FEBS Lett. 33 (1973) 109.
[36] J. Cartaud, E. L. Benedetti, A. Sobel and J.-P. Changeux, J. Cell Sci. 29 (1978) 313.
[37] C. Chagas, E. Penna-Franca, K. Nishie and E. J. Garcia, Arch. Biochem. Biophys. 75 (1958) 251.
[38] H. W. Chang, Proc, Nat. Acad. Sci. USA 71 (1974) 2113.
[39] H. W. Chang and E. Bock, Biochemistry 16 (1977) 4513.
[40] R. S. L. Chang, L. T. Potter and D. S. Smith, Tissue Cell 9 (1977) 623.
[41] J.-P. Changeux, in: Handbook of Psychopharmacology, eds. S. Snyder and L. Iversen, vol. 6 (1975) pp. 235–301.
[42] J.-P. Changeux, in: The Neurosciences, Fourth Study Program, (The MIT Press, Cambridge and London, 1979) pp. 749–778.

[43] J.-P. Changeux, L. Benedetti, J.-P. Bourgeois, A. Brisson, J. Cartaud, P. F. Devaux, H. H. Grünhagen, M. Moreau, J.-L. Popot, A. Sobel and M. Weber, in: The Synapse, Cold Spring Harbor Symp. Quant. Biol. 40 (1976) 203.
[44] J.-P. Changeux and A. Danchin, Nature 264 (1976) 705.
[45] J.-P. Changeux, T. Heidmann, J.-L. Popot and A. Sobel, FEBS Lett. 105 (1979) 181.
[46] J.-P. Changeux, M. Huchet and J. Cartaud, C. R. Acad. Sci. Paris 274 (1972) 122.
[46b] J.-P. Changeux, M. Kasai, M. Huchet and J.-C. Meunier, C. R. Acad. Sci. Paris 270 D (1970) 2864.
[47] J.-P. Changeux, M. Kasai and C. Y. Lee, Proc. Nat. Acad. Sci. USA 67 (1970) 1241.
[48] J.-P. Changeux, J.-C. Meunier and M. Huchet, Mol. Pharmacol. 7 (1971) 538.
[49] J.-P. Changeux, T. Podleski and L. Wofsy, Proc. Nat. Acad. Sci. 58 (1967) 2063.
[50] J. B. Cohen and N. D. Boyd, in: Catalysis in Chemistry and Biochemistry, eds. B. Pulman and D. Ginsburg (Reidel, 1980) in press.
[53] J. B. Cohen and J.-P. Changeux, Biochemistry 12 (1973) 4855.
[54] J. B. Cohen and J.-P. Changeux, Ann. Rev. Pharmacol. 15 (1975) 83.
[55] J. B. Cohen, M. Weber and J.-P. Changeux, Mol. Pharmacol. 10 (1974) 904.
[56] J. B. Cohen, M. Weber, M. Huchet and J.-P. Changeux, FEBS Lett. 26 (1972) 43.
[57] D. Colquhoun and H. P. Rang, Mol. Pharmacol. 12 (1976) 519.
[58] D. Cooper and E. Reich, J. Biol. Chem. 247 (1972) 3008.
[59] J. W. Daly, I. Darle, C. W. Myers, T. Tokuyama, J. A. Waters and B. Witkop, Proc. Nat. Acad. Sci. USA 68 (1971) 1870.
[60] V. N. Damle and A. Karlin, Biochemistry 17 (1978) 2039.
[61] V. N. Damle, M. McLaughlin and A. Karlin, Biochem. Biophys. Res. Comm. 84 (1978) 845.
[62] J. Del Castillo and G. D. Webb, J. Physiol. 270 (1977) 271.
[63] J. W. Deutsch and M. Raftery, Arch. Biochem. Biophys. 197 (1979) 503.
[64] A. Devillers-Thiéry, J.-P. Changeux, P. Paroutaud and A. D. Strosberg, FEBS Lett. 104 (1979) 99.
[65] O. J. Dolly, E. Barnard and R. G. Shorr, Biochem. Soc. Trans. 5 (1977) 168.
[66] D. B. Drachman, New Engl. J. Med. 298 (1978) 136.
[67] J. R. Duguid and M. A. Raftery, Biochemistry 12 (1973) 3593.
[68] Y. Dupont, J. B. Cohen and J.-P. Changeux, FEBS Lett. 40 (1974) 130.
[69] M. E. Eldefrawi and A. T. Eldefrawi, in: Receptors and Recognition, vol. A4, eds. P. Cuatrecasas and L. P. Greaves (Excerpta Medica, 1977) pp. 73–84.
[70] M. E. Eldefrawi and A. T. Eldefrawi, in: Advances in Cytopharmacology, vol. 3, eds. B. Ceccarelli and F. Clementi (Raven Press, New York, 1979) pp. 213–223.
[71] A. T. Eldefrawi, M. E. Eldefrawi, E. X. Albuquerque, A. C. Oliveira, N. Mansour, M. Adler, J. W. Daly, G. B. Brown, W. B. Burgermeister and B. Witkop, Proc. Nat. Acad. Sci. USA 74 (1977) 2172.
[72] M. E. Eldefrawi, A. T. Eldefrawi, N. A. Mansour, J. W. Daly, B. Witkop and E. X. Albuquerque, Biochemistry 17 (1978) 5474.
[73] J. Elliott, S. M. J. Dunn, S. G. Blanchard and M. A. Raftery, Proc. Nat. Acad. Sci. USA 76 (1979) 2576.
[74] J. Elliott and M. A. Raftery, Biochemistry 18 (1979) 1868.
[75] M. Epstein and E. Racker, J. Biol. Chem. 253 (1978) 6660.
[76] D. M. Fambrough, Physiol. Rev. 59 (1979) 165.

[77] H. C. Fertuck and M. M. Salpetier, J. Cell. Biol. 69 (1976) 144.
[78] A. Fessard, in: Traité de Zoologie, ed. P. P. Grassé, vol. 13A (Masson, Paris, 1958) pp. 1143–1238.
[79] S. D. Flanagan, S. H. Barondes and P. Taylor, J. Biol. Chem. 251 (1976) 858.
[80] G. Q. Fox and G. P. Richardson, J. Comp. Neurol. 179 (1978) 677.
[81] E. Frank, K. Gautvik and H. Sommerschild, Acta. Physiol. Scand. 95 (1975) 66.
[82] G. I. Franklin and L. T. Potter, FEBS Lett. 28 (1972) 101.
[83] S. C. Froehner, A. Karlin and Z. W. Hall, Proc. Nat. Acad. Sci. USA 74 (1977) 4685.
[84] S. C. Froehner and S. Rafto, Biochemistry 18 (1979) 301.
[85] S. C. Froehner, C. G. Reiness and Z. W. Hall, J. Biol. Chem. 252 (1977) 8589.
[86] J. H. Gaddum, J. Physiol. 89 (1937) 7P.
[87] J. Giraudat and J.-P. Changeux, TIPS 1(1980) 198.
[88] C. Goulon, B. Estournet, A. Sobel and M. Goulon, Rev. Prat. Paris 29 (1979) 2774.
[89] H. Grundfest, in: Sharks, Skates and Rays, eds. P. W. Gilbert, R. F. Mathewson and D. P. Rall (Johns Hopkins Press, Baltimore, 1967) pp. 399–432.
[90] H. H. Grünhagen and J.-P. Changeux, J. Mol. Biol. 106 (1976) 497.
[91] H. H. Grünhagen and J.-P. Changeux, J. Mol. Biol. 106 (1976) 517.
[92] H. H. Grünhagen, M. Iwatsubo and J.-P. Changeux, Eur. J. Biochem. 80 (1977) 225.
[93] M. R. Hanley, Biochem. Biophys. Res. Comm. 82 (1978) 392.
[94] G. L. Hazelbauer and J.-P. Changeux, Proc. Nat. Acad. Sci. USA 71 (1974) 1479.
[95] T. Heidmann and J.-P. Changeux, Ann. Rev. Biochem. 47 (1978) 371.
[96] T. Heidmann and J.-P. Changeux, Eur. J. Biochem. 94 (1979) 255.
[97] T. Heidmann and J.-P. Changeux, Eur. J. Biochem. 94 (1979) 281.
[98] T. Heidmann, A. Sobel and J.-P. Changeux, FEBS Lett. 94 (1978) 397.
[99] T. Heidmann, A. Sobel, J.-L. Popot and J.-P. Changeux, Eur. J. Biochem. (1980) submitted for publication.
[100] E. Heilbronn, in: Motor Innervation of Muscle, ed. S. Thesleff (Acad. Press, London 1976) pp. 177–212.
[101] E. Heilbronn, C. Bjork, L. Elfman, A. Hartman and C. Mattson, in: Advances in Cytopharmacology, vol. 3, eds. B. Ceccarelli and F. Clementi (Raven Press, New York, 1979) pp. 151–158.
[102] G. P. Hess, J. P. Andrews, G. E. Struve and S. E. Coombs, Proc. Nat. Acad. Sci. USA 72 (1975) 4371.
[103] G. P. Hess, J. P. Andrews and G. E. Struve, Biochem. Biophys. Res. Comm. 69 (1976) 830.
[104] G. P. Hess, and J. P. Andrews, Proc. Nat. Acad. Sci. USA 74 (1977) 482.
[105] G. P. Hess, D. J. Cash and H. Aoshima, Nature 282 (1979) 329.
[106] J. E. Heuser and S. R. Salpeter, J. Cell Biol. 82 (1979) 150.
[107] H. Higman, T. R. Podleski and E. Bartels, Biochim. Biophys. Acta 79 (1964) 138.
[108] F. Hucho, FEBS Lett. 103 (1979) 27.
[109] F. Hucho, G. Bandini and B. A. Suarez-Islá, Eur. J. Biochem. 83 (1978) 335.
[110] F. Hucho, P. Layer, H. Kiefer and G. Bandini, Proc. Nat. Acad. Sci. USA 73 (1976) 2624.
[111] R. Jürss, H. Prinz and A. Maelicke, Proc. Nat. Acad. Sci. USA 76 (1979) 1064.
[112] A. Karlin and E. Bartels, Biochim. Biophys. Acta 126 (1966) 525.
[113] A. Karlin and D. Cowburn, Proc. Nat. Acad. Sci. USA 70 (1973) 3636.

[114] A. Karlin, V. N. Damle, S. Hamilton, M. McLaughlin, R. Valderrama and D. Wise, in: Advances in Cytopharmacology, vol. 3, eds. B. Ceccarelli and F. Clementi (Raven Press, New York, 1979) pp. 183–188.
[115] A. Karlin, C. Weill, M. McNamee and R. Valderrama, in: The Synapse, Cold Spring Harbor Symp. Quant. Biol. 40 (1976) 203.
[116] A. Karlin and M. Winnik, Proc. Nat. Acad. Sci. USA 60 (1968) 668.
[117] M. Kasaï and J.-P. Changeux, J. Memb. Biol. 6 (1971) 1.
[118] G. Kato and J.-P. Changeux, Mol. Pharmacol. 12 (1976) 92.
[119] B. Katz and S. Thesleff, J. Physiol. 138 (1957) 63.
[120] R. D. Keynes, in: Bioelectrogenesis, eds. C. Chagas and P. de Carvalho (Elsevier, Amsterdam, 1961) pp. 14–19.
[121] M. W. Klymkowsky and R. M. Stroud, J. Mol. Biol. 128 (1979) 319.
[122] D. K. Koblin and H. A. Lester, Mol. Pharmacol. 15 (1979) 559.
[123] R. Kohanski, J. P. Andrews, P. Wins, M. Eldefrawi and G. P. Hess, Anal. Biochem. 80 (1977) 531.
[124] J. I. Korenbrot, Ann. Rev. Physiol. 39 (1977) 19.
[125] E. K. Krodel, R. A. Beckman and J. B. Cohen, Mol. Pharmacol. 15 (1979) 294.
[126] C. Y. Lee, Ann. Rev. Pharmacol. 12 (1972) 265.
[127] C. Y. Lee, in: Pharmacology and the Future of Man, Proc. 5th Int. Congr. Pharmacology, San Francisco 1972, vol. 2 (Karger, Basel, 1979) pp. 210–232.
[128] C. Y. Lee and C. C. Chang, Mem. Inst. Butantan Simp. Int. 33 (1966) 555.
[129] C. Y. Lee and L. F. Tseng, Toxicon 3 (1966) 281.
[130] T. Lee, V. Witzemann, M. Schimerlik and M. A. Raftery, Arch. Biochem. Biophys. 183 (1977) 57.
[131] A. K. Lefvert and K. Bergström, Scand. J. Immunol. 8 (1978) 525.
[132] T. L. Lentz, J. E. Mazurkiervicz and J. Rosenthal, Brain Res. 132 (1977) 423.
[133] H. A. Lester, J. Gen. Physiol. 72 (1978) 847.
[134] H. A. Lester and H. W. Chang, Nature 266 (1977) 373.
[135] H. A. Lester, J.-P. Changeux and R. E. Sheridan, J. Gen. Physiol. 65 (1975) 797.
[136] H. A. Lester, D. D. Koblin and R. E. Sheridan, Biophys. J. 21 (1978) 181.
[137] J. Lindstrøm, in: Advances in Cytopharmacology, vol. 3, eds. B. Ceccarelli and F. Clementi (Raven Press, New York, 1979) pp. 245–253.
[138] J. Lindstrøm, B. Einarson and J. Merlie, Proc. Nat. Acad. Sci. USA 75 (1978) 769.
[138b] J. Lindstrøm and J. Patrick, in: Synaptic transmission and nerve interaction, ed. M. V. L. Bennett (Raven Press, New York, 1974) pp. 191–216.
[139] J. M. Lindstrøm, M. E. Seybold, V. A. Lennon, S. Whittingham and D. D. Duane, Neurology Minneap. 26 (1976) 1054.
[140] T. Lømo, in: Motor Innervation of Muscle, ed. S. Thesleff (Acad. Press, London, 1976) pp. 177–212.
[141] B. W. Low, in: Advances in Cyto. vol. 3 eds. B. Ceccarelli and F. Clementi (Raven Press, New York, 1979) pp. 141–147.
[142] L. G. Magazanik and F. Vyskočil, in: Motor Innervation of Muscle, ed. S. Thesleff (Acad. Press, London, 1976) pp. 151–176.
[143] D. Marsh and F. J. Barrantes, Proc. Nat. Acad. Sci. USA 75 (1978) 4329.
[144] M. Martinez-Carrión and M. A. Raftery, Biochem. Biophys. Res. Comm. 55 (1973) 1156.
[145] L. M. Masukawa and E. X. Albuquerque, J. Gen. Physiol. 72 (1978) 351.
[146] A. Menez, J. L. Morgat, P. Fromageot, A. M. Ronseray, P. Boquet and J.-P. Changeux, FEBS Lett. 17 (1971) 333.

[147] J. Merlie, J.-P. Changeux and F. Gros, J. Biol. Chem. 253 (1978) 2882.
[147b] J.-C. Meunier, R. W. Olsen, A. Menez, J. L. Morgat, P. Fromageot, A. M. Ronseray, P. Boquet and J.-P. Changeux, C. R. Acad. Sci. Paris 273 D (1971) 595.
[148] J.-C. Meunier, R. Sealock, R. Olsen and J.-P. Changeux, Eur. J. Biochem. 45 (1974) 371.
[149] D. M. Michaelson and M. A. Raftery, Proc. Nat. Acad. Sci. USA 71 (1974) 4768.
[150] R. Miledi, P. Molinoff and L. T. Potter, Nature 229 (1971) 554.
[151] R. Miledi and L. T. Potter, Nature 233 (1971) 599.
[152] D. L. Miller, H.-P. H. Moore, P. R. Hartig and M. A. Raftery, Biochem. Biophys. Res. Comm. 85 (1978) 632.
[153] J. Miller, V. Witzemann, U. Quast and M. A. Raftery, Proc. Nat. Acad. Sci. USA 76 (1979) 3580.
[154] H.-P. H. Moore, P. R. Hartig, W. C. S. Wu and M. A. Raftery, Biochem. Biophys. Res. Comm. 88 (1979) 735.
[155] H.-P. H. Moore and M. A. Raftery, Biochemistry 18 (1979) 1862.
[156] M. Moreau and J.-P. Changeux, J. Mol. Biol. 106 (1976) 457.
[157] D. Nachmansohn, Chemical and Molecular Basis of Nerve Activity (Academic Press, New York, 1959).
[158] D. Nachmansohn and E. Neumann, Chemical and Molecular Basis of Nerve Activity, rev. ed. (Academic Press, New York, 1975).
[159] R. R. Neubig and J. B. Cohen, Biochemistry (1980) in press.
[160] R. R. Neubig, E. K. Krodel, N. D. Boyd and J. B. Cohen, Proc. Nat. Acad. Sci. USA 76 (1979) 690.
[161] E. Nickel and L. T. Potter, Brain Res. 57 (1973) 508.
[162] N. Orida and M. M. Poo, Nature 275 (1978) 31.
[163] J. Patrick, J. Boulter and J. C. O'Brien, Biochem. Biophys. Res. Comm. 64 (1975) 219.
[164] J. Patrick and J. Lindstrøm, Science 180 (1973) 871.
[165] J.-L. Popot, J. Cartaud, and J.-P. Changeux, Eur. J. Biochem. (1980) submitted for publication.
[166] J.-L. Popot, A. Demel, A. Sobel, L. L. M. Van Deenen and J.-P. Changeux, Eur. J. Biochem. 85 (1978) 27.
[167] J.-L. Popot, H. Sugiyama and J.-P. Changeux, C. R. Acad. Sci. 279 D (1974) 1721.
[168] J.-L. Popot, H. Sugiyama and J.-P. Changeux, J. Mol. Biol. 106 (1976) 469.
[169] C. W. Porter, E. A. Barnard and T. H. Chiu, J. Memb. Biol. 14 (1973) 383.
[170] C. W. Porter and E. A. Barnard, J. Memb. Biol. 20 (1975) 31.
[170b] L. Potter, in: Drug Receptors, ed. H. P. Rang (MacMillan, London, 1973) pp. 295–312.
[171] U. Quast, M. I. Schimerlik and M. A. Raftery, Biochemistry 18 (1979) 1891.
[172] M. A. Raftery, S. Blanchard, J. Elliott, P. Hartig, H. Moore, U. Quast, M. Schimerlik, V. Witzemann and W. Wu, in: Advances in Cytopharmacology, vol. 3, eds. B. Ceccarelli and F. Clementi (Raven Press, New York, 1979) pp. 159–182.
[173] M. A. Raftery, J. Bode, R. Vandlen, D. Michaelson, J. Deutsch, T. Moody, M. J. Ross and R. M Stroud, in: Protein–Ligand Interactions, eds. H. Sund, and G. Blauer (W. de Gruyter, Berlin/New York, 1975) pp. 328–355.
[173b] M. A. Raftery, J. Schmidt, D. G. Clark and R. G. Wolcott, Biochem. Biophys. Res. Commun. 45 (1971) 1622.
[174] H. P. Rang, Quart. Rev. Biophys. 7 (1975) 283.
[175] H. P. Rang and J. M. Ritter, Mol. Pharmacol. 5 (1969) 394.

[176] H. P. Rang and J. M. Ritter, Mol. Pharmacol. 6 (1970) 357.
[177] (a) H. P. Rang and J. M. Ritter, Mol. Pharmacol. 6 (1970) 383; (b) J. A. Reynolds and A. Karlin, Biochemistry 17 (1978) 2035.
[178] M. Ross, M. Klymkowsky, D. Agard and R. Stroud, J. Mol. Biol. 116 (1977) 635.
[179] A. Rousselet, J. Cartaud and P. F. Devaux, C. R. Acad. Sci. Série D (1979) in press.
[180] A. Rousselet and P. F. Devaux, Biochem. Biophys. Res. Comm. 78 (1977) 448.
[181] A. Rousselet, P. F. Devaux and K. W. Wirtz, Biochem. Biophys. Res. Comm. 90 (1979) 871.
[182] H. Rübsamen, G. R. Hess, A. T. Eldefrawi and M. E. Eldefrawi, Biochem. Biophys. Res. Comm. 68 (1976) 56.
[183] F. Ruiz-Manresa and H. Grundfest, J. Gen. Physiol. 57 (1971) 71.
[184] T. Saitoh and J.-P. Changeux, Eur. J. Biochem. 105 (1980) 51.
[185] T. Saitoh, L. Wennogle and J.-P. Changeux, FEBS Lett. 108 (1979) 489.
[186] M. M. Salpeter and M. Szabo, J. Histochem. Cytochem. 20 (1972) 425.
[187] W. Schiebler and F. Hucho, Eur. J. Biochem. 85 (1978) 55.
[187b] W. Schiebler, L. Lauffer and F. Hucho, FEBS Lett. 81 (1977) 39.
[188] M. Schimerlik, U. Quast and M. A. Raftery, Biochemistry 18 (1979) 1884.
[189] M. I. Schimerlik, U. Quast and M. A. Raftery, Biochemistry 18 (1979) 1902.
[190] J. Schmidt and M. A. Raftery, Anal. Biochem. 52 (1973) 349.
[191] E. Schoffeniels, Biochim. Biophys. Acta 26 (1957) 585.
[192] E. Schoffeniels and D. Nachmansohn, Biochim. Biophys. Acta 26 (1957) 1.
[193] A. E. Shamoo and D. A. Goldstein, Biochim. Biophys. Acta 472 (1977) 13.
[194] R. E. Sheridan and H. A. Lester, J. Gen. Physiol. 70 (1977) 187.
[195] R. G. Shorr, J. O. Dolly and E. A. Barnard, Nature 274 (1978) 283.
[196] I. Silman and A. Karlin, Science 164 (1969) 1420.
[197] A. Sobel, T. Heidmann, J. Cartaud and J.-P. Changeux, Eur. J. Biochem., submitted for publication.
[198] A. Sobel, T. Heidmann, J. Hofler and J.-P. Changeux, Proc. Nat. Acad. Sci. USA 75 (1978) 510.
[199] A. Sobel, M. Weber and J.-P. Changeux, Eur. J. Biochem. 80 (1977) 215.
[200] H. Sugiyama, P. Benda, J.-C. Meunier and J.-P. Changeux, FEBS Lett. 35 (1973) 124.
[201] H. Sugiyama and J.-P. Changeux, Eur. J. Biochem. 55 (1975) 505.
[202] H. Sugiyama, J.-L. Popot, J. B. Cohen, M. Weber and J.-P. Changeux, in: Protein–Ligand Interactions, eds. H. Sund and G. Blauer (Walter de Gruyter, New York, 1975) pp. 289–305.
[203] H. Sugiyama, J.-L. Popot and J.-P. Changeux, J. Mol. Biol. 106 (1976) 485.
[204] M.-C. Tsai, A. C. Oliveira, E. X. Albuquerque, M. E. Eldefrawi and A. T. Eldefrawi, Mol. Pharmacol. 16 (1979) 382.
[205] D. Tsernoglou and G. A. Petsko, Proc. Nat. Acad. Sci. USA 74 (1977) 971.
[206] V. I. Tsetlin, E. Karlsson, A. S. Arseniev, Yu. N. Utkin, A. M. Surin, V. S. Pashkov, K. A. Pluzhnikov, V. T. Ivanov, V. F. Bystrov and Yu. A. Ovchinnikov, FEBS Lett. 106 (1979) 47.
[207] A. T. Tu, Ann. Rev. Biochem. 42 (1973) 235.
[207b] R. L. Vandlen, J. Schmidt and M. A. Raftery, J. Macromol. Chem. A 10 (1976) 73.
[208] R. L. Vandlen, W. C. S. Wu, J. C. Eisenach and M. A. Raftery, Biochemistry 18 (1979) 1845.

[209] G. Waksman, M. C. Fournié-Zaluski, B. Roques, T. Heidmann, H. H. Grünhagen and J.-P. Changeux, FEBS Lett. 67 (1976) 335.
[210] M. Weber and J.-P. Changeux, Mol. Pharmacol. 10 (1974) 1.
[211] M. Weber, M. T. David-Pfeuty and J.-P. Changeux, Proc. Nat. Acad. Sci. USA 72 (1975) 3443.
[212] G. Weiland, B. Georgia, S. Lappi, C. F. Chignell and P. Taylor, J. Biol. Chem. 252 (1977) 7648.
[213] G. Weiland, D. Frisman and P. Taylor, Mol. Pharmacol. 15 (1979) 213.
[214] G. Weiland, B. Georgia, V. T. Wee, C. F. Chignell and P. Taylor, Mol. Pharmacol. 12 (1976) 1091.
[215] G. Weiland and P. Taylor, Mol. Pharmacol. 15 (1979) 197.
[216] C. L. Weill, M. G. McNamee and A. Karlin, Biochem. Biophys. Res. Comm. 61 (1974) 997.
[217] L. P. Wennogle and J.-P. Changeux, Eur. J. Biochem. 106 (1980) 381.
[218] V. Witzemann and M. A. Raftery, Biochem. Biophys. Res. Comm. 85 (1978) 623.
[219] W. C. S. Wu and M. A. Raftery, Biochem. Biophys. Res. Comm. 89 (1979) 26.

Collective Books:

[220] Cold Spring Harbor Symposia on Quantitative Biology, vol. 40: The Synapse (1976).
[221] "Myasthenia gravis," Ann. NY Acad. Sci. 274 (1976) 1.
[222] Pathogenesis of Human Muscular Dystrophies, ed. L. P. Rowland, (Excerpta Medica, Amsterdam, 1977).

COURSE 10

GENETIC AND "EPIGENETIC" FACTORS REGULATING SYNAPSE FORMATION IN MOUSE CEREBELLUM AND DEVELOPING NEUROMUSCULAR JUNCTION

Jean-Pierre CHANGEUX

Institut Pasteur, Unité de Neurobiologie Moléculaire,
25 rue du Docteur Roux, 75724 Paris Cedex 15, France

(Lecture notes written by a participant, Jean Davoust)

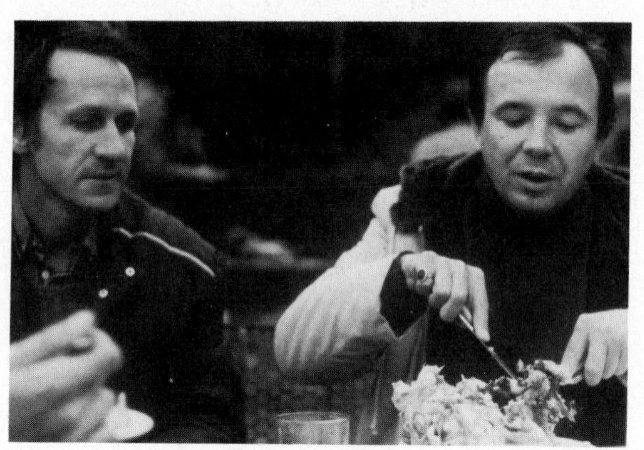

Contents

R. Balian et al., eds.
Les Houches, Session XXXIII, 1979 – Membranes et Communication Intercellulaire / Membranes and Intercellular Communication

1. Cerebellum

1.1. Introduction

The neuron. The nervous system is formed by a set of specialized cells, the neurons, connected in specific ways and surrounded with the glial cells, the function of which is certainly underestimated and will not be discussed in the present lecture.

Like other cells, the neurons have a cell soma but they can expand into very long cytoplasmic filaments characteristic of the nervous tissue: the dendrites and the axons. The dendrites receive signals not only from sensory cells, but also from other nerve cells while the axons are the main output way for action potentials emitted by given neurons. This classification also corresponds to some morphological criteria visualized on histological preparations stained for the neurons (see for instance the Purkinje cell from the cerebellar cortex (fig. 1, in the following subsection). In fact, the description of these neurites is far from being sufficient to understand the "circuitry" of the nervous system where they are not distributed at random: these intricate dendrites and axons create, between neurons, many contacts having a great functional significance.

The synapse. The information flows through connections fom one neuron to the other, or between one neuron and another class of cell. Sherrington first introduced, in 1897, the term synapse to account for the region in which an individual neuron established special contact and communicated with another cell. The term communication is more general than the so-called synaptic transmission and it will prove itself to be a very useful one as soon as we are interested in the functional organization of the nervous system.

It is, of course, a major challenge for the neurobiologist to give a molecular description for the structural organization of synapses. Later in this chapter, we will see how molecular interactions could be involved in the development and the stabilization of synaptic contact. For that purpose, we will choose the neuromuscular junction where the motor neuron contacts a muscle fiber and which has been studied for a long time: it possesses many other advantages, one of which is its relative simplicity and accessibility as compared to other synapses found in the brain, imbedded inside a very complex environment of neurites and connections. In this latter case, the information is not necessarily restrained to some local "circuit" but can diffuse through large subsets of neurons, as a result of their characteristic ability to establish synaptic contacts, not only with adjacent cells, but also with more distant ones.

Neuronal networks. Consequently, the nervous system looks more like a complex and highly organized network of interneuronal connections than any other organ. This view has been introduced very early, since histological and cytochemical methods have been able to give structural information about the "circuitry" of the system. Moreover, electrophysiological measurements were able to test the functional importance of main pathways within the nervous system. Many hypotheses have been formulated to account for complex networks formation. In this first section, we give a short presentation of the cerebellum and pay particular attention to its genetic determinism, trying to elucidate the development of the neuronal networks, which is obviously one of the most intriguing problems that ever arose in neuroscience.

1.2. Complexity of the nervous system

A special case, the cerebellum. The cerebellum is involved in coordination of motor behavior. There are two main classes of cells located in two different layers, the Purkinje cell layer and the granular cell layer (see fig. 2, in the following subsection). The first layer represents 30 million cells and the second 30 billion cells. Therefore, we face an incredible complexity even within a single class of cells.

1.2.1. The complexity within a given class of cells: the Purkinje cell

The organization of the neurites within one Purkinje cell is rather complex. The surface of its dendritic arborisation (spines together with primary and secondary dendrites) is very large as compared to the cell soma surface (see fig. 1). The same being true for the axonal arborisation. So, one aspect of the nervous system complexity lies in its neurite arborisation. The connectivity of which seems to be absolutely characteristic of each class of nerve cells. But even within one of these classes, there is very little true redundancy as determined from intracellular potential recordings. For instance, identical Purkinje cells, in a

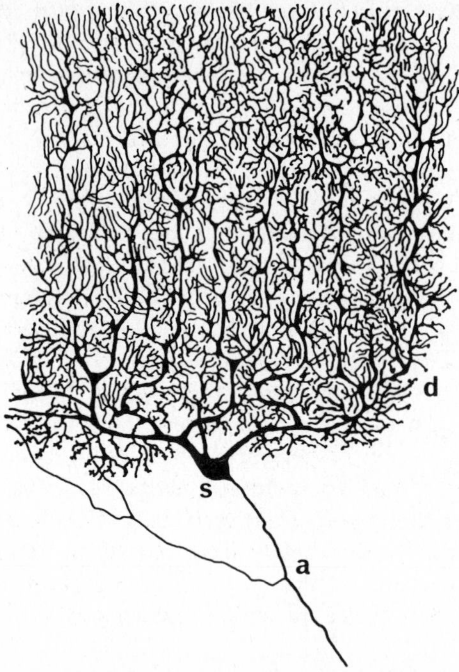

Fig. 1. Cerebellar Purkinje cell in Golgi stain by light microscopy (Cajal 1911). The dendritic arbor is a broad flat plane of richly branched dendrites: a-axon, s-soma, and d-dendrite.

morphological point of view, are different in their firing activity. Thus, the complexity of the nervous system lies not only in the connectivity of a given cell, but also in the absolute number of neurons since each nerve cell is different from its neighbours.

1.2.2. *Complexity of interneuronal connections*

The only exit from the cerebellum is the axon of the Purkinje cell but this unique cell also receives a very large number of synaptic contacts, for instance from the granular cells. The spines from the dendritic arborisation of the Purkinje cell contact the parallel fibers (axons of the granular cells). It forms the main class of synapses which is found in the molecular layer of the cerebellum. So there are in this cerebellar cortex both a convergence of inputs on a given Purkinje cell and a divergent pathway, where one given granular cell can establish contacts with many Purkinje cells (see fig. 2).

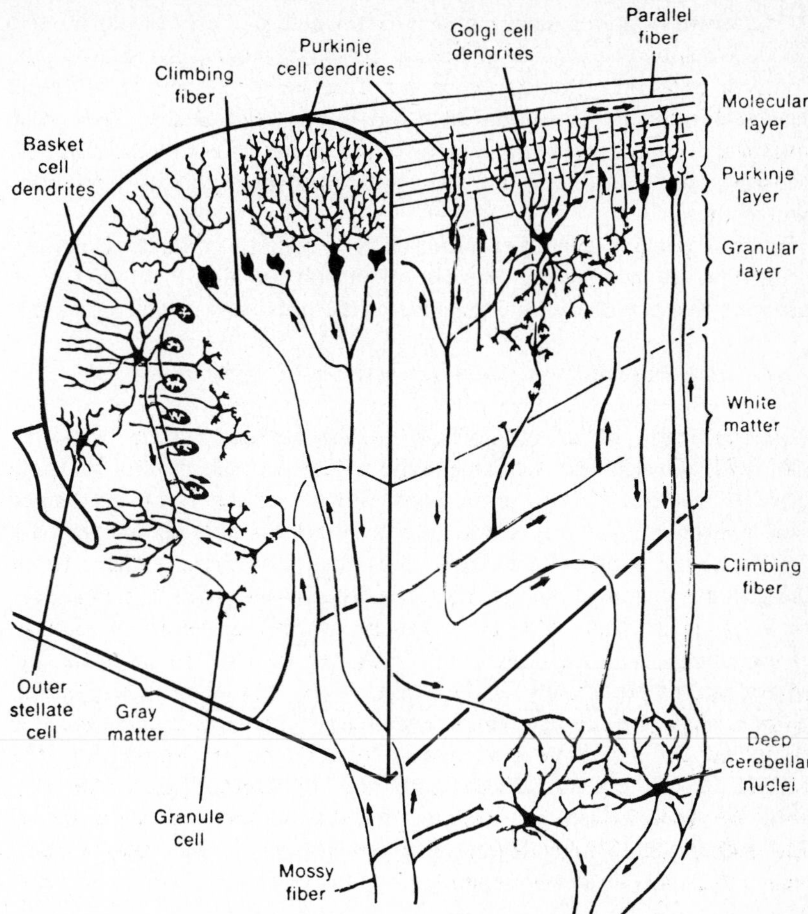

Fig. 2. Stereodiagram illustrating the principal neuronal types in the cerebellar cortex, the two afferent systems, and the interconnections between these elements. The mossy fiber afferents innervate granular cells and Golgi cells in complex synaptic glomeruli. The granular cell axons then rise toward the surface of the cerebellum, where they branch to form parallel fibers that excite Purkinje cells, Golgi cells, basket cells, and stellate cells. The Purkinje cell axons constitute the only output from the cerebellar cortex. (Eccles et al. 1967.)

The entries coming from sensory pathways of the brain cortex are divided into two categories of fibers: the mossy fibers, giving divergent contacts onto 600 granular cells per fiber, and the climbing fibers, innervating the Purkinje cells in a one-to-one relationship. This latter situation is rather interesting since we can precisely count the number-per-Purkinje cell and there are some situations where this strict relationship is altered.

Even if we add some other minor class of synaptic contacts effectively present in the cerebellum (see fig. 2), it still remains a rather simple network of connections as compared to the neocortex itself.

1.2.3. Complexity of the nervous system and of the genome

Any evaluation of the complexity of the nervous system could be criticized. Nevertheless, we can use the number of neurons and compare it within species. It is a rather poor estimate of the complexity since each neuron is able to give and to receive a large number of synapses.

Clearly, the number of neurons does not follow linearly the mass of the genome but increases dramatically from Drosophilia to mouse (see table 1). It increases also from mouse or early ancestor of man to Homosapiens, but the weight of DNA per nucleus, to code for the corresponding complexity of the brain, is very similar in mouse and in Homosapiens. Of course, these evaluations are very crude, and the complexity of the nervous system is certainly underestimated but the complexity of the genome is certainly not overestimated (see table 1).

So we face a very interesting paradox as soon as we want to understand such a high degree of complexity of the nervous system in terms of its genetic determinism.

Table 1
Complexity of the nervous system and of the genome

Estimated number of neurones	Mass of the brain (g)	Content of DNA (pg per nucleus)
Drosophilia 10^5		0.18
Mouse 5.5×10^6	0.45	2.3
Chimpanzee	400	
Homosapiens $2–16 \times 10^9$	1 400	2.8[a)]

[a)]This amount of DNA, assuming an average protein weight of 50 000 Daltons, can code for 10^6 different structural genes as a maximum. In fact, the number of structural genes is only of 10^5 or less.

1.3. How to create such a complex nervous system

1.3.1. Embryonic development of the nervous system

As for the other organs of the body, the starting point for the embryonic development of the nervous system is the fertilized egg, afterwards come the segmentation and the differentiation of cells into distinct tissues. An interesting hypothesis postulates that this process of cell diversification and differentiation occurs sequentially. Each stage would correspond to a state of expression of a limited number of genes of the genome at a given time. Therefore this theory proposes transitions between a few distinct states of expression for a given structural gene. They are visualized as switches between alternative states: a limited number of "yes or no" signals, combined for instance in the cytoplasm of the fertilized egg, would be able to determine a rather large number of differentiate stages for a given cell, depending on its location in the embryo.

This model has been proposed in the case of the development of the nervous system. Experimental evidence comes from abnormal embryos of mouse mutated for their ability to develop or differentiate their tissues. The mechanism of gene action during early development of mouse is not really known in great detail, but this kind of scheme may have some validity for embryonic development in general and of course for the development of the nervous system. But one has to keep in mind that the cellular organization of the brain is a more complex structure and has more categories of cells than any other organ.

1.3.2. How to code for the complexity of the brain

One could argue that we have no good reason to make a particular case for the nervous system except again our previous remark about the number of different classes of cells. In fact, what is much more characteristic of the nervous system is of course that these cells established connections once they have been positioned. We have shown that, in the case of Purkinje cell, they create this complex neuronal network which is found nowhere else in the body. Not only the connections themselves, but also the maps of somatic projections on the cortex are specified. How can we create this complexity, this regular pattern of connections of maps having such limited genetic information?

The following discussion essentially concerns this very interesting question. Classical answers that have been proposed are presented.

The chemoaffinity hypothesis. In order to explain this complexity, Sperry proposed a model, many years ago, which is the so-called chemoaffinity hypothesis.

According to Sperry's model, growing nerve fibers would bear chemical labels complementary to those present on the target cell. The hooking of a given axon with its specific partner, for instance the granular cell axon contacting the Purkinje cell dendrite, would be due to the mutual affinity of chemical present on the two surfaces. Following the same model, the genome would have to code for all these chemical labels and it is clearly not the case because of the enormous number of synapses (10^{14}) present in the brain. So this hypothesis, at least as it was proposed by Sperry to explain specificity, is not valid.

Looking at the 80 000 synapses which are present on the dendritic tree of a single Purkinje cell, the most plausible guess is that basically there are no chemical differences relevant for a specific recognition within this class of synaptic contacts. However, this theory might be responsible for the recognition between main classes of cells which could bear complementary cell surface determinants.

The timing hypothesis. Another mechanism proposed is the so-called timing hypothesis advocated by Levinthal et al. This theory proposes that the nerve terminals reaching the target neurons at different moments number them sequentially and thus bring order in the pattern of connections. Taking the visual system as an example, the growth of a nerve terminal from the retina starts with a leading fiber which first reaches the optic ganglia. Maybe, some chemical diffusible signal is responsible for this oriented growth. Once this leader has reached any cell located in the central region of the ganglia, then each contact is numbered. This timing can create a kind of differentiation in each cell and in each axon and may even create a given map when the visual field of the retina project on the visual cortex.

Therefore, aside from cell division, cell migration, and growth of neurites, we may have specific surface determinants involved in the recognition of the main classes of cells and this timing could bring order into the pattern of connections.

The selective stabilization hypothesis. The two former theories do not discuss the possibility that some regulatory signal could specify the final connectivity starting from a transient stage of multiinnervation which is found very frequently in the immature nervous system. Moreover, experimental evidence has shown that neuronal activity takes place at a very early stage in the embryo.

In the selective stabilization hypothesis, we propose that the activity of developing neuronal networks could act as a regulatory signal responsible for the final choice in the connections. According to this view, there would be stabilization of some synapses and regression of others from a critical stage of transient redundancy. The characteristic connectivity of each neurone would be achieved through some kind of regulatory mechanism taking place via the activity of the developing neuronal network. Therefore, the striking diversity between neighbouring cells could be explained through this kind of scheme. The selective stabilization hypothesis brings additional order and might be responsible for the final connectivity of each individual nerve cell (see fig. 3). Moreover, biochemical prediction of this model could be tested as we shall see in the case of the neuromuscular junction.

1.4. Genetic analysis of the nervous system

One way to analyze these kind of hypotheses is to study the genetic analysis of the development of the nervous system. Mutations of neurological origin can be extensively studied in the mouse and more than 700 pure strains of mice having a given neurological defect have been isolated up to now!

1.4.1. Mutations affecting the cerebellum

Among many genetic mutations of the mouse which create defects in the cerebellum, four of them are rather well known because of the known abnormality in the cerebellum circuitry they give.

In the case of the weaver mouse or nervous mouse, one of the main classes of cells is missing: respectively the granular cell and the Purkinje cell. None of these two classes are missing in the staggerer mouse, where the motor behavior is abnormal. But slices in the cerebellum demonstrate the absence of synapses between spines of the Purkinje cell dendritic tree and parallel fibers from the granular cells. In the reeler mouse, not only the cerebellum, but all the nervous system is affected. Looking at the cerebellum, one step in its differentiation is missing: the

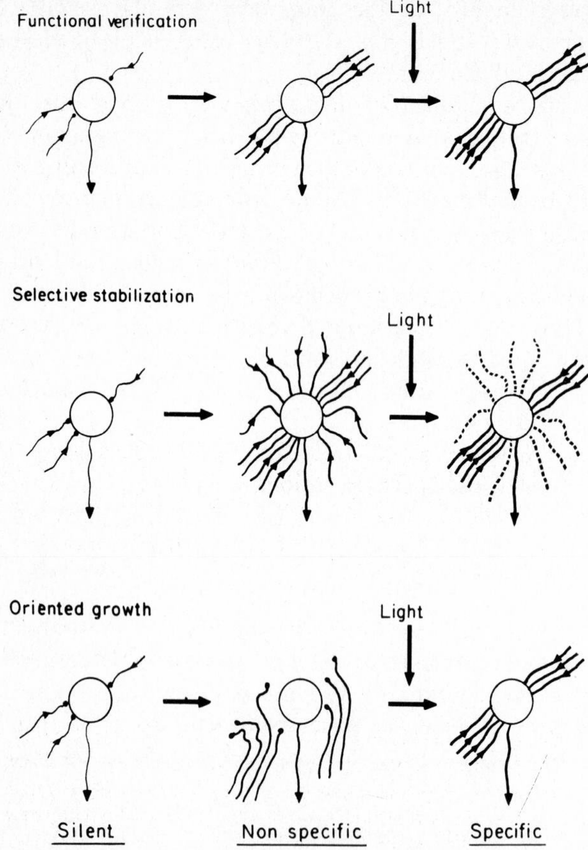

Fig. 3. Hypotheses regarding the effect of functional activity on the specification of a neuronal network. The three possibilities considered deal with changes in connectivity, but alternative (or additional) mechanisms may take place such as changes of efficacy or excitory and/or inhibitory synapses, growth of new sets of connections and so on (adapted from Changeux and Danchin 1976). The vertical arrow indicates the onset of spontaneous or evoked activity.

Purkinje cells remain close to the deep cerebellar nucleus: their position is abnormal because they do not migrate.

Clearly, these defects concern some basic feature of the organization of the cerebellum: cell type, cell migration, and main classes of synapses (see fig. 4). They originate from a mutated target cell, the knowledge of which is required to examine the influence of each class of cells on the final connectivity in the cerebellum.

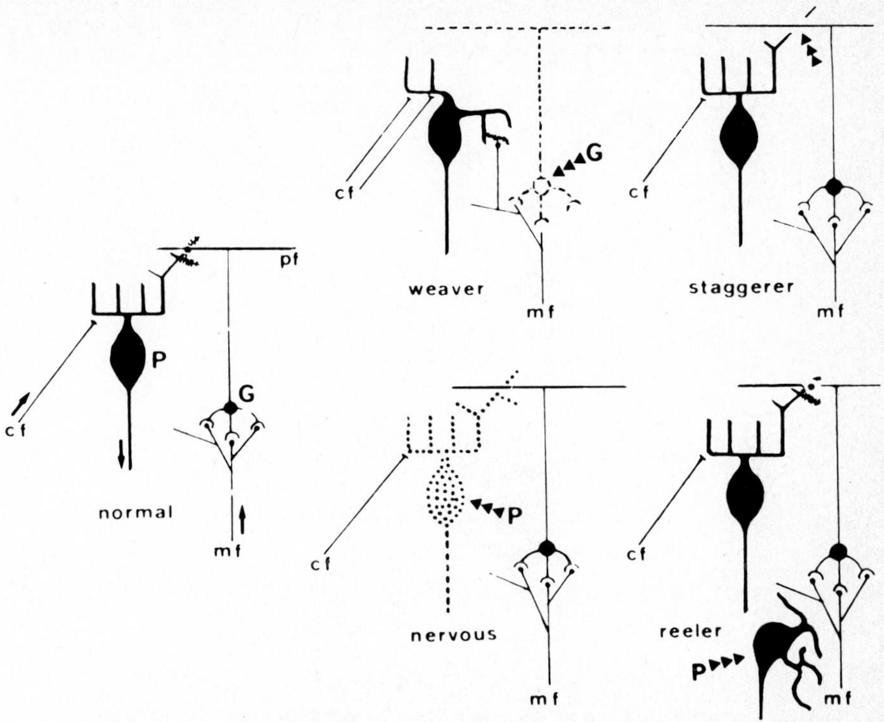

Fig. 4. Diagrammatic representation of the connectivity of the cerebellum from the homozygous mutant mice: weaver, stagger, nervous, and reeler. P, Purkinje cell; G, Granular cell; mf, mossy fiber; cf, climbing fiber; pf, parallel fiber (axons of granular cells). → indicates the direction of the nerve impulse; →→→→→ indicates the site of the lesion.

1.4.2. Use of mosaics to analyse mutations

The mosaic method could solve the search of the primary target cell responsible for a given phenotypic mutation. It is possible to obtain a tetraparental chimera from a black homozygous strain of mice and an albino one (see fig. 5). It looks like a "zebra" with 34 white or black patches on the skin. Each patch comes from a single cell having one of the parental phenotype. In that case, each cell expresses its own genotype into the black or white phenotype in an autonomous manner for each one.

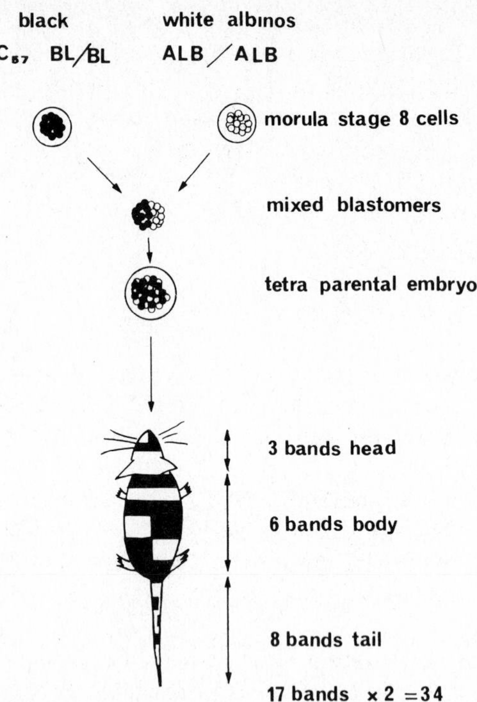

Fig. 5. The method of the mosiac. Each band results from one clone of melanoblast (derives from one cell). Therefore 34 melanoblasts are responsible for the phenotypic color of the mouse. (See Cerebellum – Mullen, 1977 – and refs. cited therein.)

This kind of methodology is suitable to determine to what extent the phenotype of a given neuron depends only on its own genotype or on other cell genotypes (glial cell, hormone secreting cell, etc.).

1.4.3. Analysis of the migration of the Purkinje cell

Let us consider the case of the reeler mutation and determine whether a wild type Purkinje cell would be normally located or not in a mosaic cerebellum of reeler and wild.

A neutral marker (here the gene coding for the β glucuronidase) not essential for the cell is used in order to visualize the genotype of the cells after the proper staining making a chimera with (wild, β glucuronidase +) and (Reeler, β glucuronidase −) each Purkinje cell genotype can be known and be correlated or not with a normal or an abnormal position.

The absence of correlation clearly demonstrates that the primary locus of the mutation is not lying in the Purkinje cell. Otherwise, none of the genetically mutated Purkinje cells would have been normally located.

So in the particular case of the reeler mutation, the control of migration of Purkinje cell is determined by some kind of organ or a group of cells which are not the neurones themselves. A plausible explanation would be that the glial cells are responsible for the migration of other classes of cells.

1.4.4. Analysis of the growth of neurites

The staggerer mutation is particularly interesting because only one class of synapses is missing: here, the granular cell and/or the Purkinje cell could be involved for the genetical determinism of the parallel fiber-dendritic spines.

One method uses a quantitative analysis of the branching pattern of the dendritic arborisation of a given Purkinje cell. There are striking differences between a wild mouse and a staggerer one. For sure one of the partners is modified, but the lesion could not be intrinsic only to the Purkinje cell.

The mosaic method gives a clear issue on this problem: here, all the abnormal Purkinje cells (they receive no contact from granular cells) have the staggerer genotype as determined by the looking at preparations stained for β glucuronidase. So the absence of synapses in the staggerer mutation originates in an intrinsic defect in the Purkinje cell manifesting itself by the branching pattern of the dendrites. Moreover, a few genes may regulate this branching pattern common for all Purkinje cells in the cerebellum.

Looking at abnormally located Purkinje cells in the Reeler mouse, Sotelo used the same quantitative analysis of their dendritic arborisation. He found that, even if the dendritic tree is abnormal for those Purkinje cells located close to the deep cerebellum nucleus, their branching pattern is not modified.

Therefore, the growth branching rules still hold true but they apply themselves in different environment. The final solutions of this application are different depending on the presence of the partner or not. Fo instance, when one of the partners is absent, the granular cell in the weaver mouse (see fig. 6) then heterologous synapses form between Mossy fibers and Purkinje cell soma (this synapse should never form according to the chemoaffinity hypothesis). Moreover, the deficit in

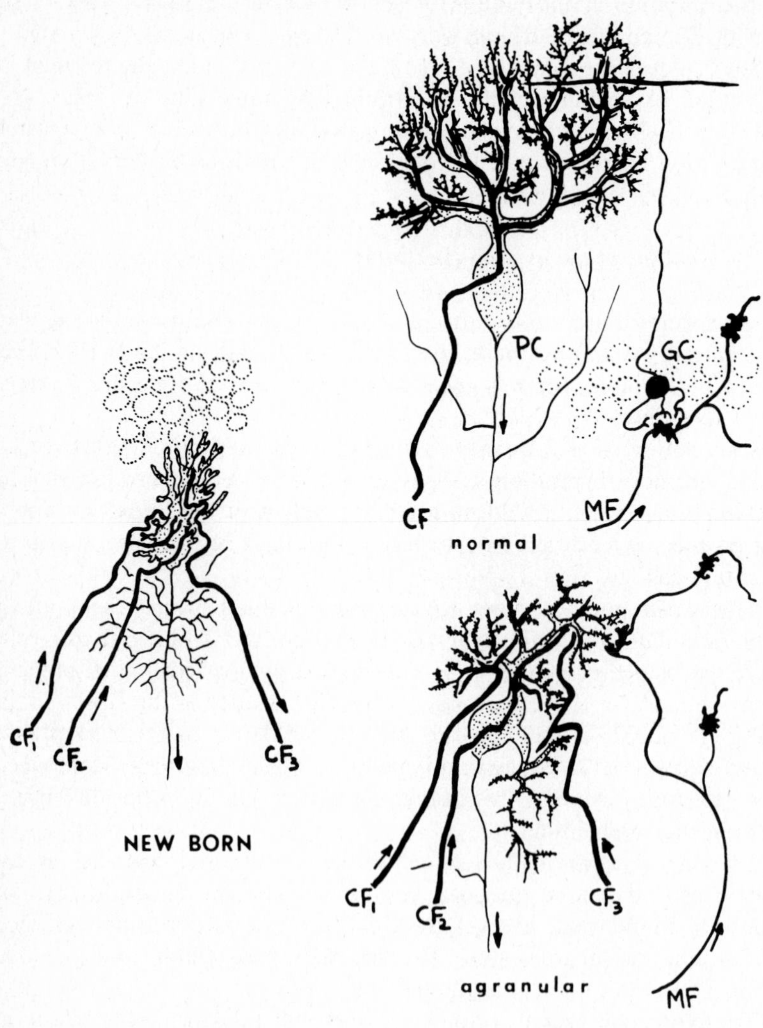

Fig. 6. The innervation of the Purkinje cell in normal and agranular cerebella from newborn and adult mouse or rat.

behavior is more pronounced with this kind of heterologous synapses than even without cerebellum! It shows how blind the system is and how these growth rules have to fit with each other in order to create a functional organization.

1.4.5. Selective stabilization of synaptical contacts

Aside from these genetic factors regulating cell migration and branching of neurites, we can take advantage of these mutants to test an eventuality proposed in the beginning: could the activity be involved in the stabilization of some contacts and the regression of others?

Indeed, the adult cerebellum offers a rather unique situation: a one-to-one relationship between the climbing fibers and the Purkinje cell they innervate. Here electrophysiological criteria together with some morphological ones clearly demonstrate that several climbing fibers do converge on the same Purkinje cell in the newborn cerebellum and establish several functional synapses. These evidences of transient redundancy are in good agreement with predictions from the selective stabilization theory. Moreover, synapse elimination is taking place at this stage leading to a one-to-one relationship (see fig. 6).

Looking at the Reeler mutation, Mariani has shown that, even though Purkinje cells are genetically identical, the abnormally located ones have preserved in the adult their multiple innervations while those which have the normal position only have a single afferent climing fiber. Thus, the environment of a given Purkinje cells commands the elimination of multiple innervation. And there are factors which regulate the evolution of this multiple innervation.

As in the case of the sequential expression of genes, a few genetic determinants are certainly coding for cell division, cell migration, neurite growth, branching pattern of main classes of cell. But the number of genes is small to account for a one-to-one relationship between synaptic partners in a unique manner. Therefore, some additional elements are necessary to explain the regression of multiple innervation, that gives the final connectivity as a function of cellular environment. Here the activity of developing neuronal network would be involved at least in the regulation of ultimate levels of development which would create a specification of the final connectivity of the neuronal network.

The most simple example of neuronal network is the neuromuscular junction and still some specification of the pattern of innervation is found during embryogenesis.

2. Neuromuscular junction

2.1. Introduction

The neuromuscular junction is a synapse hooking the motor axon with the muscle fiber (see Ascher in this volume). But a given motor neuron of the spinal cord can innervate a limited number of muscle fibers and then the muscle is divided into corresponding motor units the size of which is constant for each muscle. So, at this ultimate level, the pattern of innervation is not at random, moreover, it develops from embryogenesis and becomes specific for each muscle or at least for each class of muscles.

As pointed out in section 1, the neuromuscular junction begins to be well understood even at the molecular level. This situation is a rather unique one for the detailed study of a given synapse development and stabilization.

2.1.1. Spontaneous activity in the neuromuscular junction

Actually, the neuromuscular junctions present in the embryo are not only in a functional state, but they do function. For instance, even at a very early stage ($3\frac{1}{2}$ days of incubation), the chick embryo is mobile in the egg and this motion is triggered by the spinal cord which is, of course, very immature. This activity which is the motor activity is present during all the embryonic development (21 days), but reaches a maximum before hatching.

This spontaneous activity during the development of neuronal networks is a very general phenomenon which is also true for mammals. It is not restricted to the motor behavior. Electrophysiological recording in the central nervous system, even when the system is immature, already indicates spontaneous activity of nervous cells. Indeed molecular interactions are involved in the specification of neuronal networks. The neuromuscular junction provides us with a good chance to study the molecular basis of the effect of the activity during the embryogenesis. The following section will present together with the well known hisology and cytochemistry of the adult neuromuscular junction, some of the experimental evidence concerning molecular interactions taking place in the subsynaptic membrane at a very early stage of development.

2.2. Synaptogenesis

Obviously the functional capacity of the nervous system remains rather stable during the adult life. But in fact, we face a dynamical process where synaptogenesis could compensate synaptolysis to some extent. Therefore, the factors of stability of the synapse are of crucial importance not only because they have to correlate the establishment of a given contact, but also because they trigger some regression, and influence, as the synaptogenesis does, the evolution of neuronal networks. Here too, the subsynaptic membrane from the neuromuscular junction gives experimental support both for studying the stability and the formation of the endplate (See fig. 7).

2.2.1. Stability of the adult subsynaptic membrane

The direct stability of the adult subsynaptic membrane is checked after the denervation. Despite the fact that the blood vessel is also cut with the nerve, the nerve terminal degenerates, but the muscle does not. Moreover, the very concentrate acetylcholine receptor molecules keep their previous position on the fold tips of the subsynaptic membrane (see fig. 7) with a similar density. Their half life time remains very long (5–7 d).

Finally, the adult subsynaptic membrane remains stable up to 7 months. Thus an interesting question concerns the formation of such a stable structure.

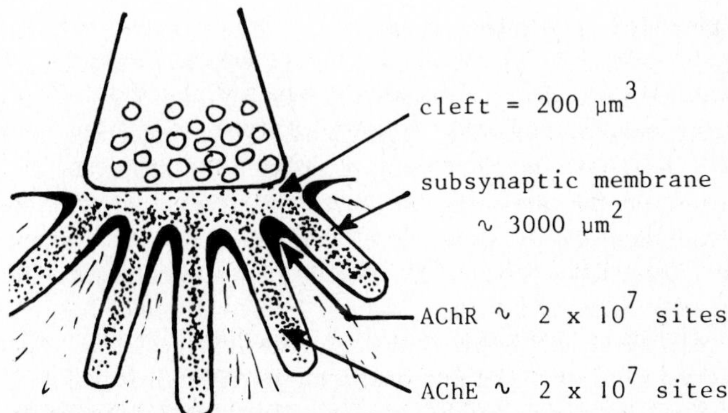

Fig. 7. Schematic drawing of the neuromuscular junction indicating the location and the number of acetylcholine receptors and acetylcholine esterases.

Table 2

Structural differences between extrasynaptic and subsynaptic acetylcholine receptors[a)]

(1) Binding properties	No differences	
(2) Lateral diffusion coefficient	7×10^{-11} cm^2/s (35° C)	Extra Ach R
	Non-diffusible	Sub Ach R
(3) Metabolic stability (half life)	10–18	Extra Ach R
	5–7 d	Sub Ach R

[a)](See *Neuromuscular Junction* – Changeux, 1979 – and refs. cited therein.)

2.2.2. *End-plate formation*

On the contrary, looking at the embryonic muscle fiber, called myotube, even before the nerve arrival, the entire plasma membrane is covered with acetylcholine receptor. It corresponds to about 300 α toxin sites per μ^2. Its properties compared to those of the junctional one present in the adult subsynaptic membrane (see table 2) indicate large differences for the lateral diffusion constant, and also for the mean half life time. So that the extrajunctional receptor molecules contrast with those present in the subsynaptic membrane in the sense that they are both mobile and labile. Therefore, the growth cone from the exploratory motor axon, as soon as it reaches the muscle fiber, elicits a drastic change in the membrane.

Experimental evidences show that the growth cone releases acetylcholine from several contacts, one of which is stabilized further. The nerve terminal does not select patches which already preexist, but causes the two dimensional aggregation of the receptor molecules. Further events take place making a rather long sequence of events: localisation of the acetylcholine receptor esterase of the basement membrane, then one the spot of acetylcholine and acetycholine esterase has been formed the subsynaptic membrane area increases with a very significant enlargement of the number of receptor molecules.

The generalisation of this scheme to the interneuronal connections establishment has not been demonstrated yet. Even if it is not identical, it may still have some validity. In this latter case, biochemical techniques are not as effective as in the neuromuscular junction where the arrival of the nerve terminal induces such dramatic changes in the subsynaptic membrane.

2.3. *Molecular basis of the end-plate formation*

2.3.1. *Two forms for the acetylcholine receptor?*

The striking differences between the two categories of receptors mentioned above can support two interpretations: (a) either we deal with completely different molecules coded by different genes or (b) the subsynaptic receptor derives from the extrasynaptic one and some kind of covalent modification is postulated to account for physico-chemical discrepancies (see table 2).

Unambiguously, some fluorescent extra synaptic receptor becomes patched as soon as the nerve terminal reaches the muscle fiber, but subsequently, newly synthetized receptors get incorporated. So the second hypothesis is a plausible one but the controversy is not settled.

2.3.2. *Patching and stabilization of the receptor*

The patching itself is taking place in less than 12 h for the chick embryo where the patch receptor is still labile. The stabilisation process that follows is distinct from the patching.

Recently, rats have been investigated: as soon as the receptor is patched, it becomes stabilized. So the stabilization may be correlated to the patching in the rat, but it is not the case for the chicken. In general a complex sequence of chemical reactions certainly takes place. Moreover, the mean opening time of the ionic gate changes as soon as the receptors aggregate in the myotubes. So, the post transcriptional model proposes an interconversion of already existing molecules which changes their properties as a consequence of a chemical modification. But definite proof against the idea of two distinct genes coding for these two receptors may still be lacking for a long time.

Whatever the valid hypothesis is, some regulatory signals are certainly involved in the aggregation process triggered by the nerve terminal and then in further steps of endplate formation as the stabilization and the accumulation of junctional receptors.

2.4. *Regulatory factors of the end-plate formation*

2.4.1. *How to control the location of the acetylcholine receptor*

Some attempts are performed to isolate a factor that we refer to as an anterograde signal coming from the nerve terminal. Although, the acetylcholine itself is not completely excluded as an anterograde signal, its effect via the binding to the acetyl receptor toxin site excluded since the receptor is patched together with its fluorescent toxin. So a definite answer for the anterograde factor that induces aggregation in the postsynaptic membrane is not accessible yet. But other phenomena take place as the localisation of the acetylcholine esterase and the disappearance of extra synaptic receptor.

2.4.2. Shut-off of acetylcholine receptor synthesis at the onset of the muscle activity

Upon arrival of the nerve terminal, the total content of receptor molecule in muscle markedly decreases, and clearly the nerve induces a loss in the density of the only extrasynaptic receptor. The receptor close to the nerve terminal persists and its aggregation in the synaptic membrane is not sufficient to account for a loss of 90% of the total receptor molecules. This decline may result from two mechanisms: either the half life of the receptor molecule is enhanced, or its synthesis is turned off upon arrival of the nerve terminal.

Several experimental observations support the second hypothesis in the chick embryo where the rate of the receptor molecule remains unambiguously constant upon arrival of the developing nerve terminal (usually between day 10 and 19). Moreover, chronic blocking of embryonic muscle activity by the injection of flaxedil which is a curare-like agent gives a relatively high content in muscle acetylcholine receptor site. This observation strongly supports the conclusion that in ovo the spontaneous activity of embryonic muscles shuts off the synthesis of the extra-synaptic receptor protein.

In muscle cultures from a dystrophic strain of mouse, a similar regulation is observed in the absence of mechanical contraction. Finally, addition of dibutyryl cyclic GMP slows down acetylcholine receptor synthesis indicating that cyclic GMP might be one of the signals involved in the coupling between electrical activity and acetylcholine receptor synthesis.

2.4.3. Location of acetylcholine esterase

At a very early stage of embryonic development *in vivo* the appearance of acetylcholine esterase in skeletal muscle closely parallels that of acetylcholine receptor. But denervation does not cause a spread of acetylcholine esterase as found for the acetylcholine receptor, it induces a decrease of acetylcholine esterase. The same acetylcholine esterase depletion is found under chronic blocking with the flaxedil of neuromuscular transmission during development. Yet the localisation of acetylcholine receptor still takes place. The activity therefore regulates the localisation of acetylcholine esterase but this behavior again markedly differs from that of the acetylcholine receptor.

2.5. *Presynaptic stabilization of the motor nerve ending*

2.5.1. *Formation of end-plate pattern*

The internal machinery of the developing neuromuscular junctions is able to regulate the metabolism of various crucial receptors after the proper interaction with their direct environment. But there are still some other "degrees of freedom" unspecified in the system. One of which is obviously the number of end-plates per muscle fiber that we consider as representative of a higher degree of organization. The corresponding experimental situation is found in the chick whose *anterior latissimus dorsi* (ALD) and *posterior latissimus dorsi* (PLD) muscles markedly differ in their innervation pattern. There are around 15 end plates-per-muscle fiber in ALD vs in a single one-per-muscle fiber of PLD. Again we may ask about the effect of the firing activity on the end plate pattern specification (see fig. 8).

Interesting spontaneous activity takes place in the embryo: the firing pattern of ALD presents a low frequency (0.2–1 Hz) of action potentials

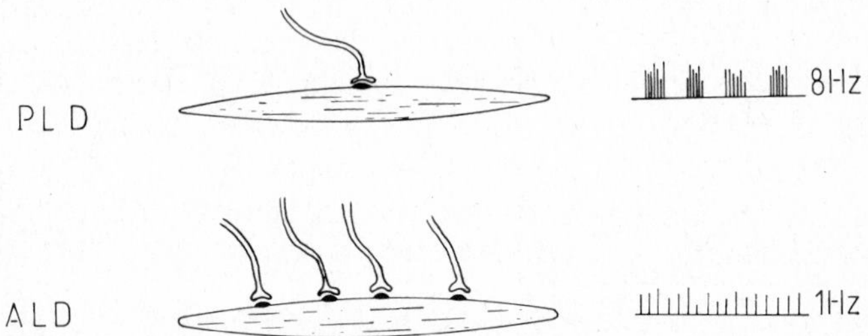

Fig. 8. Schematic representation of the topology of synaptical contacts on single muscle fiber from chick embryo (17 d). Top = PLD fiber foccally innervated, the electromyographic activity presents sporadic high frequency bursts. Bottom = ALD fiber with multiple innervation, the electromyographic activity is continuous and corresponds to a low frequency.

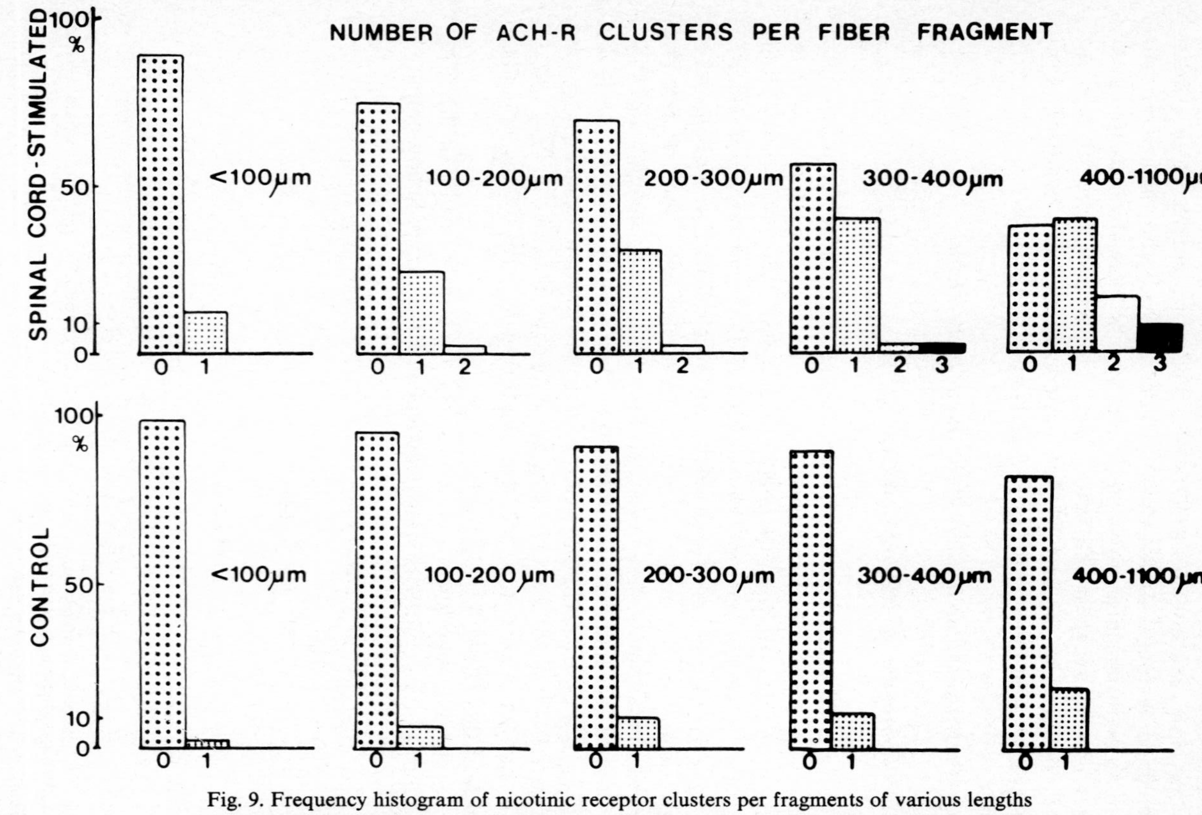

Fig. 9. Frequency histogram of nicotinic receptor clusters per fragments of various lengths from single fiber of PLD muscle. (Top) control chick embryo of 17 d, (bottom) chronically cord stimulated (0.5 Hz from day 5–10) embryo of 17 d.

while PLD receives some burst of high frequency (8 Hz) interrupted by silence. Furthermore, an electrode implanted in the spinal cord adds a sustained activity of 0.5 Hz to the spontaneous one from the 10th to the 15th day. Under such conditions, quantitative measurements with isolated fiber or PLD muscle indicate a significant increase in the number of receptor clusters per muscle fiber, while control muscle fibers remain focally innervated (see fig. 9). Although the distribution of acetylcholine receptor molecules clusters in chronically stimulated PLD is not as regular as the control ALD muscle, perhaps because of the imperfect mimic of the physiological stimulation, one can create to some extent a geometrical organization from a purely temporal signal.

2.5.2. *Transient polyneuronal innervation*

A second regressive phase occurs during the first weeks following hatching (chick) or birth (rat) and affects primarily motor-axon collaterals without making significant changes in cell number (see fig. 10)

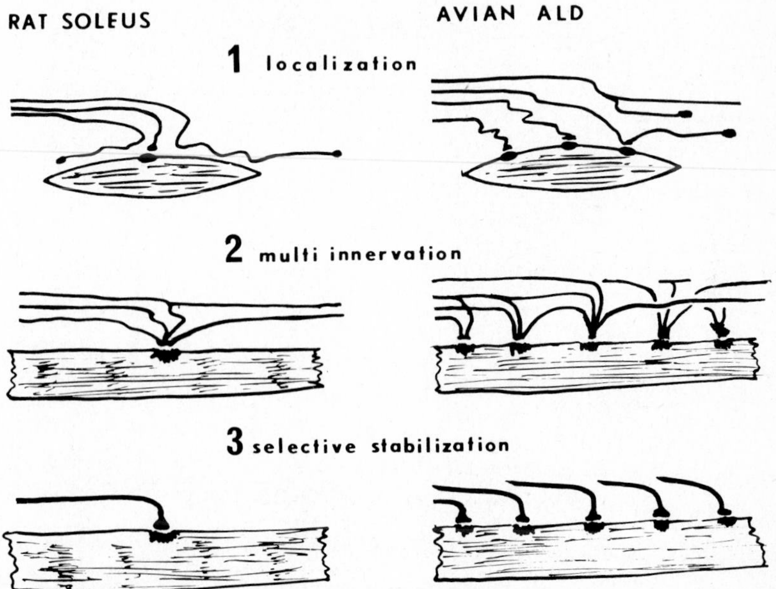

Fig. 10. Diagrammatic representation of these important steps in the development of the neuromuscular junction in skeletal muscles with focal and distributed innervation. (1) postsynaptic localization of the acetylcholine receptor; (2) transient polyneural innervation; (3) selective stabilization of a single nerve terminal per end plate.

For example, in a fetal rat diaphragm at day 17, electron microscopy confirms that several synaptic profiles are in contact with the same synaptic fold. The postsynaptic potentials of individual muscle fibers recorded with intracellular microelectrodes exhibit unusual features: the amplitude increases discontinuously through successive steps (three or more) as a function of stimulus strength, instead of jumping in a single

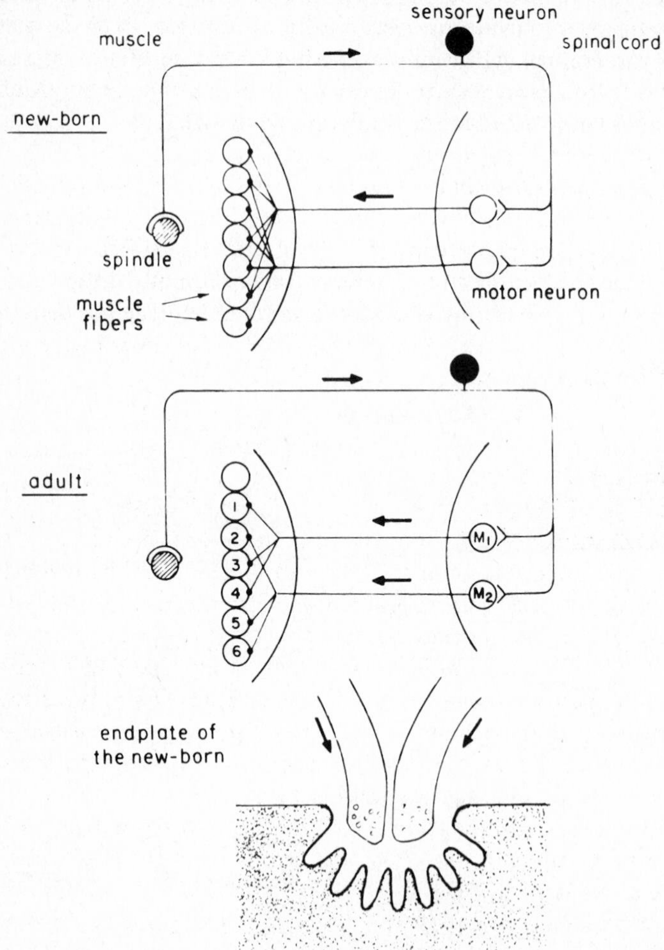

Fig. 11. The differentiation of motor units in a skeletal fast muscle by retrograde selective stabilization of nerve terminals. In the neonate one motor neuron innervates many more muscle fibers than in the adult, and each muscle fiber receives several nerve terminal. A few weeks after birth only one nerve terminal persists per muscle, the others having regressed (Changeux and Danchin 1976).

step as in adult muscle fibers. Analysis of this complex end plate potential shows that it is due not to electrical coupling between muscle fibers, but to the presence of several functional axon terminals from different neurons at the same end plate; this explains the difference in threshold. A considerable redundancy therefore exists in the innervation of the muscle fiber. Then, retraction of axon collaterals, rather than a degeneration, takes place. These observations have been repeated with various muscles, in particular, avian ALD, in which each of the several endplates present per muscle fiber becomes innervated by several axon terminals. The transient polyneuronal innervation seems to be an obligatory step of endplate formation. Indeed, during postnatal development, the average size of the motor unit decreases (see fig. 11)

To test the possibility that regression of polyneuronal innervation is regulated by the state of activity of the muscle, one of the tendons of the sartorius muscle was sectioned in infant rats. It is not yet known whether neonatal tenotomy modifies the chronic firing of the motoneurons, but it certainly changes the state of mechanical activity of the muscle. In any case, the regression of the polyneuronal innervation was significantly delayed.

3. Conclusion

The main purpose of this course has been to present a cellular mechanism that might account for the "specification" of the cerebellum neuronal network and even molecular mechanism accounting for the neuromuscular junction development.

Many elements are still missing, in particular the chemical identification of the diffusible signals involved. Nevertheless, these mechanisms make plausible the hypothesis that during development a selection of synapses takes place that is directly or indirectly, regulated by the state of activity of the developing neuronal network.

One of the main advantages of this selective-stabilization hypothesis is that it affords an economy of genes. Some of the genes that dictate, for example, the general rules of growth, the stability properties of the immature synapses, the regulation of their stability by the activity of the immature synapse, and the integrative properties of the postsynaptic neuron may be shared by different categories of neurons or even be common to all neurons. The set of genes involved (the genetic envelope) should therefore be smaller than it would have to be if each synapse were determined individually.

Another advantage of the hypothesis is that it provides a plausible mechanism for learning. It illustrates how a given temporal pattern of activity might transcribed into a particular three-dimensional topology of synapses. According to this theory "to learn" becomes "to eliminate". It is radically different from so-called instructive theories, which postulate, for example, that a particular nervous activity directs the growth of nerve endings toward the suitable target or causes the appearance of new molecular species.

An interesting prediction of the formalized model of selective synapse stabilization in a developing neuronal network is that the same final learned output might be achieved through stabilization of different pathways (Changeux and Danchin 1976). In other words, it allows for what is referred to as a "variability" of the connectional organization, which is indeed observed in isogenic organisms. According to this view, the "degeneracy" of the code for behavior appears as a consequence (and not as a prerequisite) of the selection.

For reasons that are not yet clear, the total stock of genes remains almost constant throughout the evolution of vertebrates (mammals in particular). Despite this, the complexity of the nervous system and the correlative behaviorial competences continue to increase. As the autonomous programming of the system becomes increasingly difficult, the genetic determinism must break down and the redundancy of the connectivity become amplified. The ability to learn might thus be viewed as the evolutionary result of an increased complexity of neuronal networks based on a constant number of genes.

Reading list

General references

C. S. Sherrington, The Integrative Action of the Nervous System (Yale Univ. Press, New Haven, 1906).

S. Ramon y Cajal, Histologie du Système nerveux de l'Homme et des Vertébrés (Maloine, Paris, 1911).

S. Ramon y Cajal, Studies on Vertebrate Neurogenesis (Charles C. Thomas, Springfield, IL, 1929).

R. Sperry, Proc. Natl. Acad. Sci. USA 50 (1963) 703.

L. C. Dunn and D. Bennett, Science 144 (1964) 260.

J. C. Eccles, M. Ito and J. Szentagothai, The Cerebellum as a Neuronal Machine (Springer, Berlin, 1967).

J. C. Eccles, in: The Understanding of the Brain (McGraw-Hill, New York, 1972).

J. P. Changeux, Ph Courrege and A. Danchin Proc. Natl. Acad. Sci USA 70 (1973) 2974.

M. Prestige and D. Willshaw, Proc. R. Soc. B 190 (1975) 77.

L. Wolpert and J. H. Lewis, Fed. Proc. 34 (1975). 14.

J. P. Changeux and A. Danchin Nature 264 (1976) 705.

V. Hamburger, Neurosci Res. Program Bull. 15 suppl. (1976).

F. Levinthal E. Macagno and C. Levinthal Cold Spring Harbor Symp. Quant. Biol. 40 (1976) 321.

J. P. Changeux and K. Mikoshiba, Brain Res. 48 (1978) 43.

P. Patterson, Ann Rev. Neurosci 1 (1978) 1.

P. Patterson, Epigenetic in Nuences in Neuronal Development, pp. 929–936,

D. A. McClain and G. M. Edelman, The Dynamic of the Cell Surface: Modulation and Transmembrane Control, pp. 675–690,

W. M. Cowan Selection and Control in Neurogenesis, pp. 59–79, and

P. Rakic, Genetic and Epigenetic Determinants of Local Neuronal Circuits in the Mammalian Central Nervous System, pp. 109–128, in: The Neuroscience Fourth Study Program F. O. Schmitt, M. I. T. Press (1979).
The Brain, Scientific American (Sept. 1979).

Cerebellum

F. Crepel, J. Mariani and N. Delhaye-Bouchaud, J. Neurobiol. 7, no. 6 (1976) 567.

P. Rakic, Cold Spring Harb. Symp. Quant. Biol. 40 (1976) 333.

J. Mariani, F. Crepel, K. Mikoshiba, J. P. Changeux and C. Sotelo, Phil. Trans. R. Soc. London B 281 (1977) 1.

R. J. Mullen, Genetic Dissection of the Central Nervous System With Mutant-Normal Mouse and Rat Chimeras, in: W. M. Cowan and J. A. Ferrendelli, eds. Society for Neuroscience Symposia, vol. 2. (Soc. for Neuroscience Bethesda, MD, 1977) pp. 47–65.

V. S. Jor Caviness, and P. Rakic, Ann. Rev. Neuroscience 1 (1978) 297.

C. Sotelo and A. Privat, Acta Neuropathol. Berl. 43 (1978) 19.

J. Mariani and J. P. Changeux, J. Neurobiology 11 (1980) 41.

Neuromuscular junction

G. D. Fischbach, D. K. Berg, S. A. Cohen and E. Frank, Cold Spring Harb. Symp. Quant. Biol. 40 (1976) 347.

S. Burden, Dev. Biol. 57 (1977) 317.

J. P. Changeux, Molecular Interactions in Adult and Developing Neuromuscular Junction, in: The Neuroscience Fourth Study Program, ed. F. O. Schmitt (M. I. T. Press, 1979) pp. 749–778.

M. Toutant, J. P. Bourgeois, D. Renaud, G. Le Douarin and J. P. Changeux, Devel. Biol. 76 (1980) 384.

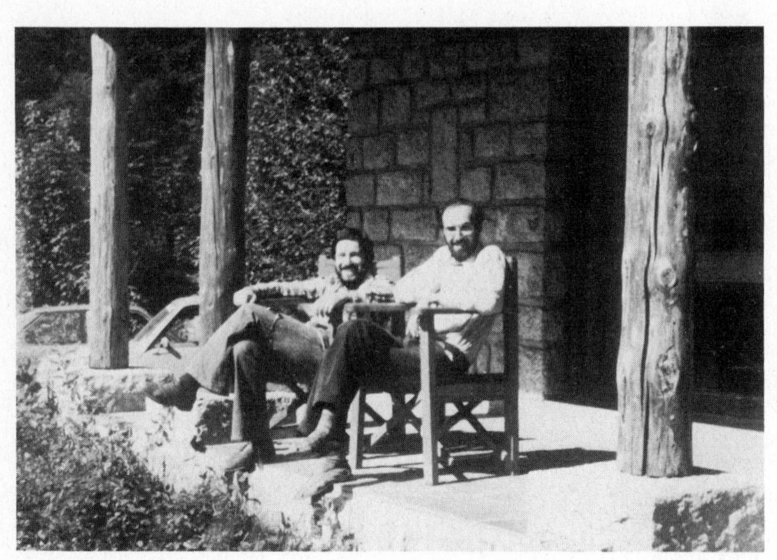